Applied and Numerical Harmonic Analysis

Advances in Discrete Tomography and Its Applications

Gabor T. Herman
Attila Kuba
Editors

Birkhäuser
Boston • Basel • Berlin

Gabor T. Herman
Ph.D. Program in Computer Science
The Graduate Center
The City University of New York
365 Fifth Avenue
New York, NY 10016
U.S.A.

Attila Kuba[†]
Department of Image Processing
    and Computer Graphics
University of Szeged
Árpád tér 2.
H-6720 Szeged
Hungary

Cover design by Joseph Sherman.

Mathematics Subject Classification (2000): 05-04, 06-04, 15A29, 52-04, 65K10, 68U10, 90C05, 92-08

Library of Congress Control Number: 2006937473

ISBN-10: 0-8176-3614-5   e-ISBN-10: 0-8176-4543-8
ISBN-13: 978-0-8176-3614-2   e-ISBN-13: 978-0-8176-4543-4

Printed on acid-free paper.

9 8 7 6 5 4 3 2 1

www.birkhauser.com   (KeS/SB)

To the memory of Alberto Del Lungo

ANHA Series Preface

The *Applied and Numerical Harmonic Analysis (ANHA)* book series aims to provide the engineering, mathematical, and scientific communities with significant developments in harmonic analysis, ranging from abstract harmonic analysis to basic applications. The title of the series reflects the importance of applications and numerical implementation, but richness and relevance of applications and implementation depend fundamentally on the structure and depth of theoretical underpinnings. Thus, from our point of view, the interleaving of theory and applications and their creative symbiotic evolution is axiomatic.

Harmonic analysis is a wellspring of ideas and applicability that has flourished, developed, and deepened over time within many disciplines and by means of creative cross-fertilization with diverse areas. The intricate and fundamental relationship between harmonic analysis and fields such as signal processing, partial differential equations (PDEs), and image processing is reflected in our state-of-the-art *ANHA* series.

Our vision of modern harmonic analysis includes mathematical areas such as wavelet theory, Banach algebras, classical Fourier analysis, time-frequency analysis, and fractal geometry, as well as the diverse topics that impinge on them.

For example, wavelet theory can be considered an appropriate tool to deal with some basic problems in digital signal processing, speech and image processing, geophysics, pattern recognition, biomedical engineering, and turbulence. These areas implement the latest technology from sampling methods on surfaces to fast algorithms and computer vision methods. The underlying mathematics of wavelet theory depends not only on classical Fourier analysis, but also on ideas from abstract harmonic analysis, including von Neumann algebras and the affine group. This leads to a study of the Heisenberg group and its relationship to Gabor systems, and of the metaplectic group for a meaningful interaction of signal decomposition methods. The unifying influence of wavelet theory in the aforementioned topics illustrates the justification for providing a means for centralizing and disseminating information from the broader, but still focused, area of harmonic analysis. This will be a key role of *ANHA*. We intend to publish with the scope and interaction that such a host of issues demands.

Along with our commitment to publish mathematically significant works at the frontiers of harmonic analysis, we have a comparably strong commitment to publish major advances in the following applicable topics in which harmonic analysis plays a substantial role:

Antenna theory	*Prediction theory*
Biomedical signal processing	*Radar applications*
Digital signal processing	*Sampling theory*
Fast algorithms	*Spectral estimation*
Gabor theory and applications	*Speech processing*
Image processing	*Time-frequency and*
Numerical partial differential equations	*time-scale analysis*
	Wavelet theory

The above point of view for the *ANHA* book series is inspired by the history of Fourier analysis itself, whose tentacles reach into so many fields.

In the last two centuries Fourier analysis has had a major impact on the development of mathematics, on the understanding of many engineering and scientific phenomena, and on the solution of some of the most important problems in mathematics and the sciences. Historically, Fourier series were developed in the analysis of some of the classical PDEs of mathematical physics; these series were used to solve such equations. In order to understand Fourier series and the kinds of solutions they could represent, some of the most basic notions of analysis were defined, e.g., the concept of "function." Since the coefficients of Fourier series are integrals, it is no surprise that Riemann integrals were conceived to deal with uniqueness properties of trigonometric series. Cantor's set theory was also developed because of such uniqueness questions.

A basic problem in Fourier analysis is to show how complicated phenomena, such as sound waves, can be described in terms of elementary harmonics. There are two aspects of this problem: first, to find, or even define properly, the harmonics or spectrum of a given phenomenon, e.g., the spectroscopy problem in optics; second, to determine which phenomena can be constructed from given classes of harmonics, as done, for example, by the mechanical synthesizers in tidal analysis.

Fourier analysis is also the natural setting for many other problems in engineering, mathematics, and the sciences. For example, Wiener's Tauberian theorem in Fourier analysis not only characterizes the behavior of the prime numbers, but also provides the proper notion of spectrum for phenomena such as white light; this latter process leads to the Fourier analysis associated with correlation functions in filtering and prediction problems, and these problems, in turn, deal naturally with Hardy spaces in the theory of complex variables.

Nowadays, some of the theory of PDEs has given way to the study of Fourier integral operators. Problems in antenna theory are studied in terms of unimodular trigonometric polynomials. Applications of Fourier analysis abound in signal processing, whether with the Fast Fourier transform (FFT), or filter design, or the adaptive modeling inherent in time-frequency-scale methods such as wavelet theory. The coherent states of mathematical physics are translated and modulated Fourier transforms, and these are used, in conjunction with the uncertainty principle, for dealing with signal reconstruction in communications theory. We are back to the raison d'être of the *ANHA* series!

John J. Benedetto
Series Editor
University of Maryland
College Park

Preface

Seven years have passed since we finished editing the first book on discrete tomography: *Discrete Tomography: Foundations, Algorithms, and Applications* (Birkhäuser, Boston, 1999). There has been a flowering of the field since that time. New research groups have started, new theoretical and practical results have been presented, and new applications have developed. There have been about 200 papers published on discrete tomography since 1999.

The current book reports on present advances in discrete tomography. Its structure is the same as that of the previous one: after an introduction (Chapter 1) there are chapters on new theoretical foundations (Chapters 2–7), reconstruction algorithms (Chapters 8–11), and selected applications (Chapters 12–16). The level of presentation aims at a potential readership of mathematicians, programmers, engineers, researchers working in the application areas, and students in applied mathematics, computer imaging, biomedical imaging, computer engineering, and/or image processing.

Acknowledgments

We thank the National Science Foundation and the Graduate Center of City University of New York for sponsoring the 2005 Workshop on Discrete Tomography and Its Applications, June 13–15, New York City. We wish to thank the Electronic Notes on Discrete Mathematics, its publisher (Elsevier, Inc.), and its editors (P.L. Hammer and V. Lozin) for publishing a special issue based on the presentations given at the workshop and for giving permission to extend some of that material into this book.

We are grateful to a number of people for technical help; among them we wish to mention Lajos Rodek, László Csernetics, László G. Nyúl, Antal Nagy, Kálmán Palágyi, Stuart Rowland, and Alain Daurat.

Gabor T. Herman   *Attila Kuba*
New York, New York   Szeged, Hungary

August 2006

Contributors

Andreas Alpers
School of Operations Research and Industrial Engineering, Cornell University
414 Rhodes Hall, Ithaca, NY 14853, USA
alpers@orie.cornell.edu

Péter Balázs
Dept. of Computer Algorithms and Artificial Intelligence, University of Szeged
Árpád tér 2., Szeged, H-6720, Hungary
pbalazs@inf.u-szeged.hu

Elena Barcucci
Dipartimento di Sistemi e Informatica, Universitá degli Studi di Firenze
Via Lombroso 6/17, 50134 Firenze, Italy
barcucci@dsi.unifi.it

Kees Joost Batenburg
CWI, Amsterdam and Mathematical Institute, Leiden University
P.O. Box 9512, 2300 RA Leiden, The Netherlands
kbatenbu@math.leidenuniv.nl

Joachim Baumann
Corporate Technology PS 9, Siemens AG
Otto-Hahn-Ring 6, D-81730 Munich, Germany
Joachim.Baumann@siemens.com

Richard A. Brualdi
Department of Mathematics, University of Wisconsin
Madison, Wisconsin 53706, USA
brualdi@math.wisc.edu

Sara Brunetti
Dipartimento di Scienze Matematiche e Informatiche, Università di Siena
Pian dei Mantellini 44, 53100, Siena, Italy
sara.brunetti@unisi.it

Thomas David Capricelli
Lab. Jacques-Louis Lions – UMR 7598, Univ. Pierre et Marie Curie – Paris 6
75005 Paris, France
capricelli@ann.jussieu.fr

Patrick Louis Combettes
Lab. Jacques-Louis Lions – UMR 7598, Univ. Pierre et Marie Curie – Paris 6
75005 Paris, France
plc@math.jussieu.fr

Marie-Christine Costa
Conservatoire National des Arts et Métiers, Laboratoire CEDRIC
292 rue Saint Martin, 75003, Paris, France
costa@cnam.fr

Geir Dahl
Center of Mathematics for Applications, University of Oslo
P.O. Box 1053 Blindern, NO-0316 Oslo, Norway
geird@math.uio.no

Alain Daurat
LSIIT UMR 7005 CNRS, Pôle API, Université Louis Pasteur (Strasbourg 1)
Boulevard Sébastien Brant, 67400, Illkirch-Graffenstaden, France
daurat@dpt-info.u-strasbg.fr

Paolo Dulio
Dipartimento di Matematica "F. Brioschi," Politecnico di Milano
Piazza Leonardo da Vinci 32, I-20133, Milano, Italy
paolo.dulio@polimi.it

Fabien Feschet
University of Auvergne 1 - IUT/LAIC Laboratory
Campus des Cezaux, BP 86, 63172, Aubiere Cedex, France
feschet@laic.u-clermont1.fr

Andrea Frosini
Dip. di Scienze Matematiche e Informatiche, Univ. degli Studi di Siena
Pian dei Mantellini 44, 53100, Siena, Italy
frosini@unisi.it

Richard J. Gardner
Department of Mathematics, Western Washington University
Bellingham WA 98225-9063, USA
Richard.Gardner@wwu.edu

Yan Gerard
University of Auvergne 1 - IUT/LAIC Laboratory
Campus des Cezaux, BP 86, 63172, Aubiere Cedex, France
gerard@laic.u-clermont1.fr

Lajos Hajdu
Institute of Mathematics, University of Debrecen
P.O. Box 12, 4032, Debrecen, Hungary
hajdul@math.klte.hu

Gabor T. Herman
Dept. of Computer Science, The Graduate Center, City Univ. of New York
365 Fifth Avenue, New York, NY 10016, USA
gabortherman@yahoo.com

Fethy Jarray
Conservatoire National des Arts et Métiers, Laboratoire CEDRIC
292 rue Saint Martin, 75003, Paris, France
Fethy.Jarray@cnam.fr

Zoltán Kiss
Dept. of Image Processing and Computer Graphics, University of Szeged
Árpád tér 2., Szeged, H-6720, Hungary
kissz@inf.u-szeged.hu

Erik Knudsen
Materials Research Department, Risø National Laboratory
P.O. Box 49, DK-4000 Roskilde, Denmark
erik.knudsen@risoe.dk

Sven Krimmel
Physik Department E 21, Technical University Munich,
D-85747 Garching, Germany
xray.external@mchp.siemens.de

Attila Kuba
Dept. of Image Processing and Computer Graphics, University of Szeged
Árpád tér 2., Szeged, H-6720, Hungary
kuba@inf.u-szeged.hu

Hstau Y. Liao
Institute for Mathematics and Its Applications, University of Minnesota
Minnesota, USA
liao@ima.umn.edu

Antal Nagy
Dept. of Image Processing and Computer Graphics, University of Szeged
Árpád tér 2., Szeged, H-6720, Hungary
nagya@inf.u-szeged.hu

Carla Peri
Università Cattolica S.C.
Largo Gemelli 1, I-20123, Milano, Italy
carla.peri@unicatt.it

Christophe Picouleau
Conservatoire National des Arts et Métiers, Laboratoire CEDRIC
292 rue Saint Martin, 75003, Paris, France
chp@cnam.fr

Henning F. Poulsen
Materials Research Department, Risø National Laboratory
P.O. Box 49, DK-4000 Roskilde, Denmark
henning.friis.poulsen@risoe.dk

Simone Rinaldi
Dip. di Scienze Matematiche e Informatiche, Univ. degli Studi di Siena
Pian dei Mantellini 44, 53100, Siena, Italy
rinaldi@unisi.it

Lajos Rodek
Dept. of Image Processing and Computer Graphics, University of Szeged
Árpád tér 2., Szeged, H-6720, Hungary
rodek@inf.u-szeged.hu

Martin Šámal
Dept. of Nuclear Medicine, First Faculty of Medicine, Charles Univ. Prague
Salmovska 3, CZ-120 00 Praha 2, Czech Republic
samal@cesnet.cz

Burkhard Schillinger
FRM-II, Technical University Munich,
D-85747 Garching, Germany
burkhard.schillinger@frm2.tum.de

Christoph Schnörr
Dept. M&CS, CVGPR-Group, University of Mannheim
D-68131 Mannheim, Germany
schnoerr@uni-mannheim.de

Thomas Schüle
Dept. M&CS, CVGPR-Group, University of Mannheim
D-68131 Mannheim, Germany
schuele@uni-mannheim.de

Jürgen Stephan
Corporate Technology PS 9, Siemens AG
Otto-Hahn-Ring 6, D-81730, Munich, Germany
Juergen.Stephan@siemens.com

Robert Tijdeman
Mathematical Institute, Leiden University
P. O. Box 9512, 2300 RA Leiden, The Netherlands
tijdeman@math.leidenuniv.nl

Ernesto Vallejo
Instituto de Matemáticas, Unidad Morelia, UNAM
Apartado Postal 61-3, Santa María, 58089, Morelia, Michoacon, Mexico
vallejo@matmor.unam.mx

Stefan Weber
Dept. M&CS, CVGPR-Group, University of Mannheim
D-68131 Mannheim, Germany
sweber@uni-mannheim.de

Steffen Zopf
Dept. of Image Processing and Computer Graphics, University of Szeged
Árpád tér 2., Szeged, H-6720, Hungary
Steffen.Zopf@sick.de

Contents

Part II Discrete Tomography Reconstruction Algorithms

Part III Applications of Discrete Tomography

1

Introduction

A. Kuba and G.T. Herman

Summary. This chapter discuses the excellent progress made in discrete tomography (DT) during the last seven years and includes a comprehensive bibliography illustrating this progress. It also presents some of the fundamental definitions relevant to DT.

1.1 Discrete Tomography since 1999

In the historical overview of discrete tomography (DT) [123] that was presented in the predecessor [106] of this book, the earliest reference is to an 1838 paper of J. Steiner. This is because much work that is now considered relevant to DT had been done, in mathematical analysis, combinatorics, and geometry, even before the idea of DT occurred. The first papers explicitly dealing with DT, in the sense that their titles contained the phrase "reconstruction of binary patterns," appeared in the early 1970s (e.g., by S.K. Chang and G.T. Herman). However, it was not until 1994 that a scientific meeting devoted to DT took place. That year L. Shepp organized the DIMACS Mini-Symposium on Discrete Tomography, where the participants discussed problems related mostly to the reconstruction of finite lattice sets from their projections taken along straight lines. In the following five years, DT had an explosive development; several workshops were held and many relevant papers were published. The first book devoted to DT appeared in 1999 [106] and contained a collection of papers on DT foundations, algorithms, and applications, based on earlier presentations at a DT workshop. Its first chapter [123] provided an overview of DT up to the time of its publication. In the current book we do not repeat material that already appeared [106] but concentrate on advances that have taken place since 1999.

During this period, several meetings devoted entirely to DT have been organized:

(a) Meeting on the Mathematics of Discrete Tomography, December 3–9, 2000, Oberwolfach, Germany (organizers: P. Gritzmann and R.J. Gardner).

(b) Workshop on Discrete Tomography: Algorithms and Applications, 2001, Certosa di Pontignano, Italy (organizers: A. Del Lungo, P. Gronchi, and G.T. Herman).
(c) Workshop on Discrete Tomography and Its Applications, June 13–15, 2005, New York City, USA (organizers: G.T. Herman and A. Kuba).

Furthermore, there were meetings, such as the International Conferences on Discrete Geometry for Computer Imagery (DGCI 2000, 2002, 2003, 2005, 2006) and the International Workshops on Combinatorial Image Analysis (IW-CIA 2001, 2003, 2004, 2005) at which many papers on DT were presented, sometimes in special sessions devoted to this topic. Special issues of journals were also devoted to DT:

(a) *Linear Algebra and Its Applications* **339**, 2001 (special issue editors: A. Del Lungo, P. Gronchi, and G.T. Herman).
(b) *Electronic Notes on Discrete Mathematics* **12**, 2005 (special issue editors: G.T. Herman and A. Kuba).

Due to all this activity, as well as an impressive number of papers that have been published on DT independently of the above-mentioned workshops and special issues, we find that the last seven years have produced in the order of 200 publications [1–191] relevant to our topic. The current book is the culmination of some of this activity. Its chapters were invited by the editors based on the presentations that were given at the Workshop on Discrete Tomography and Its Applications, June 13–15, 2005, in New York City. They were refereed, revised, and edited with the aim of producing between them a cohesive coverage of some of the important advances in DT since 1999. The book is divided into three parts: Foundations of DT; DT Reconstruction Algorithms; and Applications of DT.

1.2 Definitions

The introductory chapter [123] of [106] starts with the following definition of DT:

> We assume that there is a domain, which may itself be discrete (such as a set of ordered pairs of integers) or continuous (such as Euclidean space). We further assume that there is an unknown function f whose range is known to be a given discrete set (usually of real numbers). The problems of *discrete tomography*, as we perceive the field, have to do with determining f (perhaps only partially, perhaps only approximately) from weighted sums over subsets of its domain in the discrete case and from weighted integrals over subspaces of its domain in the continuous case.

This definition is much more general in scope than how DT had been considered by some practitioners, namely that it focuses on subsets of the integer lattice. Our definition includes, for example, problems involving the recovery of planar convex sets from their integrals. Since neither the statements nor the solution of such problems involve much discrete mathematics, the definition is debatable. Of course, the word "discrete" in the definition is not referring to the nature of the methods to be used, but rather to the nature of the range of the function to be recovered. Approached this way, planar convex sets are represented by their characteristic functions, which are of course binary-valued. As we explain below, the tomography of measurable sets and the tomography of finite sets overlap somewhat, and we find it convenient to bring both under the same heading.

In fact, the tomography of planar measurable sets is subsumed under the already established field of geometric tomography. This term was introduced by R.J. Gardner at the 1990 Oberwolfach meeting on tomography and is defined in his book [90] as the area of mathematics dealing with the retrieval of information about a geometric object from data about its sections, or projections, or both. The term "projection" here means orthogonal projection, and according to Gardner, the phrase "geometric object" is deliberately vague: a convex polytope or body would certainly qualify, as would a star-shaped body, or even, when appropriate, a compact set or measurable set.

Clearly, then, the tomography of measurable sets falls under both DT, as we define it, and geometric tomography. Researchers should be aware of this and choose whichever term they feel more suitable as a general description.

It is a characteristic property of all young fields of research that the terminology is not yet settled. DT is no exception and in some cases different names are used for the same things. For example, some people use "X-ray," others "marginal," and yet others "discrete Radon-transform" to refer to the weighted sums mentioned in the definition above; here we selected to use the term "projection."

There are many different kinds of objects studied in DT, e.g., lattice sets, binary matrices, digital or label images, measurable sets, dominoes, etc. In general, they can be represented as functions with a domain X and with a given discrete range (of real numbers). Let us denote the class of functions to be studied by $\mathcal{E}$. Let $\mathcal{S}$ be a collection of subsets of the domain (X) of the functions in $\mathcal{E}$ (e.g., lines, strips, hyperplanes). The *projection* of a function in $\mathcal{E}$ onto a subset S in $\mathcal{S}$ is the weighted sum (alternatively, integral)

$$[\mathcal{P}f](S) = \sum_{x \in S} w(x, S) \cdot f(x) \left(= \int_S w(x, S) \cdot f(x) \right), \qquad (1.1)$$

where $w : X \times \mathcal{S} \longrightarrow \mathbb{R}$ is a given weight function. (The weight function is often chosen, in particular in the examples below, to have the constant value 1. However, this is not always the case; see Chapters 13 and 16 of this book for examples.) With this notation, the uniqueness, existence, and reconstruction problems can be stated as follows.

UNIQUENESS($\mathcal{E}$, $\mathcal{S}$).

Given: A function $f \in \mathcal{E}$.

Question: Does there exist a function $f' \in \mathcal{E}$ different from f such that f and f' have the same projections onto S "for all" S in $\mathcal{S}$?

EXISTENCE($\mathcal{E}$, $\mathcal{S}$).

Given: A real-valued function g defined on $\mathcal{S}$.

Question: Does there exist a function $f \in \mathcal{E}$ such that $[\mathcal{P}f](S) = g(S)$ "for all" S in $\mathcal{S}$?

RECONSTRUCTION($\mathcal{E}$, $\mathcal{S}$).

Given: A real-valued function g defined on $\mathcal{S}$.

Task: Construct a function $f \in \mathcal{E}$ such that $[\mathcal{P}f](S) = g(S)$ "for all" S in $\mathcal{S}$.

The reason for putting "for all" into quotes, is that sometimes things are known to us only partially; we now give two illustrations of the general terminology, the second of which makes essential use of partial information.

In the first example, $X = \mathbb{Z}^2$, where $\mathbb{Z}$ denotes the set of integers. $\mathcal{E}$ is the set of $\{0,1\}$-valued functions on X, such that the number elements of X for which the value is 1 is finite. (These are the characteristic functions of finite lattice sets.) The elements of $\mathcal{S}$ are the horizontal and vertical lattice lines; i.e., sets of the form $\{(i,j) \mid j = j_0\}$ or $\{(i,j) \mid i = i_0\}$. The weight w is always 1, and so the projections are just sums of the function values on a horizontal or a vertical lattice line. For this example, "for all" really means for all. A *switching component* of an $f \in \mathcal{E}$ is a set of four points in X of the form $x_1 = (i_1, j_1)$, $x_2 = (i_2, j_1)$, $x_3 = (i_1, j_2)$ and $x_4 = (i_2, j_2)$, such that $f(x_1) \neq f(x_2)$, but $f(x_1) = f(x_3)$ and $f(x_2) = f(x_4)$. It is a well-known result of DT (published in 1957 by H.J. Ryser) that under the definitions of this paragraph, a function f is not unique (according to the definition given above) if, and only if, f has a switching component (see Theorem 1.4 of [123]).

In the second example, $X = \mathbb{R}^2$, the Euclidean plane, and $\mathcal{E}$ is the set of $\{0,1\}$-valued functions f on X, such that the set of elements of X for which the value is 1 (the *support* of f) is of a finite Lebesgue measure. More precisely, elements of $\mathcal{E}$ are equivalence classes of such functions: two functions are considered equivalent if the symmetric difference between their supports is of measure zero. The elements of $\mathcal{S}$ are the horizontal and vertical lines (i.e., the lines parallel to the axes of $\mathbb{R}^2$); there are uncountably many such lines. Selecting the weight w to again be always 1, the natural interpretation of the integral in (1.1) is that it is a line integral of f along S, providing us with two functions of one variable each (one for the horizontal and one for the vertical lines). However, either of these two functions may be undefined on a set of measure zero (hence the quotes on "for all"). Having the same projections, in this context, is to be interpreted as the same everywhere except on a set of measure zero. In a 1988 paper, A. Kuba and A. Volčič introduced the notion of a switching component in this context as well (essentially, it consists of four vertexes of a rectangle defined by two horizontal and two vertical lines in $\mathbb{R}^2$ and a set of positive measure that is shifted to each of the four points, such that points that belong to the sets that are shifted to diagonally opposing vertexes of the rectangle are either all in the support of f or none are in the support of f, with the opposite being the case for the points of the sets that are shifted to the other two vertexes; see, e.g., Chapter 5 of [106]) and proved that a function f is not unique if, and only if, f has a switching component. It is interesting to observe that the theorem of Ryser mentioned in the previous paragraph is, in fact, derivable from this result (by defining for a function over a lattice set another one over the Euclidean plane by making it piecewise constant in the interiors of the Voronoi neighborhoods of the lattice points).

This discussion is a minor illustration (using the uniqueness problem) of our viewpoint that the tomography of measurable planar sets and the tomography of lattice sets share some basic ideas and methods of proof. Another example (which we do not discuss in detail) is provided by the relationship between the existence problems for measurable planar sets and lattice sets, as characterized by the theorems of Lorentz and Gale–Ryser (both mentioned later on in this book), respectively. It is therefore our terminological preference to consider both the tomography of measurable planar sets and the tomography of lattice sets to be areas of discrete tomography as defined in the first paragraph of this section.

1.3 Conclusions

The material presented in this chapter clearly demonstrates that DT is an extremely active field of research. In recent years it has been producing new and powerful results not only in its theoretical foundations and reconstruction algorithms, but also in new and previously proposed applications. An argument has been put forth that the field of DT should be considered to include not only problems capable of being treated by discrete methods, but also those that require continuous treatment, as long as their subject matter is the recovery of functions with a discrete range.

Acknowledgments

The research of the authors in DT is supported in part by the grants DMS 0306215 (National Science Foundation, USA) and T 048476 (Hungarian Research Foundation, OTKA). The authors are grateful to R.J. Gardner for suggestions on a preliminary version of this chapter.

References

1. Alpers, A.: *Instability and Stability in Discrete Tomography*. Ph.D. Thesis, Technical Univ. of Munich, Shaker Verlag, Germany (2004).
2. Alpers, A., Brunetti, S.: On the stability of reconstructing lattice sets from X-rays along two directions. In: Andres, É., Damiand, G., Lienhardt, P. (eds.), *Digital Geometry for Computer Imagery*, Springer, Berlin, Germany, pp. 92–103 (2005).
3. Alpers, A., Gritzmann, P.: On stability, error correction, and noise compensation in discrete tomography. *SIAM J. Discr. Math.*, **20**, 227–239 (2006).
4. Alpers, A., Gritzmann, P., Thorens, L.: Stability and instability in discrete tomography. In: Bertrand, G., Imiya, A., Klette, R. (eds.), *Digital and Image Geometry*, Springer, Berlin, Germany, pp. 175-186 (2001).
5. Alpers, A., Knudsen, E., Poulsen, H., Herman, G.: Resolving ambiguities in reconstructed grain maps using discrete tomography. *Electr. Notes Discr. Math.*, **20**, 419–437 (2005).
6. Alpers, A., Poulsen, H., Knudsen, E., Herman, G.: A discrete tomography algorithm for improving the quality of 3DXRD grain maps. *J. Appl. Crystallography*, **39**, 281–299 (2006).
7. Autrusseau, F., Guédon, J.: Chiffrement Mojette d'images médicales. *Systèmes d'Information de Santé (Ingénierie des Systèmes d'Information-RSTI Série ISI)*, **8**, 113–134 (2003).
8. Baake, M., Gritzmann, P., Huck, C., Langfeld, B., Lord, K.: Discrete tomography of planar model sets. *Acta Crystallographica Section A.*, **62**, 419–433 (2006).
9. Bakirov, V.F., Kline, R.A., Winfree, W.P.: Discrete variable thermal tomography. In: Thompson, D.O., Chimenti, D.E. (eds.): *Review of Quantitative Nondestructive Evaluation*, American Institute of Physics, **23**, pp. 469–476 (2004).
10. Balaskó, M., Kuba, A., Nagy, A., Kiss, Z., Rodek, L., Ruskó, L.: Neutron-, gamma- and X-ray three-dimensional computer tomography at the Budapest research reactor, *Nucl. Inst. & Meth.*, *A*, **542**, 22–27 (2005).
11. Balaskó, M., Sváb, E., Kuba, A., Kiss, Z., Rodek, L., Nagy, A.,: Pipe corrosion and deposit study using neutron- and gamma- radiation sources, *Nucl. Inst. & Meth.*, *A*, **542**, 302–308 (2005).
12. Balázs, P.: Reconstruction of decomposable discrete sets from four projections: Strong decomposability. In: Andres, É., Damiand, G., Lienhardt, P. (eds.), *Discrete Geometry in Computer Imagery*, Springer, Berlin, Germany, pp. 104–114 (2005).
13. Balázs, P.: Reconstruction of discrete sets from four projections: Strong decomposability. *Electr. Notes Discr. Math.*, **20**, 329–345 (2005).
14. Balázs, P., Balogh, E., Kuba, A.: A fast algorithm for reconstructing hv-convex 8-connected but not 4-connected discrete sets. In: Nyström, I., Sanniti di Baja, G., Svenson, S. (eds.), *Discrete Geometry for Computer Imagery*, Springer, Berlin, Germany, pp. 388–397 (2003).
15. Balázs, P., Balogh, E., Kuba, A.: Reconstruction of 8-connected but not 4-connected hv-convex discrete sets. *Discr. Appl. Math.*, **147**, 149–168 (2005).
16. Balogh, E., Kuba, A.: Reconstruction algorithms for hv-convex 4- and 8-connected discrete sets. In: Loncaric, S., Babic, H. (eds.), *Proc. 2nd Intl. Symp. on Image and Signal Processing and Analysis, ISPA 2001*, Pula, Croatia, pp. 49-54 (2001).

17. Balogh, E., Kuba, A., Del Lungo, A., Nivat, M.: Reconstruction of binary matrices from absorbed projections. In Braquelaire, A., Lachaud, J.-O., Vialard, A. (eds.), *Discrete Geometry for Computer Imagery*, Springer, Berlin, Germany, pp. 392–403 (2002).

18. Balogh, E., Kuba, A., Dévényi, C., Del Lungo, A.: Comparison of algorithms for reconstructing *hv*-convex discrete sets. *Lin. Algebra Appl.*, **339**, 23–35 (2001).

19. Barcucci, E., Brunetti, S., Del Lungo, A., Nivat, M.: Reconstruction of discrete sets from three or more X-rays. In: Bongiovanni, G., Gambosi, G., Petreschi, R. (eds.), *Algorithms and Complexity*, Springer, Berlin, Germany, pp. 199–210 (2000).

20. Barcucci, E., Brunetti, S., Del Lungo, A., Nivat, M.: Reconstruction of lattice sets from their horizontal, vertical and diagonal X-rays. *Discr. Math.*, **241**, 65–78 (2001).

21. Barucci, E., Del Lungo, A., Nivat, M., Pinzani, R.: X-rays characterizing some classes of discrete sets. *J. Linear Algebra*, **339**, 3–21 (2001).

22. Barcucci, E., Frosini, A., Rinaldi, S.: Reconstruction of discrete sets from two absorbed projections: An algorithm. *Electr. Notes Discr. Math.*, **12** (2003).

23. Barcucci, E., Frosini, A., Rinaldi, S.: An algorithm for the reconstruction of discrete sets from two projections in presence of absorption. *Discr. Appl. Math.*, **151**, 21–35 (2005).

24. Batenburg, K.J.: Analysis and optimization of an algorithm for discrete tomography. *Electr. Notes Discr. Math.*, **12** (2003).

25. Batenburg, K.J.: A new algorithm for 3D binary tomography. *Electr. Notes Discr. Math.*, **20**, 247–261 (2005).

26. Batenburg, K.J.: An evolutionary algorithm for discrete tomography. *Discr. Appl. Math.*, **151**, 36–54 (2005).

27. Batenburg, K.J.: *Network Flow Algorithms for Discrete Tomography*. Ph.D. Thesis, Leiden Univ., The Netherlands (2006).

28. Batenburg, K.J., Kosters, W.A.: A discrete tomography approach to Japanese Puzzles. In: Verbrugge, R., Taatgen, N., Schomaker, L. (eds.), *Proc. 16th Belgian-Dutch Conf. Artificial Intelligence*, Groningen, The Netherlands, pp. 243–250 (2004).

29. Batenburg, K.J., Kosters, W.A.: Neural networks for discrete tomography. In: Verbeeck, K., Tuyls, K., Nowé, A., Manderick, B., Kuijpers, B. (eds.), *Proc. 17th Belgian-Dutch Conf. Artificial Intelligence*, Brussels, Belgium, pp. 21–27 (2005).

30. Batenburg, K.J., Palenstijn, W.J.: On the reconstruction of crystals through discrete tomography. In: Reulke, R., Eckardt, U., Flach, B., Knauer, U., Polthier, K. (eds.), *Combinatorial Image Analysis*, Springer, Berlin, Germany, pp. 23–37 (2006).

31. Batenburg, K.J., Sijbers, J.: Discrete tomography from micro-CT data: Application to the mouse trabecular bone structure. *Proc. SPIE*, **6142**, pp. 1325–1335 (2006).

32. Battle, X.L., Bizais, Y.: 3D attenuation map reconstruction using geometrical models and free-form deformations. In: Beekman, F., Defrise, M., Viergever, M. (eds.), *Proc. Fully Three-Dimensional Image Reconstruction in Radiology and Nuclear Medicine*, Egmond aan Zee, The Netherlands, pp. 181–184 (1999).

33. Battle, X.L., Bizais, Y., Le Rest, C., Turzo, A.: Tomographic reconstruction using free-form deformation models.*Proc. SPIE*, **3661**, 356–367 (1999).

34. Battle, X.L., Le Rest, A., Turzo, C., Bizais, Y.: Three-dimensional attenuation map reconstruction using geometrical models and free-form deformations. *IEEE Trans. Med. Imag.*, **19**, 404–411 (2000).

35. Battle, X.L., Le Rest, A., Turzo, C. Bizais, Y.: Free-form deformation in tomographic reconstruction. Application to attenuation map reconstruction. *IEEE Trans. Nucl. Sci.*, **47**, 1065–1071 (2000).

36. Bebeacua, C., Mansour, T., Postnikov, A., Severini, S.: On the X-rays of permutations. *Electr. Notes Discr. Math.*, **20**, 193–203 (2005).

37. Beldiceanu, N., Katriel, I., Thiel, S.: Filtering algorithms for the Same and UsedBy constraints. In: Regin, J.C., Rueher, M. (eds.), *Integration of AI and OR Techniques in Constraint Programming for Combinatorial Optimisation Problems*, Springer, Berlin, Germany, pp. 65–79 (2004).

38. Boufkhad, Y., Dubois, O., Nivat, M.: Reconstructing (h,v)-convex 2-dimensional patterns of objects from approximate horizontal and vertical projections. *Theor. Comput. Sci.*, **290**, 1647–1664 (2003).

39. Brewbaker, C.R.: *Lonesum (0,1)-Matrices and Poly-Bernoulli Numbers of Negative Index*. MSc. Thesis, Iowa State Univ. (2005).

40. Brimkov, V.E., Barneva, R.P.: Exact image reconstruction from a single projection through real computation. *Electr. Notes Discr. Math.*, **20**, 233–246 (2005).

41. Brualdi, R.A.: Minimal nonnegative integral matrices and uniquely determined (0,1)-matrices. *Lin. Algebra Appl.*, **341**, 351–356 (2002).

42. Brualdi, R.A., Dahl, G.: Matrices of zeros and ones with given line sums and a zero block. *Lin. Algebra Appl.*, **371**, 191–207 (2003).

43. Brualdi, R.A., Hwang, S.-G.: A Bruhat order for the class of (0,1)-matrices with row sum vector R and column sum vector S. *Electr. J. Linear Algebra*, **12**, 6–16 (2004).

44. Bruandet, J.P., Peyrin, F., Dinten, J.M., Amadieu, O., Barlaud, M.: Binary objects tomographic reconstruction from few noisy X-ray radiographs using a region based curve evolution method. *IEEE Nuclear Science Symposium Conference Record*, San Diego, USA, pp. 1717–1719 (2001).

45. Brunetti, S.: *Convexity and Complexity in Discrete Tomography*. Ph.D. Thesis, Univ. of Florence, Italy (2001).

46. Brunetti, S., Daurat, A.: Reconstruction of discrete sets from two or more X-rays in any direction. *Proc. 7th Intl. Workshop on Combinatorial Image Analysis*, Caen, France, pp. 241–258 (2000).

47. Brunetti, S., Daurat, A.: An algorithm reconstructing lattice convex sets. *Theoret. Comput. Sci.*, **304**, 35–57 (2003).

48. Brunetti, S., Daurat, A.: Stability in discrete tomography: Linear programming, additivity and convexity. In: Nyström, I., Sanniti di Baja, G., Svensson, S. (eds.), *Discrete Geometry for Computer Imagery*, Springer, Berlin, Germany, pp. 398–407 (2003).

49. Brunetti, S., Daurat, A.: Determination of Q-convex bodies by X-rays. *Electr. Notes Discr. Math.*, **20**, pp. 67–81 (2005).

50. Brunetti, S., Daurat, A.: Stability in discrete tomography: Some positive results. *Discr. Appl. Math.*, **147**, pp. 207–226 (2005).

51. Brunetti, S., Daurat, A., Del Lungo, A.: Approximate X-rays reconstruction of special lattice sets. *Pure Math. Appl.*, **11**, 409–425 (2000).

52. Brunetti, S., Daurat, A., Del Lungo, A.: An algorithm for reconstructing special lattice sets from their approximate X-rays, In: Borgefors, G., Nyström, I.,

Sanniti di Baja, G. (eds.), *Discrete Geometry for Computer Imagery*, Springer, Berlin, Germany, pp. 113–125 (2000).

53. Brunetti, S., Del Lungo, A., Gerard, Y.: On the computational complexity of reconstructing three-dimensional lattice sets from their two dimensional X-rays. *Lin. Algebra Appl.* **339**, 59–73 (2001).

54. Brunetti, S., Del Lungo, A., Del Ristoro, F., Kuba, A., Nivat, M.: Reconstruction of 4- and 8-connected convex discrete sets from row and column projections. *Lin. Algebra Appl.*, **339**, 37–57 (2001).

55. Capricelli, T.D., Combettes, P.L.: Parallel block-iterative reconstruction algorithms for binary tomography. *Electr. Notes Discr. Math.*, **20**, 263–280 (2005).

56. Carvalho, B.M., Herman, G.T., Matej, S., Salzberg, C., Vardi, E.: Binary tomography for triplane cardiography. In: Kuba, A., Sámal, M., Todd-Pokropek, A. (eds.), *Information Processing in Medical Imaging*, Springer, Berlin, Germany, pp. 29–41 (1999).

57. Castiglione, G., Frosini, A., Restivo, A., Rinaldi, S.: A tomographical characterization of L-convex polyominoes. In: Rangarajan, A., Vemuri, B.C., Yuille, A.L. (eds.), *Discrete Geometry in Computer Imagery*, Springer, Berlin, Germany, pp. 115–125 (2005).

58. Castiglione, G., Restivo, A.: Reconstruction of L-convex polyominoes. *Electr. Notes Discr. Math.*, **12** (2003).

59. Censor, Y.: Binary steering in discrete tomography reconstruction with sequential and simultaneous iterative algorithms. *Lin. Algebra Appl.*, **339**, 111–124 (2001).

60. Chrobak, M., Couperus, P., Dürr, C., Woeginger, G.: On tiling under tomographic constraints. *Theor. Comp. Sci.*, **290**, 2125-2136 (2003).

61. Chrobak, M., Dürr, C.: Reconstructing *hv*-convex polyominoes from orthogonal projections. *Inform. Process. Lett.*, **69**, 283–289 (1999).

62. Chrobak, M., Dürr, C.: Reconstructing polyatomic structures from X-rays: NP-completeness proof for three atoms. *Theor. Comp. Sci.*, **259**, 81–98 (2001).

63. Costa, M. C., Jarray, F., Picouleau, C.: Reconstruction of binary matrices under adjacency constraints. *Electr. Notes Discr. Math.*, **20**, 281–297 (2005).

64. Costa, M. C., de Werra, D., Picouleau, C.: Using graphs for some discrete tomography problems. *Discr. Appl. Math.*, **154**, 35–46 (2006).

65. Costa, M. C., de Werra, D., Picouleau, C., Schindl, D.: A solvable case of image reconstruction in discrete tomography. *Discr. Appl. Math.*, **148**, 240–245 (2005).

66. Dahl, G., Brualdi, R.A.: Matrices of zeros and ones with given line sums and a zero block. *Electr. Notes Discr. Math.*, **20**, 83–97 (2003).

67. Dahl, G., Flatberg, T.: Optimization and reconstruction of *hv*-convex (0, 1)-matrices. *Electr. Notes Discr. Math.*, **12** (2003).

68. Dahl, G., Flatberg, T.: Optimization and reconstruction of *hv*-convex (0, 1)-matrices. *Discr. Appl. Math.*, **151**, 93–105 (2005).

69. Daurat, A.: *Convexité dans le Plan Discret. Application à la Tomographie.* Ph.D. Thesis, LLAIC1, and LIAFA, Université Paris 7, France (2000).

70. Daurat, A.: Determination of Q-convex sets by X-rays. *Theoret. Comput. Sci.*, **332**, 19–45 (2005).

71. Daurat, A., Del Lungo, A., Nivat, M.: Medians of discrete sets according to a linear distance. *Discrete Comput. Geom.*, **23**, 465–483 (2000).

72. Debled-Rennesson, I., Remy, J.-L., Rouyer-Degli, J.: Detection of the discrete convexity of polyominoes. In: Borgefors, G., Nyström, I., Sanniti di Baja, G. (eds.), *Disc. Geometry in Computer Imagery*, Springer, Berlin, Germany, pp. 491–504 (2000).
73. Debled-Rennesson, I., Remy, J.-L., Rouyer-Degli, J.: Detection of the discrete convexity of polyominoes. *Discr. Appl. Math.*, **125**, 115–133 (2003).
74. Del Lungo, A.: Reconstructing permutation matrices from diagonal sums. *Theor. Comput. Sci.*, **281**, 235–249 (2002).
75. Del Lungo, A., Frosini, A., Nivat, M., Vuillon, L.: Discrete tomography: Reconstruction under periodicity constraints. In: Widmayer, P., Triguero, F., Morales, R., Hennessy, M., Eidenbenz, S., Conejo, R. (eds.), *Automata, Languages and Programming*, Springer, Berlin, Germany, pp. 38–56 (2002).
76. Del Lungo, A., Gronchi, P., Herman, G.T. (eds.): *Proceedings of the Workshop on Discrete Tomography: Algorithms and Applications.* Lin. Algebra Appl., **339**, 1–219 (2001).
77. Di Gesu, V.D., Valenti, C.: The stability problem and noisy projections in discrete tomography. *J. Visual Languages and Computing*, **15**, 361–371 (2004).
78. Dulio, P., Gardner, R.J., Peri, C.: Discrete point X-rays of convex lattice sets. *Electronic Notes in Discrete Math.*, **20**, 1–13 (2005).
79. Dulio, P., Gardner, R.J., Peri, C.: Discrete point X-rays. *SIAM J. Discrete Math.*, **20**, 171–188 (2006).
80. Dürr, C., Goles, E., Rapaport, I., Remila, E.: Tiling with bars under tomographic constraints. *Theor. Comput. Sci.*, **290**, 1317–1329 (2003).
81. Frosini, A.: *Complexity Results and Reconstruction Algorithms for Discrete Tomography.* Ph.D. Thesis, Univ. of Siena, Italy (2003).
82. Frosini, A., Barcucci, E., Rinaldi, S.: An algorithm for the reconstruction of discrete sets from two projections in present of absorption. *Disc. Appl. Math.*, **151**, 21–35 (2005).
83. Frosini, A., Nivat, M.: Binary matrices under the microscope. A tomographical problem. In: Klette, R, Zunic, J.D. (eds.), *Combinatorial Image Analysis*, Springer, Berlin, Germany, pp. 1–22 (2004).
84. Frosini, A., Nivat, M., Vuillon, L.: An introductive analysis of periodical discrete sets from a tomographical point of view. *Theor. Comput. Sci.*, **347**, 370–392 (2005).
85. Frosini, A., Rinaldi, S.: The complexity of the reconstruction of (r,h,v) from two projections and an approximation algorithm. *Pure Math. Appl.*, **11**, 485–496 (2000).
86. Frosini, A., Rinaldi, S., Barcucci, E., Kuba, A.: An efficient algorithm for reconstructing binary matrices from horizontal and vertical absorbed projections. *Electr. Notes Discr. Math.*, **20**, 347–363 (2005).
87. Frosini, A., Simi, G.: The reconstruction of a bicolored domino tiling from two projections. In: Widmayer, P., Triguero, F., Morales, R., Hennessy, M., Eidenbenz, S., Conejo, R. (eds.), *Automata, Languages and Programming*, Springer, Berlin, Germany, pp. 136–144 (2002).
88. Frosini, A., Simi, G.: Reconstruction of low degree domino tilings. *Electr. Notes Discr. Math.*, **12** (2003).
89. Frosini, A., Simi, G.: The NP-completeness of a tomographical problem on bicolored domino tilings. *Theor. Comput. Sci.*, **319**, 447–454 (2004).
90. Gardner, R.J.: *Geometric Tomography*, 2nd edition, Cambridge University Press, New York, NY (2006).

91. Gardner, R.J., Gritzmann, P.: Discrete tomography: Determination of finite sets by X-rays. *J. Linear Algebra*, **339**, 3–21 (2001).

92. Gardner, R.J., Gritzmann, P., Prangenberg, D.: On the computational complexity of reconstructing lattice sets from their X-rays. *Discrete Math.*, **202**, 45–71 (1999).

93. Gardner, R.J., Gritzmann, P., Prangenberg, D.: On the computational complexity of determining polyatomic structures from by X-rays. *Theor. Comput. Sci.*, **233**, 91–106 (2000).

94. Gerard, Y.: Reduction from three-dimensional discrete tomography to multicommodity flow problem. *Theor. Comput. Sci.*, **346**, 300–306 (2005).

95. Gerard, Y., Feschet, F.: Application of a discrete tomography algorithm to computerized tomography. *Electr. Notes Discr. Math.*, **20**, 501–517 (2005).

96. Gębala, M.: The reconstruction of polyominoes from approximately orthogonal projections. In: Pacholski, L., Ruika, P. (eds.), *Current Trends in Theory and Practice of Informatics*, Springer, Berlin, Germany, pp. 253–260 (2001).

97. Gębala, M.: The reconstruction of some 3D convex polyominoes from orthogonal projections. In: Grosky, W.I., Plásil, F. (eds.), *Current Trends in Theory and Practice of Informatics*, Springer, Berlin, Germany, pp. 262–272 (2002).

98. Gritzmann, P., de Vries, S.: On the algorithmic inversion of the discrete Radon transform. *Theor. Comp. Science*, **281**, 455–469 (2001).

99. Gritzmann, P., de Vries, S.: Reconstructing crystalline structures from few images under high resolution transmission electron microscopy. In: Jäger, W.(ed.), *Mathematics: Key Technology for the Future*, Springer, Berlin, Germany, pp. 441–459 (2003).

100. Gritzmann, P, de Vries, S., Wiegelmann, M.: Approximating binary images from discrete X-rays. *SIAM J. Optim.*, **11**, 522–546 (2000).

101. Guédon, J., Normand, N.: The mojette transform: The first ten years. In: Andres, É., Damiand, G., Lienhardt, P. (eds.), *Discrete Geometry for Computer Imagery*, Springer, Berlin, Germany, pp. 79–91 (2005).

102. Hajdu, L.: Unique reconstruction of bounded sets in discrete tomography. *Electr. Notes Discr. Math.*, **20**, 15–25 (2005).

103. Hajdu, L., Tijdeman, R.: Algebraic aspects of discrete tomography. *J. Reine Angew. Math.*, **534**, 119–128 (2001).

104. Hajdu, L., Tijdeman, R.: An algorithm for discrete tomography. *J. Linear Algebra*, **339**, 147–169 (2001).

105. Hajdu, L., Tijdeman, R.: Algebraic aspects of emission tomography with absorption. *Theoret. Comput. Sci.*, **290**, 2169–2181 (2003).

106. Herman, G.T., Kuba, A. (eds.): *Discrete Tomography: Foundations, Algorithms, and Applications*. Birkhäuser, Boston, MA (1999).

107. Herman, G.T., Kuba, A.: Discrete tomography in medical imaging. *Proc. IEEE*, **91**, 380–385 (2003).

108. Herman, G.T., Kuba, A. (eds.): *Proceedings of the Workshop on Discrete Tomography and Its Applications*. Electronic Notes in Discrete Math., **20**, 1–622 (2005).

109. Huck, C., Baake, M., Langfeld, B., Gritzmann, P., Lord, K.: Discrete tomography of mathematical quasicrystals: A primer. *Electr. Notes Discr. Math.*, **20**, 179–191 (2005).

110. Imiya, A., Tirii, A., Sato, K.: Tomography on finite graphs. *Electr. Notes Discr. Math.*, **20**, 217–232 (2005).

111. Jarray F.: *Résolution de Problèmes de Domographie Discrète. Applications à la Planification de Ppersonnel.* Ph.D. Thesis, CNAM, Paris, France (2004).
112. Jinschek, J.R., Batenburg, K.J., Calderon, H.A., Van Dyck, D., Chen, F.R., Kisielowski, C.: Prospects for bright field and dark field electron tomography on a discrete grid. *Microscopy and Microanalysis; Cambridge J. Online*, **10**, Suppl. 3 (2004).
113. Jinschek, J.R., Calderon, H.A., Batenburg, K.J., Radmilovic, V., Kisielowski, C.: Discrete tomography of Ga and InGa particles from HREM image simulation and exit wave reconstruction. In: Martin, D.C., Muller, D.A., Midgley, P.A., Stach, E.A. (eds.), *Electron Microscopy of Molecular and Atom-Scale Mechanical Behavior, Chemistry and Structure*, Materials Research Society, Warrendale, PA, pp. 4.5.1–4.5.6 (2004).
114. Kaneko, A., Nagahama, R: Structure of total reconstructed sets from given two projection data. *Electr. Notes Discr. Math.*, **20**, 27–46 (2005).
115. Kaneko, A., Nagahama, R: Switching graphs and digraphs associated with total reconstructed sets from two projection data. *Nat. Sci. Report Ochanomizu Univ.*, **56**, 33–45 (2005).
116. Kingston, A.M.: *Extension and Application of Finite Discrete Radon Projection Theory.* Ph.D. Thesis, Monash Univ., Australia (2005).
117. Kingston, A., Svalbe, I.: A discrete modulo N projective Radon transform for $N \times N$ images. In: Andres, É., Damiand, G., Lienhardt, P. (eds.), *Discrete Geometry for Computer Imagery*, Springer, Berlin, Germany, pp. 136–147 (2005).
118. Kiss, Z., Rodek, L., Kuba, A.: Image reconstruction and correction methods in neutron and X-ray tomography. Simulation and physical experiments, *Acta Cybernetica*, **17**, 557–587 (2006).
119. Kiss, Z., Rodek, L., Nagy, A., Kuba, A., Balaskó, M.: Reconstruction of pixel-based and geometric objects by discrete tomography. Simulation and physical experiments, *Electr. Notes Discr. Math.*, **20**, 475–491 (2005).
120. Krimmel, S., Baumann, J., Kiss, Z., Kuba, A., Nagy, A., Stephan, J.: Discrete tomography for reconstruction from limited view angles in non-destructive testing. *Electr. Notes Discr. Math.*, **20**, 455–474 (2005).
121. Kuba, A.: Reconstruction in different classes of 2D discrete sets. In: Bertrands, G., Couprie, M., Perroton, L. (eds.): *Discrete Geometry for Computer Imagery*, Springer, Berlin, Germany, pp. 1153–1163 (1999).
122. Kuba, A., Balogh, E.: Reconstruction of convex 2D discrete sets in polynomial time. *Theor. Comput. Sci.*, **283**, 223–242 (2002).
123. Kuba, A., Herman, G.T.: Discrete tomography: A historical overview. In: Herman, G.T., Kuba, A. (eds.), *Discrete Tomography: Foundations, Algorithms, and Applications*, Birkhäuser, Boston, MA, pp. 3–34 (1999).
124. Kuba, A., Herman, G.T., Matej, S., Todd-Pokropek, A.: Medical applications of discrete tomography. In: Du, D.Z., Pardalos, P.M., Wang, J. (eds.), *Discrete Mathematical Problems in Medical Applications; DIMACS Series in Discrete Mathematics and Theoretical Computer Science.* AMS, Providence, RI, **55**, pp. 195–208 (2000).
125. Kuba, A., Nagy, A.: Reconstruction of hv-convex binary matrices from their absorbed projections. *Electr. Notes Theor. Comput. Sci.*, **46** (2001).
126. Kuba, A., Nagy, A., Balogh, E.: Reconstruction of hv-convex binary matrices from their absorbed projections. *Discr. Appl. Math.*, **139**, 137–148 (2004).

127. Kuba, A., Nivat, M.: Reconstruction of discrete sets with absorption. In: Borgefors, G., Nyström, I., Sanniti di Baja, G. (eds.), *Discrete Geometry in Computed Imagery*, Springer, Berlin, Germany, pp. 137–148 (2000).

128. Kuba, A., Nivat, M.: Reconstruction of discrete sets with absorption. *Lin. Algebra Appl.*, **339**, 171–194 (2001).

129. Kuba, A., Nivat, M.: A sufficient condition for non-uniqueness in binary tomography with absorption. *Discr. Appl. Math.*, **346**, 335–357 (2005).

130. Kuba, A., Rodek, L., Kiss, Z., Ruskó, L., Nagy, A., Balaskó, M.: Discrete tomography in neutron radiography. *Nucl. Inst. & Meth., A*, **542**, 376–382 (2005).

131. Kuba, A., Ruskó, L., Kiss, Z., Nagy, A.: Discrete reconstruction techniques, *Electr. Notes Discr. Math.*, **20**, 385–398 (2005).

132. Kuba, A., Ruskó, L., Rodek, L., Kiss, Z.: Preliminary studies of discrete tomography in neutron imaging, *IEEE Trans. Nuclear Sci.*, **52**, 380–385 (2005).

133. Kuba, A., Ruskó, L., Rodek, L., Kiss, Z.: Application of discrete tomography in neutron imaging, In: Chirco, P. et al. (eds.): *Proc. 7th World Conf. Neutron Radiography*, Rome, Italy, pp. 361–371 (2005).

134. Kuba, A., Woeginger, G.: Two remarks on reconstructing binary matrices from their absorbed projections. In: Andres, É., Damiand, G., Lienhardt, P. (eds.), *Discrete Geometry for Computer Imagery*, Springer, Berlin, Germany, pp. 79–91 (2005).

135. Kudo, H., Nakamura, H.: A new approach to SPECT attenuation correction without transmission measurements. In: *Proc. IEEE Nuclear Sci. Symp. and Medical Imaging Conf.*, pp. 13.58–13.62 (2000).

136. Liao, H.Y.: *Reconstruction of Label Images Using Gibbs Priors*. Ph.D. Thesis, City University of New York, New York, USA (2005).

137. Liao, H.Y., Herman, G.T.: Automated estimation of the parameters of Gibbs priors to be used in binary tomography. *Electr. Notes Theor. Comput. Sci.*, **46** (2001).

138. Liao, H.Y., Herman, G.T.: Reconstruction of label images from a few projections as motivated by electron microscopy. In: *IEEE 28th Annual Northeast Bioengineering Conf.*, Philadephia, PA, pp. 205–206 (2002).

139. Liao, H.Y., Herman, G.T.: Tomographic reconstruction of label images from a few projections. *Electr. Notes Discr. Math.*, **12** (2003).

140. Liao, H.Y., Herman, G.T.: Automated estimation of the parameters of Gibbs priors to be used in binary tomography. *Discr. Appl. Math.*, **139**, 149–170 (2004).

141. Liao, H.Y., Herman, G.T.: A method for reconstructing label images from a few projections, as motivated by electron microscopy. *Proc. IEEE Intl. Symp. on Biomedical Imaging*, Arlington, VA, pp. 551–554 (2004).

142. Liao, H.Y., Herman, G.T.: Discrete tomography with a very few views, using Gibbs priors and a marginal posterior mode. *Electr. Notes Discr. Math.*, **20**, 399–418 (2005).

143. Liao, H.Y., Herman, G.T.: Reconstruction by direct labeling in discrete tomography, using Gibbs priors and a marginal posterior mode approach. *Proc. IEEE 31st Northeast Bioengineering Conf.*, Philadelphia, PA, pp. 134–135 (2005).

144. Liao, H.Y., Herman, G.T.: A coordinate ascent approach to tomographic reconstruction of label images from a few projections. *Discr. Appl. Math.*, **139**, 184–197 (2005).

145. Masilamani, V., Dersanambika, K.S., Krithivasan, K.: Binary 3D matrices under the microscope: A tomographical problem. *Electr. Notes Discr. Math.*, **20**, 573–586 (2005).
146. Masilamani, V., Krithivasan, K.: An efficient reconstruction of 2D-tiling with $t_{1,2}$, $t_{2,1}$, $t_{1,1}$ tiles. In: Eckardt, U., Flach, B., Knauer, U., Polthier, K. (eds.), *Combinatorial Image Analysis*, Springer, Berlin, Germany, pp. 474–480 (2006).
147. Movassaghi, B., Rasche, V., Grass, M., Viergever, M.A., Niessen, W.J.: A quantitative analysis of 3-D coronary modeling from two or more projection images. *IEEE Trans. Medical Imaging*, **23**, 1517–1531 (2004).
148. Nagy, A., Kuba, A.: Reconstruction of binary matrices from fan-beam projections. *Acta Cybernetica*, **17**, 359–385 (2005).
149. Nagy, A., Kuba, A.: Parameter settings for reconstructing binary matrices from fan-beam projections. *J. Comput. Info.Tech.*, **14**, 101–110 (2006).
150. Nagy, A., Kuba, A., Samal, M.: Reconstruction of factor structures using discrete tomography method. *Electr. Notes Comput. Sci.*, **20**, 519–534 (2005).
151. Nam, Y.: Integral matrices with given row and column sums. *Ars Combinatorica*, **52**, 141–151 (1999).
152. Nivat, M.: On a tomographic equivalence between (0,1)-matrices. In: Karhumäki, J., Maurer, H., Paun, G., Rozenberg, G. (eds.), *Theory Is Forever*, Springer, Berlin, Germany, pp. 216–234 (2004).
153. Normand, N., Guédon, J.: Spline mojette transform. Application in tomography and communication. *Proc. EUSIPCO*, **2**, 407–410 (2002).
154. Picouleau, C.: Reconstruction of domino tiling from its two orthogonal projections. *Theor. Comp. Sci.*, **255**, 437–447 (2001).
155. Picouleau, C., Brunetti, S., Frosini, A.: Reconstructing a binary matrix under timetabling constraints. *Electr. Notes Discr. Math.*, **20**, 99–112 (2005).
156. Popa, C., Zdunek, R.: Penalized least-squares image reconstruction for borehole tomography. *Proc. ALGORITMY 2005*, Podbanske, Slovakia, pp. 407–410 (2005).
157. Rodek, L., Knudsen, E., Poulsen, H., Herman, G.: Discrete tomographic reconstruction of 2D polycrystal orientation maps from X-ray diffraction projections using Gibbs priors. *Electr. Notes Discr. Math.*, **20**, 439–453 (2005).
158. Ruskó, L., Kuba, A.: Multi-resolution method for binary tomography. *Electr. Notes Discr. Math.*, **20**, 299–311 (2005).
159. Schillinger, B.: Proposed combination of CAD data and discrete tomography for the detection of coking and lubricants in turbine blades or engines. *Electr. Notes Discr. Math.*, **20**, 493–499 (2005).
160. Schüle, T., Schnörr, C., Weber, S., Hornegger, J.: Discrete tomography by convex-concave regularization and D.C. programming. *Discr. Appl. Math.*, **151**, 229–243 (2005).
161. Schüle, T., Weber, S., Schnörr, C.: Adaptive reconstruction of discrete-valued objects from few projections. *Electr. Notes in Discr. Math.*, **20**, 365–384 (2005).
162. Sensali, M., Gamero, L., Herment, A., Mousseaux, E.: 3D reconstruction of vessel lumen from very few angiograms by dynamic contours using a stochastic approach, *Graph. Models*, **62**, 105–127 (2000).
163. Servières, M.: *Reconstruction Tomographique Mojette*. Thèse de doctorat, Université de Nantes, France (2005).
164. Servières, M., Guédon, J., Normand, N.: A discrete tomography approach to PET reconstruction. In: Bizais, Y.J. (ed.), *Proc. Fully 3D Reconstruction in Radiology and Nuclear Medicine*, University of Brest, Brest, France (2003).

165. Sharif, B., Sharif, B.: Discrete tomography in discrete deconvolution: Deconvolution of binary images using Ryser's algorithm. *Electr. Notes in Discr. Math.*, **20**, 555–571 (2005).

166. Soussen, C.: *Reconstruction 3D d'un Objet Compact en Tomographie.* Ph.D. Thesis, Université de Paris-Sud, France, (2000).

167. Soussen, C., Muhammad-Djafari, A.: Contour-based models for 3D binary reconstruction in X-ray tomography. In: *AIP Conference Proceedings*, Gif-sur-Yvette, France, **568**, pp. 543–554 (2001).

168. Soussen, C., Muhammad-Djafari, A.: Polygonal and polyhedral contour reconstruction in computed tomography. *IEEE Trans. Image Processing*, **13**, 1507–1523 (2004).

169. Takiguchi, T.: Reconstruction of measurable plane sets from their orthogonal projections. *Contemporary Math.*, **348**, 199–208 (2004).

170. Valenti, C.: *An Experimental Study of the Stability Problem in Discrete Tomography.* Ph.D. Thesis, Univ. of Palermo, Italy (2002).

171. Valenti, C.: Discrete tomography from noisy projections. In: *Series on Software Engineering and Knowledge Engineering*, World Scientific Publishing, **15**, 38–45 (2003).

172. Valenti, C.: An experimental study of the stability problem in discrete tomography. *Electr. Notes Discr. Math.*, **20**, 113–132 (2005).

173. Vallejo, E.: Plane partitions and characters of the symmetric group. *J. Algebraic Comb.*, **11**, 79–88 (2000).

174. Vallejo, E.: The classification of minimal matrices of size $2 \times q$. *Lin. Algebra Appl.*, **340**, 169–181 (2002).

175. Vallejo, E.: A characterization of additive sets. *Discr. Math.*, **259**, 201–210 (2002).

176. Vallejo, E.: Minimal matrices and discrete tomography. *Electr. Notes in Discr. Math.*, **20**, 113-132 (2005).

177. Vardi, E., Herman, G.T., Kong, T.Y.: Speeding up stochastic reconstructions of binary images from limited projection directions. *Lin. Algebra Appl.*, **339**, 75–89 (2001).

178. Venere, M., Liao, H., Clausse, A.: A genetic algorithm for adaptive tomography of elliptical objects. *IEEE Signal Processing Letters*, **7**, 176–178 (2000).

179. de Vries, S.: *Discrete Tomography, Packing and Covering, and Stable Set Problems: Polytopes and Algorithms.* Ph.D. Thesis, Technical Univ. of Munich, Germany (1999).

180. Weber, S., Schnörr, C., Hornegger, J.: A linear programming relaxation for binary tomography with smoothness priors. *Electr. Notes Discr. Math.*, **12** (2003).

181. Weber, S., Schüle, T., Hornegger, J., Schnörr, C.: Binary tomography by iterating linear programs from noisy projections. In: Klette, R, Zunic, J.D. (eds.), *Combinatorial Image Analysis*, Springer, Berlin, Germany, pp. 38–51 (2004).

182. Weber, S., Schüle, T., Kuba, A., Schnörr, C.: Binary tomography with deblurring. In: Reulke, R., Eckardt, U., Flach, B., Knauer, U., Polthier, K. (eds.), *Combinatorial Image Analysis*, Springer, Berlin, Germany, pp. 375–388 (2006).

183. Weber, S., Schüle, T., Schnörr, C.: Prior learning and convex-concave regularization of binary tomography. *Electr. Notes Discr. Math.*, **20**, 313–327 (2005).

184. Weber, S., Schüle, T., Schnörr, C., Hornegger, J.: A linear programming approach to limited angle 3D reconstruction from DSA projections. *Methods of Information in Medicine*, **43**, 320–326 (2003).

185. Weber, G.-W., Yasar, Ö.: Discrete tomography: A modern inverse problem reconsidered by optimization. *J. Comp. Tech.*, **9**, 115–121 (2004).
186. Woeginger, G.J.: The reconstruction of polyominoes from their orthogonal projections. *Inform. Process. Lett.*, **77**, 225–229 (2001).
187. Yagle, A.: A convergent composite mapping Fourier domain iterative algorithm for 3-D discrete tomography. *Lin. Algebra Appl.*, **339**, 91–109 (2001).
188. Yasar, Ö., Diner, C., Dogan, A., Weber, G.-W., Özbudak, F., Tiefenbach, A.: On the applied mathematics of discrete tomography. *J. Comp. Tech.*, **9**, 14–32 (2004).
189. Ye, Y., Wang, G., Zhu, J.: Linear diophantine equations for discrete tomography. *J. X-Ray Sci. Tech.*, **10**, 59–66 (2001).
190. Zdunek, R., Pralat, A.: Detection of subsurface bubbles with discrete electromagnetic geotomography. *Electr. Notes Discr. Math.*, **20**, 535–553 (2005).
191. Zopf, S., Kuba, A.: Reconstruction of measurable sets from two generalized projections. *Electr. Notes Discr. Math.*, **20**, 47–66 (2005).

Part I

Foundations of Discrete Tomography

2

An Introduction to Discrete Point X-Rays

P. Dulio, R.J. Gardner, and C. Peri

Summary. A discrete point X-ray of a finite subset F of $\mathbb{R}^n$ at a point p gives the number of points in F lying on each line passing through p. We survey the known results on discrete point X-rays, which mostly concern uniqueness issues for subsets of the integer lattice.

2.1 Introduction

The (continuous) *parallel X-ray* of a convex body K in n-dimensional Euclidean space $\mathbb{R}^n$ in a direction u gives the lengths of all the intersections of K with lines parallel to u, and the (continuous) *point X-ray* of K at a point $p \in \mathbb{R}^n$ gives the lengths of all the intersections of K with lines passing through p. (See Section 2.2 for all terminology.) In 1963, P.C. Hammer asked: How many parallel (or point) X-rays are needed to determine any convex body among all convex bodies? Answers to these questions are now known and are surveyed in [8, Chapters 1 and 5]. The topic of determining convex bodies and more general sets by their X-rays forms part of a larger area of inverse problems called *geometric tomography*, which concerns the retrieval of information about a geometric object (for example, a convex body, star-shaped body, or compact set) via measurements of its sections by lines or planes or its orthogonal projections on lines or planes.

Around 1994, Larry Shepp introduced the term *discrete tomography*. Here the focus is on determining finite subsets of the n-dimensional integer lattice $\mathbb{Z}^n$ by means of their discrete parallel X-rays. A *discrete parallel X-ray* of a finite subset F of $\mathbb{Z}^n$ in the direction of a vector $v \in \mathbb{Z}^n$ gives the number of points in F lying on each line parallel to v.

By now there are many results available on continuous parallel or point X-rays of sets and on discrete parallel X-rays of finite subsets of the integer lattice. Here we consider the obvious remaining category of X-rays, namely, discrete point X-rays. The definition is the natural one: A *discrete point X-ray* of a finite subset F of $\mathbb{R}^n$ at a point $p \in \mathbb{R}^n$ gives the number of points in F

lying on each line passing through p. Note that the above definition of discrete parallel X-ray also extends readily to finite subsets of $\mathbb{R}^n$, but as in that case, the main interest here is with discrete point X-rays of finite subsets of $\mathbb{Z}^n$ at points in $\mathbb{Z}^n$.

In order to describe our results, it is useful to briefly recall the corresponding results for discrete parallel X-rays. First, given any finite set U of lattice directions in $\mathbb{Z}^2$, there are different finite subsets of $\mathbb{Z}^2$ with equal discrete parallel X-rays in the directions in U (see [8, Lemma 2.3.2] or [10, Theorem 4.3.1]). In view of this, Gardner and Gritzmann [9] focused on convex lattice sets, employing the notion of a U-polygon in $\mathbb{R}^2$ for a given set U of directions. Roughly speaking, a U-polygon is a nondegenerate convex polygon whose vertices line up in pairs when viewed from a direction in U; see Section 2.2 for the formal definition. When a lattice U-polygon exists, it is easy to construct two different convex lattice sets with equal discrete parallel X-rays in the directions in U. In [9] it was proved that in fact the nonexistence of a lattice U-polygon is necessary and sufficient for the discrete parallel X-rays in the directions in U to determine convex lattice sets (provided U has at least two nonparallel directions). It is easy to see that when $|U| = 3$, lattice U-polygons always exist. With tools from p-adic number theory, it was shown in [9] that they do not exist for certain sets of four lattice directions and *any* set of at least seven lattice directions, but can exist for certain sets of six lattice directions. Corresponding uniqueness results for discrete parallel X-rays follow immediately.

For discrete point X-rays, there is also a general lack of uniqueness: Given any finite set P of points in $\mathbb{Z}^2$, there are different finite subsets of $\mathbb{Z}^2$ with equal discrete point X-rays at the points in P. The proof, given in [7, Theorem 3.1], is much more involved than for parallel X-rays, requiring an unexpected use of the existence of arbitrarily long arithmetic progressions of relatively prime numbers. With this nonuniqueness result in hand, we focus on convex lattice sets in $\mathbb{Z}^2$. In Section 2.3, we provide a rather complete analysis when discrete point X-rays are taken at two points. We also note that it is hopeless to obtain uniqueness results unless the class of convex lattice sets is restricted to those not meeting any line through two of the points at which the X-rays are taken, a condition that we shall assume for the remainder of this introduction.

Lemma 2 shows that, as with parallel discrete X-rays, uniqueness results for point discrete X-rays hinge on the nonexistence of special lattice polygons we call lattice P-polygons, for finite subsets P of $\mathbb{Z}^2$. (However, the connection is less clear than in the parallel case.) An example of a lattice P-polygon is shown in Figure 2.1, where $P = \{(0,0), (210,0), (0,210)\}$ and the P-polygon is the hexagon of the other labelled lattice points. In [7, Theorem 5.1], the existence of lattice P-polygons for sets of three collinear lattice points is established. It follows that for uniqueness when the points in P are collinear, P must contain at least four points. In Section 2.4, the above results on discrete parallel X-rays are combined with the use of a new measure and projective transformations to prove that when the points in P are collinear, uniqueness is obtained for certain sets of four points and any set of at least seven points, while six points are generally not enough.

Some results on noncollinear sets P are summarized in Section 2.5. For example, there are sets P with as many as six noncollinear points in $\mathbb{Z}^2$ such that the corresponding discrete point X-rays do not determine convex lattice sets.

The development of the paper through Section 2.5 follows the extended abstract [6] of the full article [7] in which the authors introduce point X-rays. To this is added here a final Section 2.6, containing brief remarks about instability results due to Katja Lord (to whom we are grateful for permission to include this summary), the possibility of measuring discrete point X-rays in practice, and our ideas for future work.

2.2 Definitions and Preliminaries

As usual, S^{n-1} denotes the unit sphere and o the origin in Euclidean n-space $\mathbb{R}^n$. If $u \in \mathbb{R}^n$, we denote by $u^\perp$ the $(n-1)$-dimensional subspace orthogonal to u. The standard orthonormal basis for $\mathbb{R}^n$ will be $\{e_1, \ldots, e_n\}$. The line segment with endpoints x and y is denoted by $[x, y]$, and we write $L[x, y]$ for the line through x and y.

If A is a set, we denote by $|A|$, ∂A, and conv A the *cardinality, boundary,* and *convex hull* of A, respectively. The notation for the usual orthogonal *projection* of A on a subspace S is $A|S$. The *symmetric difference* of two sets A_1 and A_2 is $A_1 \triangle A_2 = (A_1 \setminus A_2) \cup (A_2 \setminus A_1)$.

We denote n-dimensional projective space by $\mathbb{P}^n$, and regard it as $\mathbb{R}^n \cup H_\infty$, where H_∞ is the hyperplane at infinity. Points in H_∞ can be associated with a pair $\{u, -u\}$ of directions in S^{n-1}. If ϕ is a projective transformation from $\mathbb{P}^n$ onto $\mathbb{P}^m$ mapping a point p in H_∞ to a finite point ϕp in $\mathbb{P}^m$ (i.e., a point in $\mathbb{R}^m$), then lines in $\mathbb{R}^n$ parallel to a direction u associated with p map to lines passing through ϕp. If $E \subset \mathbb{P}^n$ is such that $\phi E \subset \mathbb{R}^m$ (i.e., ϕE does not meet the hyperplane at infinity in $\mathbb{P}^m$), then ϕ is called *permissible* for E. Note that ϕ preserves the convexity of sets in $\mathbb{R}^n$ for which it is permissible. See [8, pp. 2, 7] for more details.

The *cross ratio* $\langle p_1, p_2, p_3, p_4 \rangle$ of four points p_i, $i = 1, \ldots, 4$, in a line L is given by

$$\langle p_1, p_2, p_3, p_4 \rangle = \frac{(x_3 - x_1)(x_4 - x_2)}{(x_4 - x_1)(x_3 - x_2)}, \tag{2.1}$$

where x_i is the coordinate of p_i, $i = 1, \ldots, 4$, in some fixed Cartesian coordinate system in L. See, for example, [3, Section 6.2].

A *convex polytope* is the convex hull of a finite subset of $\mathbb{R}^n$. We sometimes refer to a finite subset of the n-dimensional integer lattice $\mathbb{Z}^n$ as a *lattice set*. A *convex lattice set* is a finite subset F of $\mathbb{Z}^n$ such that $F = (\text{conv } F) \cap \mathbb{Z}^n$.

A *lattice polygon* is a convex polygon with its vertices in $\mathbb{Z}^2$. A polygon is called *rational* if its vertices have rational coordinates. A *lattice line* is a line containing at least two points in $\mathbb{Z}^2$.

Call a vector $u \in \mathbb{Z}^n$ *primitive* if the line segment $[o, u]$ contains no lattice points other than o and u.

Let F be a finite subset of $\mathbb{R}^n$ and let $u \in \mathbb{R}^n \setminus \{o\}$. The *discrete parallel X-ray of F parallel to u* is the function $X_u F$ defined by

$$X_u F(v) = |F \cap (L[o, u] + v)| , \tag{2.2}$$

for each $v \in u^\perp$. The function $X_u F$ is in effect the projection, counted with multiplicity, of F on $u^\perp$. For an introduction to the many known results on discrete parallel X-rays and their applications, see [4], [9], [10], and [11].

Let F be a finite subset of $\mathbb{R}^n$ and let $p \in \mathbb{R}^n$. The *discrete point X-ray of F at p* is the function $X_p F$ defined by

$$X_p F(u) = |F \cap (L[o, u] + p)| , \tag{2.3}$$

for each $u \in \mathbb{R}^n \setminus \{o\}$.

Let U be a finite set of vectors in $\mathbb{R}^2$. We call a nondegenerate convex polygon Q a U-*polygon* if it has the following property: If v is a vertex of Q, and $u \in U$, then the line $v + L[o, u]$ meets a different vertex v' of Q.

Let P be a finite set of points in $\mathbb{R}^2$. A nondegenerate convex polygon Q is a P-*polygon* if it satisfies the following property: If v is a vertex of Q, and $p \in P$, then the line $L[p, v]$ meets a different vertex v' of Q.

Note that in view of these definitions, a lattice P-polygon is a convex subset of $\mathbb{R}^2$, while a convex lattice polygon is a finite subset of $\mathbb{Z}^2$.

There is a convenient common generalization of the previous two definitions. Consider $\mathbb{P}^2 = \mathbb{R}^2 \cup H_\infty$ and let P be a finite set of points in $\mathbb{P}^2$. A nondegenerate convex polygon Q in $\mathbb{R}^2$ is a P-*polygon* if it satisfies the following property: If v is a vertex of Q, and $p \in P$, then the line $L[p, v]$ in $\mathbb{P}^2$ meets a different vertex v' of Q. Note that if $P \subset H_\infty$, then the P-polygon Q is also a U-polygon for the set U of unit vectors associated with points in P.

Let $\mathcal{F}$ be a class of finite sets in $\mathbb{R}^n$ and P a finite set of points in $\mathbb{R}^n$. We say that $F \in \mathcal{F}$ is *determined* by the discrete point X-rays at the points in P if whenever $F' \in \mathcal{F}$ and $X_p F = X_p F'$ for all $p \in P$, we have $F = F'$.

2.3 Discrete Point X-Rays at Two Points

Theorem 1. *Let p_1 and p_2 be distinct points in $\mathbb{Z}^2$. Then there are different convex lattice sets that meet $L[p_1, p_2]$ and have equal discrete point X-rays at p_1 and p_2.*

Proof. Without loss of generality, let $p_1 = (0, 0)$ and $p_2 = (k, 0)$ for some $k > 0$. Suppose that $m \in \mathbb{N}$. Then the sets $K_1 = \{(k + i, 0) \mid i = 1, \ldots, m\}$

and $K_2 = \{(k+i, 0) \mid i = 2, \ldots, m+1\}$ have equal discrete point X-rays at p_1 and p_2. By adjoining the point $(k+m, 1)$ to both sets, we can obtain two-dimensional examples with the same property. □

Note that the sets K_1 and K_2 in the previous theorem also have the same discrete point X-rays at any lattice point on the x-axis.

Theorem 2. *Let K_i, $i = 1, 2$ be convex lattice sets in $\mathbb{Z}^2$ with equal discrete point X-rays at distinct points $p_1, p_2 \in \mathbb{Z}^2$. Suppose that*

(a) $L[p_1, p_2] \cap K_i = \emptyset$, $i = 1, 2$, and
(b) conv K_1 and conv K_2 either both meet $[p_1, p_2]$ or both meet $L[p_1, p_2] \setminus [p_1, p_2]$.

Then $K_1 = K_2$.

Proof. By (a) and the fact that K_i, $i = 1, 2$ are convex lattice sets, we have $p_i \notin \text{conv } K_1 \cup \text{conv } K_2$, $i = 1, 2$. Suppose that conv K_1 and conv K_2 both meet $L[p_1, p_2] \setminus [p_1, p_2]$. If p_1 and p_2 lie between conv K_1 and conv K_2, these sets cannot have equal supporting lines from p_1 and p_2, contradicting the equality of the discrete point X-rays of K_1 and K_2 at p_1 and p_2. Then we may assume that p_1, p_2, and $L[p_1, p_2] \cap \text{conv } K_i$, $i = 1, 2$ are in that order on $L[p_1, p_2]$. Suppose that $K_1 \neq K_2$. Without loss of generality, we may assume that $L[p_1, p_2]$ is the x-axis. Then by (a), we can assume that $(K_1 \triangle K_2) \cap \{y > 0\} \neq \emptyset$. Let L_1 be the line through p_2 and containing a point of $K_1 \triangle K_2$, with minimal positive angle with the x-axis. Since K_1 and K_2 have equal discrete point X-rays at p_2, there are points $v_1 \in K_1 \setminus K_2$ and $v_2 \in K_2 \setminus K_1$ on L_1, and we can assume that p_2, v_1, and v_2 are in that order on L_1. Since K_1 and K_2 have equal discrete point X-rays at p_1, the line L_2 through p_1 and v_1 must meet $K_2 \setminus K_1$ in a point v_3. If p_1, v_1, and v_3 are in that order on L_2, then the line through p_2 and v_3 has a smaller positive angle with the x-axis than L_1. Therefore, $v_3 \in [p_1, v_1]$. Assumptions (a) and (b) imply that there is a point $c \in K_2 \cap \{y < 0\}$, but then $v_1 \notin K_2$ lies in the interior of the triangle with vertices v_2, v_3, and c, all of which lie in K_2. This contradicts the fact that K_2 is a convex lattice set, and proves that $K_1 = K_2$.

The case when conv K_1 and conv K_2 both meet $[p_1, p_2]$ is proved in similar fashion. □

The next result shows that the assumption (b) in Theorem 2 is necessary.

Theorem 3. *Let p_1 and p_2 be distinct points in $\mathbb{Z}^2$. Then there are different convex lattice sets K_1 and K_2 such that $L[p_1, p_2] \cap K_i = \emptyset$ and $L[p_1, p_2] \cap \text{conv } K_i \neq \emptyset$, $i = 1, 2$, and with equal discrete point X-rays at p_1 and p_2.*

Proof. Let $p_1 = (0, 0)$, and let $p_2 = ku$, where $u \in \mathbb{Z}^2$ is primitive and $k \in \mathbb{N}$. Then there is a $v \in \mathbb{Z}^2$ such that $\{u, v\}$ is a basis in $\mathbb{R}^2$. The unimodular affine transformation mapping $\{u, v\}$ to $\{e_1, e_2\}$ is a bijection of $\mathbb{Z}^2$ onto itself preserving convexity and incidence. Therefore, we may, without loss of generality, take $p_1 = (0, 0)$ and $p_2 = (k, 0)$ for some $k > 0$.

Suppose that $k = 1$. Then the sets $K_1 = \{(2,3),(-1,-2)\}$ and $K_2 = \{(3,6),(-2,-3)\}$ fulfill the requirements of the theorem.

Now suppose that $k > 1$. Let $a = (k,k)$, $b = (k,k+1)$, $c = (-k(k-1),1-k^2)$, and $d = (-k(k^2-1),-k(k^2-1))$. Let $K_1 = \{a,c\}$ and $K_2 = \{b,d\}$. It is easy to check that $L[p_1,p_2] \cap \operatorname{conv} K_i \neq \emptyset$, $i = 1,2$ and that the sets K_1 and K_2 have equal discrete point X-rays at p_1 and p_2. It remains to show that K_1 and K_2 are convex lattice sets. To this end, note that the line $L[a,c]$ has slope $(k^2+k-1)/k^2$. Moreover, k^2+k-1 and k^2 are relatively prime; otherwise, if $p > 1$ is prime, $p|(k^2+k-1)$, and $p|k^2$, then $p|(k-1)$, so p does not divide k, contradicting $p|k^2$. It follows that $K_1 = (\operatorname{conv} K_1) \cap \mathbb{Z}^2$, as required. The line $L[b,d]$ has slope $(k^3+1)/k^3$, and since k^3 and k^3+1 are consecutive integers, they are relatively prime. Consequently, $K_2 = (\operatorname{conv} K_2) \cap \mathbb{Z}^2$, and the proof is complete. $\qquad\square$

The next two lemmas are rather general and will be useful also in subsequent sections of the paper.

Lemma 1. *If Q is a P-polygon such that $|P| \geq 2$ and $P \cap Q = \emptyset$, then Q does not meet any line through two points in P.*

Proof. Let p_1 and p_2 be different points in P, and without loss of generality, suppose that they lie on the x-axis and that Q is a P-polygon whose interior meets the upper open half-plane. Suppose that $Q \cap [p_1,p_2] \neq \emptyset$. Let L_1 be the lattice line through p_1 with minimal positive angle with the x-axis such that L_1 contains vertices v_1 and v_2 of Q. Without loss of generality suppose that p_1, v_2, and v_1 lie on L_1 in that order. Since Q meets $[p_1,p_2]$, by convexity the line L_2 through p_2 and v_2 contains a vertex v_3 of Q with p_2, v_3, and v_2 in that order on L_2. But then the line L_3 through p_1 and v_3 has a smaller positive angle with the x-axis than L_1, a contradiction. A similar argument applies to the case when Q meets the x-axis outside the segment $[p_1,p_2]$. $\qquad\square$

Lemma 2. *Let P be a set of points in $\mathbb{Z}^2$. If there is a lattice P-polygon Q, then there are different convex lattice sets K_1 and K_2 with equal discrete point X-rays at the points in P. Moreover, if $P \cap Q = \emptyset$, then in addition $\operatorname{conv} K_1$ and $\operatorname{conv} K_2$ do not meet any line through two points of P.*

Proof. Let Q be a lattice P-polygon. Partition the vertices of Q into two disjoint sets V_1 and V_2, where the members of each set are alternate vertices in a clockwise ordering around ∂Q. Let

$$C = (\mathbb{Z}^2 \cap Q) \setminus (V_1 \cup V_2), \tag{2.4}$$

and let $K_i = C \cup V_i$, $i = 1,2$. Then K_1 and K_2 are different convex lattice sets with equal discrete point X-rays at the points in P.

If $P \cap Q = \emptyset$, then by Lemma 1, Q does not meet any line through two points of P and the second statement follows immediately. $\qquad\square$

Theorem 4. *Let p_1 and p_2 be distinct points in $\mathbb{Z}^2$ and let $P = \{p_1, p_2\}$. Then there is a lattice P-polygon Q with $P \cap Q = \emptyset$, and hence two different convex lattice sets, with convex hulls disjoint from $L[p_1, p_2]$ and with equal discrete point X-rays at the points in P.*

Proof. Without loss of generality, let $p_1 = (0,0)$ and $p_2 = (k,0)$ for some $k > 0$. Then one can check that $(2k, 2k), (3k, 3k), (3k, 4k)$, and $(9k, 12k)$ are the vertices of a lattice P-quadrilateral. The conclusion follows from Lemma 2. □

2.4 Discrete Point X-Rays at Collinear Points

As we have seen, a convex lattice set is determined by its discrete point X-rays at two different points only in the situation of Theorem 2. Thus to have more general uniqueness results, we need more than two points.

In fact, for collinear sets of points, at least four points are necessary. This is a consequence of the following theorem, proved in [7, Theorem 5.1] by means of some number-theoretical computations involving the Chinese remainder theorem, and its corollary.

Theorem 5. *If P is a set of three collinear points in $\mathbb{Z}^2$, there exists a lattice P-hexagon.*

Corollary 1. *If P is a set of three collinear points in $\mathbb{Z}^2$, then convex lattice sets not meeting the line containing P are not determined by discrete point X-rays at the points in P.*

Proof. This is an immediate consequence of Theorem 5 and Lemma 2. □

To make progress, we require the following technical lemmas.

Lemma 3. *Let $p \in \mathbb{Z}^2$ and let F_1 and F_2 be finite subsets of $\mathbb{Z}^2$ such that $p \notin F_1 \cup F_2$ and $X_p F_1 = X_p F_2$. Then $|F_1| = |F_2|$.*

Proof. Since $p \notin F_1 \cup F_2$, we have for $i = 1, 2$,

$$|F_i| = \sum_{u \in S^1} |F_i \cap (L[o, u] + p)| = \sum_{u \in S^1} X_p F_i(u) . \tag{2.5}$$

□

Let L be a lattice line in $\mathbb{R}^2$, and suppose that L is taken as the x-axis in a Cartesian coordinate system. For each finite set F in $\mathbb{Z}^2$, define

$$\nu(F) = \sum_{(x,y) \in F} \frac{1}{|y|} . \tag{2.6}$$

Then ν is a measure in $\mathbb{Z}^2$, and we call L the *base line* of ν.

Lemma 4. *Let ν be a measure defined by (2) with respect to the base line L. Suppose that F_1 and F_2 are finite subsets of $\mathbb{Z}^2$ contained in one of the open half-planes bounded by L and with equal discrete point X-rays at $p \in L \cap \mathbb{Z}^2$. Then the centroids of F_1 and F_2 with respect to ν lie on the same line through p.*

Proof. Without loss of generality we may take L to be the x-axis, $p = (0,0)$, and F_1 and F_2 finite subsets of $\mathbb{Z}^2$ contained in the upper open half-plane. Let $c_i = (x_i, y_i)$ be the centroid of F_i, for $i = 1, 2$, with respect to the measure ν. Then

$$x_i = \frac{1}{\nu(F_i)} \sum_{(x,y) \in F_i} \frac{x}{y} \tag{2.7}$$

and

$$y_i = \frac{|F_i|}{\nu(F_i)}, \tag{2.8}$$

for $i = 1, 2$. Therefore,

$$\frac{y_i}{x_i} = \frac{|F_i|}{\displaystyle\sum_{(x,y) \in F_i} (x/y)} = \frac{|F_i|}{\displaystyle\sum_{u \in S^1} (X_p F_i(u)) \cot \theta(u)}, \tag{2.9}$$

for $i = 1, 2$, where $\theta(u)$ denotes the angle between the x-axis and a line parallel to u. Since $X_p F_1 = X_p F_2$ and $p \notin F_1 \cup F_2$, we have $|F_1| = |F_2|$ by Lemma 3, and hence $y_1/x_1 = y_2/x_2$, as required. $\qquad\square$

Theorem 6. *Let P be a set of at least three points in $\mathbb{Z}^2$ lying in a line L. If there are different convex lattice sets not meeting L with equal discrete point X-rays at the points in P, then there is a rational P-polygon disjoint from L.*

Proof. Let K_1 and K_2 be different convex lattice sets not meeting L and with equal discrete point X-rays at the points in P. If $L \cap \operatorname{conv} K_1 \neq \emptyset$, then clearly $L \cap \operatorname{conv} K_2 \neq \emptyset$. Then either for some $1 \leq i \neq j \leq 3$, $\operatorname{conv} K_1$ and $\operatorname{conv} K_2$ both meet $[p_i, p_j]$, or for some $1 \leq i \neq j \leq 3$, $\operatorname{conv} K_1$ and $\operatorname{conv} K_2$ both meet $L[p_i, p_j] \setminus [p_i, p_j]$, contradicting Theorem 2.

Consequently, $L \cap \operatorname{conv} K_1 = \emptyset$ and therefore $L \cap \operatorname{conv} K_2 = \emptyset$. Then we can follow exactly the proof of [9, Theorem 5.5] for discrete parallel X-rays, on replacing lattice lines parallel to directions in a set with lattice lines through points in P, replacing ordinary centroids with centroids with respect to the measure ν defined by (2.6) with base line L, and using Lemma 4 instead of [9, Lemma 5.4]. Note that this argument uses only cardinality and collinearity properties and the fact that the centroid of a finite set of lattice points is a point with rational coordinates, a fact that still holds when centroids are taken with respect to ν. Also, note that the observation that $|U| \geq 4$ in the second paragraph of the proof of [9, Theorem 5.5] is not needed. The conclusion is that there is a rational P-polygon disjoint from L. $\qquad\square$

Theorem 7. (i) *Let U be a set of mutually nonparallel vectors in $\mathbb{Z}^2$ such that there exists a lattice U-polygon and let L be a lattice line. Then for some set P of $|U|$ points in L, there exists a lattice P-polygon disjoint from L.*

(ii) *Let P be a set of at least two points in $\mathbb{Z}^2$ in line L such that there exists a rational P-polygon disjoint from L. Let ϕ be a projective transformation of $\mathbb{P}^2$ taking L to the line at infinity, and let $U = \phi P$. Then there exists a lattice U-polygon.*

Proof. (i) Let Q be a lattice U-polygon and suppose that L is a lattice line. Let ϕ be a nonsingular projective transformation of $\mathbb{P}^2$ such that $\phi H_\infty = L$, where H_∞ is the line at infinity in $\mathbb{P}^2$, so that $L \cap \phi Q = \emptyset$. If $p \in \mathbb{P}^2$ has rational coordinates (rational slope if $p \in H_\infty$), then ϕp also has rational coordinates. By translating Q, if necessary, we may assume that $Q \cap \phi^{-1} H_\infty = \emptyset$. Then $(\phi Q) \cap H_\infty = \emptyset$, so ϕ is permissible for Q and hence ϕQ is a rational ϕU-polygon, where ϕU is a set of $|U|$ points in L with rational coordinates. Choose an $m \in \mathbb{N}$ so that the $|U|$ points in $m\phi U$ and the vertices of $m\phi Q$ belong to $\mathbb{Z}^2$. Then $m\phi Q$ is a lattice $m\phi U$-polygon, and $m\phi U$ is a subset of the line mL. Let ψ be a translation taking mL onto L and let $P = \psi(m\phi U)$. Then $\psi(m\phi Q)$ is the required lattice P-polygon.

(ii) Let Q be a rational P-polygon disjoint from L. Since the hypotheses ensure that Q is permissible for ϕ and L is a lattice line, ϕQ is a rational U-polygon. Then there is an $m \in \mathbb{N}$ such that $m\phi Q$ is a lattice U-polygon.   □

Corollary 2. *Let P be a set of points in $\mathbb{Z}^2$ in a line L. Then convex lattice sets in $\mathbb{Z}^2$ not meeting L are determined by discrete point X-rays at the points in P if either*

(a) $|P| \geq 7$, or
(b) $|P| = 4$ and there is no ordering of points in P such that their cross ratio is 2, 3, or 4.

On the other hand, it is possible that $|P| = 6$ and there exist different convex lattice sets with convex hulls disjoint from L and equal discrete point X-rays at points in P.

Proof. Suppose that P is a set of points in $\mathbb{Z}^2$ in a line L, such that convex lattice sets in $\mathbb{Z}^2$ not meeting L are not determined by discrete point X-rays at the points in P. Then, by Theorem 6, there is a rational P-polygon disjoint from L. Theorem 7(ii) implies that there is a set U of $|P|$ mutually nonparallel vectors such that there exists a lattice U-polygon. By [9, Theorem 4.5], we have $|U| \leq 6$, so $|P| \leq 6$ and (a) is proved. Moreover, if $|P| = |U| = 4$, [9, Theorem 4.5] implies that there is an ordering of the vectors in U such that their cross ratio is 2, 3, or 4. Since U is obtained from P by a projective transformation, and such transformations preserve the cross ratio, the same is true for P. Therefore, (b) is established.

By [9, Example 4.3], there is a set U of six mutually nonparallel vectors such that there exists a lattice U-polygon. It follows from Theorem 7(i) that there is a set P of six points in $L \cap \mathbb{Z}^2$ such that there is a lattice P-polygon disjoint from L. The proof is completed by an application of Lemma 2.   □

In particular it follows from the previous result that convex lattice sets not meeting the x-axis are determined by their discrete point X-rays at points in the set $\{(0,0),(1,0),(2,0),(5,0)\}$.

2.5 Discrete Point X-Rays at Noncollinear Points

Volčič (see [12] or [8, Chapter 5]) proved that planar convex bodies are determined by their continuous point X-rays at any set of four points, no three of which are collinear. We see in this section that the situation is somewhat different for discrete point X-rays.

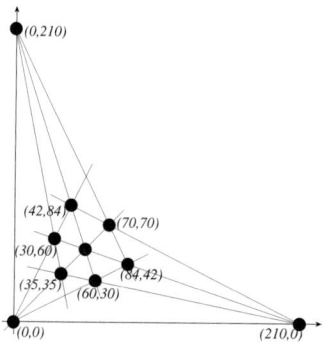

Fig. 2.1. A lattice P-hexagon for three noncollinear points.

In [7, Theorem 7.1], Pappus' theorem is used to prove that there are sets $P = \{p_1, p_2, p_3\}$ of three noncollinear points in $\mathbb{Z}^2$, such that there exists a lattice P-hexagon Q with $P \cap Q = \emptyset$. An example is depicted in Figure 2.1, where $p_1 = (0,0)$, $p_2 = (210,0)$, and $p_3 = (0,210)$. The "center" c of this hexagon, that is, the common intersection of the lines through pairs of opposite vertices, has coordinates $(105/2, 105/2)$, so on multiplying each coordinate by 2, we obtain an example where c is also a lattice point. The hexagon is then a lattice P'-polygon for a set $P' = \{p_1, p_2, p_3, c\}$ of four noncollinear points. By Lemma 2, there are different convex lattice sets with equal discrete point X-rays from the points in P'. Such examples show that the results of Volčič (see [12] or [8, Theorems 5.3.6 and 5.3.7]) do not hold in the discrete case.

A more elaborate construction in [7, Theorem 7.5] provides sets P of four noncollinear points in $\mathbb{Z}^2$ such that there exists a lattice P-octagon Q with $P \cap Q = \emptyset$. This and Lemma 2 show that another result of Volčič (see [12] or [8, Theorem 5.3.8]) also does not hold in the discrete case.

Theorem 8. *There is a set P of four points in $\mathbb{Z}^2$, no three of which are collinear, such that convex lattice sets not meeting any line joining two points in P are not determined by discrete point X-rays at the points in P.*

Finally, it is demonstrated in [7, Theorem 7.6] that there exists a set P of six points, no four of which are collinear, for which there is a lattice P-dodecagon Q with $P \cap Q = \emptyset$. This can be combined with Lemma 2 to yield the following result.

Theorem 9. *There is a set P of six points in $\mathbb{Z}^2$, no four of which are collinear, such that convex lattice sets not meeting any line joining two points in P are not determined by discrete point X-rays at the points in P.*

2.6 Concluding Remarks

At present, so far as we are aware, the only results on discrete point X-rays in the integer lattice beyond those in [7] are contained in as yet unpublished work by Katja Lord, who has obtained some instability results for discrete point X-rays analogous to those found by Alpers and Gritzmann [2] for discrete parallel X-rays. Suppose that $m \geq 3$, that $p_1, \ldots, p_m$ are distinct lattice points in $\mathbb{Z}^2$, and that $n \in \mathbb{N}$. Lord proves that there are disjoint finite subsets F_1 and F_2 of $\mathbb{Z}^2$, of cardinality at least n, such that (i) both F_1 and F_2 are uniquely determined by their discrete point X-rays at the points $p_1, \ldots, p_m$, (ii) $\sum_{i=1}^{m} |X_{p_i} F_1 - X_{p_i} F_2| = 2(m-1)$, and (iii) $|F_1 \cap \phi(F_2)| \leq 3$ (or ≤ 4) for any affine transformation $\phi : \mathbb{R}^2 \to \mathbb{R}^2$ (or projective transformation $\phi : \mathbb{P}^2 \to \mathbb{P}^2$, respectively). Thus there is an even worse instability for discrete point X-rays than for discrete parallel X-rays, for which the results are the same except that in (iii) the bounds depend on m. She also extends these results to higher dimensions.

According to a couple of experts in electron microscopy (private communications), there might be a chance to realize discrete point X-rays experimentally for small samples. Apparently the STEM (scanning transmission microscopy) (also called Z-contrast) technique lends some hope for this, though there would be some extra technical challenges.

For the moment, however, discrete point X-rays lack the application in the material sciences enjoyed by discrete parallel X-rays. Nevertheless, the theory of discrete point X-rays seems worthy of study as interesting in its own right. In particular, lattice P-polygons, and indeed P-polygons generally, are fundamental incidence objects whose structure remains quite mysterious when the points in P are not collinear.

In future work, the authors hope to tackle the obvious open questions concerning uniqueness: Are convex lattice sets in $\mathbb{Z}^2$ determined by their discrete point X-rays at *some* set of three noncollinear points, or at *any* set of seven or more noncollinear lattice points in $\mathbb{Z}^2$? Complexity issues and reconstruction algorithms, both for general lattice sets and special ones such as polyominoes, need to be addressed. Algebraic methods might also be applicable. Generally, it is likely that while some results will transfer from parallel to point X-rays by appropriate use of projective transformations, especially when the points at which the X-rays are taken are collinear, the noncollinear case may well require new techniques.

We remark that the notion of a point X-ray in a graph has been introduced and studied from a similar point of view (questions of uniqueness and so on). The concept is, however, quite different from the discrete point X-rays considered in this article. For more details, see the work of Dulio [5].

Acknowledgments

Supported in part by U.S. National Science Foundation Grant DMS-0203527.

References

1. Adler, A., Coury, J.E.: *The Theory of Numbers*. Jones and Bartlett, Boston, MA (1995).
2. Alpers, A., Gritzmann, G.: On stability, error correction and noise compensation in discrete tomography. *SIAM J. Discrete Math.*, **20**, 227–239 (2006).
3. Berger, M.: *Geometry*. Springer, Berlin, Germany (1987).
4. Brunetti, S., Daurat, A.: An algorithm reconstructing lattice convex sets. *Theoret. Comput. Sci.*, **304**, 35–57 (2003).
5. Dulio, P.: Geometric tomography in a graph. *Rend. Circ. Mat. Palermo* (2) Suppl. No. 77, to appear.
6. Dulio, P., Gardner, R.J., Peri, C.: Discrete point X-rays of convex lattice sets. *Electronic Notes in Discrete Math.*, **20**, 1–13 (2005).
7. Dulio, P., Gardner, R.J., Peri, C.: Discrete point X-rays. *SIAM J. Discrete Math.*, **20**, 171–188 (2006).
8. Gardner, R.J.: *Geometric Tomography*. Second edition, Cambridge University Press, New York, NY (2006).
9. Gardner, R.J., Gritzmann, P.: Discrete tomography: Determination of finite sets by X-rays. *Trans. Amer. Math. Soc.*, **349**, 2271–2295 (1997).
10. Gardner, R.J., Gritzmann, P.: Uniqueness and complexity in discrete tomography. In: Herman, G.T., Kuba, A. (eds.), *Discrete Tomography: Foundations, Algorithms, and Applications*. Birkhäuser, Boston, MA, pp. 85–113 (1999).
11. Herman, G.T., Kuba, A. (eds.): *Discrete Tomography: Foundations, Algorithms, and Applications*. Birkhäuser, Boston, MA (1999).
12. Volčič, A.: A three-point solution to Hammer's X-ray problem. *J. London Math. Soc.* (2), **34**, 349–359 (1986).

3

Reconstruction of Q-Convex Lattice Sets

S. Brunetti and A. Daurat

Summary. We study the reconstruction of special lattice sets from X-rays when some convexity constraints are imposed on the sets. Two aspects are relevant for a satisfactory reconstruction: the unique determination of the set by its X-rays and the existence of a polynomial-time algorithm reconstructing the set from its X-rays. For this purpose we present the notion of Q-convex lattice sets for which there are unique determination by X-rays in suitable directions, and a polynomial-time reconstruction algorithm. After discussing these results, we show that many reconstructions of sets with convexity and connectivity constraints can be seen as particular cases of the algorithm reconstructing Q-convex lattice sets.

3.1 Introduction

Let $\mathcal{D}$ be a set of directions, and $\mathcal{B}$ be a class of *lattice sets* (finite subsets of $\mathbb{Z}^2$). The main problem in discrete tomography (DT) is to reconstruct a member of $\mathcal{B}$ by its X-rays taken in the directions of $\mathcal{D}$. For applications, the retrieval of the original lattice set is of interest. This is ensured by uniqueness of the reconstruction. Therefore, the first important question is to know whether *any member of $\mathcal{B}$ is uniquely determined by its X-rays parallel to directions in $\mathcal{D}$ among the members of $\mathcal{B}$*. In case of positive answer, we say that $\mathcal{B}$ is determined by $\mathcal{D}$. In general, if no assumption is made on the set, it cannot be uniquely reconstructed [5]. On the other hand, Gardner and Gritzmann have proved that a convex lattice set is completely determined by its X-rays parallel to some sets consisting of four directions [16]. Unfortunately, the proof of this result is not constructive: It does not give an *algorithm* that reconstructs the set from the given X-rays. The second question is to know *what is the complexity of reconstructing lattice sets of $\mathcal{B}$*, that is, whether they can be computed in *polynomial time* in the size of the data. There are examples of classes of lattice sets for which there exist efficient reconstruction algorithms. In particular, in [4] it is proved that the *hv-convex polyominoes* (defined ahead) can be reconstructed from X-rays parallel to horizontal and vertical directions in polynomial time.

This result and the uniqueness theorem of Gardner–Gritzmann described above are a priori unrelated: The directions of the X-rays and the considered classes of lattice sets are different. In this chapter we introduce a third class of lattice sets, so-called *Q-convex lattice sets*, which strongly links the two results. Q-convexity, which will be defined precisely in Section 3.3, is a property of lattice sets that depends on a set of directions. Generally, the directions of Q-convexity are the same as the ones of the X-rays. In Section 3.4, we show that Q-convex lattice sets are completely determined by X-rays in the same set of directions that distinguish convex lattice sets. An algorithm that reconstructs Q-convex lattice sets is presented in Section 3.5, extending the algorithm for hv-convex polyominoes.

If we consider Q-convex lattice sets w.r.t. the directions of uniqueness, the reconstruction algorithm for Q-convex lattice sets can be exploited for reconstructing convex lattice sets. This represents one case where the fact that lattice sets of the class are uniquely determined by a set of directions can be exploited to compute members of the class in polynomial time. There are a few other classes that are both uniquely determined by X-rays and reconstructible in polynomial time: We cite the class of additive sets that are reconstructed in polynomial time by use of linear programming [15], and the class of directed column-convex polyominoes associated with the horizontal and vertical directions [13].

We conclude the chapter by showing in Section 3.6 the consequences on other computational problems in DT, and in particular how already known reconstruction results can be proved again using Q-convexity.

Where some proofs are only sketched in this chapter, the reader can refer to the cited articles for the details. Especially, the result of Section 3.4 has already been published in [11], but the proof is only sketched in this chapter. The algorithm described in Section 3.5 is the same as the one published in [6] except for the last step (reduction to 2-SAT), which is faster and simpler in this chapter.

3.2 Definitions and Preliminaries

We first give some notations and classical definitions we use in the chapter, and then we recall some known results that are relevant for our discussion.

3.2.1 Definitions

A *lattice direction* is represented by a vector $p = (a, b) \neq (0, 0)$ with a, b coprime integers. Any straight line parallel to p has equation $bx - ay = k$ where k is a constant. By convenience, we define the function $\tilde{p}$ by $\tilde{p}(x, y) = bx - ay$. So if M_1 and M_2 are two points on the same straight line parallel to the direction p, then $\tilde{p}(M_1) = \tilde{p}(M_2)$. The straight lines of direction p are called p-*lines*, and sometimes we denote by $\tilde{p} = k$ the line of equation $\tilde{p}(x, y) = k$.

The horizontal (respectively, vertical, diagonal) direction $(1,0)$ (respectively, $(0,1)$, $(1,-1)$) is denoted by h (respectively, v, d), and so, $\tilde{h}(x,y) = y$, $\tilde{v}(x,y) = x$ and $\tilde{d}(x,y) = x + y$.

If $p_i = (a_i, b_i)$, $i = 1,\ldots,4$, are four different lattice directions with slopes (possibly infinite) $\lambda_i = -b_i/a_i$, then the cross ratio of these four directions, denoted by $[p_1, p_2, p_3, p_4]$, is the quantity

$$[p_1, p_2, p_3, p_4] = \frac{(\lambda_3 - \lambda_1)(\lambda_4 - \lambda_2)}{(\lambda_3 - \lambda_2)(\lambda_4 - \lambda_1)} . \tag{3.1}$$

The *ordered cross ratio* of $p_1, \ldots, p_4$ is $[p_{\sigma(1)}, p_{\sigma(2)}, p_{\sigma(3)}, p_{\sigma(4)}]$, where σ is the permutation such that $\lambda_{\sigma(i)} < \lambda_{\sigma(i+1)}$. The ordered cross ratio of four lattice directions is always a rational number that is greater than 1.

Let E be a lattice set. The *X-ray of E parallel to a direction p* is the function $X_p E : \mathbb{Z} \to \mathbb{N}_0$ defined by $X_p E(k) = |\{M \in E \mid \tilde{p}(M) = k\}|$, where $|S|$ denotes the cardinality of a set S.

Let $\mathcal{B}$ be a class of lattice sets and $\mathcal{D}$ be a set of directions. We say that $\mathcal{D}$ *determines* the class $\mathcal{B}$ of lattice sets if for every sets E_1 and E_2 of $\mathcal{B}$, we have

$$(\forall p \in \mathcal{D}, \ X_p E_1 = X_p E_2) \implies E_1 = E_2 . \tag{3.2}$$

In this chapter we deal with special lattice sets having convexity and connectivity constraints. Let us recall some basic definitions.

A lattice set is *convex* if it is the intersection between a convex polygon and $\mathbb{Z}^2$. We denote the class of convex lattice sets by $\mathcal{C}$. A lattice set E is *line-convex* along a direction p if the intersection of any line parallel to p and E is empty or it is the set of the points with integer coordinates in a straight line segment. So, a convex lattice set is also line-convex along all directions. The class of line-convex sets along the directions in $\mathcal{D}$ is denoted by $\mathcal{L}(\mathcal{D})$. A lattice set that is line-convex along the horizontal and vertical directions is said to be *hv-convex*. A *4-path* (respectively, an *8-path*, a *6-path*) is a finite sequence $(M_0, M_1, \ldots, M_n)$ of points of $\mathbb{Z}^2$ such that $M_{i+1} - M_i$ is in the set $\{(\pm 1, 0), (0, \pm 1)\}$ (respectively, $\{(\pm 1, 0), (0, \pm 1), (\pm 1, \pm 1)\}$, $\{(\pm 1, 0), (0, \pm 1), (1, 1), (-1, -1)\}$). For $k = 4, 6, 8$, a lattice set E is said to be *k-connected* if, for any A, B in E, there is a k-path from A to B. The class of the k-connected lattices sets is denoted by $\mathcal{P}_k$. So we have that $\mathcal{P}_4 \subsetneq \mathcal{P}_6 \subsetneq \mathcal{P}_8$. A 4-connected lattice set is also called a *polyomino*.

3.2.2 Previous Results

Here are two important theorems that are the bases of the results of this chapter.

Theorem 1. *[16] A set $\mathcal{D}$ of lattice directions determines the class $\mathcal{C}$ if, and only if, it contains four directions whose ordered cross ratio is not in $\{4/3, 3/2, 2, 3, 4\}$. In particular, any set of seven different lattice directions determines the convex lattice sets.*

For example, the set of directions $\{(1,0),(0,1),(2,1),(1,-2)\}$ determines the convex lattice sets.

Theorem 2. *[4] Let* $\mathcal{D} = \{h,v\}$*. The reconstruction problem for* $\mathcal{P}_4 \cap \mathcal{L}(\mathcal{D})$ *(hv-convex polyominoes) can be solved in polynomial time.*

The following sections generalize these results to a common class of lattice sets. A natural candidate is the class of *line-convex* sets; unfortunately, neither of the two theorems holds for this class:

(a) *No* finite set of lattice directions determines $\mathcal{L}(\mathcal{D})$, for any fixed $\mathcal{D}$. This result is a simple consequence of Proposition 3.6 of [5].
(b) The reconstruction of an *hv*-convex set from the horizontal and vertical X-rays is NP-hard [23].

3.3 Q-Convexity

If $p = (a,b)$ and $q = (c,d)$ define two lattice directions and M is a point of $\mathbb{R}^2$, then the lines of directions p and q through M determine the following four quadrants (see Fig. 3.1):

$$Z_0^{pq}(M) = \{M' \in \mathbb{Z}^2 \mid \tilde{p}(M') \leq \tilde{p}(M) \text{ and } \tilde{q}(M') \leq \tilde{q}(M)\} , \qquad (3.3)$$
$$Z_1^{pq}(M) = \{M' \in \mathbb{Z}^2 \mid \tilde{p}(M') \geq \tilde{p}(M) \text{ and } \tilde{q}(M') \leq \tilde{q}(M)\} , \qquad (3.4)$$
$$Z_2^{pq}(M) = \{M' \in \mathbb{Z}^2 \mid \tilde{p}(M') \geq \tilde{p}(M) \text{ and } \tilde{q}(M') \geq \tilde{q}(M)\} , \qquad (3.5)$$
$$Z_3^{pq}(M) = \{M' \in \mathbb{Z}^2 \mid \tilde{p}(M') \leq \tilde{p}(M) \text{ and } \tilde{q}(M') \geq \tilde{q}(M)\} . \qquad (3.6)$$

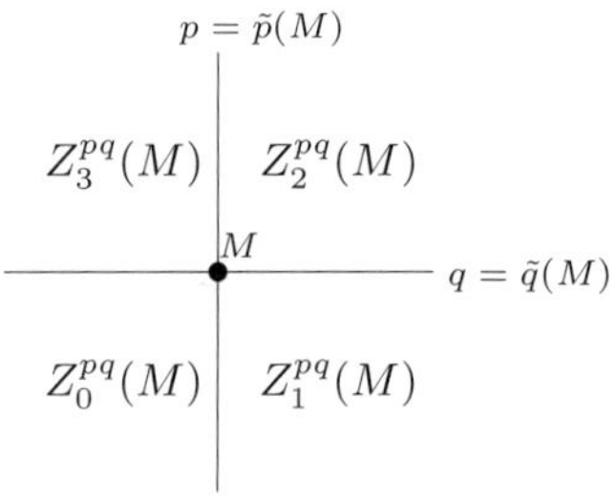

Fig. 3.1. The four quadrants around a point M w.r.t. the vertical and horizontal directions $(\tilde{p}(x,y) = x, \tilde{q}(x,y) = y)$.

Definition 1. *A lattice set E is Q-convex (quadrant-convex) w.r.t.* $\mathcal{D} = \{p,q\}$ *if* $Z_k^{pq}(M) \cap E \neq \emptyset$*, for* $k \in \{0,1,2,3\}$*, implies that* $M \in E$.

Definition 2. *A lattice set is Q-convex w.r.t. a set $\mathcal{D}$ of directions if it is Q-convex w.r.t. every pair of directions included in $\mathcal{D}$.*

We denote the class of the Q-convex sets w.r.t. $\mathcal{D}$ by $\mathcal{Q}(\mathcal{D})$. Figure 3.2 illustrates some examples of Q-convex lattice sets. The following proposition shows the links between the different notions of convexity.

Proposition 1. *Let E be a lattice set.*

(a) If E is convex, then E is Q-convex w.r.t. any set of directions.
(b) If E is Q-convex w.r.t. $\mathcal{D}$, then it is line-convex along $\mathcal{D}$.
(c) If E is hv-convex and 8-connected, then it is Q-convex w.r.t. the horizontal and vertical directions.

This can be summarized by

$$\mathcal{C} \subseteq \mathcal{Q}(\mathcal{D}) \subseteq \mathcal{L}(\mathcal{D}) \,, \qquad \mathcal{P}_8 \cap \mathcal{L}(\{h, v\}) \subseteq \mathcal{Q}(\{h, v\}) \,. \tag{3.7}$$

Proof. (a) Suppose that E is convex, and p, q are two lattice directions. Let M be such that each $Z_i^{pq}(M)$ contains a point N_i of E. As the point M is in the convex hull of the N_i, by convexity it is in E.

(b) Suppose that E is Q-convex w.r.t. $\mathcal{D}$ and M is in a segment $[A, B]$ parallel to a direction $p \in \mathcal{D}$ with $A, B \in E$. Let q be another direction of $\mathcal{D}$, and suppose for example that $\tilde{q}(A) \leq \tilde{q}(M) \leq \tilde{q}(B)$. Then we have $A \in Z_3^{pq}(M) \cap Z_0^{pq}(M)$ and $B \in Z_1^{pq}(M) \cap Z_2^{pq}(M)$, so by Q-convexity $M \in E$.

(c) Suppose now that E is hv-convex and 8-connected. Let M be such that each $Z_i^{hv}(M)$ contains a point N_i of E. For each i there is an 8-path joining N_i and N_{i+1} included in E, and so there is a point A_i in $Z_i^{hv}(M)$ that satisfies $\tilde{h}(A_i) = \tilde{h}(M)$ or $\tilde{v}(A_i) = \tilde{v}(M)$. Then it is easy to see that M lies in a horizontal or vertical segment $[A_i A_j]$, and so M is in E by hv-convexity. $\qquad \square$

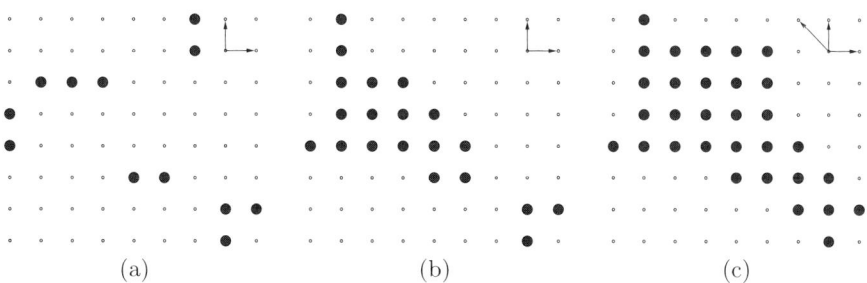

Fig. 3.2. (a) A set that is line-convex but not Q-convex w.r.t. $\{h, v\}$. (b) A Q-convex lattice set w.r.t. $\{h, v\}$. (c) A Q-convex lattice set w.r.t. $\{h, v, d\}$.

3.4 Uniqueness Result

The aim of this section is to explain and sketch the proof of the following result extending Theorem 1 to Q-convex lattice sets.

Theorem 3. *[11] Let $\mathcal{D}$ be a set of lattice directions. Then $\mathcal{D}$ determines the class $\mathcal{Q}(\mathcal{D})$ if, and only if, it contains four different directions whose ordered cross ratio is not in $\{4/3, 3/2, 2, 3, 4\}$.*

Proof. By Proposition 1(a), $\mathcal{C} \subseteq \mathcal{Q}(\mathcal{D})$. Hence, if $\mathcal{D}$ determines $\mathcal{Q}(\mathcal{D})$, then it determines $\mathcal{C}$. By Theorem 1, the set $\mathcal{D}$ contains four different directions whose ordered cross ratio is not in $\{4/3, 3/2, 2, 3, 4\}$. This completes the proof of the "only if" part. The proof of the "if" part is sketched out in the rest of this section.   □

To describe the fundamental steps of the proof, we need some definitions, which are based on the ideas from [16].

Definition 3. *A $\mathcal{D}$-polygon P is a convex polygon such that any line of direction in $\mathcal{D}$ contains either no or two vertices of P.*

Definition 4. *Let $\mathbb{Z}_m$ denote the set of integers modulo m. A $\mathcal{D}$-sequence is a sequence $(A_k)_{k \in \mathbb{Z}_m}$ of m points of $\mathbb{R}^2$ such that m is even and for any p in $\mathcal{D}$ there is an $s \in \mathbb{Z}_m$ such that*

$$\tilde{p}(A_{s-1}) < \tilde{p}(A_{s-2}) < \cdots < \tilde{p}(A_{s-\frac{m}{2}}),$$
$$\text{||} \qquad\qquad \text{||} \qquad\qquad\qquad \text{||} \qquad\qquad\qquad (3.8)$$
$$\tilde{p}(A_s) \; < \tilde{p}(A_{s+1}) < \cdots < \tilde{p}(A_{s+\frac{m}{2}-1}) \,.$$

Notice that the vertices of a $\mathcal{D}$-polygon always form a $\mathcal{D}$-sequence, but the converse is not true: Fig. 3.3 shows a $\mathcal{D}$-sequence, with $\mathcal{D} = \{(1, 0), (0, 1), (1, 1), (1, -1)\}$, which is not a convex polygon, because the point A_2 is in the interior of the convex hull of the points $A_0, A_1, \ldots, A_{15}$.

The "if" part of Theorem 3 is a consequence of the following three lemmas.

Lemma 1. *If two distinct Q-convex lattice sets have the same X-rays in $\mathcal{D}$, then there exists a $\mathcal{D}$-sequence.*

Proof (sketch). Let us assume that two distinct Q-convex lattice sets E_1 and E_2 have the same X-rays in $\mathcal{D}$. Let $F_1 = E_1 \setminus E_2$ and $F_2 = E_2 \setminus E_1$. We say that two points A and B of F_1 are related by $\sim$ (which is denoted by $A \sim B$) if there exist two directions $p, q \in \mathcal{D}$ and a quadrant $Z_i^{pq}(N)$ with $N \in \mathbb{R}^2$ containing A and B and such that $Z_i^{pq}(N) \cap F_2 = \emptyset$. Similarly, we define the relation $\sim$ on the points of F_2. Then the following properties can be proved in this order:

(a) The relation $\sim$ is an equivalence relation on $F_1 \cup F_2$.
(b) If $A, B \in F_1$, $A', B' \in F_2$ and $p \in \mathcal{D}$ are such that $\tilde{p}(A) = \tilde{p}(A')$, $\tilde{p}(B) = \tilde{p}(B')$, then $A \sim B$ implies $A' \sim B'$.

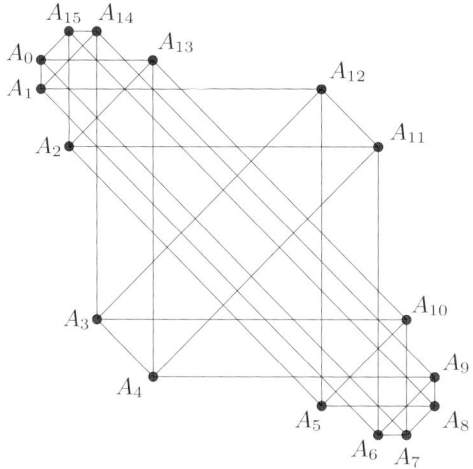

Fig. 3.3. A $\mathcal{D}$-sequence that is not a $\mathcal{D}$-polygon.

(c) The set of the centroids of the equivalence classes of $\sim$ can be ordered in a $\mathcal{D}$-sequence.

This construction is illustrated in Fig. 3.4 (for details, see Section 3.3 of [11].)   ☐

For the two next lemmas we need another definition:

Definition 5. *An affinely regular polygon is the image of a regular polygon by an affine transformation of the plane.*

Lemma 2. *If there exists a $\mathcal{D}$-sequence, then there exists an affinely regular $\mathcal{D}$-polygon.*

Proof (sketch). If $(M_k)_{k \in \mathbb{Z}_m}$ is sequence of points, we define the midpoint sequence $\phi((M_k))$ as the sequence $((M_k + M_{k+1})/2)_{k \in \mathbb{Z}_m}$ formed by midpoints of consecutive points of M_k.

To prove the lemma we suppose that there exists a $\mathcal{D}$-sequence $(A_k)_{k \in \mathbb{Z}_m}$. We can suppose that the centroid of $(A_k)_{k \in \mathbb{Z}_m}$ is $(0,0)$. Then we consider the sequence $(P_n) = \phi^{2n}((A_k))$ of sequences of points obtained by iterating the transformation ϕ^2 to (A_k). Classical linear algebra shows that $\cos^{-2n}(\frac{\pi}{n})(P_n)$ converges to an affinely regular polygon P. Moreover, as each P_n satisfies (3.8), the polygon P also satisfies it and so is a $\mathcal{D}$-sequence. Thus, finally P is an affinely regular $\mathcal{D}$-polygon.   ☐

Lemma 3. *Let $\mathcal{D}$ be a set of* lattice *directions. If there exists an affinely regular $\mathcal{D}$-polygon, then four directions of $\mathcal{D}$ have a cross ratio in $\{4/3, 3/2, 2, 3, 4\}$.*

This lemma was already used for the proof of Theorem 1 (see Lemma 4.3.7 of [17]). Its proof, which is omitted in this chapter, uses the complex roots of the unity and p-adic analysis. It achieves the proof of Theorem 3.

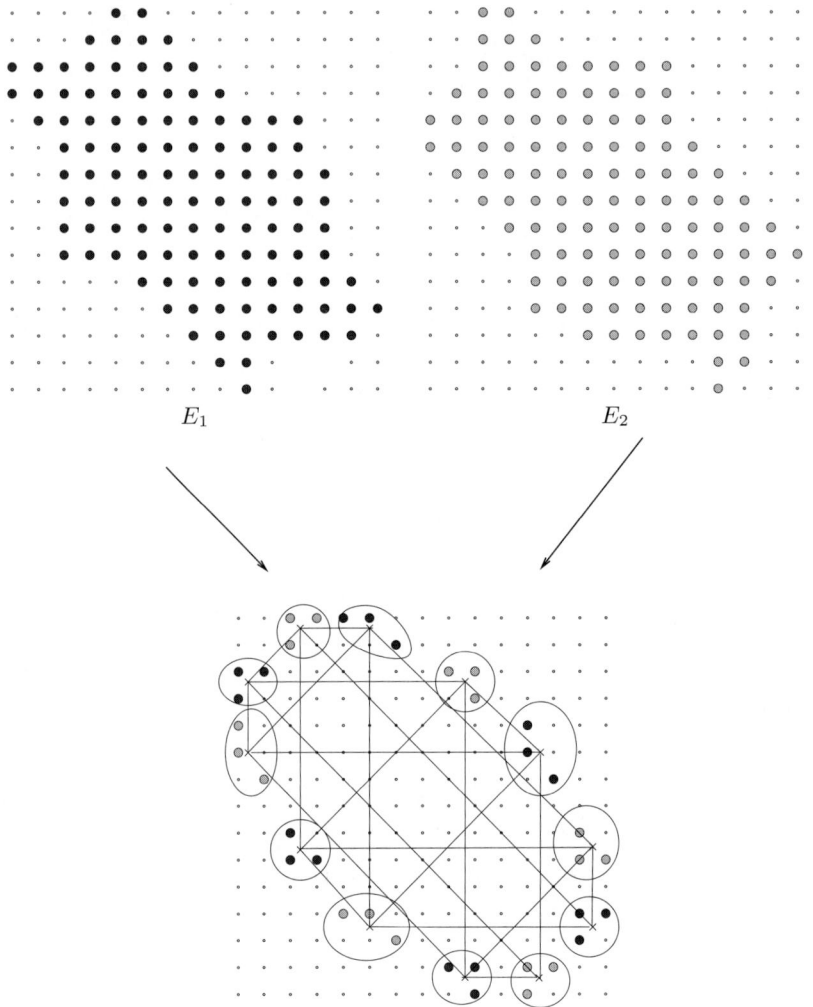

Fig. 3.4. The construction of a $\mathcal{D}$-sequence from two Q-convex sets that have the same X-rays. ($\mathcal{D} = \{(1,0),(0,1),(1,1),(1,-1)\}$.)

3.5 Complexity Result

Let $\mathcal{D}$ be a set of directions, and $\mathcal{B}$ be a class of lattice sets. Now we introduce the reconstruction problem for $\mathcal{B}$ and $\mathcal{D}$.

RECONSTRUCTION$_{\mathcal{B}}(\mathcal{D})$

Input: A map $f : \mathcal{D} \times \mathbb{Z} \to \mathbb{N}_0$ with finite support.

Output: A set $E \in \mathcal{B}$, if it exists, which satisfies

$$X_p E(k) = f(p,k), \quad \text{for all } (p,k) \in \mathcal{D} \times \mathbb{Z} . \tag{3.9}$$

This section focuses on the reconstruction problem for the class $\mathcal{Q}(\mathcal{D})$ of Q-convex lattice sets w.r.t. $\mathcal{D}$.

3.5.1 Reconstruction from Exact X-Rays in Two Directions

In this subsection the set of directions $\mathcal{D}$ consists of two directions: $p = (a, b)$ and $q = (c, d)$.

If M is a point of $\mathbb{Q}^2$ such that $\tilde{p}(M) = i$ and $\tilde{q}(M) = j$, we represent it by $\langle i, j \rangle_{p,q}$. (We sometimes omit the index, when the context is clear.) Let us emphasize that $\langle i, j \rangle_{p,q}$ is not always a lattice point. More precisely, there exists $\kappa \in \{0, \dots, \delta - 1\}$ such that $\langle i, j \rangle_{p,q} \in \mathbb{Z}^2$ if, and only if, $j \equiv \kappa i \pmod{\delta}$, δ denoting $|\det(p, q)| = |ad - bc|$ (see, for example, [12]).

We are going to describe a polynomial-time algorithm that solves RECONSTRUCTION$_{\mathcal{Q}(\{p,q\})}(\{p, q\})$. Given a function f in input, let $pmin = \min\{k \mid f(p, k) > 0\}$, $pmax = \max\{k \mid f(p, k) > 0\}$, $qmin = \min\{k \mid f(q, k) > 0\}$, $qmax = \max\{k \mid f(q, k) > 0\}$. We can easily compute the grid

$$\mathcal{G} = \{M \in \mathbb{Z}^2 \mid pmin \leq \tilde{p}(M) \leq pmax, \quad qmin \leq \tilde{q}(M) \leq qmax\} \quad (3.10)$$

in polynomial time by the input data. Notice that any solution to the reconstruction problem is a subset of $\mathcal{G}$ and has the cardinality:

$$S = \sum_{pmin \leq i \leq pmax} f(p, i) = \sum_{qmin \leq j \leq qmax} f(q, j). \quad (3.11)$$

If this last equality is not satisfied by f, then there is no solution to the reconstruction problem, so we can assume it.

Let α and β be two subsets of $\mathcal{G}$, and let us denote the set of all elements $E \in \mathcal{Q}(\{p, q\})$ that satisfy (3.9) and $\alpha \subseteq E \subseteq \beta$ by $\mathcal{E}(\alpha, \beta)$. The reconstruction problem consists in determining whether $\mathcal{E}(\emptyset, \mathcal{G})$ is empty or not, and in reconstructing a member of it in the latter case.

In the algorithm we use two variable sets α and β satisfying $\alpha \subseteq \beta \subseteq \mathcal{G}$ and such that $\mathcal{E}(\alpha, \beta)$ is invariant. The general sketch of the algorithm is the following:

1. We choose two points $U_1, U_2 \in \mathcal{G}$ such that $\tilde{p}(U_1) = pmin$ and $\tilde{p}(U_2) = pmax$, and the set α is initiated to $\alpha_0 = \{U_1, U_2\}$. These points are called the p-bases.
2. We compute a set β_0 such that $\mathcal{E}(\alpha_0, \mathcal{G}) = \mathcal{E}(\alpha_0, \beta_0)$ and each p-line $p = i$ has less than $2f(p, i)$ points of β_0. The variable set β is initiated to β_0.
3. We iterate some "filling operations" that add points to α and delete points to β but let $\mathcal{E}(\alpha, \beta)$ invariant.
4. Finally, the special form of the obtained α, β permits us to use a 2-SAT algorithm to compute an element of $\mathcal{E}(\alpha, \beta)$ if the latter is not empty.

Because the choice of the p-bases, which is done in step 1, is completely arbitrary, steps 2, 3, and 4 must be repeated for all the possible positions of the p-bases.

The rest of the section is devoted to the detailed description of steps 2, 3, and 4 of the algorithm.

Computation of the Initial Set β_0

At this step we suppose that $\alpha_0 = \{U_1, U_2\} \subset \mathcal{G}$, $\tilde{p}(U_1) = pmin$ and $\tilde{p}(U_2) = pmax$ and we will compute a suitable β_0 such that $\mathcal{E}(\alpha_0, \beta_0) = \mathcal{E}(\alpha_0, \mathcal{G})$. We also make the hypothesis that $\tilde{q}(U_1) \leq \tilde{q}(U_2)$. (The case $\tilde{q}(U_1) \geq \tilde{q}(U_2)$ would be studied in an analogous way.)

First, we present some lemmas that give sufficient conditions for a quadrant to contain a point of any Q-convex lattice set E that satisfies (3.9).

For this we define the four partial sums:

$$S_0(i) = \sum_{pmin \leq i' \leq i} f(p, i'); \qquad S_2(i) = \sum_{i \leq i' \leq pmax} f(p, i');$$

$$S_1(j) = \sum_{qmin \leq j' \leq j} f(q, j'); \qquad S_3(j) = \sum_{j \leq j' \leq qmax} f(q, j'); \tag{3.12}$$

for $i = pmin, \ldots, pmax$ and $j = qmin, \ldots, qmax$. If M is a point of $\mathbb{Q}^2$, $S_k(M)$ will denote $S_k(\tilde{p}(M))$ if $k = 0, 2$ and $S_k(\tilde{q}(M))$ if $k = 1, 3$. These sums satisfy the following easy but fundamental lemma:

Lemma 4. Let $M = \langle i, j \rangle_{p,q}$ with $i, j \in \mathbb{Z}$ (notice that M is, in general, in $\mathbb{Q}^2$). If $S_k(M) + S_{k+1}(M) > S$, then $E \cap Z_k(M) \neq \emptyset$ for any $E \in \mathcal{E}(\emptyset, \mathcal{G})$, where $k = 0, 1, 2, 3$, and $k + 1 = 0$ for $k = 3$.

Proof. At first we take $k = 0$ into consideration. If $E \cap Z_0(M) = \emptyset$, then $S_0(M) + S_1(M) = |E \cap (Z_3(M) \cup Z_1(M))| \leq S$. Cases $k = 1, 2, 3$ can analogously be proven. $\qquad \square$

For each i such that $f(p, i) > 0$, we can define two q-indices, as follows:

$$a_i = \min\{j \mid S_1(j) + S_2(i) > S\}; \tag{3.13}$$

$$b_i = \max\{j \mid S_3(j) + S_0(i) > S\}. \tag{3.14}$$

Lemma 5. If $f(p, i) > 0$, then $a_i \leq b_i$, for $i = pmin, \ldots, pmax$.

Proof. By (3.13) we have that $S_1(a_i - 1) + S_2(i) \leq S$. Since $S_1(a_i - 1) = S - S_3(a_i)$ and $S_2(i) = S - S_0(i - 1)$, the inequality can be rewritten as $S_3(a_i) + S_0(i - 1) \geq S$. If $f(p, i) > 0$, then $S_0(i - 1) < S_0(i)$ and therefore, $S_3(a_i) + S_0(i) > S$. In view of (3.14), this implies $a_i \leq b_i$. $\qquad \square$

Now we can define a third index c_i as follows:

(a) If $a_i < \tilde{q}(U_1)$, then $c_i = \tilde{q}(U_1)$.
(b) If $\tilde{q}(U_1) \leq a_i \leq b_i \leq \tilde{q}(U_2)$, then $c_i = a_i$.
(c) If $b_i > \tilde{q}(U_2)$, then $c_i = \tilde{q}(U_2)$.

Let C be the point $\langle i, c_i \rangle_{p,q}$.

Lemma 6. *Let $E \in \mathcal{E}(\{U_1, U_2\}, \mathcal{G})$. If $f(p, i) > 0$, then*

$$Z_k(C) \cap E \neq \emptyset, \ \forall k \in \{0, \ldots, 3\} . \tag{3.15}$$

Proof. (a) If $a_i < \tilde{q}(U_1)$, we have $C = \langle i, \tilde{q}(U_1) \rangle_{p,q}$ and so $U_1 \in Z_0(C) \cap Z_3(C)$ and $U_2 \in Z_2(C)$ because $\tilde{q}(U_1) < \tilde{q}(U_2)$. Moreover, by the definition of a_i it follows that $S_1(C) + S_2(C) > S$ and then, by Lemma 4, we conclude that $Z_1(C) \cap E \neq \emptyset$.

(b) If $\tilde{q}(U_1) \leq a_i \leq b_i \leq \tilde{q}(U_2)$, then $C = \langle i, a_i \rangle_{p,q}$. So, $U_1 \in Z_0(C)$ and $U_2 \in Z_2(C)$. By the definition of a_i, $S_1(C) + S_2(C) > S$ and therefore $Z_1(C) \cap E \neq \emptyset$. Finally, we use the fact that $\tilde{q}(C) = a_i \leq b_i$ and $S_3(C) + S_0(C) > S$ to conclude that $Z_3(C) \cap E \neq \emptyset$.

(c) If $b_i > \tilde{q}(U_2)$, then we have $C = \langle i, \tilde{q}(U_2) \rangle_{p,q}$. It follows that $U_2 \in Z_1(C) \cap Z_2(C)$ and $U_1 \in Z_0(C)$. By the definition of b_i, $S_3(C) + S_0(C) > S$ and so $Z_3(C) \cap E \neq \emptyset$. $\qquad\square$

If C is a point of $\mathbb{Z}^2$, Lemma 6 proves that C belongs to E, and we could add the point C to the set α. It is in fact the strategy used for the reconstruction of hv-convex polyominoes from horizontal and vertical X-rays in [14]. But for general directions, C can be outside $\mathbb{Z}^2$, and we must consider the set β instead of α. Let us define:

$$\beta_0 = \{\langle i, j \rangle \mid f(p, i) > 0, f(q, j) > 0 \text{ and } c_i - \delta f(p, i) < j \leq c_i + \delta f(p, i)\} . \tag{3.16}$$

Lemma 7. $\mathcal{E}(\{U_1, U_2\}, \mathcal{G}) = \mathcal{E}(\{U_1, U_2\}, \beta_0)$.

Proof. Let $E \in \mathcal{E}(\{U_1, U_2\}, \mathcal{G})$ and $i \in \{pmin, \ldots, pmax\}$ such that $f(p, i) > 0$. Define $c'_i = \max\{j \equiv \kappa i \pmod{\delta} \mid j \leq c_i\}$, $A = \langle i, c'_i \rangle_{p,q}$ and $B = \langle i, c'_i + \delta \rangle_{p,q}$; we have $c'_i \leq c_i \leq c'_i + \delta$ and $A, B \in \mathbb{Z}^2$. We are going to show that $E \cap \{A, B\} \neq \emptyset$. Lemma 6 states that $Z_k(C) \cap E \neq \emptyset$, for any k. Since $f(p, i) > 0$, there exists a point $N \in E$ such that $\tilde{p}(N) = i$.

(a) If $\tilde{q}(N) \leq \tilde{q}(C)$, then $N \in Z_0(A) \cap Z_1(A)$. We have $Z_2(C) \subseteq Z_2(A)$, $Z_3(C) \subseteq Z_3(A)$, and therefore $Z_2(A) \cap E \neq \emptyset$, $Z_3(A) \cap E \neq \emptyset$. By the Q-convexity of F, we deduce $A \in E$.

(b) If $\tilde{q}(N) \geq \tilde{q}(C)$, then $N \in Z_2(B) \cap Z_3(B)$. Since $Z_0(C) \subseteq Z_0(B), Z_1(C) \subseteq Z_1(B)$, by the same arguments as above we can conclude that $B \in E$.

So $\{A, B\} \cap E \neq \emptyset$, then $\{j \mid \langle i, j \rangle \in E\} \subset [q(A) - \delta(f(p, i) - 1), q(B) + \delta(f(p, i) - 1)] \subseteq [c_i - \delta f(p, i) + 1, c_i + \delta f(p, i)]$. As this property is true for any i such that $f(p, i) > 0$, it proves that $E \in \mathcal{E}(\{U_1, U_2\}, \beta_0)$. $\qquad\square$

By the definition of β_0, we also have:

Lemma 8. $|\{M \in \beta_0 \mid \tilde{p}(M) = i\}| \leq 2f(p, i)$.

The Filling Operations

An operation that transforms α, β into α', β' such that $\mathcal{E}(\alpha, \beta) = \mathcal{E}(\alpha', \beta')$ and $\alpha \subseteq \alpha' \subseteq \beta' \subseteq \beta$ is called a *filling operation* (see [4, 14, 22]).

In this section we define some filling operations that will be iteratively applied to $\alpha = \{U_1, U_2\}$ and $\beta = \beta_0$, where β_0 satisfies Lemmas 7 and 8.

Denote the set of points of β on the *ith* p-line (*jth* q-line) of $\mathcal{G}$ by β_p^i (β_q^j), and the set of points of α on the *ith* p-line (*jth* q-line) of $\mathcal{G}$ by α_p^i (α_q^j). We also define

$$l(\alpha_p^i) = \min_{M \in \alpha_p^i} \tilde{q}(M), \quad r(\alpha_p^i) = \max_{M \in \alpha_p^i} \tilde{q}(M) , \tag{3.17}$$

$$l(\beta_p^i) = \min_{M \in \beta_p^i} \tilde{q}(M), \quad r(\beta_p^i) = \max_{M \in \beta_p^i} \tilde{q}(M) . \tag{3.18}$$

We list here the four operations $\oplus, \otimes, \ominus, \odot$ already described in [4], adapted to any direction p.

(a) If $\alpha_p^i \neq \emptyset$, then $\oplus \alpha_p^i = \{\langle i, j \rangle \mid l(\alpha_p^i) \leq j \leq r(\alpha_p^i)\}$.
(b) $\otimes \alpha_p^i = \{\langle i, j \rangle \mid r(\beta_p^i) - \delta f(p, i) < j < l(\beta_p^i) + \delta f(p, i)\}$.
(c) If $\alpha_p^i \neq \emptyset$, $\langle i, j' \rangle \notin \beta_p^i$ with $j' \leq l(\alpha_p^i)$, then $\ominus \beta_p^i = \{\langle i, j \rangle \in \beta_p^i \mid j > j'\}$.
   If $\alpha_p^i \neq \emptyset$, $\langle i, j' \rangle \notin \beta_p^i$ with $j' \geq r(\alpha_p^i)$, then $\ominus \beta_p^i = \{\langle i, j \rangle \in \beta_p^i \mid j < j'\}$.
(d) If $\alpha_p^i \neq \emptyset$, then $\odot \beta_p^i = \{\langle i, j \rangle \in \beta_p^i \mid r(\alpha_p^i) - \delta f(p, i) < j < l(\alpha_p^i) + \delta f(p, i)\}$.

To these four operations we add a further operation denoted by $\odot'$, which allows us to delete in β a sequence of consecutive indeterminate points of the *ith* p-line, when the sequence is shorter than $f(p, i)$:

$$\odot' \beta_p^i = \beta_p^i \setminus \bigcup_{\substack{\langle i,j' \rangle, \langle i,j'' \rangle \in \mathbb{Z}^2 \setminus \beta \\ 0 < j'' - j' \leq \delta f(p,i)}} \{\langle i, j \rangle \in \beta_p^i \mid j' < j < j''\} . \tag{3.19}$$

The filling operations on the q-lines are defined analogously. Figure 3.5 illustrates an application of these operations.

The algorithm performs all these operations on the p-lines and on the q-lines, and repeats this procedure until $\alpha \not\subseteq \beta$ or no further changes in α and β are produced. If we obtain $\alpha \not\subseteq \beta$, then $\mathcal{E}(\{U_1, U_2\}, \mathbb{Z}^2) = \emptyset$. Therefore, the algorithm chooses two different p-bases and tries again. If $\alpha = \beta$, then $\mathcal{E}(\{U_1, U_2\}, \mathbb{Z}^2) = \mathcal{E}(\alpha, \beta) \subseteq \{\alpha\}$, and so, in order to conclude, it only remains to check if α is Q-convex. Besides we can obtain the case in which α and β are invariant with respect to the filling operations and $\alpha \subset \beta$, so that $\beta \setminus \alpha$ is not empty.

The Types of Lines

In the previous section we have obtained two sets α, β, which are invariant by the filling operations and which satisfy:

$$\{U_1, U_2\} \subseteq \alpha \subseteq \beta \subseteq \beta_0 . \tag{3.20}$$

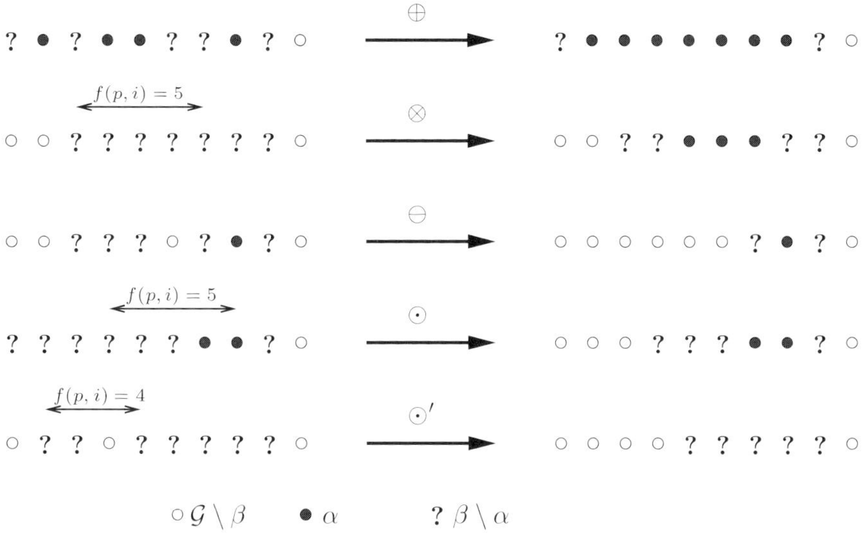

Fig. 3.5. The filling operations.

It is possible to show that α and β have very particular forms on the p-lines and q-lines.

More precisely, the line $\tilde{p} = i$ is of type

(a) t_0 if $\beta_p^i = \emptyset$,
(b) t_1 if $\alpha_p^i \neq \emptyset$; then we have:

$$\alpha_p^i = \{\langle i, j\rangle \mid l(\alpha_p^i) \leq j \leq r(\alpha_p^i)\} \,, \tag{3.21}$$
$$\beta_p^i = \{\langle i, j\rangle \mid l(\alpha_p^i) - \delta(f(p,i) - |\alpha_p^i|) \leq j \leq r(\alpha_p^i) + \delta(f(p,i) - |\alpha_p^i|)\} \,;$$

(c) t_2 if $\alpha_p^i = \emptyset$ and β_p^i is composed of $2f(p,i)$ consecutive points. So we have

$$\beta_p^i = \{\langle i, j\rangle \mid l(\beta_p^i) \leq j < l(\beta_p^i) + 2\delta f(p,i)\} \,; \tag{3.22}$$

(d) t_3 if $\alpha_p^i = \emptyset$ and β_p^i consists of two separated sequences of $f(p,i)$ points. So:

$$\beta_p^i = \{\langle i, j\rangle \mid \; l(\beta_p^i) \leq j \leq l(\beta_p^i) + \delta(f(p,i) - 1) \quad \text{or} \atop r(\beta_p^i) - \delta(f(p,i) - 1) \leq j \leq r(\beta_p^i)\} \tag{3.23}$$

and

$$r(\beta_p^i) - l(\beta_p^i) \geq 2\delta f(p,i). \tag{3.24}$$

Since we know that $\beta \subseteq \beta_0$, thanks to Lemma 8 we can claim that:

Proposition 2. *After performing the filling operations, every p-line is of type either t_0 or t_1 or t_2.*

By Proposition 2, we deduce that

$$|\beta_p^i| = 2f(p, i) - |\alpha_p^i| \text{ for all } i = pmin, \ldots, pmax . \tag{3.25}$$

By summing over i, we have

$$|\beta| = 2S - |\alpha| . \tag{3.26}$$

Consider now the q-lines, and suppose that the jth q-line contains indeterminate points. Thanks to the operations $\otimes$ and $\odot'$, we have

$$|\beta_q^j| \geq 2f(q, j) - |\alpha_q^j|, \tag{3.27}$$

and, therefore,

$$|\beta| = \sum_j |\beta_q^j| \geq \sum_j (2f(q, j) - |\alpha_q^j|) = 2S - |\alpha| . \tag{3.28}$$

By (3.26), we deduce

$$|\beta_q^j| = 2f(q, j) - |\alpha_q^j| \text{ for all } j = qmin, \ldots, qmax . \tag{3.29}$$

We note that this result permits to determine the type of the q-lines. Indeed, when $|\alpha_q^j| > 0$, we know that the ith q-line is a line of type t_1. If $|\alpha_q^j| = 0$, then we have $|\beta_q^j| = 2f(q, j)$; thanks to the operation $\odot'$, this means that the set β_q^j is made up of two sequences having the same length, being either consecutive (in this case the ith q-line is of type t_2) or separated (in this case the ith q-line is of type t_3):

Proposition 3. *After performing the filling operations, every q-line is of type either t_0 or t_1 or t_2 or t_3.*

Reduction to a 2-SAT Formula

In the previous subsections we have found two sets α and β such that $E(\{U_1, U_2\}, \mathbb{Z}^2) = \mathcal{E}(\alpha, \beta)$, and every p-line and q-line is of type $t_i, i = 0, \ldots, 3$. We are going to see that this last property allows us to find an element of $\mathcal{E}(\alpha, \beta)$ by reducing the problem to 2-SAT. We present here a new assignment of variables to points that permits us to have a lower complexity for this reduction to 2-SAT than in [6].

We first recall the 2-SAT problem. Given n_v Boolean variables $V_1, \ldots, V_{n_v}$, a 2-SAT formula is a conjunction of clauses, where each clause is a disjunction of two variables or negations of variables, so it has the form

$$\bigwedge_{k=1}^{n_e} (W_{2k-1} \vee W_{2k}), \tag{3.30}$$

where $\wedge$ (respectively, $\vee$) denotes the **and** (respectively, **or**) operator and W_k is a variable V_i or a negation of variable $\overline{V_i}$. In fact, a clause of a 2-SAT formula can also be a single variable, a negation of variable, an implication, or an equivalence of variables because we have the equalities: $W = (W \vee W)$, $(W \Rightarrow W') = (\overline{W} \vee W')$, $(W \Leftrightarrow W') = ((W \Rightarrow W') \wedge (W' \Rightarrow W))$. The 2-SAT problem is the following.

Input: A 2-SAT formula $\mathcal{F}$ of the form (3.30).
Output: If it exists, an assignment of the variables V_i satisfying $\mathcal{F}$.

Theorem 4 ([1]). 2-SAT *problem can be solved in* $O(n_e + n_v)$-*time, where* n_e *is the number of clauses of* $\mathcal{F}$, *and* n_v *is the number of Boolean variables of* $\mathcal{F}$.

We will use this result to solve our problem. For it, we associate five Boolean variables to each point M of $\mathcal{G}$.

(a) $W(M)$ expresses the presence of M in the final solution. Hence $W(M)$ is true if M is a point of the solution.
(b) $V_i(M)$ expresses the presence of points of the final solution in $Z_i^{pq}(M)$, for $i = 0, \ldots, 3$. Hence $V_i(M)$ is true if the intersection of the solution with $Z_i^{pq}(M)$ is not empty.

Each instantiation of the Boolean variables $W(M)$ gives a set $\alpha \subseteq F(W) \subseteq \beta$ where

$$F(W) = \{M \in \mathcal{G} \mid W(M) = \mathbf{true}\} . \tag{3.31}$$

Now we construct a 2-SAT formula $\mathcal{F}$ whose variables are $(W(M))_{M \in \mathcal{G}}$ and $(V_i(M))_{i=0\ldots3, M \in \mathcal{G}}$ such that the truth of $\mathcal{F}$ implies that $F(W)$ is a Q-convex lattice set having the given X-rays.

Now we describe the different steps of the construction of this formula.

Coherence

As we want $\alpha \subseteq F(W) \subseteq \beta$, we impose that the following variables are true:

$$W(M) \quad \text{for} \quad M \in \alpha; \tag{3.32}$$
$$\overline{W(M)} \quad \text{for} \quad M \notin \beta . \tag{3.33}$$

Besides, for every M and N such that $M \in Z_i(N)$ as $Z_i(M) \subseteq Z_i(N)$, we must express the formulas

$$V_i(M) \Rightarrow V_i(N) . \tag{3.34}$$

Formulas (3.34) can be imposed by the $O(n^2)$-long following formulas:

$$\bigwedge_{\substack{M,N\in\mathcal{G} \\ \tilde{p}(N)-\delta\leq\tilde{p}(M)\leq\tilde{p}(N) \\ \tilde{q}(N)-\delta\leq\tilde{q}(M)\leq\tilde{q}(N)}} V_0(M) \Rightarrow V_0(N) \ ;$$

$$\bigwedge_{\substack{M,N\in\mathcal{G} \\ \tilde{p}(N)-\delta\geq\tilde{p}(M)\geq\tilde{p}(N) \\ \tilde{q}(N)-\delta\leq\tilde{q}(M)\leq\tilde{q}(N)}} V_1(M) \Rightarrow V_1(N) \ ;$$

$$\bigwedge_{\substack{M,N\in\mathcal{G} \\ \tilde{p}(N)-\delta\geq\tilde{p}(M)\geq\tilde{p}(N) \\ \tilde{q}(N)-\delta\geq\tilde{q}(M)\geq\tilde{q}(N)}} V_2(M) \Rightarrow V_2(N) \ ;$$

$$\bigwedge_{\substack{M,N\in\mathcal{G} \\ \tilde{p}(N)-\delta\leq\tilde{p}(M)\leq\tilde{p}(N) \\ \tilde{q}(N)-\delta\geq\tilde{q}(M)\geq\tilde{q}(N)}} V_3(M) \Rightarrow V_3(N) \ .$$

$$(3.35)$$

Additionally, since if M is in $F(V)$, then $Z_i(M)$ contains a point of $F(V)$, we also impose the following formulas:

$$W(M) \Rightarrow V_i(M) \ . \tag{3.36}$$

Formulas (3.35) and (3.36) imply that

$$\left(\bigvee_{N\in Z_i(M)} W(N) \right) \Rightarrow V_i(M) \ , \tag{3.37}$$

and so $\overline{V_i(M)}$ implies $F(W)\cap Z_i(M) = \emptyset$. (Notice that the converse is generally not true.)

Expression of the Q-Convexity

Now we impose that the set $F(W)$ is Q-convex. We could express it directly by $V_0(M)\wedge V_1(M)\wedge V_2(M)\wedge V_3(M) \Rightarrow V(M)$, but it is not a 2-SAT formula.

Remark 1. Let $M = \langle i,j\rangle_{p,q}$ be a point of $\mathbb{Z}^2 \setminus \alpha$ that verifies one of the following properties:

(a) $\tilde{q} = j$ (respectively, $\tilde{p} = i$) is a t_1 line or a t_2 line.
(b) $\tilde{q} = j$ is a t_3 line such that $r(\beta_q^j) - \delta(f(q,j) - 1) \leq i$ or $i \leq l(\beta_q^j) + \delta(f(q,j) - 1)$.

Then, one of the two semi-lines $\Lambda_q^-(M) = \{\langle i',j\rangle \mid i' \leq i\}$ and $\Lambda_q^+(M) = \{\langle i',j\rangle \mid i' \geq i\}$ (respectively, $\Lambda_p^-(M) = \{\langle i,j'\rangle \mid j' \leq j\}$ and $\Lambda_p^+(M) = \{\langle i,j'\rangle \mid j' \geq j\}$) contains a point of E for any $E \in \mathcal{E}(\alpha,\beta)$. We denote this semi-line by $\Lambda_q(M)$ (respectively, $\Lambda_p(M)$). Indeed, under the previous hypothesis:

(a) if the line is of type t_1, then $\Lambda_q(M)$ is the semi-line containing a point of α_q^j;

(b) if the line is of type t_2 or t_3 and $M \notin \beta$, then $\Lambda_q(M)$ is the semi-line containing all the points of β_q^j;

(c) if the line is of type t_2 or t_3 and $M \in \beta$, then we have $\Lambda_q^-(M) \cap \Lambda_q^+(M) = \{M\} \subseteq \beta_q^j$ and $|\beta_q^j| = 2f(q, j)$. So, one of the semi-lines verifies $|\Lambda_q^-(M) \cap \beta_q^j| > f(q, j)$. This semi-line contains at least one point of any $E \in \mathcal{E}(\alpha, \beta)$.

As a summary, if $l(\beta_q^j) + \delta(f(q, j) - 1) \geq i$, then $\Lambda_q(M) = \Lambda_q^+(M)$, whereas if $r(\beta_q^j) - \delta(f(q, j) - 1) \leq i$, then $\Lambda_q(M) = \Lambda_q^-(M)$.

Now we can express the Q-convexity of $F(W)$ around any $M \in \mathcal{G}$ by means of a 2-SAT Boolean formula.

(a) If $M \in \alpha$, then there is nothing to express.

(b) If $M \notin \beta$, let $Z_{i_1}(M)$ and $Z_{i_2}(M)$ contain neither U_1 nor U_2. Then the Q-convexity is simply expressed by

$$\overline{V_{i_1}(M)} \vee \overline{V_{i_2}(M)} . \qquad (3.38)$$

(c) If $M \in \beta \setminus \alpha$, then we are under the hypothesis of Remark 1 and so only one quadrant $Z_i(M)$ exists that contains neither $\Lambda_p(M)$ nor $\Lambda_q(M)$. Therefore, Q-convexity is expressed by:

$$V_i(M) \Rightarrow W(M) . \qquad (3.39)$$

Expression of $X_q E(j) = f(q, j)$

Fix the q-line $\tilde{q} = j$. This line is of type t_i with $i \in \{0, \ldots, 3\}$ and, so, there are exactly $2(f(q, j) - |\alpha_p^i|)$ unknown points on jth q-line. If the line is of type t_1 or t_2, and $A = \langle i, j \rangle_{p,q}, B = \langle i + \delta f(p, i), j \rangle_{p,q} \in \beta \setminus \alpha$, then for any set $E \in \mathcal{E}(\alpha, \beta)$, we have

$$A \in E \text{ if, and only if, } B \notin E , \qquad (3.40)$$

and so we can express $X_q E(j) = f(q, j)$ by the formula

$$EQ_j = \bigwedge_{\substack{\langle i,j \rangle, \langle i',j \rangle \in \beta \setminus \alpha \\ i' - i = \delta f(q,j)}} W(\langle i, j \rangle) \Longleftrightarrow \overline{W(\langle i', j \rangle)} . \qquad (3.41)$$

If the line is of type t_3, then this line is made up of two sequences of consecutive indeterminate points. Since we know that each set $E \in \mathcal{E}(\alpha, \beta)$ contains exactly one of these sequences, in this case we can express $X_q E(j) = f(q, j)$ by the formula

$$\bigwedge_{\substack{\langle i,j \rangle, \langle i',j \rangle \in \beta \setminus \alpha \\ i' - i > \delta f(q,j)}} W(\langle i, j \rangle) \Longleftrightarrow \overline{W(\langle i', j \rangle)}, \qquad (3.42)$$

which is equivalent to the shortest formula

$$EQ_j = \left(W(\langle l(\beta_q^j), j \rangle) \Longleftrightarrow \overline{W(\langle r(\beta_q^j), j \rangle)} \right)$$

$$\wedge \bigwedge_{\langle i,j \rangle, \langle i+\delta, j \rangle \in \beta \backslash \alpha} (W(\langle i, j \rangle) \Longleftrightarrow W(\langle i+\delta, j \rangle)) . \quad (3.43)$$

In the same way we can express that $X_p E(i) = f(p, i)$ by a similar formula EP_i.

Final Reduction

Let $\mathcal{F}$ be the conjunction of the formulas (3.35), (3.36), (3.38), (3.39), EP_i, EQ_j. By construction, we have

Lemma 9. *If $E \in \mathcal{E}(\alpha, \beta)$, then $W(M) =$ "$M \in E$" and $V_i(M) =$ "$Z_i(M) \cap E \neq \emptyset$" satisfy $\mathcal{F}$. Conversely, if $W(M), V_i(M)$ satisfy $\mathcal{F}$, then $F(W) \in \mathcal{E}(\alpha, \beta)$.*

We can use the algorithm of Theorem 4 to check if $\mathcal{E}(\alpha, \beta)$ is not empty, and if this is the case to compute a solution of the reconstruction problem.

Complexity

The complexity of the algorithm depends on the cost of the following steps.

(a) There are $O(n^2)$ choices for the base points.
(b) The computation of β_0 can be done in $O(n^2)$-time.
(c) The filling operations can be implemented in $O(n^3)$ (see [6, Section 6.1]).
(d) The reduction to 2-SAT takes $O(n^2)$-time, since the formula $\mathcal{F}$ has the form (3.30) with $n_v = O(n^2)$ and $n_e = O(n^2)$.
(e) Finally, the assignment of the variables can be done in $O(n^2)$-time by Theorem 4.

Theorem 5. RECONSTRUCTION$_{\mathcal{Q}(\{p,q\})}(\{p, q\})$ *can be solved in $O(n^5)$-time, where $n = \max(pmax - pmin + 1, qmax - qmin + 1)$.*

Remark 2. In [19] the author gives an algorithm that applies the filling operations $\oplus, \ominus, \otimes, \odot$ until invariance in time $O(n^2 \log(n))$. Unfortunately, this algorithm cannot be easily extended to the operation $\odot'$.

3.5.2 Reconstruction from Exact X-Rays in More Than Two Directions

The reconstruction algorithm for Q-convex lattice sets w.r.t. two directions can be easily extended to any set $\mathcal{D}$ of cardinality greater than two. In this case, the solutions to the problem are subsets of the grid

$$\mathcal{G} = \{ M \in \mathbb{Z}^2 \mid \forall p \in \mathcal{D} \quad \min\{k \mid f(p, k) > 0\} \leq \tilde{p}(M) \leq \quad (3.44)$$
$$\max\{k \mid f(p, k) > 0\} \} .$$

We list here the steps to be performed.

(a) We choose the direction minimizing $\max\{k \mid f(p,k) > 0\} - \min\{k \mid f(p,k) > 0\}$. Suppose it is p: We fix the p-bases U_1, U_2. We also fix another arbitrary direction q.

(b) We compute the set β_0 exactly by the same method described above. So we only consider the data corresponding to the directions p and q in f.

(c) We apply the filling operations for all the directions of $\mathcal{D}$. At the end, all the lines parallel to any direction of $\mathcal{D} \setminus p$ are of type t_i, $i = 0, 1, 2, 3$ by Proposition 3, and p-lines are of type t_0, t_1, t_2 by Proposition 2.

(d) The problem is reduced to 2-SAT by using $1 + 4\binom{n}{2}$ variables for each point M: $W(M)$ and $V_i^{q_1 q_2}(M)$ for $i = 0, \ldots, 3$, $q_1, q_2 \in \mathcal{D}$. The formulas are almost the same, but we must consider all the couples of directions. The only formulas that cannot be generalized to any couple of directions are the formulas (3.38). So suppose that M is a point of $\mathcal{G} \setminus \beta$. We have to express the Q-convexity around M w.r.t. two directions q_1, q_2. There is at least a quadrant $Z_i^{q_1 q_2}(M)$ that contains U_1 or U_2, and hence it cannot be empty. Consider all the q_1-lines and q_2-lines that do not pass by this quadrant. If one of these lines has a strict majority of its unknown points in a quadrant, then we have found another quadrant that cannot be empty. So in this case we can find i_1 and i_2 such that (3.38) expresses the Q-convexity around M. In the other case, it is easy to see that the formula $V_{i+1}^{q_1 q_2}(M) \Leftrightarrow V_{i-1}^{q_1 q_2}(M)$ holds, and so we can express the Q-convexity by

$$\left(\overline{V_{i+1}^{q_1 q_2}(M)} \vee \overline{V_{i+2}^{q_1 q_2}(M)} \right) \wedge \left(\overline{V_{i-1}^{q_1 q_2}(M)} \vee \overline{V_{i+2}^{q_1 q_2}(M)} \right) . \tag{3.45}$$

Theorem 6. RECONSTRUCTION$_{\mathcal{Q}(\mathcal{D})}(\mathcal{D})$ *can be solved in $O(n^5)$-time, where* $n = \max_{p \in \mathcal{D}}(\max\{k \mid f(p,k) > 0\} - \min\{k \mid f(p,k) > 0\})$.

Remark 3. RECONSTRUCTION$_{\mathcal{Q}(\{p,q\}) \cap \mathcal{L}(\mathcal{D})}(\mathcal{D})$ *can also be solved in $O(n^5)$ time*. Indeed, we can generalize the algorithm to reconstruct sets that are only Q-convex in two directions p, q and line-convex w.r.t. the other directions. To this goal, the set β_0 is computed using the directions p and q, and the filling operations are executed exactly as before, since they only use line-convexity. For the reduction to 2-SAT, we use five variables by point $W(M)$ and $V_i^{pq}(M)$, and we can express Q-convexity in the same way, whereas we express line-convexity on the line $\tilde{r} = k$ by adding the formulas $W(\langle i, k-\delta \rangle_{p,r}) \Rightarrow W(\langle i, k \rangle)$ for $k < g(\beta_r^k) + f(r,k)$ and $W(\langle i, k+\delta \rangle) \Rightarrow W(\langle i, k \rangle)$ for $k > r(\beta_r^k) - f(r,k)$.

3.6 Further Remarks

In this section we present some remarks about complexity results that can be obtained by the algorithm described in the previous section.

First we show that the algorithm can be applied to solve a more general problem, and then we see how it generalizes some known algorithms previously designed for the reconstruction of special classes of lattice sets having convexity and/or connectivity properties.

3.6.1 Other Algorithmic Problems

Consider the following problem:

PRESCRIBED_RECONSTRUCTION$_{\mathcal{Q}(\mathcal{D})}(\mathcal{D})$

Input: A map $f : \mathcal{D} \times \mathbb{Z} \to \mathbb{N}_0$ with finite support, and two sets A and B.

Output: A set $E \in \mathcal{Q}(\mathcal{D})$, if it exists, that satisfies $A \subset E \subset B$ and (3.9).

To solve this problem, we can use the algorithm of Section 3.5 with a little modification: The initial α and β are settled to $\{U_1, U_2\} \cup A$ and $\beta_0 \cap B$, which results in

Theorem 7. PRESCRIBED_RECONSTRUCTION$_{\mathcal{Q}(\mathcal{D})}(\mathcal{D})$ *can be solved in $O(n^5)$-time.*

Notice that the corresponding problem for the class of all the lattice sets is NP-complete when $|\mathcal{D}| \geq 3$, even if A contains almost all the points of the solutions ([18, Theorem 5.1]).

We can also consider the following algorithmic problem:

UNIQUENESS$_{\mathcal{Q}(\mathcal{D})}(\mathcal{D})$

Input: A lattice set $E \in \mathcal{Q}(\mathcal{D})$.

Question: Does there exist another set $E' \in \mathcal{Q}(\mathcal{D})$ that has the same X-rays in $\mathcal{D}$?

The corresponding problem for the class of all the lattice sets has been proved to be NP-complete for $|\mathcal{D}| \geq 3$ ([18, Theorem 4.3]). In Section 3.4 we have characterized the sets of directions of uniqueness, that is, for which sets $\mathcal{D}$ the answer to UNIQUENESS$_{\mathcal{Q}(\mathcal{D})}(\mathcal{D})$ is always negative. For the other sets of directions, the answer depends on the X-rays of the set E in input. We can give the following result.

Theorem 8. UNIQUENESS$_{\mathcal{Q}(\mathcal{D})}(\mathcal{D})$ *can be solved in $O(n^6)$-time, where $n = \max_{p \in \mathcal{D}}(\max\{k \mid X_p E(k) > 0\} - \min\{k \mid X_p E(k) > 0\})$.*

Proof. Consider a set $E \in \mathcal{Q}(\mathcal{D})$ and choose an arbitrary direction $p \in \mathcal{D}$. Let $\mathcal{G}$ be defined by (3.44). If there exists a set E' that has the same X-rays in $\mathcal{D}$ as E, then there is an integer k such that $E \cap \{\tilde{p} = k\}$ and $F \cap \{\tilde{p} = k\}$ are different. Hence to solve the problem, we only have to apply the following algorithm:

(a) For all k such that $X_p E(k) > 0$, do the following:
  a) Let I, J be the endpoints of $E \cap \{\tilde{p} = k\}$.
  b) Apply an algorithm solving PRESCRIBED_RECONSTRUCTION$_{\mathcal{Q}(\mathcal{D})}(\mathcal{D})$ with $f(p, i) = X_p E(i)$ for all $(p, i) \in \mathcal{D} \times \mathbb{Z}$, $A = \emptyset$, $B = \mathcal{G} \setminus \{I\}$. If the algorithm finds a solution, then return the answer "yes."
  c) Same as above with I replaced by J.
(b) Return the answer "no."

By Theorem 7 the complexity of this algorithm is $O(n^6)$. $\qquad\square$

3.6.2 Reconstruction of Lattice Sets with Line-Convexity and Connectivity Constraints

Consider the problem of reconstructing hv-convex 8-connected lattice sets from the horizontal and vertical directions.

Lemma 10. *A lattice set E is hv-convex 8-connected if, and only if, the two following assertions are true:*

1. *E is Q-convex w.r.t. $\{h, v\}$.*
2. *$\{k \in \mathbb{Z} \mid X_h E(k) > 0\}$ and $\{k \in \mathbb{Z} \mid X_v E(k) > 0\}$ are sets of consecutive integers.*

Proof. The direct sense is a consequence of Proposition 1.

Conversely, suppose that E satisfies conditions 1 and 2. By Proposition 1 we know that E is hv-convex. Let $A = (x_A, y_A)$ and $B = (x_B, y_B)$ be two points of E. We suppose that $x_A < x_B$ and $y_A < y_B$ (the other cases are similar). Let $A_1 = A + (0, 1)$, $A_2 = A + (1, 0)$, $A_3 = A + (1, 1)$, and suppose that none of these points is in E. By Q-convexity we have $Z_3^{vh}(A_1) \cap E = \emptyset$, and $Z_1^{vh}(A_2) \cap E = \emptyset$. Moreover, $Z_3^{vh}(A_3) \cap E = \emptyset$ or $Z_1^{vh}(A_3) \cap E = \emptyset$, but the first case implies $X_v E(x_A + 1) = 0$ and the second one implies $X_h E(y_A + 1) = 0$. So one of the points A_1, A_2, A_3 is in E. So, by a recurrence on $(x_B - x_A) + (y_B - y_A)$ we can prove that there is a 8-path from A to B. □

Since condition 2 concerns the X-rays only, by Theorem 5 it follows that:

Theorem 9. *If $\mathcal{D}$ is a set of directions containing the horizontal and vertical directions, then* RECONSTRUCTION$_{\mathcal{P}_8 \cap \mathcal{L}(\mathcal{D})}(\mathcal{D})$ *can be solved in $O(n^5)$-time.*

To extend this result to 4-connected lattice sets, we need the following lemma:

Lemma 11. *A lattice set E is an hv-convex polyomino if, and only if, E is hv-convex 8-connected and for any integers j and k such that $X_v E(j) > 0$, $X_v E(j + 1) > 0$, $X_h E(k) > 0$, $X_h E(k + 1) > 0$, we have that E is not a subset of either $Z_0^{vh}(j, k) \cup Z_2^{vh}(j + 1, k + 1)$ or $Z_1^{vh}(j + 1, k) \cup Z_3^{vh}(j, k + 1)$.*

Proof. The direct sense is clear.

Conversely, suppose that E satisfies the conditions about the quadrants. If E is not 4-connected, it means that there exist two points A and B that are not connected by a 4-path. As E is 8-connected, we can suppose that the difference $A - B$ is in $\{(\pm 1, \pm 1)\}$. Suppose, for example, that $B = A + (1, 1)$, but $A + (1, 0)$ and $A + (0, 1)$ are not in E; we have $E \subseteq Z_0^{vh}(A) \cup Z_2^{vh}(B)$, which contradicts the hypothesis on E. □

Theorem 10. *If $\mathcal{D}$ is a set of directions containing the horizontal and vertical directions, then* RECONSTRUCTION$_{\mathcal{P}_4 \cap \mathcal{L}(\mathcal{D})}(\mathcal{D})$ *can be solved in $O(n^5)$-time.*

Proof. Let f be the function given in $\text{RECONSTRUCTION}_{\mathcal{P}_4 \cap \mathcal{L}(\mathcal{D})}(\mathcal{D})$. We can suppose that $\{k \in \mathbb{Z} \mid f(x, k) > 0\}$ and $\{k \in \mathbb{Z} \mid f(y, k) > 0\}$ are made up of consecutive integers, since otherwise the problem has no solution.

Then we can apply the algorithm outlined in Remark 3, where we add the formulas

$$V_1(j+1, k) \vee V_3(j, k+1), V_0(j, k) \vee V_2(j+1, k+1) \qquad (3.46)$$

to the final 2-SAT formula $\mathcal{F}$.

We must check that if the truth assignment to variables W satisfies $\mathcal{F}$, then $F(W)$ is a polyomino. As there is no horizontal or vertical lines with null X-ray, for any point $M \in \mathcal{G}$ such that $\overline{W(M)}$, exactly one $V_i(M)$ is set to false. It corresponds to the only quadrant such that $Z_i(M) \cap F(W) \neq \emptyset$. It follows that $V_i(M)$ is set to true if, and only if, $F(W) \cap Z_i(M) \neq \emptyset$, and, by the previous lemma, $F(W)$ is a polyomino. □

Lemma 12. *A lattice set E is line-convex w.r.t. $\{h, v, d\}$ and 6-connected if, and only if, the following assertions are true:*

1. *E is Q-convex w.r.t. $\{h, v, d\}$.*
2. *$\{k \in \mathbb{Z} \mid X_h E(k) > 0\}$, $\{k \in \mathbb{Z} \mid X_v E(k) > 0\}$, $\{k \in \mathbb{Z} \mid X_d E(k) > 0\}$ are sets of consecutive integers.*

The proof of this lemma is left to the reader, as it follows the same ideas as the one of Lemma 10 (see [10, Proposition 2.5.10]).

We deduce the following:

Theorem 11. *If $\mathcal{D}$ is a set of directions containing the horizontal, vertical, and diagonal directions, then $\text{RECONSTRUCTION}_{\mathcal{P}_6 \cap \mathcal{L}(\mathcal{D})}(\mathcal{D})$ can be solved in $O(n^5)$-time.*

Remark 4. The algorithms presented [3, 8] also solve the problems of Theorems 9, 10 and 11. The complexity given in these papers is $O(n^4 \log(n))$, but these complexities were based on the hypothesis that the operation $\odot'$ is applied only one time. This cannot be supposed in the general case.

Remark 5. In [9] the authors give an algorithm that solves $\text{RECONSTRUCTION}_{\mathcal{P}_4 \cap \mathcal{L}(\{h,v\})}(\{h, v\})$ in $O(n^4)$ time. So it has a better worst-case computational complexity than the algorithm presented here. The algorithm can also be generalized to Q-convex lattice sets (see [7]) and more than two directions, but its complexity grows exponentially with the cardinality of $\mathcal{D}$. A comparison of the algorithms presented in [8] and [9] is given in [2], where the authors show that the algorithm of [8] is better from the viewpoint of average time complexity and memory requirements.

Remark 6. In [14, Section 7.3] are collected intractability results for the reconstruction of the polyomino and/or convexity property.

3.6.3 Reconstruction of Convex Lattice Sets

By combining Proposition 1 and Theorems 3 and 6, we obtain

Theorem 12. *If $\mathcal{D}$ is a set of directions containing four directions whose ordered cross ratio is not in $\{4/3, 3/2, 2, 3, 4\}$, then* RECONSTRUCTION$_\mathcal{C}(\mathcal{D})$ *can be solved in $O(n^5)$-time, where $n = \max_{p \in \mathcal{D}}(\max\{k \mid f(p,k) > 0\} - \min\{k \mid f(p,k) > 0\})$.*

We still do not know the computational complexity of RECONSTRUCTION$_\mathcal{C}(\mathcal{D})$ when $\mathcal{D}$ does not uniquely determine $\mathcal{C}$ and, for example, when $\mathcal{D}$ consists of the horizontal and vertical directions.

3.6.4 Practical Considerations

If we want to solve RECONSTRUCTION$_{\mathcal{Q}(\mathcal{D})}(\mathcal{D})$ in practice, it seems that the choices of the base points are often unnecessary (see [10, Annexe B], [2] for the two-directions case).

Indeed with three directions or more, the filling operations and an exceptional use of 2-SAT (when there are more than one solution) seem to be almost always sufficient, but no theoretical result justifies this fact.

In practice, reconstruction from approximate X-rays must also certainly be considered. There are theoretical results about reconstruction of sets that have a convexity property from approximate X-rays ([20, 7]). The algorithms are straightforward extensions of the exact case of [9]: [20] considers the case of two directions, while [7] works with more directions, but the obtained theoretical and experimental time-complexities are worse than in the exact case.

References

1. Aspvall, B., Plass, M.F., Tarjan, R.E.: A linear-time algorithm for testing the truth of certain quantified boolean formulas. *Inform. Process. Lett.*, **8**, 121–123 (1979).
2. Balogh, E., Kuba, A., Dévényi, C., Del Lungo, A.: Comparison of algorithms for reconstructing hv-convex discrete sets. *Linear Algebra Appl.*, **339**, 23–35 (2001).
3. Barcucci, E., Brunetti, S., Del Lungo, A., Nivat, M.: Reconstruction of lattice sets from their horizontal, vertical and diagonal X-rays. *Discr. Math.*, **241**, 65–78 (2001).
4. Barcucci, E., Del Lungo, A., Nivat, M., Pinzani, R.: Reconstructing convex polyominoes from horizontal and vertical projections. *Theor. Comput. Sci.*, **155**, 321–347 (1996).
5. Barcucci, E., Del Lungo, A., Nivat, M., Pinzani, R.: X-rays characterizing some classes of discrete sets. *Linear Algebra Appl.*, **339**, 3–21 (2001).
6. Brunetti, S., Daurat, A.: An algorithm reconstructing convex lattice sets. *Theor. Comput. Sci.*, **304**, 35–57 (2003).
7. Brunetti, S., Daurat, A., Del Lungo, A.: Approximate X-rays reconstruction of special lattice sets. *Pure Math. Appl.*, **11**, 409–425 (2000).

8. Brunetti, S., Del Lungo, A., Del Ristoro, F., Kuba, A., Nivat, M.: Reconstruction of 4- and 8-connected convex discrete sets from row and column projections. *Linear Algebra Appl.*, **339**, 37–57 (2001).

9. Chrobak, M., Dürr, C.: Reconstructing hv-convex polyominoes from orthogonal projections. *Inform. Process. Lett.*, **69**, 283–289 (1999).

10. Daurat, A.: *Convexité dans le plan discret. Application à la tomographie.* Ph.D. thesis, LLAIC1, and LIAFA. Université Paris 7 (2000).

11. Daurat, A.: Determination of Q-convex sets by X-rays. *Theor. Comput. Sci.*, **332**, 19–45 (2005).

12. Daurat, A., Del Lungo, A., Nivat, M.: Medians of discrete sets according to a linear distance. *Discr. Comput. Geom.*, **23**, 465–483 (2000).

13. Del Lungo, A.: Polyominoes defined by two vectors. *Theor. Comput. Sci.*, **127**, 187–198 (1994).

14. Del Lungo, A., Nivat, M.: Reconstruction of connected sets from two projections. In: Herman and Kuba [21], pp. 163–188.

15. Fishburn, P.C., Shepp, L.A.: Sets of uniqueness and additivity in integer lattices. In: Herman and Kuba [21], pp. 35–58.

16. Gardner, R.J., Gritzmann, P.: Discrete tomography: Determination of finite sets by X-rays. *Trans. Amer. Math. Soc.*, **349**, 2271–2295 (1997).

17. Gardner, R.J., Gritzmann, P.: Uniqueness and complexity in discrete tomography. In: Herman and Kuba [21], pp. 88–90.

18. Gardner, R.J., Gritzmann, P., Prangenberg, D.: On the computational complexity of reconstructing lattice sets from their X-rays. *Discr. Math.*, **202**, 45–71 (1999).

19. Gębala, M.: The reconstruction of convex polyominoes from horizontal and vertical projections. In: Rovan, B. (ed.), *Theory and Practice of Informatics*, Springer, Berlin, Germany, pp. 350–359 (1998).

20. Gębala, M.: The reconstruction of polyominoes from approximately orthogonal projections. In: Pacholski, L., Ruika, P. (eds.), *Current Trends in Theory and Practice of Informatics*, Springer, Berlin, Germany, pp. 253–260 (2001).

21. Herman, G.T., Kuba, A. (eds.): *Discrete Tomography: Foundations, Algorithms, and Applications.* Birkhäuser, Boston, MA (1999).

22. Kuba, A.: Reconstruction of two-directionally connected binary patterns from their two orthogonal projections. *Comput. Vis. Graph. Image Process.*, **27**, 249–265 (1984).

23. Woeginger, G.J.: The reconstruction of polyominoes from their horizontal and vertical projections. *Inform. Process. Lett.*, **77**, 225–229 (2001).

4

Algebraic Discrete Tomography

L. Hajdu and R. Tijdeman

Summary. In this chapter we present an algebraic theory of patterns that can be applied in discrete tomography for any dimension. We use that the difference of two such patterns yields a configuration with vanishing line sums. We show by introducing generating polynomials and applying elementary properties of polynomials that such so-called switching configurations form a linear space. We give a basis of this linear space in terms of the so-called switching atom, the smallest nontrivial switching configuration. We do so both in case that the material does not absorb light and absorbs light homogeneously. In the former case we also show that a configuration can be constructed with the same line sums as the original and with entries of about the same size, and we provide a formula for the number of linear dependencies between the line sums. In the final section we deal with the case that the transmitted light does not follow straight lines.

4.1 Introduction

One of the basic problems of discrete tomography is to reconstruct a function $f : A \rightarrow \{0,1\}$, where A is a finite subset of $\mathbb{Z}^n$ ($n \geq 2$), if the sums of the function values (the so-called X-rays) along all the lines in a finite number of directions are given. A related problem on emission tomography is to reconstruct f if it represents (radioactive) material emitting radiation. If $f(\underline{i}) = 1$ for some $\underline{i} \in A$, then there is a unit of radiating material at $\underline{i}$; otherwise, $f(\underline{i}) = 0$ and there is no such material at $\underline{i}$. The radiation is partially absorbed by the medium, such that its intensity is reduced by a factor β for each unit line segment in the given direction (with some real number $\beta \geq 1$).

As an illustration we include an example. In Fig. 4.1 the row sums of f (the number of particles in each row, from top to bottom) are given by $[4, 4, 2, 5, 1, 2]$, while the column sums (the number of particles in each column, from left to right) are $[2, 3, 2, 1, 2, 3, 2, 3]$. Further, taking the line sums of f in the direction $(1, -1)$, i.e., the sums of elements lying on the same lines of slope -1, we get (from the bottom-left corner to the top-right corner)

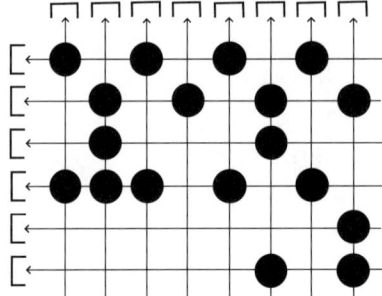

$$
\begin{array}{l}
1\,0\,1\,0\,1\,0\,1\,0\\
0\,1\,0\,1\,0\,1\,0\,1\\
0\,1\,0\,0\,0\,1\,0\,0\\
f:\;1\,1\,1\,0\,1\,0\,1\,0\\
0\,0\,0\,0\,0\,0\,0\,1\\
0\,0\,0\,0\,0\,1\,0\,1
\end{array}
$$

Fig. 4.1. The symbols • denote particles on a grid that are represented in the table f on the right by 1's. In the classical case the light is going horizontally and vertically, resulting in row and column sums. In the emission case the particles emit radiation, which is partially absorbed by the material surrounding the particles. The intensity of the radiation is measured by detectors, denoted by [signs.

$[0,0,1,1,2,3,1,3,3,2,0,2,0]$. Finally, suppose that the particles emit radiation in the directions $(-1,0)$ and $(0,1)$. If β is the absorption coefficient in these directions, i.e., the absorption on a line segment of unit length is proportional with β, then the "absorption row sums" (measured at the detectors) from top to bottom are

$$[\beta^{-1}+\beta^{-3}+\beta^{-5}+\beta^{-7}, \beta^{-2}+\beta^{-4}+\beta^{-6}+\beta^{-8}, \beta^{-2}+\beta^{-6}, \tag{4.1}$$

$$\beta^{-1}+\beta^{-2}+\beta^{-3}+\beta^{-5}+\beta^{-7}, \beta^{-8}, \beta^{-6}+\beta^{-8}], \tag{4.2}$$

and the "absorption column sums" from left to right are given by

$$[\beta^{-1}+\beta^{-4}, \beta^{-2}+\beta^{-3}+\beta^{-4}, \beta^{-1}+\beta^{-4}, \beta^{-2}, \beta^{-1}+\beta^{-4}, \tag{4.3}$$

$$\beta^{-2}+\beta^{-3}+\beta^{-6}, \beta^{-1}+\beta^{-4}, \beta^{-2}+\beta^{-5}+\beta^{-6}]. \tag{4.4}$$

In the past decade considerable attention has been given to this type of problems; see, e.g., [6, 7, 15, 16] and especially [19] for a historical overview. Many papers investigate the problem under which circumstances the line sums determine the original set uniquely; see, e.g., [1, 8, 9, 11, 25] for the nonabsorption and [20, 21] for the absorption case. However, in many cases more than one configuration yields the same line sums. Observe that the "difference" of two configurations with equal line sums has zero line sums. Such a difference is called a switching configuration. In the case of row and column sums they were already studied by Ryser [23] in 1957. We refer to [17, 18] for the case of two general directions and for the investigation of so-called switching chains. Shliferstein and Chien [25] studied switching configurations in situations with more than two directions. Switching configurations play a role in solution methods of, e.g., [1, 13, 17, 18, 20, 21, 25]. Already Ryser [23] showed in the case of row and column sums that every switching configuration can be composed of simple switching components

$$\begin{pmatrix} -1 & 1 \\ 1 & -1 \end{pmatrix}. \tag{4.5}$$

An algebraic theory on their structure was developed by the authors [12, 14] based on switching components of minimal size, so-called switching atoms. In order to reconstruct the original itself, one can use additional known properties of the original object to favor some inverse images above the others, such as convexity (see, e.g., [1]) or connectedness (see, e.g., [3, 4, 13]). For an extensive study on the computational complexity of discrete tomographical problems, see [10].

In this chapter we describe a general algebraic framework for switching configurations. We collect and at certain points generalize some of our previous results. We show that our method can be applied to more general problems than only the classical ones in discrete tomography. We mention that, though we focus on $\mathbb{Z}^n$ only, the results presented below can be generalized to any integral domain R such that $R[x_1, \ldots, x_n]$ is a unique factorization domain. We recommend the book of Lang [22] as a general reference for algebra.

To formulate the above problems in a precise way, we introduce some definitions and notation that we use throughout this chapter without any further reference. Let n be a positive integer. The jth coordinate of a point $\underline{v} \in \mathbb{Z}^n$ will be denoted by v_j $(j = 1, \ldots, n)$, that is, $\underline{v} = (v_1, \ldots, v_n)$. Let m_j $(j = 1, \ldots, n)$ denote positive integers, and put

$$A = \{\underline{i} \in \mathbb{Z}^n \mid 0 \le i_j < m_j \text{ for } j = 1, \ldots, n\}. \tag{4.6}$$

Let d be a positive integer, and suppose that $\overset{k}{\sim}$ are equivalence relations on A for $k = 1, \ldots, d$. (For example, points are equivalent if they are on a line in some direction characterized by k.) Let $H_1^{(k)}, \ldots, H_{t_k}^{(k)}$ denote the equivalence classes of $\overset{k}{\sim}$. Finally, let $\varrho_k : A \to \mathbb{R}_{>0}$ be so-called weight functions for $k = 1, \ldots, d$, and set $\varrho = \sum_{k=1}^{d} \varrho_k$. Now the above-mentioned problems can be formulated in the following more general way.

Problem 1. Let c_{kl} be given real numbers for $k = 1, \ldots, d$ and $l = 1, \ldots, t_k$. Construct a function $g : A \to \{0, 1\}$ (if it exists) such that

$$\sum_{\underline{i} \in H_l^{(k)}} g(\underline{i}) \varrho_k(\underline{i}) = c_{kl} \quad (k = 1, \ldots d; \ l = 1, \ldots t_k). \tag{4.7}$$

It is important to note that Eq.(4.7) is certainly underdetermined with respect to functions $g : A \to \mathbb{Z}$. Moreover, the same may be true for solutions $g : A \to \{0, 1\}$. For example, the function g given by

$$g: \begin{array}{c} 0\,1\,1\,0\,1\,0\,1\,0 \\ 1\,0\,0\,0\,1\,1\,0\,1 \\ 0\,1\,0\,0\,0\,1\,0\,0 \\ 1\,1\,1\,1\,0\,0\,0\,1 \\ 0\,0\,0\,0\,0\,0\,1\,0 \\ 0\,0\,0\,0\,0\,1\,0\,1 \end{array} \tag{4.8}$$

has the same row and column sums as f from Fig. 4.1. Consequently, $h := f - g$ has zero row and column sums. Vice versa, having a function $h : A \to \mathbb{Z}$ with zero line sums, the line sums of $g + h$ will coincide with those of g. It turns out that the study of switching configurations over $\mathbb{Z}$ is much simpler than that over $\{0, 1\}$. It is therefore important to note that the solutions to Problem 1 can be characterized as the solutions of the following optimization problem over $\mathbb{Z}$.

Problem 2. Construct a function $g : A \to \mathbb{Z}$ (if it exists) such that (4.7) holds, and

$$\sum_{i \in A} g(i)^2 \varrho(i) \text{ is minimal .} \tag{4.9}$$

Remark 1. If g is a solution to Problem 1, then g is a solution to Problem 2. To show this, let $f : A \to \mathbb{Z}$ be any other solution to (4.7). Then we have

$$\sum_{i \in A} g(i)^2 \varrho(i) = \sum_{i \in A} g(i)\varrho(i) = \sum_{i \in A} f(i)\varrho(i) \le \sum_{i \in A} f(i)^2 \varrho(i) . \tag{4.10}$$

The idea used here, that a binary solution has small "length," has been used in several papers; see, e.g., [3, 4, 13].

Remark 2. We also mention that when the equivalence relations $\overset{k}{\sim}$ mean that the corresponding points are on the same lines in given directions, and the weight functions ϱ_k are defined as certain powers of some real numbers $\beta_k \ge 1$, then in view of Remark 1, our problems just reduce to the classical problem of emission tomography with absorption. In particular, when $\beta_k = 1$ ($\varrho_k = 1$ for every k), we get back the classical problem on discrete tomography.

As we indicated, we will study the structure of the set of integral solutions of Eq.(4.7). It turns out that in case of line sums there exists a minimal configuration (the so-called switching atom) such that every integral solution of the homogenized equation (4.7) (i.e., with $c_{kl} = 0$) can be expressed as a linear combination of shifts of one of the switching atoms. For the case of row and column sums, the switching atom is

$$\begin{pmatrix} -1 & 1 \\ 1 & -1 \end{pmatrix} . \tag{4.11}$$

In this chapter we characterize and derive properties of switching configurations.

The structure of this chapter is as follows. In the next section we briefly outline the main principles of our method. In Section 4.3 we give a complete description of the set of integral solutions of (4.7) in case of the classical problem of discrete tomography, for arbitrary dimension (see Theorem 1). Theorem 2 shows that if Problem 2 admits a solution, then a relatively small solution can be found in polynomial time. In Section 4.4 we derive similar results for the case of emission tomography with absorption, also for any dimension n. Finally, in Section 4.5 we consider a new type of tomographical problems. Instead of lines, the X-rays (in $\mathbb{Z}^2$) are assumed to be parallel broken lines or parallel shifts of the graph of a function $G : \mathbb{Z} \to \mathbb{Z}$. It turns out that our machinery is applicable in this case, as well.

4.2 The Main Principles of the Method

In this section we summarize the main principles of our approach. Our method relies on the following four fundamental observations.

1) If both functions $f, g : A \to \mathbb{Z}$ are solutions to Eq. (4.7), then the difference $h := f - g$ is a solution to (4.7) with $c_{kl} = 0$ for all k, l, that is, to

$$\sum_{\underline{i} \in H_l^{(k)}} h(\underline{i}) \varrho_k(\underline{i}) = 0 \quad (k = 1, \ldots d; \; l = 1, \ldots t_k) . \qquad (4.12)$$

So to characterize the set of integral solutions of (4.7), it is sufficient to know one particular solution g together with all the solutions of (4.12).

2) Suppose that $H_1, \ldots, H_t$ is a partition of A. Let $f : A \to \mathbb{Z}$ and $f_l : H_l \to \mathbb{Z}$ ($l = 1, \ldots, t$) be given functions and write $\chi_f(\underline{x}) = \sum_{\underline{i} \in A} f(\underline{i}) \underline{x}^{\underline{i}}$ for the generating polynomial of f. Suppose that $\chi_{f_l}(\underline{x}) = \sum_{\underline{i} \in H_l} f_l(\underline{i}) \underline{x}^{\underline{i}}$ vanishes for $l = 1, \ldots, t$, and that $\chi_f(\underline{x}) = \sum_{l=1}^{t} \chi_{f_l}(\underline{x})$. Then $\chi_f(\underline{x})$ vanishes.

3) If $\chi_f(\underline{x})$ is divisible by polynomials $P_1(\underline{x}), \ldots, P_s(\underline{x}) \in \mathbb{Z}[\underline{x}]$, then $\chi_f(\underline{x})$ is divisible by $\mathrm{lcm}(P_1(\underline{x}), \ldots, P_s(\underline{x}))$ in $\mathbb{Z}[\underline{x}]$.

4) Let f be a solution to Eq.(4.12). Then in the cases investigated in this chapter we have $\chi_f(\underline{x}) = P(\underline{x})Q(\underline{x})$, where P corresponds to a "minimal" solution M to (4.12), and Q indicates which combination of the translates of M yields f.

To illustrate how these principles work, we exhibit some examples.

Example 1 (row sums). Let $n = 2$, $A = \{(i, j) \mid 0 \leq i < m_1, \; 0 \leq j < m_2\}$, and $H_l = \{(i, l) \mid 0 \leq i < m_1\}$ for $l = 0, \ldots, m_2 - 1$. Let $f : A \to \mathbb{Z}$ be a given function. Define $f_l : H_l \to \mathbb{Z}$ for $l = 0, \ldots, m_2 - 1$ by $f_l(i, l) = f(i, l)$ ($i = 0, \ldots, m_1 - 1$). Then

$$\chi_f(x,y) = \sum_{l=0}^{m_2-1} \chi_{f_l}(x,y) \text{ and } \chi_{f_l}(x,y) = y^l \sum_{i=0}^{m_1-1} f_l(i,l)x^i . \qquad (4.13)$$

(i) Suppose $\sum_{i=0}^{m_1-1} f(i,l) = 0$ for $l = 0, \ldots, m_2 - 1$. Then

$$\chi_{f_l}(1,y) = y^l \sum_{i=0}^{m_1-1} f_l(i,l) = y^l \sum_{i=0}^{m_1-1} f(i,l) = 0 \text{ for } l = 0, \ldots, m_2 - 1 . \qquad (4.14)$$

Hence

$$\chi_{f_l}(x,y) = \sum_{(i,j)\in H_l} f_l(i,j)x^i y^j = y^l \sum_{i=0}^{m_1-1} f_l(i,l)x^i \qquad (4.15)$$

is divisible by $x - 1$ for $l = 0, \ldots, m_2 - 1$. Thus $\chi_f(x,y) = \sum_{l=0}^{m_2-1} \chi_{f_l}(x,y)$ is divisible by $x - 1$.

(ii) Let $\beta \in \mathbb{C}$, and suppose that $\sum_{i=0}^{m_1-1} f(i,l)\beta^i = 0$ for $l = 0, \ldots, m_2 - 1$. Then

$$\chi_{f_l}(\beta,y) = y^l \sum_{i=0}^{m_1-1} f_l(i,l)\beta^i = y^l \sum_{i=0}^{m_1-1} f(i,l)\beta^i = 0 \text{ for } l = 0, \ldots, m_2 - 1 .$$

$$(4.16)$$

Hence $\chi_{f_l}(x,y)$ is divisible by $x - \beta$ over $\mathbb{C}$ for $l = 0, \ldots, m_2 - 1$. Then $\chi_f(x,y)$ is divisible by $x - \beta$ over $\mathbb{C}$. Since $\chi_f(x,y) \in \mathbb{Z}[x,y]$, this implies that $\chi_f = 0$ if β is a transcendental number and that $\chi_f(x,y)$ is divisible by the minimal defining polynomial of β if it is an algebraic number. The above argument can be given for columns, as well.

Barcucci, Frosini, and Rinaldi [2] treated the binary case (i.e., only coefficients 0 or 1) where the row sums are measured in both directions for the absorption coefficient $\beta = (1 + \sqrt{5})/2$. They proved that in that case the row sums determine the configuration uniquely. Since it is a good illustration of our approach, we show how this conclusion follows from the above considerations. Suppose there are two distinct binary solutions. Then the polynomial f, defined as the difference of both characteristic polynomials, has only coefficients 1, 0, and -1 and vanishing row sums into both directions. The polynomial $\sum_{i=0}^{m-1} f(i,l)x^i$ is therefore divisible by both the minimal polynomial $x^2 - x - 1$ of β and the minimal polynomial $x^2 + x - 1$ of β^{-1} for all l. Hence both $\sum_{i=0}^{m-1} f(i,l)\beta^i = 0$ and $\sum_{i=0}^{m-1} f(i,l)(-\beta)^i = 0$. By addition and subtraction we find that both $\sum_{i \text{ even}} f(i,l)\beta^i = 0$ and $\sum_{i \text{ odd}} f(i,l)\beta^i = 0$. Since the nonzero coefficients have modulus 1 and $\beta^2 > 2$, the first nonzero term of each expression exceeds the sum of the remaining terms. We conclude that all the coefficients of f are 0 and therefore the solution is unique.

Example 2 (row and column sums). On combining Example 1 with β_1 to the row sums and with β_2 to the column sums, we obtain that if $\sum_{i=0}^{m_1-1} f(i,l)\beta_1^i = 0$ for $l = 0, \ldots, m_2-1$ and $\sum_{j=0}^{m_2-1} f(l,j)\beta_2^j = 0$ for $l = 0, \ldots, m_1-1$, then $\chi_f = 0$ if β_1 or β_2 is transcendental and that otherwise χ_f is divisible by the product of the minimal defining polynomials $P_1(x,1)$ of β_1 and $P_2(1,y)$ of β_2 (as $P_1(x,1)$ and $P_2(1,y)$ are coprime).

Kuba and Nivat [20] studied the special case of row and column sums for $\beta_1 = \beta_2 = (1 + \sqrt{5})/2$ (cf., Example 4 in Section 4.4.1). The situation of having different absorption coefficients in different directions was studied by Zopf and Kuba [26] in another context.

Example 3 (line sums). Let n and A be as in Example 1 and $a, b \in \mathbb{Z}$. Without loss of generality, we may assume that $a > 0$. Suppose first that we have $b \leq 0$. Put $H_l = \{(i,j) \mid aj = bi+l\}$ for $l = 0, \ldots, m$ with $m = (m_1-1)b+(m_2-1)a$. Hence A is the disjoint union of the H_l. Define the functions $f_l : H_l \to \mathbb{Z}$ for the above values of l by $f_l(i,j) = f(i,j)$ $((i,j) \in H_l)$, where $f : A \to \mathbb{Z}$ is a given function. Then

$$\chi_f(x,y) = \sum_{l=0}^{m} \chi_{f_l}(x,y) \text{ where } \chi_{f_l}(x,y) = \sum_{(i,j)\in H_l} f_l(i,j)x^i y^j . \quad (4.17)$$

Let $\beta \in \mathbb{C}$, and suppose that $\sum_{(i,j)\in H_l} f_l(i,j)\beta^i = 0$ for $l = 0, \ldots, m$. Then

$$\chi_{f_l}(x,y) = \sum_{(i,j)\in H_l} f_l(i,j)x^i y^{(bi+l)/a} = y^{l/a} \sum_{(i,j)\in H_l} f_l(i,j)(xy^{b/a})^i = 0 \quad (4.18)$$

for $x = \beta y^{-b/a}$ and $l = 0, \ldots, m$. It follows that $\chi_f(\beta y^{-b/a}, y) \equiv 0$. Equivalently, $\chi_f(\beta y^{-b}, y^a) = 0$. We conclude that $\chi_f = 0$ if β is transcendental and that otherwise χ_f is divisible by the minimal defining polynomial of $x^{a/d} - \beta^{a/d}y^{-b/d}$, where $d = \gcd(a,b)$, if β is algebraic. Similarly we find in case $b > 0$ that χ_f is divisible by the minimal polynomial of $x^{a/d}y^{b/d} - \beta^{a/d}$.

Combine Example 1 with $\beta = \beta_1$ and Example 3 with $a = 1$, $b = -1$, $\beta = \beta_1^{\sqrt{2}}$. Suppose $\sum_{i=0}^{m_1-1} f(i,l)\beta_1^i = 0$ for $l = 0, \ldots, m_2-1$ and $\sum_{j=-i+l} f(i,j)\beta_1^{\sqrt{2}i} = 0$ for $l = 0, \ldots, m_1 + m_2 - 2$. Then χ_f is divisible by both polynomials $x - \beta_1$ and $x - \beta_1^{\sqrt{2}}y$ over $\mathbb{C}$. By the theorem of Gelfond–Schneider, we know that if $\beta_1 \neq 0, 1$, then $\beta_1^{\sqrt{2}}$ is transcendental if β_1 is algebraic. Hence either $\beta_1 = 0$

and χ_f is divisible by x, or $\beta_1 = 1$ and χ_f is divisible by $(x-1)(x-y)$, or $\chi_f = 0$.

Combine Example 3 with $a = 1$, $b = -1$, $\beta \neq 0$ arbitrary and Example 3 with $a = b = 1$, and β^{-1} in place of β. Suppose $\sum\limits_{j=-i+l} f(i,j)\beta^i = 0$ for $l = 0, \ldots, m_1 + m_2 - 2$ and $\sum\limits_{j=i+l} f(i,j)\beta^{-i} = 0$ for $l = -m_1 + 1, \ldots, m_2 - 1$. Then χ_f is divisible by both polynomials $x - \beta y$ and $xy - \beta^{-1}$ over $\mathbb{C}$. Hence χ_f is identically zero if β is transcendental. If β is algebraic, then χ_f is divisible by the product of the minimal polynomials of $x - \beta y$ and $xy - \beta^{-1}$.

Finally, combine Example 3 with $a = 1$, $b = -1$, $\beta \neq 0$ arbitrary and Example 3 with $a = 1$, $b = -1$, β^{-1} in place of β. (The latter condition is equivalent with $a = -1$, $b = 1$, absorption coefficient β.) Suppose $\sum\limits_{j=-i+l} f(i,j)\beta^i = \sum\limits_{j=-i+l} f(i,j)\beta^{-i} = 0$ for $l = 0, \ldots, m_1 + m_2 - 2$. Then $\chi_f = 0$ if β is transcendental. If β is algebraic, then $\chi_f(x,y)$ is divisible by the minimal polynomial of $xy - \beta$, and, if the minimal polynomial of β is nonreciprocal, even by the product of the minimal polynomials of $x - \beta y$ and $x - \beta^{-1}y$.

4.3 Discrete Tomography in nD

In [12] we developed a theory on switching configurations in case $n = 2$. In this section we generalize it to arbitrary n.

4.3.1 Some Notation

Let $\underline{a} \in \mathbb{Z}^n$ with $\gcd(a_1, \ldots, a_n) = 1$, such that $\underline{a} \neq \underline{0}$, and for the smallest j with $a_j \neq 0$ we have $a_j > 0$. We call $\underline{a}$ a *direction*. By lines with direction $\underline{a}$, we mean lines of the form $\underline{b} + t\underline{a}$ ($\underline{b} \in \mathbb{R}^n$, $t \in \mathbb{R}$) in $\mathbb{R}^n$. Let A be as in the Introduction. By the help of a direction $\underline{a}$, we can define an equivalence relation on A as follows. We call two elements of A *equivalent* if they are on the same line with direction $\underline{a}$. If $g : A \to \mathbb{Q}$ is a function, then the line sum of g along the line $T = \underline{b} + t\underline{a}$ is defined as $\sum\limits_{\underline{i} \in A \cap T} g(\underline{i})$. Note that the line sums are in fact the "class sums" from (4.7), corresponding to the above-defined equivalence.

We will work with polynomials $F \in \mathbb{Q}[x_1, \ldots, x_n]$. For brevity we write $\underline{x} = (x_1, \ldots, x_n)$ and $\underline{x}^{\underline{i}} = \prod\limits_{j=1}^{n} x_j^{i_j}$ ($\underline{i} \in \mathbb{Z}^n$). The generating polynomial of a function $g : A \to \mathbb{Q}$ is defined as

$$\chi_g(\underline{x}) = \sum_{\underline{i} \in A} g(\underline{i})\underline{x}^{\underline{i}} . \tag{4.19}$$

A set $S = \{\underline{a}_k\}_{k=1}^d$ of directions is called *valid* for A if $\sum_{k=1}^d |a_{kj}| < m_j$ for any $j = 1, \ldots, n$. Suppose that S is a valid set of directions for A. For $\underline{a} \in S$, put $f_{\underline{a}}(\underline{x}) = (\underline{x}^{\underline{a}} - 1) \prod_{a_j < 0} x_j^{-a_j}$ and set $F_S(\underline{x}) = \prod_{k=1}^d f_{\underline{a}_k}(\underline{x})$. Let

$$U = \left\{ \underline{u} \mid 0 \le u_j < m_j - \sum_{k=1}^d |a_{kj}| \ (j = 1, \ldots, n) \right\}. \tag{4.20}$$

For $\underline{u} \in U$, put $F_{(\underline{u};S)}(\underline{x}) = \underline{x}^{\underline{u}} F_S(\underline{x})$ and define the functions $M_{(\underline{u};S)} : A \to \mathbb{Z}$ by

$$M_{(\underline{u};S)}(\underline{i}) = \text{coeff}(\underline{x}^{\underline{i}}) \text{ in } F_{(\underline{u};S)}(\underline{x}) \text{ for } \underline{i} \in A. \tag{4.21}$$

The $M_{(\underline{u};S)}$'s are called the switching atoms corresponding to the direction set S. By the minimal corner of the switching atom $M_{(\underline{0};S)}$, we mean the element $\underline{i}^* \in A$ for which $M_{(\underline{0};S)}(\underline{i}^*) \ne 0$, but $M_{(\underline{0};S)}(\underline{i}) = 0$ whenever $\underline{i} \in A$ lexicographically precedes $\underline{i}^*$. That is, $\underline{i}^*$ is lexicographically the first element of A for which the function value of $M_{(\underline{0};S)}$ is nonzero. It follows from the definitions of $f_{\underline{a}}$ and F_S that

$$M_{(\underline{0};S)}(\underline{i}^*) = \pm 1. \tag{4.22}$$

Since it corresponds with the minimal corner of $M_{(\underline{0};S)}$, for every $\underline{u} \in U$ we define the minimal corner of $M_{(\underline{u};S)}$ as $\underline{i}^* + \underline{u}$. Again, the minimal corner of $M_{(\underline{u};S)}$ is lexicographically the first element of A for which the function value of $M_{(\underline{u};S)}$ is nonzero, and we also have

$$M_{(\underline{u};S)}(\underline{i}^* + \underline{u}) = \pm 1. \tag{4.23}$$

It is clear that a function g defined on A can be considered as a vector (a $\prod_{j=1}^n m_j$-tuple). If we want to emphasize this, we write $\mathbf{g}$ instead of g. We always assume that the entries of these vectors are arranged according to elements of A in lexicographical order. The length of $\mathbf{g}$ (or g) is $|g| = |\mathbf{g}| = \sqrt{\sum_{\underline{i} \in A} g(\underline{i})^2}$.

4.3.2 The Structure of the Switching Configurations

Our main result shows that every switching configuration is a linear combination of translates of the switching atom $M_{(\underline{0};S)}$.

Theorem 1. *Let A be as before, let $S = \{\underline{a}_k\}_{k=1}^d$ be a valid set of directions for A, and let R be either $\mathbb{Z}$ or $\mathbb{Q}$. Then any function $g : A \to R$ with zero line sums along the lines corresponding to S can be uniquely written in the form*

$$g = \sum_{\underline{u} \in U} c_{\underline{u}} M_{(\underline{u};S)} \tag{4.24}$$

with some $c_{\underline{u}} \in R$ ($\underline{u} \in U$). Moreover, every such function g has zero line sums along the lines corresponding to S.

Remark 3. As one can easily see from the proofs, if S is not valid for A, then the only function having all its line sums zero is the identically zero function on A.

To prove the theorem, we need the following lemma.

Lemma 1. *Assume that $\underline{a}$ is a valid direction for A, and let R be either $\mathbb{Z}$ or $\mathbb{Q}$. Then a function $g : A \to R$ has zero line sums along the lines with direction $\underline{a}$ if, and only if, $f_{\underline{a}}(\underline{x})$ divides $\chi_g(\underline{x})$ in $R[\underline{x}]$.*

Proof. We give the proof only when $a_j > 0$ ($j = 1, \ldots, n$); the proof is similar in all the other cases. Put $B = \{\underline{b} \mid \underline{b} \in A, \; \underline{b} - \underline{a} \notin A\}$, and for $\underline{b} \in B$ set $I_{\underline{b}} = \max\{t \in \mathbb{Z} \mid \underline{b} + t\underline{a} \in A\}$. Observe that we can write

$$\chi_g(\underline{x}) = \sum_{\underline{b} \in B} \sum_{t=0}^{I_{\underline{b}}} g(\underline{b} + t\underline{a})\underline{x}^{\underline{b}+t\underline{a}} = \sum_{\underline{b} \in B} \underline{x}^{\underline{b}} \sum_{t=0}^{I_{\underline{b}}} g(\underline{b} + t\underline{a})\underline{x}^{t\underline{a}} \tag{4.25}$$

$$= (\underline{x}^{\underline{a}} - 1) \sum_{\underline{b} \in B} \underline{x}^{\underline{b}} \sum_{t=0}^{I_{\underline{b}}} g(\underline{b} + t\underline{a}) \sum_{s=0}^{t-1} \underline{x}^{s\underline{a}} + \sum_{\underline{b} \in B} \underline{x}^{\underline{b}} \sum_{t=0}^{I_{\underline{b}}} g(\underline{b} + t\underline{a}) . \tag{4.26}$$

As $f_{\underline{a}}(\underline{x}) = \underline{x}^{\underline{a}} - 1$ and the line sums of g in the direction $\underline{a}$ are given by $\sum_{t=0}^{I_{\underline{b}}} g(\underline{b} + t\underline{a})$, the lemma follows. $\square$

Proof (of Theorem 1). By definition, for every $\underline{u} \in U$, the function $F_{(\underline{u};S)}$ is divisible by $f_{\underline{a}_k}$ for any k with $1 \leq k \leq d$. Hence by Lemma 1, $M_{(\underline{u};S)}$ has zero line sums along all the lines corresponding to S. This proves the second statement of Theorem 1.

Now let

$$H = \{f : A \to R \mid f \text{ has zero line sums corresponding to } S\} . \tag{4.27}$$

We first prove that the switching atoms generate H. Suppose that $g \in H$. Lemma 3 (from Section 4.4) implies that the polynomials $f_{\underline{a}_k}(\underline{x})$ are pairwise nonassociated irreducible elements of the unique factorization domain $R[\underline{x}]$. Hence by Lemma 1, we obtain

$$F_S(\underline{x}) \mid \chi_g(\underline{x}) \quad \text{in} \quad R[\underline{x}] . \tag{4.28}$$

Hence there exists a polynomial $h(\underline{x}) = \sum_{\underline{u} \in U} c_{\underline{u}} \underline{x}^{\underline{u}}$ in $R[\underline{x}]$ such that $\chi_g(\underline{x}) = h(\underline{x}) F_S(\underline{x})$. We rewrite this equation as

$$\chi_g(\underline{x}) = \sum_{\underline{u} \in U} c_{\underline{u}} F_{(\underline{u};S)}(\underline{x}) . \tag{4.29}$$

Now by the definitions of $\chi_g(\underline{x})$ and the switching atoms $M_{(\underline{u};S)}$, we immediately obtain

$$g = \sum_{\underline{u} \in U} c_{\underline{u}} M_{(\underline{u};S)} \, , \tag{4.30}$$

which proves that the functions $M_{(\underline{u};S)}$ generate H.

Suppose now that for some coefficients $l_{\underline{u}} \in R$ $(\underline{u} \in U)$ we have

$$\sum_{\underline{u} \in U} l_{\underline{u}} M_{(\underline{u};S)}(\underline{i}) = 0 \text{ for all } \underline{i} \in A \, . \tag{4.31}$$

By the definitions of the switching atoms, at the minimal corner of $M_{(\underline{0};S)}$ all the other switching atoms vanish. This immediately implies $l_{\underline{0}} = 0$. Running through the switching atoms $M_{(\underline{u};S)}$ with $\underline{u} \in U$ in increasing lexicographical order, we conclude that all the coefficients $l_{\underline{u}}$ are zero. This shows that the switching atoms are linearly independent, which completes the proof of the theorem. $\qquad\square$

The following result is a consequence of Theorem 1.

Corollary 1. *Let A, S, and R be as in Theorem 1. Let C be the set of those elements of A that are the minimal corners of the switching atoms. Then for any $f : A \to R$ and for any prescribed values from R for the elements of C, there exists a unique $g : A \to R$ having the prescribed values at the elements of C and having the same line sums as f along the lines corresponding to S.*

Proof. As every switching atom takes value ± 1 at its minimal corner, we obtain unique coefficients $c_{\underline{u}} \in R$ $(\underline{u} \in U)$ such that

$$g := f + \sum_{\underline{u} \in U} c_{\underline{u}} M_{(\underline{u};S)} \tag{4.32}$$

has the prescribed values at the element of C. By the second statement of Theorem 1, the line sums of f and g corresponding to S coincide. $\qquad\square$

4.3.3 Existence of "Small" Solutions

We provide a polynomial-time algorithm for finding an approximation to f having the required line sums. We first compute a function $q : A \to \mathbb{Q}$ having the same line sums as f in the given directions by solving a system of linear equations. Subsequently, we use the structure of switching configurations to find a function $g : A \to \mathbb{Z}$ that is not far from q and f. The general result is given in Theorem 2. It follows that in case when f has $\{0, 1\}$ values, the algorithm provides a solution $g : A \to \mathbb{Z}$ satisfying (4.7) with $|g(\underline{i})| \leq 2^{d-1} + 1$ on average, where d is the number of directions involved. The function obtained by replacing all function values of q greater than $1/2$ by 1 and all others by 0 provides a good first approximation to f in practice. In [13] an algorithm is given that relies on this principle.

Theorem 2. *Let A, d, and S be as in Theorem 1. Let all the line sums in the directions of S of some unknown function $f : A \to \mathbb{Z}$ be given. Then there exists an algorithm that is polynomial in $\max\limits_{j=1,\ldots,n} \{m_j\}$, providing a function $g : A \to \mathbb{Z}$ such that f and g have the same line sums corresponding to S. Moreover,*

$$|g| \le |f| + 2^{d-1} \sqrt{\prod_{j=1}^{n} m_j} . \tag{4.33}$$

Proof. Put $N_j = \sum\limits_{k=1}^{d} |a_{kj}|$ for $j = 1, \ldots, n$. First, compute some function $q : A \to \mathbb{Q}$ having the same line sums as f. It can be done by solving the system of linear equations provided by the line sums. This step is known to be polynomial in $\max\limits_{j=1,\ldots,n} \{m_j\}$ (see, e.g., [5], p. 48). We construct a function $s : A \to \mathbb{Z}$ with the same line sums as f. We follow the procedure used in the second part of the proof of Theorem 1 and start with the minimal corner $\underline{i}^*$ of $M_{(\underline{0};S)}$. With an appropriate rational coefficient $r_{\underline{0}}$ with $|r_{\underline{0}}| \le 1/2$, the value $(q + r_{\underline{0}} M_{(\underline{0};S)})(\underline{i}^*)$ will be an integer. We now continue in increasing lexicographical order in $\underline{i}$ and choose coefficients $r_{\underline{i}}$ subject to $|r_{\underline{i}}| \le 1/2$ such that the value of $(q + \sum\limits_{\underline{i}' \le \underline{i}} r_{\underline{i}'} M_{(\underline{i}';S)})(\underline{i})$ is an integer. (Here $\le$ under the $\sum$ refers to the lexicographical ordering.) Observe that the values at $\underline{i}'$ ($\underline{i}' < \underline{i}$) are not changed in the $\underline{i}$th step. After executing this procedure for the whole set C of the minimal corners of the switching atoms, we obtain a function s having integer values on C. By a similar process (taking the switching atoms one by one, in increasing lexicographical order) we get that there exist integers $t_{\underline{u}}$ ($\underline{u} \in U$) such that the values of $f + \sum\limits_{\underline{u} \in U} t_{\underline{u}} M_{(\underline{u};S)}$ and s coincide on C. As these functions have the same line sums corresponding to S, applying Corollary 1 with $R = \mathbb{Q}$, we conclude that they are equal; hence s takes integer values on the whole set A. Clearly, this construction of s needs only a polynomial number of steps in $\max\limits_{j=1,\ldots,n} \{m_j\}$.

Consider now all the functions as vectors ($\prod\limits_{j=1}^{n} m_j$-tuples), and solve over $\mathbb{Q}$ the following system of linear equations:

$$(\mathbf{s}, \mathbf{M}_{(\underline{v};S)}) = \sum_{\underline{u} \in U} c_{\underline{u}}^* (\mathbf{M}_{(\underline{u};S)}, \mathbf{M}_{(\underline{v};S)}) \tag{4.34}$$

in $c_{\underline{u}}^*$, where $(.,.)$ denotes the inner product of vectors and $\underline{v}$ runs through the elements of U. As the switching atoms are linearly independent according to Theorem 1, this system of equations has a unique solution. This can be computed again in time that is polynomial in $\max\limits_{j=1,\ldots,n} \{m_j\}$. Put $\mathbf{g} = \mathbf{s} - \sum\limits_{\underline{u} \in U} ||c_{\underline{u}}^*|| \mathbf{M}_{(\underline{u};S)}$, where $||\alpha||$ denotes the nearest integer to α. Observe that

$\mathbf{s} - \sum_{\underline{u} \in U} c_{\underline{u}}^* \mathbf{M}_{(\underline{u};S)}$ is just the projection of $\mathbf{f}$ (but also of $\mathbf{q}$ and $\mathbf{s}$) onto the orthogonal complement of the linear subspace generated by the switching atoms. This implies

$$|\mathbf{g}| \leq |\mathbf{f}| + \left| \sum_{\underline{u} \in U} (c_{\underline{u}}^* - ||c_{\underline{u}}^*||) \mathbf{M}_{(\underline{u};S)} \right| . \tag{4.35}$$

There are at most 2^d switching atoms that contribute to the value of any fixed point, each with a contribution at most $1/2$ in absolute value in the above equation. Thus, we may conclude $|\mathbf{g}| \leq |\mathbf{f}| + 2^{d-1} \sqrt{\prod_{j=1}^{n} m_j}$.

Finally, notice that all the steps of the above algorithm are polynomial in $\max_{j=1,\ldots,n} \{m_j\}$. Thus, the proof of Theorem 2 is complete. $\quad\square$

Remark 4. We mention that if we know that Problem 1 admits a solution, i.e., f has $\{0, 1\}$ values in the above theorem, then $|f| = \sqrt{\sum_{l=1}^{t_k} c_{kl}}$ (for any $k = 1, \ldots, d$), whence we get $|\mathbf{g}| \leq (2^{d-1} + 1)\sqrt{\prod_{j=1}^{n} m_j}$. Moreover, as noted in the proof of Theorem 2, we can replace $|f|$ with $|q|$ (or with $|s|$) in the upper bound (4.33). Therefore, an upper bound for $|g|$ can be given that only depends on the line sums and the directions.

4.3.4 Dependencies Among the Line Sums

Obviously, the sum of all row sums of a function $f : A \to \mathbb{Z}$ coincides with the sum of all column sums of f. In this subsection we give a simple formula for the number of dependencies among the line sums corresponding to S.

Let A, S, and $F_S(\underline{x})$ be as above, and write N_j for the degree of F_S in x_j ($j = 1, \ldots, n$). Then by Theorem 1, the switching atoms form a basis of a module of dimension $\prod_{j=1}^{n} (m_j - N_j)$ over $\mathbb{Z}$. Suppose that L_S denotes the number of line sums for A corresponding to the directions in S, and let D_S denote the number of dependencies among these line sums. Then as the number of unknowns is $\prod_{j=1}^{n} m_j$, elementary linear algebra tells us that

$$D_S = L_S + \prod_{j=1}^{n} (m_j - N_j) - \prod_{j=1}^{n} m_j . \tag{4.36}$$

In particular, if $n = 2$, then there are $a_k m_2 + |b_k| m_1 - a_k |b_k|$ line sums belonging to a direction $(a_k, b_k) \in S$. Hence in this case, as $a_k \geq 0$ we have

$$D_S = m_2 \sum_{k=1}^{d} a_k + m_1 \sum_{k=1}^{d} |b_k| - \sum_{k=1}^{d} a_k |b_k| \tag{4.37}$$

$$+ \left(m_1 - \sum_{k=1}^{d} a_k \right) \left(m_2 - \sum_{k=1}^{d} |b_k| \right) - m_1 m_2 = \sum_{k=1}^{d} a_k \sum_{k=1}^{d} |b_k| - \sum_{k=1}^{d} a_k |b_k| . \tag{4.38}$$

4.4 Emission Tomography with Absorption

In this section we generalize the results from [14], which were presented for dimension 2, to the case of general dimension.

To model the physical background of emission tomography with absorption, consider a ray (such as light or X-ray) transmitting through homogeneous material. Let I_0 and I denote the initial and the detected intensities of the ray. Then

$$I = I_0 \cdot e^{-\mu x} , \tag{4.39}$$

where $\mu \geq 0$ denotes the absorption coefficient of the material, and x is the length of the path of the ray in the material. We put $\beta = e^{\mu}$, and we call β the exponential absorption coefficient. We mention that as $\mu \geq 0$, we have $\beta \geq 1$. Note that by the absorption we have to work with directed line sums that do depend not only on the line, but also on the direction of the radiation through that line.

We further assume that g represents (radioactive) material that is emitting radiation. If $g(\underline{i}) = 1$, then there is a unit of radiating material at $\underline{i}$; otherwise, $g(\underline{i}) = 0$ and there is no such material at $\underline{i}$.

As we have absorption, we attach some absorption coefficient to each direction. Hence we slightly adjust our previous notation. Let d be a positive integer, and let $S = \{(\underline{a}_k, \beta_k) \mid k = 1, \ldots, d\}$ be a set, where $\underline{a}_k \in \mathbb{Z}^n$ with $\gcd(a_{k1}, \ldots, a_{kn}) = 1$ for $k = 1, \ldots, d$, and for the real numbers β_k we have $\beta_k \geq 1$. For $k = 1, \ldots, d$, put $B_k = \{\underline{b} \in A \mid \underline{b} + \underline{a}_k \notin A\}$, and for any $\underline{i} \in A$ let $s_{(\underline{i}, k)}$ denote the integer for which $\underline{i} = \underline{b} - (s_{(\underline{i}, k)} - 1)\underline{a}_k$ with some $\underline{b} \in B_k$. By the directed absorption line sum of g along the line $T = \underline{b} - t\underline{a}_k$ ($\underline{b} \in B_k, t \in \mathbb{Z}$), we mean

$$\sum_{\underline{i} \in T \cap A} g(\underline{i}) \beta_k^{-s_{(\underline{i}, k)}} . \tag{4.40}$$

(Here there is a hidden assumption on the shape of the absorbing material, but this is irrelevant for the switching configurations.) In Fig. 4.1 in the Introduction, we illustrated how directed absorption line sums are interpreted.

Let $\underline{i}_1 \overset{k}{\sim} \underline{i}_2$ for $\underline{i}_1, \underline{i}_2 \in A$ and $k = 1, \ldots, d$ if, and only if, $\underline{i}_1 - \underline{i}_2 = t\underline{a}_k$ for some $t \in \mathbb{Z}$, and write $H_1^{(k)}, \ldots, H_{t_k}^{(k)}$ for the equivalence classes of $\overset{k}{\sim}$. Taking arbitrary real numbers c_{kl} ($k = 1, \ldots, d; \ l = 1, \ldots, t_k$), Eq.(4.7) is just given by

$$\sum_{\underline{i} \in H_l^{(k)}} g(\underline{i}) \beta_k^{-s_{(\underline{i},k)}} = c_{kl} \qquad (k = 1, \ldots d; \ l = 1, \ldots t_k) \,. \qquad (4.41)$$

Thus, in this case Problem 1 is the standard problem in emission tomography with absorption. (See also the DA2D(β) reconstruction problem in [20] for the two-dimensional case.)

If the absorption is independent of the direction, then $\beta_k = e^{\mu|\underline{a}|}$, since $|\underline{a}|$ is the distance between consecutive lattice points on the line $\underline{b} - t\underline{a}$. However, we prefer to leave the possibility open that the absorption coefficient depends on the direction in which the medium is passed. Our definition of $s_{(\underline{i},k)}$ makes it possible to distinguish between two opposite directions. Thus, $\underline{b} - t\underline{a}$ and $\underline{b} - t(-\underline{a})$ represent the same line, but opposite directions.

Finally, we mention that in case when $\beta_k = 1$ $(k = 1, \ldots, d)$, the problem reduces to the classical problem of discrete tomography.

4.4.1 The Structure of the Switching Configurations

In this section we give a full description of the set of solutions $g : A \to \mathbb{Z}$ to (4.41). First we consider the case when $c_{kl} = 0$ for all $k = 1, \ldots, d$ and $l = 1, \ldots, t_k$, which is when all the directed absorption line sums of g are zero. For this purpose we need some further notation.

First we note that if any of the β_k-s are transcendental, then f is uniquely determined by its directed absorption line sums in the corresponding direction $\underline{a}_k$. Hence from this point on, we assume that all the exponential absorption coefficients are algebraic.

Let $\underline{a} \in \mathbb{Z}^n$ be a direction (i.e., $\gcd(a_1, \ldots, a_n) = 1$). Let β be a nonzero algebraic number of degree r, and let $P_\beta(z)$ be the defining polynomial of β having coprime integral coefficients. Put

$$f_{(\underline{a},\beta)}(\underline{x}) = P_\beta(\underline{x}^{\underline{a}}) \prod_{a_j < 0} x_j^{-ra_j} \,. \qquad (4.42)$$

Hence $f_{(\underline{a},\beta)}(\underline{x}) \in \mathbb{Z}[\underline{x}]$.

In the proof we shall make use of a fundamental correspondence between functions $g : A \to \mathbb{Z}$ and polynomials in n variables. Namely, to such a function g, we attach the polynomial

$$\chi_g(\underline{x}) = \sum_{\underline{i} \in A} g(\underline{i}) \underline{x}^{\underline{i}} \,. \qquad (4.43)$$

Then into direction $\underline{a}$ the line sums of g are the coefficients of $\chi_g(\underline{x})$ "modulo" $f_{(\underline{a},\beta)}$. The polynomials are pairwise coprime except for some well-described special cases, when they are conjugate. Therefore, the polynomial F_S defined below represents the least common multiple of the polynomials $f_{(\underline{a}_k,\beta_k)}$. Let $S = \{(\underline{a}_k, \beta_k) \mid k = 1, \ldots, d\}$ be a set, where for each k, $\underline{a}_k$ is a direction and β_k is a real algebraic number with $\beta_k \geq 1$ of degree r_k. Two elements $(\underline{a}_k, \beta_k)$

and $(\underline{a}_c, \beta_c)$ of S are equivalent if $\underline{a}_k = \underline{a}_c$ and β_k and β_c are algebraically conjugated elements, or $\underline{a}_k = -\underline{a}_c$ and β_k and $1/\beta_c$ are algebraically conjugated elements. Let S^* be a subset of S containing exactly one element of S from each class of this equivalence relation. Put

$$F_S(\underline{x}) = \prod_{(\underline{a}_k, \beta_k) \in S^*} f_{(\underline{a}_k, \beta_k)}(\underline{x}) \,. \tag{4.44}$$

We say that S is valid for A if $N_j := \deg_{x_j}(F_S(\underline{x})) < m_j$ $(j = 1, \ldots, n)$. Put $U = \{\underline{u} \in \mathbb{Z}^n \mid 0 \leq u_j < m_j - N_j \ (j = 1, \ldots, n)\}$. For $\underline{u} \in U$ set $F_{(\underline{u};S)}(\underline{x}) = \underline{x}^{\underline{u}} F_S(\underline{x})$, and define the functions $M_{(\underline{u};S)} : A \to \mathbb{Z}$ by

$$M_{(\underline{u};S)}(\underline{i}) = \mathrm{coeff}(\underline{x}^{\underline{i}}) \text{ in } F_{(\underline{u};S)}(\underline{x}) \text{ for } \underline{i} \in A \,. \tag{4.45}$$

The functions $M_{(\underline{u};S)}$ are called the *switching atoms* corresponding to the set S. By the minimal corner of the switching atom $M_{(\underline{0};S)}$, we mean the element $\underline{i}^*$ that is lexicographically the first element of A for which the function value of $M_{(\underline{0};S)}$ is nonzero. The minimal corner of $M_{(\underline{u};S)}$ is $\underline{i}^* + \underline{u}$.

Our main result in this section shows that switching configurations can be obtained as combinations of shifts of the switching atom $M_{(\underline{0};S)}$ also in the case of emission tomography.

Theorem 3. *Let A, S, and $M_{(\underline{u};S)}$ be as above, with the assumption that S is valid for A. Then any function $g : A \to \mathbb{Z}$ with zero directed absorption line sums corresponding to the pairs $(\underline{a}_k, \beta_k)$ of S can be uniquely written in the form*

$$g = \sum_{\underline{u} \in U} c_{\underline{u}} M_{(\underline{u};S)} \tag{4.46}$$

with $c_{\underline{u}} \in \mathbb{Z}$ $(\underline{u} \in U)$. Moreover, every such function g has zero directed absorption line sums corresponding to the elements of S.

Remark 5. Note that if S is not valid for A, then there is no nontrivial f having zero directed absorption line sums in the directions given by S. This fact simply follows from the proof of Theorem 3.

As an illustration, we give two examples (partly from [14]).

Example 4. First we consider a similar situation as Kuba and Nivat do in [20]; however, in $\mathbb{Z}^3$. Let $S = \{((-1,0,0),\beta), ((0,1,0),\beta), ((0,0,1),\beta)\}$, where $\beta = (1 + \sqrt{5})/2$. Then we have $P_\beta(z) = z^2 - z - 1$,

$$f_{((-1,0,0),\beta)}(x_1, x_2, x_3) = -x_1^2 - x_1 + 1, \ f_{((0,1,0),\beta)}(x_1, x_2, x_3) = x_2^2 - x_2 - 1, \tag{4.47}$$

and

$$f_{((0,0,1),\beta)}(x_1, x_2, x_3) = x_3^2 - x_3 - 1 \,. \tag{4.48}$$

Thus, we obtain

$$F_S(x_1, x_2, x_3) = (x_1^2 x_2^2 - x_1^2 x_2 - x_1^2 + x_1 x_2^2 - x_1 x_2 - x_1 - x_2^2 + x_2 + 1)(1 + x_3 - x_3^2),$$
$$(4.49)$$

and $N_1 = N_2 = N_3 = 2$. So if A is of type $m_1 \times m_2 \times m_3$ with $m_1, m_2, m_3 \geq 3$, then S is a valid set for A. Now $M_{(0;S)}$ is given by

0	0	0	0...0		0	0	0	0...0		0	0	0	0...0
$\vdots$	$\vdots$	$\vdots$	$\vdots$ $\vdots$		$\vdots$	$\vdots$	$\vdots$	$\vdots$ $\vdots$		$\vdots$	$\vdots$	$\vdots$	$\vdots$ $\vdots$
0	0	0	0...0		0	0	0	0...0		0	0	0	0...0
−1	1	1	0...0		−1	1	1	0...0		1	−1	−1	0...0
1	−1	−1	0...0		1	−1	−1	0...0		−1	1	1	0...0
1	−1	−1	0...0		1	−1	−1	0...0		−1	1	1	0...0

$$(4.50)$$

where these tables represent the values of $M_{(0;S)}$ on the "slices" corresponding to the coefficients of $1, x_3, x_3^2$ in F_S, respectively. (All the other values are zero.) The switching atoms $M_{(u;S)}$ ($u \in U$) form a basis of the set of functions $g : A \to \mathbb{Z}$ having zero line sums corresponding to the three elements of S.

Example 5. Now we consider an example for $n = 2$ where both opposite directions and different exponential absorption coefficients occur. Let

$$S = \{((-1,0), \beta), ((1,0), \beta), ((0,-1), \gamma), ((0,1), \delta)\}, \qquad (4.51)$$

with $\beta = (1 + \sqrt{5})/2$, $\gamma = 2 + \sqrt{2}$, and $\delta = \gamma/2$. We obtain $P_\beta(z) = z^2 - z - 1$, $P_\gamma(z) = z^2 - 4z + 2$, and $P_\delta(z) = 2z^2 - 4z + 1$. We have

$$f_{((-1,0),\beta)}(x_1, x_2) = -x_1^2 - x_1 + 1, \quad f_{((1,0),\beta)}(x_1, x_2) = x_1^2 - x_1 - 1, \quad (4.52)$$

and

$$f_{((0,-1),\gamma)}(x_1, x_2) = f_{((0,1),\delta)}(x_1, x_2) = 2x_2^2 - 4x_2 + 1, \qquad (4.53)$$

as γ and $1/\delta$ are associated elements. We get

$$F_S(x_1, x_2) = -2x_1^4 x_2^2 + 4x_1^4 x_2 - x_1^4 + 6x_1^2 x_2^2 - 12x_1^2 x_2 + 3x_1^2 - 2x_2^2 + 4x_2 - 1, \quad (4.54)$$

and $N_1 = 4$, $N_2 = 2$. So if A is of type $m_1 \times m_2$ with $m_1 \geq 5$ and $m_2 \geq 3$, then S is a valid set for A. Now $M_{(0;S)}$ is given by

0	0	0	0	0	0	...	0
$\vdots$	$\vdots$	$\vdots$	$\vdots$	$\vdots$	$\vdots$	$\vdots$	$\vdots$
0	0	0	0	0	0	...	0
−2	0	6	0	−2	0	...	0
4	0	−12	0	4	0	...	0
−1	0	3	0	−1	0	...	0

$$(4.55)$$

and the switching atoms $M_{(u;S)}$ ($u \in U$) form a basis of the set of functions $g : A \to \mathbb{Z}$ having zero line sums corresponding to the four elements of S.

To prove Theorem 3, we need several lemmas. To keep this exposition self-contained, we include their proofs. Lemma 2 shows the correspondence between zero line sums and division by polynomials. Note that line sums of functions $A \to L$ are defined in the obvious way.

Lemma 2. *Let A be as before, $\underline{a}$ a direction, and β a nonzero algebraic number. Let L be some field containing the splitting field of $P_\beta(z)$. Put*

$$\tilde{f}_{(\underline{a},\beta)}(\underline{x}) = (\underline{x}^{\underline{a}} - \beta) \prod_{a_j < 0} x_j^{-a_j} . \tag{4.56}$$

Then a function $g : A \to L$ has zero line sums corresponding to the pair $(\underline{a}, \beta)$ if, and only if, $\tilde{f}_{(\underline{a},\beta)}(\underline{x})$ divides $\chi_g(\underline{x})$ in $L[\underline{x}]$.

Proof. We prove the lemma only with $a_j > 0$ $(j = 1, \ldots, n)$, as the other cases can be treated similarly.

Put $B = \{\underline{b} \in A \mid \underline{b} + \underline{a} \notin A\}$ and let $I_{\underline{b}}$ be the number of the points of A on the line $\underline{b} - t\underline{a}$ $(\underline{b} \in B, t \in \mathbb{Z})$. Observe that we may write

$$\chi_g(\underline{x}) = \sum_{\underline{b} \in B} \sum_{s=0}^{I_{\underline{b}}-1} g(\underline{b} - s\underline{a})\underline{x}^{\underline{b}-s\underline{a}} = \sum_{\underline{b} \in B} \underline{x}^{\underline{b}} \sum_{s=0}^{I_{\underline{b}}-1} g(\underline{b} - s\underline{a})\underline{x}^{-s\underline{a}} . \tag{4.57}$$

If $\underline{x}^{\underline{a}} - \beta$ divides $\chi_g(\underline{x})$ in $L[\underline{x}]$, then after substituting $x_1 \leftarrow \beta^{1/a_1} \prod_{j=2}^{n} x_j^{a_j/a_1}$ the polynomial $\chi_g(\underline{x})$ becomes identically zero. This shows that $\sum_{s=0}^{I_{\underline{b}}-1} g(\underline{b} - s\underline{a})\beta^{-s}$ vanishes for every $\underline{b} \in B$; hence g has zero absorption line sums corresponding to $(\underline{a}, \beta)$. This proves the "if" part of the statement.

To prove the "only if" part, suppose that all the line sums

$$\sum_{s=0}^{I_{\underline{b}}-1} g(\underline{b} - s\underline{a})\beta^{-s-1} = \beta^{-I_{\underline{b}}} \sum_{s=0}^{I_{\underline{b}}-1} g(\underline{b} - (I_{\underline{b}} - s - 1)\underline{a})\beta^s \quad (\underline{b} \in B) \tag{4.58}$$

of g corresponding to $(\underline{a}, \beta)$ vanish. This means that β is a root of the polynomial $Q_{\underline{b}}(z) := \sum_{s=0}^{I_{\underline{b}}-1} g(\underline{b} - (I_{\underline{b}} - s - 1)\underline{a})z^s$ for each $\underline{b} \in B$. Thus, for every $\underline{b} \in B$, the polynomial $Q_{\underline{b}}(\underline{x}^{\underline{a}})$ is divisible by $\underline{x}^{\underline{a}} - \beta$ over L. Hence $\underline{x}^{\underline{a}} - \beta$ divides $\chi_g(\underline{x}) = \sum_{\underline{b} \in B} \underline{x}^{\underline{b}+(1-I_{\underline{b}})\underline{a}} Q_{\underline{b}}(\underline{x}^{\underline{a}})$ in $L[\underline{x}]$, and the lemma follows. $\quad\square$

Lemma 3. *Using the notation of Lemma 2, write r for the degree and $\beta^{(c)}$ $(1 \le c \le r)$ for the conjugates of β. Then the polynomials $\tilde{f}_{(\underline{a},\beta^{(c)})}(\underline{x})$ $(1 \le c \le r)$ defined in Lemma 2 are pairwise nonassociated irreducible elements in $L[\underline{x}]$.*

Proof. As $\gcd(a_1, \ldots, a_n) = 1$, the irreducibility of these polynomials is a simple consequence of Corollary 2 of [24] p. 103. The statement that the polynomials are pairwise nonassociated is trivial. $\qquad\square$

Corollary 2. *The polynomials* $P_\beta(\underline{x}^{\underline{a}}) \prod_{a_j < 0} x_j^{-ra_j}$ *are irreducible in* $\mathbb{Z}[\underline{x}]$.

Proof. We prove the statement only for $a_j > 0$ $(j = 1, \ldots, n)$; the other cases are similar.

Let $\beta^{(c)}$ $(1 \le c \le r)$ be the conjugates of β, and let L be the splitting field of P_β over $\mathbb{Q}$. Then, in view of

$$P_\beta(\underline{x}^{\underline{a}}) = c_0 \prod_{c=1}^{r} (\underline{x}^{\underline{a}} - \beta^{(c)}), \tag{4.59}$$

where c_0 is the leading coefficient of P_β, the statement immediately follows from Lemma 3. $\qquad\square$

In the next lemma we show that the divisibility property of χ_g over L in Lemma 2 implies a stronger property over $\mathbb{Z}$.

Lemma 4. *Let $\underline{a}$ and β be as in Lemma 2. Using the previous notation, a function $g : A \to \mathbb{Z}$ has zero line sums corresponding to the pair $(\underline{a}, \beta)$ if, and only if, $P_\beta(\underline{x}^{\underline{a}}) \prod_{a_j < 0} x_j^{-ra_j}$ divides $\chi_g(\underline{x})$ in $\mathbb{Z}[\underline{x}]$.*

Proof. The "if" part of the statement easily follows from Lemma 2. We prove the "only if" part only for $a_j > 0$ $(j = 1, \ldots, n)$; the other cases can be handled similarly. In this case observe that by Lemma 2, $\underline{x}^{\underline{a}} - \beta$ divides $\chi_g(\underline{x})$ over any field L that contains the splitting field of $P_\beta(z)$. However, by conjugation, for every conjugate $\beta^{(c)}$ of β, $\underline{x}^{\underline{a}} - \beta^{(c)}$ also divides $\chi_g(\underline{x})$ in $L[\underline{x}]$. By Lemma 3, this assertion immediately implies the statement. $\qquad\square$

Lemma 5. *Let $\underline{a}, \underline{a}^*$ be directions, and β, β^* be nonzero algebraic numbers of degrees r and r^*, respectively. Then the polynomials $P_\beta(\underline{x}^{\underline{a}}) \prod_{a_j < 0} x_j^{-ra_j}$ and $P_{\beta^*}(\underline{x}^{\underline{a}^*}) \prod_{a_j^* < 0} x_j^{-r^* a_j^*}$ are associated in $\mathbb{Z}[\underline{x}]$ if, and only if, either $\underline{a} = \underline{a}^*$ and β and β^* are conjugated, or $\underline{a} = -\underline{a}^*$ and β and $1/\beta^*$ are conjugated.*

Proof. The "if" part of the statement is trivial. Suppose that $P_\beta(\underline{x}^{\underline{a}}) \prod_{a_j < 0} x_j^{-ra_j}$ and $P_{\beta^*}(\underline{x}^{\underline{a}^*}) \prod_{a_j^* < 0} x_j^{-r^* a_j^*}$ are associated. Then the degrees of β and β^* must be equal, i.e., $r = r^*$. For $1 \le c \le r$, let $\beta^{(c)}$ and $\beta^{*(c)}$ be the conjugates of β and β^*, respectively. Let L be any field that contains the splitting fields of both P_β and P_{β^*}. Then we have the factorizations

$$P_\beta(\underline{x}^{\underline{a}}) \prod_{a_j < 0} x_j^{-ra_j} = \prod_{c=1}^{r} \tilde{f}_{(\underline{a}, \beta^{(c)})}(\underline{x}) \tag{4.60}$$

and

$$P_{\beta^*}(\underline{x}^{\underline{a}^*}) \prod_{a_j^* < 0} x_j^{-r^* a_j^*} = \prod_{c=1}^{r} \tilde{f}_{(\underline{a}^*, \beta^*(c))}(\underline{x}) \tag{4.61}$$

in $L[\underline{x}]$, where the polynomials on the right-hand sides are defined in Lemma 2. By our assumption and Lemma 3, we obtain that for each c_1 with $1 \le c_1 \le r$, there exists a c_2 also with $1 \le c_2 \le r$, such that $\tilde{f}_{(\underline{a}, \beta^{(c_1)})}(\underline{x})$ and $\tilde{f}_{(\underline{a}^*, \beta^*(c_2))}(\underline{x})$ are associated elements in $L[\underline{x}]$. By comparing the exponents of x_j $(j = 1, \ldots, n)$ in these polynomials, we get that $\underline{a} = \pm \underline{a}^*$ holds, and for the corresponding pairs (c_1, c_2), $\beta^{(c_1)} = \beta^*(c_2)$ or $\beta^{(c_1)} \beta^*(c_2) = 1$ is valid, respectively. This yields that $\{\beta^{(c)} \mid 1 \le c \le r\} = \{\beta^*(c) \mid 1 \le c \le r\}$ or $\{\beta^{(c)} \mid 1 \le c \le r\} = \{1/\beta^*(c) \mid 1 \le c \le r\}$, respectively, which establishes the "only if" part of the statement. The proof of the lemma is now complete. $\square$

Proof (of Theorem 3). By definition, for every $\underline{u} \in U$, the function $F_{(\underline{u};S)}$ is divisible by $f_{(\underline{a}_k, \beta_k)}$ for any k with $1 \le k \le d$. Hence by Lemma 2, $M_{(\underline{u};S)}$ has zero line sums corresponding to the pairs in S. This proves the second statement of the theorem.

Let

$$H = \{f : A \to \mathbb{Z} \mid f \text{ has zero absorption line sums for the elements of } S\} . \tag{4.62}$$

We first prove that the switching atoms $M_{(\underline{u};S)}$ $(\underline{u} \in U)$ generate H. Combining Corollary 2 and Lemmas 4 and 5, for any $g \in H$, we obtain

$$F_S(\underline{x}) \mid \chi_g(\underline{x}) \text{ in } \mathbb{Z}[\underline{x}] . \tag{4.63}$$

Hence there exists a polynomial $Q(\underline{x}) = \sum_{\underline{u} \in U} c_{\underline{u}} \underline{x}^{\underline{u}}$ with $c_{\underline{u}} \in \mathbb{Z}$ $(\underline{u} \in U)$ such that $Q(\underline{x}) F_S(\underline{x}) = \chi_g(\underline{x})$. We rewrite this equation as

$$\chi_g(\underline{x}) = \sum_{\underline{u} \in U} c_{\underline{u}} F_{(\underline{u};S)}(\underline{x}) . \tag{4.64}$$

Now by the definitions of $\chi_g(\underline{x})$ and the switching atoms $M_{(\underline{u};S)}$, we immediately obtain

$$g = \sum_{\underline{u} \in U} c_{\underline{u}} M_{(\underline{u};S)} , \tag{4.65}$$

which proves that the functions $M_{(\underline{u};S)}$ generate H.

Suppose now that for some coefficients $l_{\underline{u}} \in \mathbb{Z}$, we have

$$\sum_{\underline{u} \in U} l_{\underline{u}} M_{(\underline{u};S)}(\underline{i}) = 0 \text{ for } \underline{i} \in A . \tag{4.66}$$

By the definitions of the switching atoms, at the minimal corner of $M_{(\underline{0};S)}$ all the other switching atoms vanish. This immediately implies $l_{\underline{0}} = 0$. Considering now $M_{(\underline{u};S)}$ with $\underline{u} \in U$ in increasing lexicographical order, we conclude that all the coefficients $l_{\underline{u}}$ are zero in (4.66). This shows that the switching atoms are linearly independent, which completes the proof of the theorem. $\square$

Remark 6. Similarly as in case of the classical problem of discrete tomography in Section 4.3, it would be possible to provide an algorithm that produces a "small" integral solution to (4.7) in case of emission tomography. We omit the details.

4.5 Tomography on Curves

In this section we illustrate that our method is rather flexible in the sense that variations to other sums than line sums are possible. In this more general case, there do not exist translation-invariant switching atoms. However, our polynomial method allows us to construct nontrivial configurations with vanishing sums and characterize such configurations in Theorems 4 and 5.

We shall illustrate the method in two dimensions by examples where sums are taken over sets of the shape $H_k = \{(i, j) \in A \mid a_k j = b_k G(i) + t\}$, where $G : \mathbb{Z} \to \mathbb{Z}$, $t \in \mathbb{Z}$ and the (a_k, b_k) are distinct pairs of coprime integers for $k = 1, \ldots, d$. The basic idea is that to the given function $g : A \to \mathbb{Z}$ we adjoin the "generating" polynomial $\sum_{(i,j) \in A} g(i, j) x^{G(i)} y^j$ (instead of $\sum_{(i,j) \in A} g(i, j) x^i y^j$). Since $a_k j = b_k G(i) + t$, the exponent pairs $(G(i), j)$ for $(i, j) \in H_k$ are on the lines $a_k y = b_k x + t$. So the sums over H_k turn into line sums, and we can apply the preceding theory. Doing so, we find switching atoms. The problem is to return to the original situation, where there is no linear structure. However, by constructing polynomials with exponents of prescribed form that are multiples of the switching atom polynomial, we are able to construct configurations with vanishing sums for all given H_k. We give two examples.

Example 6 (Broken line sums). We consider the situation where light (or X-ray) entering from the left along the half-line $ay = bx + t$ ($x \leq 0$) is broken when reaching the y-axis and continues along the half-line $ay = cbx + t$ ($x > 0$), where c is a given integer.

To describe this case, we need to slightly adjust our previous settings. Let m_1, m_2 be positive integers and n_1 a negative integer. Put

$$A = \{(i, j) \in \mathbb{Z}^2 \mid n_1 \leq i < m_1, 0 \leq j < m_2\}, \tag{4.67}$$

and let a_k, b_k ($k = 1, \ldots, d$) and c be nonzero integers with $\gcd(a_k, b_k) = 1$ and $a_k \geq 0$ ($k = 1, \ldots, d$). Set

$$T_{kt} = \{(i,j) \in \mathbb{Z}^2 \mid i \le 0,\ a_k j = b_k i + t\} \cup \{(i,j) \in \mathbb{Z}^2 \mid i > 0,\ a_k j = cb_k i + t\}$$
$$(4.68)$$

for $k = 1, \ldots, d$ and $t \in \mathbb{Z}$. Let $(i_1, j_1) \overset{k}{\sim} (i_2, j_2)$ for $(i_1, j_1), (i_2, j_2) \in A$ and $k = 1, \ldots, d$ if, and only if, these points belong to the same set T_{kt} for some integer t. Write $H_1^{(k)}, \ldots, H_{t_k}^{(k)}$ for the equivalence classes of $\overset{k}{\sim}$ on A. These classes are in fact the intersections of the broken lines T_{kt} with A. By the broken line sums corresponding to (a_k, b_k) of a given function $g : A \to \mathbb{Z}$, we mean the expressions

$$c_{kl} := \sum_{(i,j) \in H_l^{(k)}} g(i,j) \quad \text{for } k = 1, \ldots, d;\ l = 1, \ldots, t_k . \tag{4.69}$$

Note that (4.69) is a special case of Eq.(4.7), with unit weights $\varrho_k = 1$ ($k = 1, \ldots, d$).

With the above modifications we can apply our machinery to the broken line case as well. First we introduce some further notation.

Let $S = \{(a_k, b_k)\}_{k=1}^{d}$ with (a_k, b_k) as above, and write $N_1 = \sum_{k=1}^{d} a_k$ and $N_2 = \sum_{k=1}^{d} |b_k|$. We say that S is valid for A if $N_1 < m_1 - n_1$ and $N_2 < m_2$. For $k = 1, \ldots, d$, put

$$f_k(x,y) = \begin{cases} x^{a_k} y^{b_k} - 1, & \text{if } b_k \ge 0, \\ x^{a_k} - y^{-b_k}, & \text{if } b_k < 0 , \end{cases} \tag{4.70}$$

and set $F_S(x,y) = \prod_{k=1}^{d} f_k(x,y)$.

In view of the broken lines, we define

$$\chi_g(x,y) = x^{-n_1} \left(\sum_{i=n_1}^{0} \sum_{j=0}^{m_2-1} g(i,j) x^i y^j + \sum_{i=1}^{m_1-1} \sum_{j=0}^{m_2-1} g(i,j) x^{ci} y^j \right) \tag{4.71}$$

as the "generating" polynomial of $g : A \to \mathbb{Z}$. Note that the factor x^{-n_1} is introduced only to keep the exposition inside $\mathbb{Z}[x,y]$.

For the solutions of (4.69), we have the following:

Theorem 4. *Let A and S be as above, with the assumption that S is valid for A. Then a function $g : A \to \mathbb{Z}$ has zero broken line sums corresponding to S if, and only if, $\chi_g(x,y)$ is divisible by $F_S(x,y)$ in $\mathbb{Z}[x,y]$.*

Proof. Let $g : A \to \mathbb{Z}$ be an arbitrary function and let $(a,b) \in S$. For simplicity we assume that $b \ge 0$; the case where $b < 0$ is similar. Observe that we can write

$$\chi_g(x,y) = x^{-n_1} \sum_{t\in\mathbb{Z}} \left(\sum_{i=n_1}^{0} \sum_{\substack{aj=bi+t \\ 0\le j<m_2}} g(i,j)x^i y^j + \sum_{i=1}^{m_1-1} \sum_{\substack{aj=cbi+t \\ 0\le j<m_2}} g(i,j)x^{ci}y^j \right)$$

$$= x^{-n_1} \sum_{b\in\mathbb{Z}} y^{t/a} \left(\sum_{i=n_1}^{0} \sum_{\substack{aj=bi+t \\ 0\le j<m_2}} g(i,j)(xy^{b/a})^i + \sum_{i=1}^{m_1-1} \sum_{\substack{aj=cbi+t \\ 0\le j<m_2}} g(i,j)(xy^{b/a})^{ci} \right) .$$

$$(4.72)$$

Now just as previously (see, e.g., the proof of Theorem 1), we obtain that g has zero broken line sums corresponding to $(a,b)\in S$ if, and only if, $x^a y^b - 1$ divides $\chi_g(x,y)$ in $\mathbb{Z}[x,y]$. Observing that the polynomials $f_k(x,y)$ ($k = 1,\ldots,d$) are pairwise coprime (in fact, prime) elements of $\mathbb{Z}[x,y]$, the theorem follows. □

We illustrate the above theory by the example when $S = \{(1,1),(3,1)\}$ and $c = 2$. In this case the broken line sums are calculated in accordance with Fig. 4.2. Moreover, we have

$$F_S(x,y) = (xy-1)(x^3 y - 1) = x^4 y^2 - x^3 y - xy + 1 . \qquad (4.73)$$

Theorem 4 shows that $g : A \to \mathbb{Z}$ has zero broken line sums corresponding to S if, and only if, F_S divides χ_g over $\mathbb{Z}$. Hence to present a nontrivial example, we should find a nonzero multiple of F_S in which all the exponents of x greater than some nonnegative integer are even. For switching configurations entirely contained in $\{(x,y) \mid x \le 0\}$ or in $\{(x,y) \mid x > 0\}$, the theory of Section 4.3

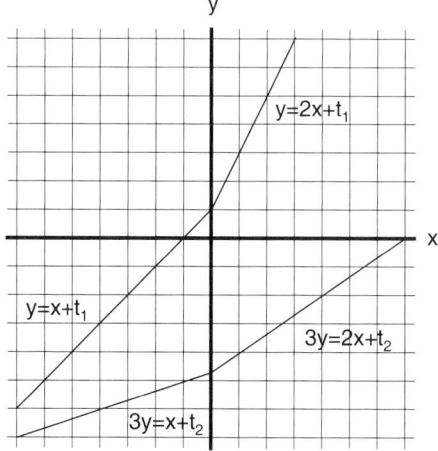

Fig. 4.2. Broken lines corresponding to $S = \{(1,1),(3,1)\}$ and $c = 2$.

applies. Suppose we want a switching configuration with "minimal corner" at $(-3, 0)$. Then all exponents of x in χ_g greater than 3 should be odd. We have

$$(xy+1)F_S(x,y) = x^5 y^3 - x^3 y - x^2 y^2 + 1 = x^3(x^2 y^3 - y - x^{-1}y^2 - x^{-3}) . \quad (4.74)$$

Hence if $n_1 \leq -3$, $m_1 \geq 3$, and $m_2 \geq 4$, then the function $g : \ A \to \mathbb{Z}$ represented by

$$
\begin{array}{ccccccccc}
0\ldots 0 & 0 & 0 & 0 & 0 & 0 & 0\ldots 0 \\
\vdots\ \vdots\ \vdots & \vdots & \vdots & \vdots & \vdots & \vdots\ \vdots\ \vdots \\
0\ldots 0 & 0 & 0 & 0 & 0 & 0 & 0\ldots 0 \\
0\ldots 0 & 0 & 0 & 0 & 0 & 1 & 0\ldots 0 \\
0\ldots 0 & 0 & 0 & -1 & 0 & 0 & 0\ldots 0 \\
0\ldots 0 & 0 & 0 & 0 & -1 & 0 & 0\ldots 0 \\
0\ldots 0 & 1 & 0 & 0 & 0 & 0 & 0\ldots 0 \\
& & & \uparrow & & &
\end{array}
\qquad (4.75)
$$

has zero broken line sums along the corresponding broken lines. Here $\uparrow$ indicates the y-axis.

Example 7 (Parabola sums). We consider the situation when the X-rays (or light) pass along parabolas $ay = bx^2 + t \ (x \geq 0)$.

Let A be as before, and let a_k, b_k be coprime nonzero integers with $a_k \geq 0$ $(k = 1, \ldots, d)$. Let $(i_1, j_1) \overset{k}{\sim} (i_2, j_2)$ for $(i_1, j_1), (i_2, j_2) \in A$ and $k = 1, \ldots, d$ if, and only if, $b_k(i_1^2 - i_2^2) = a_k(j_1 - j_2)$ (i.e., for some integer t_k, we have $b_k i_1^2 = a_k j_1 - t_k$ and $b_k i_2^2 = a_k j_2 - t_k$, that is, these points lie on the same vertical translate of the graph of the function $a_k y = b_k x^2$). Further, write $H_1^{(k)}, \ldots, H_{t_k}^{(k)}$ for the equivalence classes of $\overset{k}{\sim}$ on A. Let a function $g : A \to \mathbb{Z}$ be given. By the parabola sums of g corresponding to (a_k, b_k), we mean the expressions

$$c_{kl} := \sum_{(i,j) \in H_l^{(k)}} g(i,j) \quad \text{for } k = 1, \ldots, d; \ l = 1, \ldots, t_k . \qquad (4.76)$$

Obviously, (4.76) is a special case of Eq.(4.7) with $\varrho_k = 1 \ (k = 1, \ldots, d)$.

As it will turn out, with the modifications indicated above, we can apply our previous results to this case. We need, however, some notation. Let S, N_1, N_2, $f_k(x, y)$, and $F_S(x, y)$ be defined as in case of broken lines. We choose

$$\chi_g(x, y) = \sum_{(i,j) \in A} g(i,j) x^{i^2} y^j \qquad (4.77)$$

as the "generating" polynomial of $g : \ A \to \mathbb{Z}$.

For the solutions of (4.76), we have the following

Theorem 5. *Let A and S be as above, with the assumption that S is valid for A. Then a function $g : \ A \to \mathbb{Z}$ has zero parabola sums corresponding to S if, and only if, $\chi_g(x, y)$ is divisible by $F_S(x, y)$ in $\mathbb{Z}[x, y]$.*

Proof. Let $g : A \to \mathbb{Z}$ be an arbitrary function and let $(a, b) \in S$. For simplicity we assume that $b \geq 0$; the case where $b < 0$ is similar. Observe that we can write

$$\chi_g(x, y) = \sum_{t \in \mathbb{Z}} \sum_{\substack{aj=bi^2+t \\ (i,j) \in A}} g(i, j) x^{i^2} y^j = \sum_{t \in \mathbb{Z}} y^{t/a} \sum_{\substack{aj=bi^2+t \\ (i,j) \in A}} g(i, j)(xy^{b/a})^{i^2} . \quad (4.78)$$

Now similarly as, e.g., in the proof of Theorem 1, we can easily verify that g has zero parabola sums corresponding to $(a, b) \in S$ if, and only if, $x^a y^b - 1$ divides $\chi_g(x, y)$ in $\mathbb{Z}[x, y]$. As the polynomials $f_k(x, y)$ $(k = 1, \ldots, d)$ are pairwise coprime elements of $\mathbb{Z}[x, y]$, the theorem follows. □

We illustrate the example by analyzing two particular cases. We start with $S = \{(1, 1), (1, 2)\}$, i.e., the parabolas are given by $y = x^2 + t_1$ and $y = 2x^2 + t_2$, respectively. In this case we have

$$F_S(x, y) = (xy - 1)(xy^2 - 1) = x^2 y^3 - xy^2 - xy + 1 . \quad (4.79)$$

Theorem 5 shows that $g : A \to \mathbb{Z}$ has zero parabola sums corresponding to S if, and only if, F_S divides χ_g over $\mathbb{Z}$. The problem, however, is to find some nonzero multiple of F_S such that all the exponents of x are squares. Suppose we want a switching configuration with "minimal corner" at the origin. We can readily verify that

$$(x^2 y^4 + xy^3 + xy^2 + y^2 + y + 1)F_S(x, y) = x^4 y^7 - xy^4 - xy^3 - xy^2 - xy + y^2 + y + 1 . \quad (4.80)$$

Thus, if $m_1 \geq 2$ and $m_2 \geq 8$, then the function $g : A \to \mathbb{Z}$ represented by

$$
\begin{matrix}
0 & 0 & 0 & 0 \ldots 0 \\
\vdots & \vdots & \vdots & \vdots \; \vdots \; \vdots \\
0 & 0 & 0 & 0 \ldots 0 \\
0 & 0 & 1 & 0 \ldots 0 \\
0 & 0 & 0 & 0 \ldots 0 \\
0 & 0 & 0 & 0 \ldots 0 \\
0 & -1 & 0 & 0 \ldots 0 \\
0 & -1 & 0 & 0 \ldots 0 \\
1 & -1 & 0 & 0 \ldots 0 \\
1 & -1 & 0 & 0 \ldots 0 \\
1 & 0 & 0 & 0 \ldots 0 \\
\uparrow
\end{matrix}
\qquad (4.81)
$$

provides a nontrivial configuration having zero parabola sums along the parabolas $y = x^2 + t_1$ and $y = 2x^2 + t_1$ for any $t_1, t_2 \in \mathbb{Z}$.

Finally, we consider $S = \{(1, 1), (1, 2), (1, 3)\}$, i.e., we have three parabolas given by $y = x^2 + t_1$, $y = 2x^2 + t_2$, and $y = 3x^2 + t_3$, respectively. Now we have

$$\begin{aligned}
F_S(x,y) &= (xy-1)(xy^2-1)(xy^3-1)\\
&= x^3y^6 - x^2y^5 - x^2y^4 - x^2y^3 + xy^3 + xy^2 + xy - 1 .
\end{aligned} \tag{4.82}$$

By Theorem 5 we know that $g: A \to \mathbb{Z}$ has zero parabola sums corresponding to S if, and only if, F_S divides χ_g over $\mathbb{Z}$. The problem is again to find some nonzero multiple of F_S in which all the exponents of x are squares. We can easily check that the polynomial

$$\begin{aligned}
&(y^{26} + y^{25} + 2y^{24} + y^{23} + y^{22})x^9 - (y^{21} + y^{20} + 2y^{19} + 2y^{18} + 3y^{17} + 3y^{16}\\
&+ 4y^{15} + 4y^{14} + 4y^{13} + 3y^{12} + 3y^{11} + 2y^{10} + 2y^9 + y^8 + y^7)x^4 + (y^{15} + 2y^{14}\\
&+ 4y^{13} + 6y^{12} + 8y^{11} + 9y^{10} + 10y^9 + 10y^8 + 10y^7 + 9y^6 + 8y^5 + 6y^4 + 4y^3\\
&+ 2y^2 + y)x - (y^{12} + 2y^{11} + 4y^{10} + 5y^9 + 7y^8 + 7y^7 + 8y^6 + 7y^5 + 7y^4\\
&+ 5y^3 + 4y^2 + 2y + 1)
\end{aligned} \tag{4.83}$$

is a multiple of F_S in $\mathbb{Z}[x,y]$. Hence we obtain a nontrivial $g: A \to \mathbb{Z}$ having zero parabola sums along the three parabolas by replacing x^9 with x^3 and x^4 with x^2 and making the corresponding table.

Acknowledgments

The authors are grateful to the referee for his valuable comments and remarks. The research was supported in part by the János Bolyai Research Fellowship of the Hungarian Academy of Sciences and by the OTKA grants F43090, T42985, and T48791.

References

1. Barcucci, E., Del Lungo, A., Nivat, M., Pinzani, R.: X-rays characterizing some classes of discrete sets. *Lin. Algebra Appl.*, **339**, 3–21 (2001).
2. Barcucci, E., Frosini, A., Rinaldi, S.: Reconstruction of discrete sets from two absorbed projections: An algorithm. *Electr. Notes Discr. Math.*, **12** (2003).
3. Batenburg, K.J.: *Reconstruction of binary images from discrete X-rays*. CWI, Technical Report PNA-E0418, ftp.cwi.nl/CWIreports/PNA/PNA-E0418.pdf (2004).
4. Batenburg, K.J.: A new algorithm for 3D binary tomography. *Electr. Notes Discr. Math.*, **20**, 247–261 (2005).
5. Cohen, H.: *A Course in Computational Algebraic Number Theory*. Springer, Berlin, Germany (1993).
6. Del Lungo, A., Gronchi, P., Herman, G.T. (eds.): *Proceedings of the Workshop on Discrete Tomography: Algorithms and Applications. Lin. Algebra Appl.*, **339**, 1–219 (2001).
7. Gardner, R.J.: *Geometric Tomography*. Cambridge University Press, Cambridge, UK (1995).
8. Gardner, R.J., Gritzmann, P.: Discrete tomography: Determination of finite sets by X-rays. *Trans. Amer. Math. Soc.*, **349**, 2271–2295 (1997).

9. Gardner, R.J., Gritzmann, P.: Uniqueness and complexity in discrete tomography. In: Herman, G.T., Kuba, A. (eds.), *Discrete Tomography: Foundations, Algorithms, and Applications*. Birkhäuser, Boston, MA, pp. 85–113 (1999).

10. Gardner, R.J., Gritzmann, P., Prangenberg, D.: On the computational complexity of reconstructing lattice sets from their X-rays. *Discr. Math.*, **202**, 45–71 (1999).

11. Hajdu, L.: Unique reconstruction of bounded sets in discrete tomography. *Electr. Notes Discr. Math.*, **20**, 15–25 (2005).

12. Hajdu, L., Tijdeman, R.: Algebraic aspects of discrete tomography. *J. Reine Angew. Math.*, **534**, 119–128 (2001).

13. Hajdu, L., Tijdeman, R.: An algorithm for discrete tomography. *Lin. Algebra Appl.*, **339**, 147–169 (2001).

14. Hajdu, L., Tijdeman, R.: Algebraic aspects of emission tomography with absorption. *Theoret. Comput. Sci.*, **290**, 2169–2181 (2003).

15. Herman, G.T., Kuba, A. (eds.): *Discrete Tomography: Foundations, Algorithms, and Applications*. Birkhäuser, Boston, MA (1999).

16. Herman, G.T., Kuba, A. (eds.): *Proceedings of the Workshop on Discrete Tomography and Its Applications*. *Electr. Notes Discr. Math.*, **20**, 1–622 (2005).

17. Kong, T.Y., Herman, G.T.: On which grids can tomographic equivalence of binary pictures be characterized in terms of elementary switching operations? *Int. J. Imaging Syst. Technol.*, **9**, 118–125 (1998).

18. Kong, T.Y., Herman, G.T.: Tomographic equivalence and switching operations. In: Herman, G.T., Kuba, A. (eds.), *Discrete Tomography: Foundations, Algorithms, and Applications*. Birkhäuser, Boston, MA, pp. 59–84 (1999).

19. Kuba, A., Herman, G.T.: Discrete tomography: A historical overview. In: Herman, G.T., Kuba, A. (eds.), *Discrete Tomography: Foundations, Algorithms, and Applications*. Birkhäuser, Boston, MA, pp. 3–34 (1999).

20. Kuba, A., Nivat, M.: Reconstruction of discrete sets with absorption. In: Borgefors, G., Nystrm, I., Sanniti di Baja, G. (eds.), *Discrete Geometry in Computer Imagery*, Springer, Berlin, Germany, pp. 137–148 (2000).

21. Kuba, A., Nivat, M.: Reconstruction of discrete sets with absorption. *Lin. Algebra Appl.*, **339**, 171–194 (2001).

22. Lang, S.: *Algebra*. Addison-Wesley, Reading, MA (1984).

23. Ryser, H.J.: Combinatorial properties of matrices of zeros and ones. *Canad. J. Math.*, **9**, 371–377 (1957).

24. Schinzel, A.: *Polynomials with Special Regard to Reducibility*. Cambridge University Press, Cambridge, UK (2000).

25. Shliferstein, H.J., Chien, Y.T.: Switching components and the ambiguity problem in the reconstruction of pictures from their projections. *Pattern Recognition*, **10**, 327–340 (1978).

26. Zopf, S., Kuba, A.: Reconstruction of measurable sets from two generalized projections. *Electr. Notes Discr. Math.*, **20**, 47–66 (2005).

5

Uniqueness and Additivity for n-Dimensional Binary Matrices with Respect to Their 1-Marginals

E. Vallejo

Summary. In this chapter we deal with the question of when an n-dimensional binary matrix is uniquely determined by its 1-marginals and with the related notion of $(0, 1)$-additivity. We present a survey of known results; several of them have been considered before only in dimensions 2 and 3. Here, we show how to extend them to any dimension. The main results are characterizations of uniqueness and $(0, 1)$-additivity: one, of algebraic nature, involves matrices with integer entries; the other, of geometric nature, uses transportation polytopes and permutohedra.

5.1 Introduction

We consider the following problems from discrete tomography: When is an n-dimensional binary matrix X uniquely determined by its 1-marginals (also called Radon transforms, hyperplane sums, or $(n - 1)$-dimensional X-rays)? When is X $(0, 1)$-additive? When is there a binary matrix with prescribed 1-marginals? We present a survey of known results; several of them have been considered before only in the two and three-dimensional cases. Here we show how to extend them to any dimension. This chapter is an expanded version of [33]. Uniqueness and additivity were treated, for arbitrary n, in a slightly different but equivalent language in [9], and extended to a much more general setting in [10]. Their computational complexity has been considered in [6, 12, 23]. The problem of checking if an n-dimensional binary matrix X ($n \geq 3$) is a matrix of uniqueness is NP-complete [12, Theorem 2.7], while checking if X is $(0, 1)$-additive (at least when X is a pyramid) can be decided in polynomial time [23, Theorem 7.1]. Since $(0, 1)$-additivity implies uniqueness, determining $(0, 1)$-additivity of a binary matrix is a computationally simpler approach to uniqueness in some cases. For $n = 2$, these problems have been studied for a long time and are well understood. They coincide with the corresponding problems for one-dimensional X-rays or line sums; see [4, 18] for an overview. For $n = 3$, a different approach was followed in [5, 23, 28, 29, 31, 32]. First, one notes that uniqueness and $(0, 1)$-additivity are invariant under permutation of slices, so we can assume without loss of generality that the 1-marginals of a binary matrix are weakly decreasing. Under this assumption the matrices X uniquely determined by its 1-marginals are *pyramids* [28]; these can be identified, in a natural way, with matrices A whose entries are nonnegative integers. Thus, uniqueness and $(0, 1)$-additivity can be translated to new notions about matrices with integer entries [28, 32]. Moreover, by extending the newly found properties to matrices with nonnegative real coefficients, we obtain geometric characterizations for uniqueness and $(0, 1)$-additivity of a pyramid X by looking at the intersection of the permutohedron determined by its corresponding matrix A with the transportation polytope in which A lies [23]. The most important notions appearing from this approach are *minimality* for a matrix A with integer entries and *real-minimality* for a matrix A with real entries. The notion of minimality has applications to the representation theory of the symmetric group [1, 30]; real-minimality ends up being equivalent to additivity [23]. Both minimal and real-minimal matrices also emerge as optimal solutions of certain quadratic programming problems [23]. It would be interesting to see if our approach can be extended to other similar instances in discrete tomography (DT), such as line sums along coordinate axes.

Our motivation for dealing with notions for integer or real matrices, such as additivity, minimality, and real-minimality, is not to study similar concepts to uniqueness and $(0, 1)$-additivity on other matrix classes generalizing binary matrices. On the contrary, π-uniqueness, minimality, additivity, and real-minimality help us to understand the original notions from DT, namely uniqueness and $(0, 1)$-additivity, from a combinatorial (integer matrices) and a geometric (polytopes) point of view. In both instances, majorization plays a substantial role. The combinatorial approach provides a more economic way of representing a pyramid, namely through an integer matrix, which permits alternative descriptions of uniqueness and $(0, 1)$-additivity. In particular, testing additivity is simpler than testing $(0, 1)$-additivity. We also believe that this approach will lead to new results in the future. The geometric approach, on the other hand, yields characterizations of uniqueness and $(0, 1)$-additivity for binary matrices that make more transparent the relation between these two notions and give a new proof that $(0, 1)$-additivity implies uniqueness. Another consequence is that an algorithm from [21] can be applied to obtain a minimal matrix with a given set of 1-marginals in polynomial time.

The material is organized as follows. In Section 5.2 we recall the definitions of majorization, dominance order, and the permutohedron and review some known results. They will be essential in some characterizations of existence, uniqueness, and additivity presented here. Section 5.3 deals with the notions of uniqueness and $(0, 1)$-additivity of n-dimensional binary matrices. Section 5.4 contains a survey of results about uniqueness, existence, and $(0, 1)$-additivity in dimension 2. In Section 5.5 we introduce the notion of minimal matrix and use it to characterize uniqueness. We also explain how $(n - 1)$-dimensional matrices with nonnegative integer entries and n-dimensional binary matrices are related. This relation is also used in Section 5.6, where $(0,1)$-additivity for binary matrices is translated to a new notion, called additivity, for matrices with nonnegative integer entries. In Section 5.7 we include several results about three-dimensional binary matrices and two-dimensional integer matrices. In particular, we present a new, shorter proof that any plane partition of size $2 \times q$ is additive. In Section 5.8 we extend the notions introduced in previous sections for matrices with integer entries to matrices with real entries and describe these new notions geometrically. We also explain how minimal and real-minimal matrices appear in quadratic programming. The main tool in this section is the beautiful geometric description of majorization due to Rado, which is presented in Section 5.2. We apply this approach in Section 5.9 to show the equivalence between additivity and real-minimality.

5.2 Majorization and the Permutohedron

This section contains some standard results about majorization, dominance order, and permutohedra that will be needed in this chapter. We include Rado's original proof of his beautiful geometric description of majorization via permutohedra [24]; see also [20, p. 113].

For a vector $\boldsymbol{a} = (a_1, \ldots, a_m) \in \mathbb{R}^m$, we denote by $\boldsymbol{\pi}(\boldsymbol{a}) = (a_1^*, \ldots, a_m^*)$ the vector formed by the coordinates of $\boldsymbol{a}$ arranged in weakly decreasing order, that is, $a_1^* \geq \cdots \geq a_m^*$. The *size* of $\boldsymbol{a}$ is defined by $|\boldsymbol{a}| = \sum_{i=1}^m a_i$. We say that $\boldsymbol{a}$ is *majorized* by $\boldsymbol{b} = (b_1, \ldots, b_m)$, and denote it by $\boldsymbol{a} \preceq \boldsymbol{b}$, if

$$|\boldsymbol{a}| = |\boldsymbol{b}|, \text{ and } \sum_{i=1}^k a_i^* \leq \sum_{i=1}^k b_i^*, \text{ for all } 1 \leq k < m . \tag{5.1}$$

If $\boldsymbol{a} \preceq \boldsymbol{b}$ and $\boldsymbol{\pi}(\boldsymbol{a}) \neq \boldsymbol{\pi}(\boldsymbol{b})$, then we write $\boldsymbol{a} \prec \boldsymbol{b}$; see [15, 20].

Let $\boldsymbol{a} \in \mathbb{R}^m$ and let σ be a permutation in the symmetric group S_m. Denote by $\boldsymbol{a}_\sigma$ the vector $(a_{\sigma(1)}, \ldots, a_{\sigma(m)})$. Then the *permutohedron* determined by $\boldsymbol{a}$ is the convex hull of the set of all vectors obtained by permuting the entries of $\boldsymbol{a}$:

$$\mathsf{P}(\boldsymbol{a}) := \mathrm{conv}\{\boldsymbol{a}_\sigma \mid \sigma \in \mathsf{S}_m\} . \tag{5.2}$$

It is a convex polytope. If all the coordinates of $\boldsymbol{a}$ are equal, then, $\mathsf{P}(\boldsymbol{a})$ is a point; otherwise, it has dimension $m - 1$. Its face lattice is known, see, for example, [2] (or [13, 34] if all coordinates of $\boldsymbol{a}$ are different). Here we only need to know the description of its vertices and edges. For this we need some notation. Let $\boldsymbol{a} \in \mathbb{R}^m$ and denote by $a_1^\circ, \ldots, a_l^\circ$ the different values of the coordinates of $\boldsymbol{a}$ arranged in decreasing order. The permutation in S_m that switches s and t and fixes the remaining numbers will be denoted by $(s\, t)$; such permutations are usually called *transpositions*. We say that a transposition $(s\, t)$ is *adjacent relative to* $\boldsymbol{a}$ if there exists $1 \leq i < l$ such that $a_s = a_i^\circ$ and $a_t = a_{i+1}^\circ$.

Example 1. Let $a = (1, 1, 1)$, $b = (2, 1, 0)$, and $c = (3, 0, 0)$. Then $a \prec b \prec c$. Here $\mathsf{P}(a)$ is a point, $\mathsf{P}(b)$ is an hexagon, and $\mathsf{P}(c)$ is a triangle and one has that $\mathsf{P}(a) \subset \mathsf{P}(b) \subset \mathsf{P}(c)$; see Fig. 5.1.

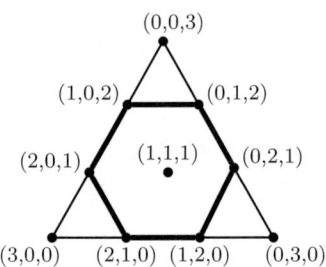

Fig. 5.1. The permutohedra $\mathsf{P}(a) \subset \mathsf{P}(b) \subset \mathsf{P}(c)$.

Theorem 1. *Let $a \in \mathbb{R}^m$. The set of vertices of $\mathsf{P}(a)$ is precisely*

$$\{a_\sigma \mid \sigma \in S_m\}. \tag{5.3}$$

If a is weakly decreasing and has at least two different coordinates, the vertices adjacent to a_σ ($\sigma \in S_m$) in $\mathsf{P}(a)$ are of the form $a_{\tau\sigma}$ for some transposition τ that is adjacent relative to a.

Theorem 2. *For any vector $a \in \mathbb{R}^m$*

$$\mathsf{P}(a) = \{x \in \mathbb{R}^m \mid x \preceq a\}. \tag{5.4}$$

Proof. Since $\mathsf{P}(a) = \mathsf{P}(\pi(a))$ and since $x \in \mathsf{P}(a)$ if, and only if, $\pi(x) \in \mathsf{P}(a)$ for all $x \in \mathbb{R}^m$, we assume without loss of generality that a and x are weakly decreasing. Let $x \in \mathsf{P}(a)$; then x is a convex combination of $\{a_\sigma \mid \sigma \in S_m\}$, that is, there are nonnegative real numbers t_σ, $\sigma \in S_m$, such that $\sum_\sigma t_\sigma = 1$ and $x = \sum_\sigma t_\sigma a_\sigma$. Let $k \in \{1, \dots, m\}$; then

$$\sum_{i=1}^k x_i = \sum_\sigma t_\sigma \sum_{i=1}^k a_{\sigma(i)} \leq \sum_\sigma t_\sigma \sum_{i=1}^k a_i = \sum_{i=1}^k a_i. \tag{5.5}$$

Therefore, $x \preceq a$.

Conversely, let $x \in \mathbb{R}^m$ be such that $x \preceq a$. Assuming that $x \notin \mathsf{P}(a)$, we obtain a contradiction: Since $\mathsf{P}(a)$ is convex, there is a hyperplane separating x and $\mathsf{P}(a)$, that is, there is some vector $u \in \mathbb{R}^m$ such that $\langle u, x \rangle > \langle u, a_\rho \rangle$ for all $\rho \in S_m$; see, for example, [14, §2.2] ($\langle \cdot, \cdot \rangle$ denotes the usual inner product in $\mathbb{R}^m$). Then $\sum_{i=1}^m u_{\sigma(i)} x_{\sigma(i)} > \sum_{i=1}^m u_{\sigma(i)} a_i$ for all $\sigma \in \mathsf{S}_m$. Choose σ such that $u_{\sigma(1)} \ge u_{\sigma(2)} \ge \cdots \ge u_{\sigma(m)}$. Then, since $\boldsymbol{x}$ is weakly decreasing,

$$\sum_{i=1}^{m-1} (u_{\sigma(i)} - u_{\sigma(i+1)})(x_1 + \cdots + x_i) + u_{\sigma(n)}(x_1 + \cdots + x_n)$$

$$\ge \sum_{i=1}^{m-1} (u_{\sigma(i)} - u_{\sigma(i+1)})(x_{\sigma(1)} + \cdots + x_{\sigma(i)}) + u_{\sigma(n)}(x_{\sigma(1)} + \cdots + x_{\sigma(n)})$$

$$= \sum_{i=1}^m u_{\sigma(i)} x_{\sigma(i)} > \sum_{i=1}^m u_{\sigma(i)} a_i$$

$$= \sum_{i=1}^{m-1} (u_{\sigma(i)} - u_{\sigma(i+1)})(a_1 + \cdots + a_i) + u_{\sigma(n)}(a_1 + \cdots + a_n) , \qquad (5.6)$$

which contradicts $\boldsymbol{x} \preceq \boldsymbol{a}$. □

Corollary 1. *Let $\boldsymbol{a}, \boldsymbol{b} \in \mathbb{R}^m$. Then*

$$\boldsymbol{a} \preceq \boldsymbol{b} \iff \mathsf{P}(\boldsymbol{a}) \subseteq \mathsf{P}(\boldsymbol{b}) . \qquad (5.7)$$

The following technical lemma can be found in [15, p. 63], [20, p. 121], or [31, Prop. 2.1]. It follows also from the face structure of $\mathsf{P}(\boldsymbol{a})$.

Lemma 1. *Let $\boldsymbol{a} \in \mathbb{R}^m$, $\boldsymbol{b} \in \mathbb{R}^k$ be such that $\boldsymbol{b} \prec (a_{i_1}, \ldots, a_{i_k})$, for some sequence $1 \le i_1 < \cdots < i_k \le m$; let $\hat{\boldsymbol{a}}$ be obtained from $\boldsymbol{a}$ by substituting a_{i_j} with b_j, $1 \le j \le k$. Then $\hat{\boldsymbol{a}} \prec \boldsymbol{a}$.*

When restricted to partitions, majorization is also known as the *dominance order*. A vector $\boldsymbol{\lambda} \in \mathbb{R}^m$ is called a *partition* if its coordinates are nonnegative integers and $\lambda_1 \ge \lambda_2 \ge \cdots \ge \lambda_m$. If $|\boldsymbol{\lambda}| = N$, we say that $\boldsymbol{\lambda}$ is a partition of N. The *Young diagram* of $\boldsymbol{\lambda}$ is the set $D(\boldsymbol{\lambda}) := \{ (i,j) \mid 1 \le j \le \lambda_i \}$. The *length* of $\boldsymbol{\lambda}$, denoted by $\ell(\boldsymbol{\lambda})$, is the number of its positive coordinates, that is, the number of rows of $D(\boldsymbol{\lambda})$. We will frequently think of $\boldsymbol{\lambda}$ as an element of $\mathbb{R}^m$, for some $m \ge \ell(\boldsymbol{\lambda})$, by adding some zeros to the right. The *conjugate* partition to $\boldsymbol{\lambda}$ is $\boldsymbol{\lambda}' = (\lambda_1', \ldots, \lambda_k')$, where $k \ge \lambda_1$ and $\lambda_j' := |\{ i \mid \lambda_i \ge j \}|$. In other words, λ_j' is the length of the jth column of $D(\boldsymbol{\lambda})$. From this observation, it follows that $\boldsymbol{\lambda}'' = \boldsymbol{\lambda}$. For example, if $\boldsymbol{\lambda} = (5, 4, 2, 2, 1, 1, 1)$, then $\boldsymbol{\lambda}' = (7, 4, 2, 2, 1)$.

Given two partitions $\boldsymbol{\lambda}, \boldsymbol{\mu}$ of N (we assume both have the same number of coordinates by adding some zeros), we say that $\boldsymbol{\lambda}$ is *dominated* by $\boldsymbol{\mu}$ if $\boldsymbol{\lambda} \preceq \boldsymbol{\mu}$. The set of all partitions of N is a lattice under the dominance order and has the property that conjugation is an antiautomorphism [3], [20, Chap. 5D], that is,

$$\boldsymbol{\lambda} \preceq \boldsymbol{\mu} \iff \boldsymbol{\mu}' \preceq \boldsymbol{\lambda}' . \qquad (5.8)$$

Let $\boldsymbol{a} \in \mathbb{R}^m$, $1 \le i < j \le m$. A *T-transform* of $\boldsymbol{a}$ is the vector

$$T_{ij}\boldsymbol{a} := (a_1, \ldots, a_i - 1, \ldots, a_j + 1, \ldots, a_m) \in \mathbb{R}^m , \qquad (5.9)$$

which only differs from a in two coordinates. We finish this section with the following result due to Muirhead [22]. The proof presented here is constructive and closely follows the proof in [20, Chap. 2B].

Lemma 2. *Let* λ, $\mu \in \mathbb{R}^m$ *be partitions of* N. *If* $\lambda \succ \mu$, *then there exist partitions* $\nu(0), \nu(1), \ldots, \nu(k) \in \mathbb{R}^m$ *such that* $\nu(0) = \lambda$, $\nu(i-1) \succ \nu(i)$, $\nu(i)$ *is a T-transform of* $\nu(i-1)$ *for all* $1 \leq i \leq k$, *and* $\nu(k) = \mu$.

Proof. Let $i = \max\{\, t \mid \lambda_t > \mu_t \,\}$. Since $\lambda \succ \mu$, $\sum_{s=1}^{i} \lambda_s > \sum_{s=1}^{i} \mu_s$. Note that $i < m$ and that $j = \min\{\, t \mid i < t$ and $\lambda_t < \mu_t \,\}$ is well defined. The inequalities $\lambda_i > \mu_i \geq \mu_j > \lambda_j$, $\lambda_i > \lambda_{i+1}$, and $\lambda_{j-1} > \lambda_j$ imply that the T-transform $T_{ij}\lambda$ is also a partition of N. Let $\nu(1) = T_{ij}\lambda$. Clearly, $\lambda \succ \nu(1)$. Finally, since $\lambda_k = \mu_k$ for all $i < k < j$, one has $\nu(1) \succeq \mu$. Either $\nu(1) = \mu$ or $\nu(1) \succ \mu$. In the latter case, we apply the previous method to obtain a T-transform $\nu(2)$ of $\nu(1)$, such that $\nu(1) \succ \nu(2) \succeq \mu$. We repeat this method until we reach μ. This is accomplished in $k = \sum(\lambda_t - \mu_t)$ steps, where the index in the sum runs over all t such that $\lambda_t > \mu_t$. □

Example 2. Let $\lambda = (6, 4, 2, 2, 2, 0, 0)$ and $\mu = (4, 3, 3, 3, 1, 1, 1)$. Then, according to the proof of the previous lemma, we require $4 = 2+1+1$ steps to go from λ to μ. The intermediate partitions obtained from the proof are $\nu(0) = \lambda$, $\nu(1) = (6, 4, 2, 2, 1, 1, 0)$, $\nu(2) = (6, 3, 3, 2, 1, 1, 0)$, $\nu(3) = (5, 3, 3, 3, 1, 1, 0)$, and $\nu(4) = \mu$.

5.3 Uniqueness and $(0, 1)$-Additivity

In this section we deal with the notions of uniqueness and $(0, 1)$-additivity for n-dimensional $(0, 1)$-matrices; these were introduced by P.C. Fishburn, J.C. Lagarias, J.A. Reeds, and L.A. Shepp [9] in a slightly different but equivalent language as the one used here. They gave characterizations of uniqueness and $(0, 1)$-additivity (Theorems 3 and 4) and used them to show that $(0, 1)$-additivity is sufficient for uniqueness (Theorem 5) but not necessary (Example 5). Later the author observed that, under the assumption that the 1-marginals are partitions, matrices of uniqueness have a *simpler* shape, namely, they are pyramids [28, 29, 32] (Theorem 6). This observation leads to the results presented in Sections 5.5 and 5.6. We also include a new elementary direct proof that $(0, 1)$-additive matrices are, up to permutation of slices, pyramids (Theorem 7).

We fix some notation that will be used throughout this paper. Let $\mathbb{N}$ denote the set of natural numbers and let $\mathbb{N}_0 := \mathbb{N} \cup \{0\}$. For a vector $q = (q_1, \ldots, q_n) \in \mathbb{N}^n$, we denote $\overline{q} = (q_1, \ldots, q_{n-1})$, $q = q_1 \cdots q_n$, and $\overline{q} = q_1 \cdots q_{n-1}$, and for $q \in \mathbb{N}$, we denote by $[q]$ the set $\{1, 2, \ldots, q\}$. Also let $\mathsf{B}(q) := [q_1] \times \cdots \times [q_n]$ denote an n-dimensional box and let $P_i : \mathsf{B}(q) \longrightarrow [q_i]$ denote the ith projection. An *n-dimensional matrix of size* $q_1 \times \cdots \times q_n$ is a map $X : \mathsf{B}(q) \longrightarrow \mathbb{R}$. A $(0, 1)$-*matrix* or *binary matrix* is a matrix whose values are zeros and ones. For any matrix X of size $q_1 \times \cdots \times q_n$, we consider its 1-*marginals*, also called *Radon transforms, hyperplane sums* or $(n-1)$-*dimensional X-rays*, $\boldsymbol{a}^i = (a_1^i, \ldots, a_{q_i}^i)$, $i \in [n]$, defined by

$$a_j^i := \sum_{\boldsymbol{k} \in P_i^{-1}(j)} X(\boldsymbol{k}), \quad j \in [q_i]. \tag{5.10}$$

Fix $N \in \mathbb{N}$. For $i \in [n]$, let $\boldsymbol{a}^i \in \mathbb{N}_0^{q_i}$ be of size N. Then we denote by $\mathsf{F}(\boldsymbol{a}^1, \ldots, \boldsymbol{a}^n)$ the set of all n-dimensional matrices with real entries having 1-marginals $\boldsymbol{a}^1, \ldots, \boldsymbol{a}^n$; by $\mathsf{T}(\boldsymbol{a}^1, \ldots, \boldsymbol{a}^n)$, the set of all matrices in $\mathsf{F}(\boldsymbol{a}^1, \ldots, \boldsymbol{a}^n)$ with nonnegative entries; by $\mathsf{M}(\boldsymbol{a}^1, \ldots, \boldsymbol{a}^n)$, the set of all matrices in $\mathsf{T}(\boldsymbol{a}^1, \ldots, \boldsymbol{a}^n)$ with integer entries; and by $\mathsf{M}^*(\boldsymbol{a}^1, \ldots, \boldsymbol{a}^n)$, the set of all binary matrices in $\mathsf{M}(\boldsymbol{a}^1, \ldots, \boldsymbol{a}^n)$. Note that $\mathsf{F}(\boldsymbol{a}^1, \ldots, \boldsymbol{a}^n)$ is an affine space, $\mathsf{T}(\boldsymbol{a}^1, \ldots, \boldsymbol{a}^n)$ is a polytope (when $n = 2$, it is usually called *transportation polytope*; see, for example, [16, 34]) and $\mathsf{M}(\boldsymbol{a}^1, \ldots, \boldsymbol{a}^n)$ is the set of lattice points in $\mathsf{T}(\boldsymbol{a}^1, \ldots, \boldsymbol{a}^n)$.

Let $X \in \mathsf{M}^*(\boldsymbol{a}^1, \ldots, \boldsymbol{a}^n)$; then X is called a *matrix of uniqueness* [9] if the set $\mathsf{M}^*(\boldsymbol{a}^1, \ldots, \boldsymbol{a}^n)$ has cardinality one; that is, if X is the only binary matrix with 1-marginals $\boldsymbol{a}^1, \ldots, \boldsymbol{a}^n$; X is called $(0, 1)$-*additive* [9] if there are maps $f_i \colon [q_i] \longrightarrow \mathbb{R}$, $i \in [n]$, such that for all $\boldsymbol{k} \in \mathsf{B}(\boldsymbol{q})$,

$$X(\boldsymbol{k}) = 1 \ \text{ if, and only if, } \ \sum_{i=1}^{n} f_i(k_i) \geq 0; \tag{5.11}$$

and X is called a *pyramid* [29, 32] if for all $\boldsymbol{k}, \boldsymbol{l} \in \mathsf{B}(\boldsymbol{q})$ such that $k_i \leq l_i$, $i \in [n]$, the condition $X(\boldsymbol{l}) = 1$ implies $X(\boldsymbol{k}) = 1$. Note that $(0, 1)$-additive matrices are called additive in [9]. We use the term $(0, 1)$-additive to distinguish it from another notion of additivity introduced in Sections 5.6, resp. 5.8, for matrices with integer, resp. real entries. A *weakly bad configuration* for X is a matrix $W \in \mathsf{F}(\boldsymbol{0}, \ldots, \boldsymbol{0})$ different from 0 with integer entries, such that if $W(\boldsymbol{k}) > 0$, then $X(\boldsymbol{k}) = 1$ and if $W(\boldsymbol{k}) < 0$, then $X(\boldsymbol{k}) = 0$. A weakly bad configuration for X is called a *bad configuration* if its entries are in $\{-1, 0, 1\}$. The *weight* of a weakly bad configuration W is the sum of its positive entries, that is, $\sum_{\boldsymbol{k}, \, W(\boldsymbol{k}) > 0} W(\boldsymbol{k})$.

Example 3. Let X be the three-dimensional binary matrix

$$\begin{bmatrix} 1 & 1 & 1 \\ 1 & 1 & 1 \\ 1 & 0 & 0 \end{bmatrix} \begin{bmatrix} 1 & 1 & 0 \\ 1 & 0 & 0 \\ 1 & 0 & 0 \end{bmatrix} \begin{bmatrix} 1 & 1 & 0 \\ 0 & 0 & 0 \\ 0 & 0 & 0 \end{bmatrix} \begin{bmatrix} 1 & 1 & 0 \\ 0 & 0 & 0 \\ 0 & 0 & 0 \end{bmatrix}. \tag{5.12}$$

Its 1-marginals are $\boldsymbol{a}^1 = (9, 4, 2)$, $\boldsymbol{a}^2 = (8, 5, 2)$, and $\boldsymbol{a}^3 = (7, 4, 2, 2)$. This matrix is a pyramid. A weakly bad configuration of weight 3 for X is the matrix W:

$$\begin{bmatrix} 0 & 0 & 0 \\ 0 & 0 & 1 \\ 0 & -1 & 0 \end{bmatrix} \begin{bmatrix} 0 & 0 & -1 \\ 0 & 0 & 0 \\ 1 & 0 & 0 \end{bmatrix} \begin{bmatrix} 0 & 0 & 0 \\ 0 & 0 & 0 \\ 0 & 0 & 0 \end{bmatrix} \begin{bmatrix} 0 & 1 & 0 \\ -1 & 0 & 0 \\ 0 & 0 & 0 \end{bmatrix}. \tag{5.13}$$

Let $Y = X - W$. Then Y has the same 1-marginals as X. This example contains the main idea behind the proof of Theorem 3. Also, note that Y is not a pyramid.

Example 4. Let $X \colon B(q, q, q) \longrightarrow \{0, 1\}$ be the binary matrix defined by $X(\boldsymbol{k}) = 1$ if, and only if, $k_1 + k_2 + k_3 \leq q + 2$. Then X is a pyramid and is $(0, 1)$-additive [29, Theorem 3.4]. Additivity can be shown as follows. Let $a = \max\{i \in [q] \mid 3i \leq q + 2\}$. Then $0 \leq q + 2 - 3a \leq 2$. Therefore, there is a unique integer b such that $\frac{4}{3}(q + 2 - 3a) < b < \frac{4}{3}(q + 3 - 3a)$. Let $f \colon [q] \longrightarrow \mathbb{R}$ be defined by $f(x) := 4a + b - 4x$ and let $f_i = f$ for $i = 1, 2, 3$. Then it follows from the inequalities satisfied by b that condition (5.11) holds for the maps f_1, f_2, and f_3. Therefore, X is $(0, 1)$-additive.

Theorem 3. *Let X be an n-dimensional binary matrix. Then X is a matrix of uniqueness if, and only if, X does not have bad configurations.*

Proof. Suppose first that X has a bad configuration W. Then $Y = X - W$ has the same 1-marginals as X, but is different from X; thus X is not a matrix of uniqueness. For the converse, suppose that X is not a matrix of uniqueness. Then there exists a binary matrix $Y \neq X$ with the same 1-marginals as X. A bad configuration W for X is obtained by letting $W = X - Y$.   □

Theorem 4. *Let X be an n-dimensional binary matrix. Then X is $(0, 1)$-additive if, and only if, X does not have weakly bad configurations.*

For a proof, see [9].

Since bad configurations are weakly bad configurations, Theorems 3 and 4 imply the following:

Theorem 5. *Every $(0, 1)$-additive matrix is a matrix of uniqueness.*

For another proof of this theorem, see the end of Section 5.9.

Example 5. It is shown in Theorem 5 of [9] that the matrix

$$\begin{bmatrix} 1&1&1&1&1 \\ 1&1&1&1&1 \\ 1&1&1&1&0 \\ 1&1&1&1&0 \\ 1&1&0&0&0 \end{bmatrix} \begin{bmatrix} 1&1&1&1&1 \\ 1&1&1&1&1 \\ 1&1&0&0&0 \\ 1&0&0&0&0 \\ 1&0&0&0&0 \end{bmatrix} \begin{bmatrix} 1&1&1&1&1 \\ 1&1&1&1&1 \\ 1&1&0&0&0 \\ 0&0&0&0&0 \\ 0&0&0&0&0 \end{bmatrix} \begin{bmatrix} 1&1&1&1&1 \\ 1&1&1&0&0 \\ 0&0&0&0&0 \\ 0&0&0&0&0 \\ 0&0&0&0&0 \end{bmatrix} \begin{bmatrix} 1&1&1&0&0 \\ 1&1&1&0&0 \\ 0&0&0&0&0 \\ 0&0&0&0&0 \\ 0&0&0&0&0 \end{bmatrix} \quad (5.14)$$

is a matrix of uniqueness that is not $(0, 1)$-additive. This is the smallest known example of a matrix of uniqueness that is not $(0, 1)$-additive. For some comments about the relation between uniqueness and $(0, 1)$-additivity, see [10, §2.5]. A weakly bad configuration of weight 6 is given by the matrix $W \colon B(5, 5, 5) \longrightarrow \mathbb{Z}$ that takes value 2 on $(4, 4, 1)$, value 1 on $(5, 1, 2)$, $(3, 2, 3)$, $(1, 5, 4)$, $(2, 3, 5)$, value -1 on $(5, 3, 1)$, $(3, 5, 1)$, $(4, 2, 2)$, $(4, 1, 3)$, $(2, 4, 4)$, $(1, 4, 5)$ and value 0 on the remaining points. The proof of uniqueness of this matrix given in [9] shows to what extent proving uniqueness for a matrix can be a daunting task and suggests to look for alternative ways of approaching uniqueness. This will be done in Sections 5.5 and 5.8.

Remark 1. A *slice in the ith direction* of an n-dimensional $(0, 1)$-matrix X of size $q_1 \times \cdots \times q_n$ is an $(n - 1)$-dimensional $(0, 1)$-matrix Y obtained by restricting X to $[q_1] \times \cdots \times \{j\} \times \cdots \times [q_n]$ for some $j \in [q_i]$. We can think of X as made of q_i slices in the ith direction; these slices can be permuted according to some permutation σ in the symmetric group S_{q_i}. The matrix obtained, denoted by σX, has the same size as X. It follows from the definitions that X is a matrix of uniqueness, resp. $(0, 1)$-additive, if, and only if, σX is a matrix of uniqueness, resp. $(0, 1)$-additive. So, when considering the properties of uniqueness and $(0, 1)$-additivity for a matrix, we can assume without loss of generality that its 1-marginals are weakly decreasing, that is, they are partitions. Then we have

Theorem 6. *Let X be an n-dimensional binary matrix whose 1-marginals are partitions. If X is a matrix of uniqueness, then X is a pyramid.*

This follows from the next lemma and Theorem 3.

Lemma 3. *Let X be an n-dimensional binary matrix whose 1-marginals are partitions. If X does not have bad configurations of weight 2, then X is a pyramid.*

Proof. Suppose X is not a pyramid. Then, there exist $\boldsymbol{k}, \boldsymbol{l} \in \mathsf{B}(\boldsymbol{q})$, and $1 \leq i \leq n$, such that $k_i < l_i$, $k_j = l_j$ for $j \neq i$, $X(\boldsymbol{k}) = 0$ and $X(\boldsymbol{l}) = 1$. Since the ith marginal $\boldsymbol{a}^i$ of X is weakly decreasing, there must exist $\boldsymbol{s}, \boldsymbol{t} \in \mathsf{B}(\boldsymbol{q})$, such that $s_i = k_i$, $t_i = l_i$, $s_j = t_j$ for $j \neq i$, $X(\boldsymbol{s}) = 1$, and $X(\boldsymbol{t}) = 0$. Let W be the matrix defined by $W(\boldsymbol{l}) = W(\boldsymbol{s}) = 1$, $W(\boldsymbol{k}) = W(\boldsymbol{t}) = -1$, and $W(\boldsymbol{r}) = 0$ for the remaining points. Then W is a bad configuration for X of weight 2.   □

Example 6. The converse of Lemma 3 is true for $n = 2, 3$ (see Sections 5.4 and 5.7). However, for $n = 4$, the converse is no longer true, as the following example from [32] shows: Let $X \colon \mathsf{B}(2, 2, 2, 2) \longrightarrow \{0, 1\}$ be the matrix that takes value 1 on the points $(1, 1, 1, 1)$, $(1, 1, 1, 2)$, $(1, 1, 2, 1)$, $(1, 2, 1, 1)$, $(2, 1, 1, 1)$, $(1, 1, 2, 2)$, $(2, 2, 1, 1)$ and value 0 on the remaining points. It is a pyramid and the matrix $W \colon \mathsf{B}(2, 2, 2, 2) \longrightarrow \{-1, 0, 1\}$ that takes value 1 on $(1, 1, 2, 2)$, $(2, 2, 1, 1)$, value -1 on $(1, 2, 2, 1)$, $(2, 1, 1, 2)$, and 0 on the remaining points is a bad configuration of weight 2 for X.

Combining Theorems 5 and 6, we obtain the following result, for which we include an elementary direct proof.

Theorem 7. *Let X be an n-dimensional binary matrix whose 1-marginals are partitions. If X is $(0, 1)$-additive, then X is a pyramid.*

Proof. Suppose X is additive, but not a pyramid. Let $f_j \colon [q_j] \longrightarrow \mathbb{R}$, $j \in [n]$, be the maps satisfying (5.11) in the definition of $(0, 1)$-additivity. Let $\boldsymbol{k}, \boldsymbol{l}, \boldsymbol{s}$, $\boldsymbol{t}$, and i be the elements constructed in the proof of Lemma 3. Since $X(\boldsymbol{k}) = 0$ and $X(\boldsymbol{l}) = 1$, we have $\sum_{j=1}^{n} f_j(k_j) < 0 \leq \sum_{j=1}^{n} f_j(l_j)$; therefore, $f_i(k_i) <$

$f_i(l_i)$. Similarly, since $X(\boldsymbol{s}) = 1$ and $X(\boldsymbol{t}) = 0$, using the identities among the coordinates of $\boldsymbol{k}$, $\boldsymbol{l}$, $\boldsymbol{s}$, $\boldsymbol{t}$, we obtain $f_i(k_i) > f_i(l_i)$, which is a contradiction. Therefore, X has to be a pyramid. □

Following constructions can be applied to the plane partitions associated to pyramids; see Remark 6.

Let $\iota\colon \mathsf{B}(\boldsymbol{q}) \longrightarrow \mathsf{B}(\boldsymbol{q})$ be the involution ($\iota^2 = 1$) defined by

$$\iota(\boldsymbol{k}) := (q_1 + 1 - k_1, \ldots, q_n + 1 - k_n), \qquad (5.15)$$

and let $\rho\colon \mathsf{B}(\boldsymbol{q}) \longrightarrow \mathsf{B}(\boldsymbol{q})$ be the rotation defined by $\rho(\boldsymbol{k}) := (k_2, \ldots, k_n, k_1)$. Then, given a $(0, 1)$-matrix $X\colon \mathsf{B}(\boldsymbol{q}) \longrightarrow \{0, 1\}$, we define the *complement* of X as the matrix X^{c} given by $X^{\mathrm{c}}(\boldsymbol{k}) = 1$ if, and only if, $X(\iota(\boldsymbol{k})) = 0$ and the *rotation* of X as the matrix X^{r} given by $X^{\mathrm{r}}(\boldsymbol{k}) = X(\rho(\boldsymbol{k}))$.

Lemma 4. *Let X be an n-dimensional binary matrix. Then X is a pyramid, resp. matrix of uniqueness, resp. $(0, 1)$-additive, if, and only if, X^{c} is a pyramid, resp. matrix of uniqueness, resp. $(0, 1)$-additive.*

Proof. The equivalence for pyramids is straightforward. The equivalence for uniqueness follows from Theorem 3: If W is a bad configuration for X, then $\overline{W}$ defined by $\overline{W}(\boldsymbol{k}) = -W(\iota(\boldsymbol{k}))$ is a bad configuration for X^{c}. Similarly, the equivalence for $(0, 1)$-additivity follows from Theorem 4. □

A similar lemma can be stated and proved for the rotation X^{r} of X.

5.4 Uniqueness and $(0, 1)$-Additivity in Dimension 2

In this section we address the problem of uniqueness and $(0, 1)$-additivity for binary matrices of dimension 2. Historically, the existence problem was considered first and independently by D. Gale [11] and H.J. Ryser [25, 26], see also [4, 18] and the references therein for other proofs. After that, H.J. Ryser gave a sufficient condition for uniqueness [26, p. 62]. E. Snapper seems to be the first to state explicitly, several years later, that the condition given by Ryser was also necessary [27, Theorem 8.1]. More recently, P.C. Fishburn, J.C. Lagarias, J.A. Reeds, and L.A. Shepp [9, §3] showed that uniqueness and $(0, 1)$-additivity coincide and that in dimension 2 it is enough to consider bad configurations of weight 2. We overview here these results, not only by of their own interest, but also because they will be used to prove their generalizations to higher dimensions.

The two classical versions of uniqueness and existence follow:

Theorem 8. *Let $\boldsymbol{\lambda}$, $\boldsymbol{\mu}$ be partitions of N. Then $|\mathsf{M}^*(\boldsymbol{\lambda}, \boldsymbol{\mu})| = 1$ if, and only if, $\boldsymbol{\lambda}' = \boldsymbol{\mu}$.*

Theorem 9 (Gale–Ryser Theorem). *Let $\boldsymbol{\lambda}$, $\boldsymbol{\mu}$ be partitions of N. Then $|\mathsf{M}^*(\boldsymbol{\lambda}, \boldsymbol{\mu})| > 0$ if, and only if, $\boldsymbol{\lambda}' \succeq \boldsymbol{\mu}$.*

Remark 2. The proof presented here for one direction of the Gale–Ryser theorem, namely that the majorization condition implies the existence of a matrix, yields an algorithm for the construction of the matrix that might be new. This algorithm depends essentially on the constructive proof of Lemma 2. Given partitions λ, μ such that $\lambda' \succeq \mu$, Lemma 2 yields an algorithm for constructing a sequence of partitions

$$\lambda' = \nu(0) \succ \nu(1) \succ \cdots \succ \nu(k) = \mu \tag{5.16}$$

such that $\nu(i)$ is a T-transform of $\nu(i-1)$ for all $1 \leq i \leq k$. Recall that the number of steps in the algorithm is

$$k = \sum_{t \in \{t | \lambda_t > \mu_t\}} \lambda_t - \mu_t . \tag{5.17}$$

For any i, let j, l be such that $T_{jl}\nu(i-1) = \nu(i)$. It is shown in the proof of Theorem 9 how to construct a matrix in $\mathsf{M}^*(\lambda, \nu(i))$ from any matrix $Y^{(i-1)} = \left(y_{st}^{(i-1)}\right)$ in $\mathsf{M}^*(\lambda, \nu(i-1))$. The choice of row r where a 1 is shifted to the right is irrelevant as long as $y_{rj}^{(i-1)} = 1$ and $y_{rl}^{(i-1)} = 0$.

The difference with other algorithms is that the choice of the columns where we shift ones to the right depends not on some matrix but only on sequence (5.16). For other algorithms, see [25, 26] as well as [18, pp. 10–14] and the references therein.

In dimension 2, all properties for a binary matrix coincide, namely

Theorem 10. *Let X be a 2-dimensional binary matrix whose 1-marginals are partitions. Then the following are equivalent:*
   (1) X is a pyramid;
   (2) X has no bad configurations of weight 2;
   (3) X is a matrix of uniqueness;
   (4) X is $(0,1)$-additive.

We conclude this section with proofs of these theorems.

Let λ be a partition and let $p = \ell(\lambda)$, $q \geq \lambda_1$. We define $X(\lambda) = (x_{ij}^\lambda)$ as the matrix of size $p \times q$ given by

$$x_{ij}^\lambda := \begin{cases} 1, & \text{if } 1 \leq j \leq \lambda_i, \\ 0, & \text{otherwise.} \end{cases} \tag{5.18}$$

Then $X(\lambda) \in \mathsf{M}^*(\lambda, \lambda')$. Observe that we use the same notation for different matrices. If $q > \lambda_1$, $X(\lambda)$ will have $q - \lambda_1$ columns of zeros. The same abuse of notation is taking place with λ'. This flexibility will be useful in the proof of Theorem 9.

Proof (of Theorem 8). Suppose first that $X \in \mathsf{M}^*(\lambda, \mu)$ is a matrix of uniqueness. Then by Theorem 6, X is a pyramid. This forces $\lambda' = \mu$. For the converse, it is enough to observe that $X(\lambda)$ is the only matrix in $\mathsf{M}^*(\lambda, \lambda')$.   □

Proof (of Theorem 9). Suppose first that there is a matrix Y in $\mathsf{M}^*(\boldsymbol{\lambda}, \boldsymbol{\mu})$. Let $X(\boldsymbol{\lambda}) \in \mathsf{M}^*(\boldsymbol{\lambda}, \boldsymbol{\lambda}')$ be of the same size as Y. Then $X(\boldsymbol{\lambda})$ is obtained from Y by shifting, along each row, ones to the left and zeros to the right. Let $1 \le j \le \ell(\boldsymbol{\mu})$. Since $\sum_{t=1}^{j} \lambda_t'$, resp. $\sum_{t=1}^{j} \mu_t$, is the number of ones in the first j columns of $X(\boldsymbol{\lambda})$, resp. Y, then, by the relation between $X(\boldsymbol{\lambda})$ and Y, $\sum_{t=1}^{j} \lambda_t' \ge \sum_{t=1}^{j} \mu_t$; that is, $\boldsymbol{\lambda}' \succeq \boldsymbol{\mu}$.

For the converse, let us assume that $\boldsymbol{\lambda}' \succeq \boldsymbol{\mu}$, and suppose that both have the same number of coordinates. Then, by Lemma 2, there are partitions $\boldsymbol{\nu}(0), \ldots, \boldsymbol{\nu}(k)$ such that $\boldsymbol{\nu}(0) = \boldsymbol{\lambda}'$, $\boldsymbol{\nu}(k) = \boldsymbol{\mu}$, $\boldsymbol{\nu}(i-1) \succ \boldsymbol{\nu}(i)$, and $\boldsymbol{\nu}(i)$ is a T-transform of $\boldsymbol{\nu}(i-1)$ for all i. We construct the desired matrix inductively. First, observe that $X(\boldsymbol{\lambda}) \in \mathsf{M}^*(\boldsymbol{\lambda}, \boldsymbol{\nu}(0))$. Let $i > 0$ and assume by induction hypothesis that there is a matrix $Y^{(i-1)} = \left(y_{st}^{(i-1)}\right)$ in $\mathsf{M}^*(\boldsymbol{\lambda}, \boldsymbol{\nu}(i-1))$. Then since $\boldsymbol{\nu}(i)$ is a T-transform of $\boldsymbol{\nu}(i-1)$, there are numbers $j < l$ such that $\boldsymbol{\nu}(i) = T_{jl}\boldsymbol{\nu}(i-1)$. Then $\boldsymbol{\nu}(i-1)_j > \boldsymbol{\nu}(i-1)_l$. Therefore, there is some r such that $y_{rj}^{(i-1)} = 1$ and $y_{rl}^{(i-1)} = 0$. Let $Y^{(i)} = \left(y_{st}^{(i)}\right)$ be obtained from $Y^{(i-1)}$ by switching the one and the zero in positions (r, j) and (r, l), that is, let

$$
y_{st}^{(i)} = \begin{cases} 0, & \text{if } (s, t) = (r, j), \\ 1, & \text{if } (s, t) = (r, l), \\ y_{st}^{(i-1)}, & \text{otherwise.} \end{cases} \tag{5.19}
$$

Thus, $Y^{(i)}$ is in $\mathsf{M}^*(\boldsymbol{\lambda}, \boldsymbol{\nu}(i))$. We conclude, by induction, that $Y^{(k)}$ is in $\mathsf{M}^*(\boldsymbol{\lambda}, \boldsymbol{\mu})$. □

Proof (of Theorem 10). Since a pyramid is of the form $X(\boldsymbol{\lambda})$, (1) $\Rightarrow$ (3) follows from Theorem 8. Theorem 3 yields (3) $\Rightarrow$ (2) and Lemma 3 yields (2) $\Rightarrow$ (1). The implication (4) $\Rightarrow$ (1) follows from Theorem 7. It remains to prove (1) $\Rightarrow$ (4). We apply a similar method to the one used in the proof of Theorem 14. Suppose X is a pyramid of size $p \times q$. Let $\lambda_1, \ldots, \lambda_p$ denote its row sums (λ_p could be zero), and let $v_1, \ldots, v_r$ denote the different values of the row sums arranged in decreasing order. Let $v_0 = q+1 > v_1$ and $v_{r+1} = -1 < v_r$. Finally, let $d_0, d_1, \ldots, d_r$ be real numbers such that $v_a > d_a > v_{a+1}$ for all $0 \le a \le r$. We now show that X is $(0, 1)$-additive. Define $f_1 \colon [p] \longrightarrow \mathbb{R}$ by $f_1(i) = \lambda_i$. Let $j \in [q]$. Then there is a unique $t(j)$ such that $v_{t(j)} \ge j > v_{t(j)+1}$. Define $f_2 \colon [q] \longrightarrow \mathbb{R}$ by $f_2(j) = -d_{t(j)}$. Let (i, j) be in $[p] \times [q]$. If $X(i, j) = 1$, then $j \le \lambda_i$ and $v_{t(j)} \le \lambda_i$. Thus, $f_1(i) + f_2(j) = \lambda_i - d_{t(j)} > \lambda_i - v_{t(j)} \ge 0$. If $X(i, j) = 0$, then $\lambda_i < j$ and $\lambda_i \le v_{t(j)+1}$. Thus, $f_1(i) + f_2(j) = \lambda_i - d_{t(j)} < \lambda_i - v_{t(j)+1} \le 0$. Therefore, X is $(0, 1)$-additive. □

We end this section with an example that shows how the algorithm contained in the proof of Theorem 9 works.

Example 7. Let $\boldsymbol{\lambda} = (5, 5, 2, 2, 1, 1)$ and $\boldsymbol{\mu} = (4, 3, 3, 3, 1, 1, 1)$. The conjugate partition to $\boldsymbol{\lambda}$ is $\boldsymbol{\lambda}' = (6, 4, 2, 2, 2)$ and $\boldsymbol{\lambda}' \succeq \boldsymbol{\mu}$. We constructed in Example 2 by means of Lemma 2 a sequence of partitions

$$\lambda' = \nu(0) \succ \nu(1) \succ \cdots \succ \nu(4) = \mu. \qquad (5.20)$$

The sequence of matrices $Y^{(i)}$ in $\mathsf{M}^*(\lambda, \nu(i))$, $0 \le i \le 4$, obtained in the proof of Theorem 9 is

$$Y^{(0)} = \begin{bmatrix} 1 & 1 & 1 & 1 & 1 & 0 & 0 \\ 1 & 1 & 1 & 1 & 1 & 0 & 0 \\ 1 & 1 & 0 & 0 & 0 & 0 & 0 \\ 1 & 1 & 0 & 0 & 0 & 0 & 0 \\ 1 & 0 & 0 & 0 & 0 & 0 & 0 \\ 1 & 0 & 0 & 0 & 0 & 0 & 0 \end{bmatrix}, \quad Y^{(1)} = \begin{bmatrix} 1 & 1 & 1 & 1 & 1 & 0 & 0 \\ 1 & 1 & 1 & 1 & 0 & 1 & 0 \\ 1 & 1 & 0 & 0 & 0 & 0 & 0 \\ 1 & 1 & 0 & 0 & 0 & 0 & 0 \\ 1 & 0 & 0 & 0 & 0 & 0 & 0 \\ 1 & 0 & 0 & 0 & 0 & 0 & 0 \end{bmatrix}, \quad Y^{(2)} = \begin{bmatrix} 1 & 1 & 1 & 1 & 1 & 0 & 0 \\ 1 & 1 & 1 & 1 & 0 & 1 & 0 \\ 1 & 1 & 0 & 0 & 0 & 0 & 0 \\ 1 & 0 & 1 & 0 & 0 & 0 & 0 \\ 1 & 0 & 0 & 0 & 0 & 0 & 0 \\ 1 & 0 & 0 & 0 & 0 & 0 & 0 \end{bmatrix},$$

$$Y^{(3)} = \begin{bmatrix} 1 & 1 & 1 & 1 & 1 & 0 & 0 \\ 1 & 1 & 1 & 1 & 0 & 1 & 0 \\ 1 & 1 & 0 & 0 & 0 & 0 & 0 \\ 1 & 0 & 1 & 0 & 0 & 0 & 0 \\ 1 & 0 & 0 & 0 & 0 & 0 & 0 \\ 0 & 0 & 0 & 1 & 0 & 0 & 0 \end{bmatrix}, \quad Y^{(4)} = \begin{bmatrix} 1 & 1 & 1 & 1 & 1 & 0 & 0 \\ 1 & 1 & 1 & 1 & 0 & 1 & 0 \\ 1 & 1 & 0 & 0 & 0 & 0 & 0 \\ 1 & 0 & 1 & 0 & 0 & 0 & 0 \\ 0 & 0 & 0 & 0 & 0 & 0 & 1 \\ 0 & 0 & 0 & 1 & 0 & 0 & 0 \end{bmatrix}. \qquad (5.21)$$

Here $Y^{(1)}$ was constructed as follows: Since $\nu(0)$ and $\nu(1)$ differ on the fifth and sixth coordinates, there must exist some i such that $Y^{(0)}_{i5} = 1$ and $Y^{(0)}_{i6} = 0$. In this example there are two such i's, namely, $i = 1, 2$. We chose the largest one (in practice, this choice is irrelevant). Proceeding in the same way, we obtain $Y^{(2)}$, $Y^{(3)}$, and $Y^{(4)}$.

5.5 Minimal Matrices and Uniqueness

In this section we give characterizations of existence and uniqueness of n-dimensional binary matrices in the same spirit as in Theorems 8 and 9. In dimension 3, a characterization for existence was given by W.B. Jurkat and H.J. Ryser (Theorem 5.5 in [19]) a long time ago. Theorem 12 generalizes their result to any dimension. A similar treatment for uniqueness in dimension 3 was given by A. Torres-Cházaro and the author [28]. Their proof uses a connection due to E. Snapper [27] between matrices and the theory of characters of the symmetric group. A combinatorial proof that closely follows the original proof in [28] was given by R. Brualdi [5] using ideas from [19]. Theorem 11 generalizes the result from [28] to any dimension. The proof presented here follows the original proof, but the crucial identity (Lemma 7), coming from character theory, is proved here combinatorially in the same way it as was done in [5] for dimension 3. It should be pointed out that the general philosophy of looking at integer matrices for characterizing uniqueness comes from the fact that matrices of uniqueness (with weakly decreasing 1-marginals) are pyramids (Theorem 6) and the observation that pyramids can be identified with integer matrices. The main notion appearing from this approach is that of a minimal matrix (to be defined below), which also has applications to Kronecker products of characters of the symmetric group [1, 30]. A third result of importance is a characterization for minimal matrices (Theorem 13) that uses the graph map. This result was first proved in dimension 3 using characters of the symmetric group [30, Proposition 3.1]. Here we extend the result to any dimension and give a new proof of combinatorial nature.

We use the notation from Section 5.3. Let $a^i \in \mathbb{N}_0^{q_i}$, $i \in [n-1]$, be a vector and $\nu \in \mathbb{N}_0^{q_n}$ be weakly decreasing, that is, a partition. Let A be a matrix in $\mathsf{M}(a^1, \ldots, a^{n-1})$ and let $k_1, \ldots, k_{\overline{q}}$ be the elements of $\mathsf{B}(\overline{q})$ arranged in lexicographic order. Then, after arranging the entries of A according to this ordering, we define a vector $\boldsymbol{\Phi}(A) := (A(k_1), \ldots, A(k_{\overline{q}}))$ in $\mathbb{N}_0^{\overline{q}}$. A second vector in $\mathbb{N}_0^{\overline{q}}$ associated to A, called the π-*sequence* of A and denoted $\boldsymbol{\pi}(A)$, is the vector formed by the entries of A arranged in weakly decreasing order. For any partition ρ in $\mathbb{N}_0^{\overline{q}}$, we denote by $\mathsf{M}_\rho(a^1, \ldots, a^{n-1})$ the set of all matrices in $\mathsf{M}(a^1, \ldots, a^{n-1})$ with π-sequence ρ. The matrix A is called π-*unique* if there is no other matrix $B \in \mathsf{M}(a^1, \ldots, a^{n-1})$ with $\boldsymbol{\pi}(B) = \boldsymbol{\pi}(A)$; A is called *minimal* if there is no other $B \in \mathsf{M}(a^1, \ldots, a^{n-1})$ with $\boldsymbol{\pi}(B) \prec \boldsymbol{\pi}(A)$; and A is called *hyperpartition of dimension $n-1$* or *$(n-1)$-dimensional partition* if for all $\overline{k}, \overline{l} \in \mathsf{B}(\overline{q})$ such that $k_i \leq l_i$, for $i \in [n-1]$, one has $A(\overline{k}) \geq A(\overline{l})$. A two-dimensional partition is usually called a *plane partition*.

In order to state the characterization for uniqueness we need the following construction: Choose any $q_n \geq \max\{ A(\overline{k}) \mid \overline{k} \in \mathsf{B}(\overline{q}) \}$. Then the *graph* $\mathsf{G}(A)$ of A is defined by

$$\mathsf{G}(A)(k) := \begin{cases} 1, & \text{if } 1 \leq k_n \leq A(k_1, \ldots, k_{n-1}), \\ 0, & \text{otherwise.} \end{cases} \tag{5.22}$$

Note that the value of q_n is unimportant; what really matters is the set of all $k \in \mathsf{B}(q)$ that satisfy $\mathsf{G}(A)(k) = 1$. The graph of A has 1-marginals $a^1, \ldots, a^{n-1}, \boldsymbol{\pi}(A)'$. So, for any partition $\rho \in \mathbb{N}_0^{\overline{q}_n}$ of N, there is an injective map

$$\mathsf{G} \colon \mathsf{M}_\rho(a^1, \ldots, a^{n-1}) \longrightarrow \mathsf{M}^*(a^1, \ldots, a^{n-1}, \rho') . \tag{5.23}$$

Example 8. Let

$$A = \begin{bmatrix} 3 & 3 & 1 \\ 2 & 1 & 1 \\ 2 & 0 & 0 \end{bmatrix}, \quad B = \begin{bmatrix} 4 & 4 & 1 \\ 2 & 1 & 1 \\ 2 & 0 & 0 \end{bmatrix}, \quad \text{and} \quad C = \begin{bmatrix} 4 & 3 & 2 \\ 3 & 1 & 0 \\ 1 & 1 & 0 \end{bmatrix}. \tag{5.24}$$

The three matrices A, B, C are plane partitions. The π-sequences of A, B, and C are, respectively, $(3, 3, 2, 2, 1, 1, 1, 0, 0)$, $(4, 4, 2, 2, 1, 1, 1, 0, 0)$, and $(4, 3, 3, 2, 1, 1, 1, 0, 0)$. Matrix A is minimal, but not π-unique [28, p. 447]. The first assertion can be checked directly by hand; for the second, just take the transpose of A. Matrix B is π-unique, but not minimal. The first assertion can be checked by hand; for the second, observe that C has the same 1-marginals as B, and $\pi(C) \prec \pi(B)$. The graph $\mathsf{G}(B)$ of B is the matrix from Example 3 with 1-marginals $a^1 = (9, 4, 2)$, $a^2 = (8, 5, 2)$, and $a^3 = (7, 4, 2, 2)$. Note that B has 1-marginals a^1 and a^2 and that $\pi(B)$ is conjugate to a^3 (zeros here are irrelevant). See Example 10 for other properties of C.

Theorem 11. *Let $X \in \mathsf{M}^*(a^1, \ldots, a^{n-1}, \nu)$. Then X is a matrix of uniqueness if, and only if, X is the graph $\mathsf{G}(A)$ of a matrix $A \in \mathsf{M}(a^1, \ldots, a^{n-1})$ that is minimal and π-unique.*

Corollary 2. *Let A be a matrix that is minimal and π-unique. If its 1-marginals are partitions, then A is a hyperpartition.*

Example 9. The graph $\mathsf{G}(D)$ of the matrix

$$D = \begin{bmatrix} 5\,5\,5\,4\,4 \\ 5\,5\,5\,3\,3 \\ 3\,3\,1\,1\,0 \\ 2\,1\,1\,1\,0 \\ 2\,1\,0\,0\,0 \end{bmatrix} \tag{5.25}$$

is the matrix of uniqueness in Example 5, which has 1-marginals

$$\boldsymbol{a}^1 = (23, 21, 8, 5, 3),\ \boldsymbol{a}^2 = (17, 15, 12, 9, 7),\ \text{and}\ \boldsymbol{a}^3 = (20, 14, 12, 8, 6). \tag{5.26}$$

The 1-marginals of D are $\boldsymbol{a}^1$ and $\boldsymbol{a}^2$; its π-sequence is precisely the partition conjugate to $\boldsymbol{a}^3$. Theorem 11 implies that D is minimal and π-unique. The graph of a matrix is customarily depicted by stacking unit cubes as shown in Fig. 5.2.

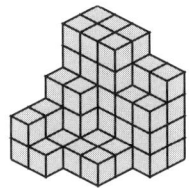

Fig. 5.2. The graph of pyramid D.

Remark 3. It should be noted that, while the property of being a matrix of uniqueness is symmetric in $\boldsymbol{a}^1, \ldots, \boldsymbol{a}^n$, the condition given in Theorem 11 is only symmetric in $\boldsymbol{a}^1, \ldots, \boldsymbol{a}^{n-1}$: If X is a matrix of uniqueness and its 1-marginals are partitions, then X is a pyramid and the matrix A such that $X = \mathsf{G}(A)$ is obtained by projecting X along the nth direction (the direction of the nth vector of the canonical basis of $\mathbb{R}^n$). In fact, a similar result holds if we choose to project X in the ith direction for any $i \in [n]$.

Theorem 12. *The set $\mathsf{M}^*(\boldsymbol{a}^1, \ldots, \boldsymbol{a}^{n-1}, \boldsymbol{\nu})$ is nonempty if, and only if, there is a matrix $A \in \mathsf{M}(\boldsymbol{a}^1, \ldots, \boldsymbol{a}^{n-1})$ such that $\pi(A)' \succeq \boldsymbol{\nu}$.*

Theorem 13. *Let $A \in \mathsf{M}_\rho(\boldsymbol{a}^1, \ldots, \boldsymbol{a}^{n-1})$. Then A is minimal if, and only if, the map*

$$\mathsf{G} \colon \mathsf{M}_\rho(\boldsymbol{a}^1, \ldots, \boldsymbol{a}^{n-1}) \longrightarrow \mathsf{M}^*(\boldsymbol{a}^1, \ldots, \boldsymbol{a}^{n-1}, \rho') \tag{5.27}$$

is bijective.

The rest of the section is devoted to the proofs. We start with a construction that is related to the graph of a matrix: The *projection* $\mathsf{Pr}(X)$ of a binary matrix X with 1-marginals $\boldsymbol{a}^1, \ldots, \boldsymbol{a}^{n-1}, \boldsymbol{\nu}$ is defined by

$$\mathsf{Pr}(X)(\overline{\boldsymbol{k}}) := \sum_{j=1}^{q_n} X(k_1, \ldots, k_{n-1}, j), \tag{5.28}$$

for all $\overline{\boldsymbol{k}} \in \mathsf{B}(\overline{\boldsymbol{q}})$. Note that $\mathsf{Pr}(X)$ is in $\mathsf{M}(\boldsymbol{a}^1, \ldots, \boldsymbol{a}^{n-1})$. So, we have a map

$$\mathsf{Pr}\colon \mathsf{M}^*(\boldsymbol{a}^1, \ldots, \boldsymbol{a}^{n-1}, \boldsymbol{\nu}) \longrightarrow \mathsf{M}(\boldsymbol{a}^1, \ldots, \boldsymbol{a}^{n-1}). \tag{5.29}$$

The π-sequence of the projection satisfies $\boldsymbol{\pi}(\mathsf{Pr}(X))' \succeq \boldsymbol{\nu}$ (the reasoning is similar to the one in the proof of Theorem 9).

A variation of the notion of pyramid will be needed below. Let $i \in [n]$. An n-dimensional binary matrix X is called *pyramid with respect to the ith direction* if for all $\boldsymbol{k}, \boldsymbol{l} \in \mathsf{B}(\boldsymbol{q})$ such that $k_i \leq l_i$ and $k_j = l_j$ for $j \neq i$, the condition $X(\boldsymbol{l}) = 1$ implies $X(\boldsymbol{k}) = 1$. Then a pyramid is a pyramid with respect to the ith direction, for all i.

The following properties of G and Pr are easy to check.

Lemma 5. *Let $A \in \mathsf{M}(\boldsymbol{a}^1, \ldots, \boldsymbol{a}^{n-1})$ and $X \in \mathsf{M}^*(\boldsymbol{a}^1, \ldots, \boldsymbol{a}^{n-1}, \boldsymbol{\nu})$. Then*
(1) A is a hyperpartition if, and only if, $\mathsf{G}(A)$ is a pyramid.
(2) If X is a pyramid, then $\mathsf{Pr}(X)$ is a hyperpartition. The converse does not hold in general.
(3) $\mathsf{Pr}(\mathsf{G}(A)) = A$.
(4) X is in the image of G if, and only if, X is a pyramid with respect to the nth direction. In this situation, $\mathsf{G}(\mathsf{Pr}(X)) = X$.

Lemma 6. *There is a bijection (the union on the right is disjoint)*

$$\beta\colon \mathsf{M}^*(\boldsymbol{a}^1, \ldots, \boldsymbol{a}^n) \longrightarrow \bigcup_{A \in \mathsf{M}(\boldsymbol{a}^1, \ldots, \boldsymbol{a}^{n-1})} \mathsf{M}^*(\boldsymbol{\Phi}(A), \boldsymbol{a}^n). \tag{5.30}$$

Proof. For $X \in \mathsf{M}^*(\boldsymbol{a}^1, \ldots, \boldsymbol{a}^n)$, let $A = \mathsf{Pr}(X)$ and $Y = (y_{ij})$ be defined by

$$y_{ij} := \begin{cases} 1, & \text{if } X(\boldsymbol{k}_i, j) = 1, \\ 0, & \text{otherwise.} \end{cases} \tag{5.31}$$

Define $\beta(X) := Y$. Then $Y \in \mathsf{M}^*(\boldsymbol{\Phi}(A), \boldsymbol{a}^n)$. It is easy to show that β is a bijection. $\qquad\square$

Lemma 7. *The following identity holds:*

$$|\mathsf{M}^*(\boldsymbol{a}^1, \ldots, \boldsymbol{a}^{n-1}, \boldsymbol{\nu})| = \sum_{\substack{B \in \mathsf{M}(\boldsymbol{a}^1, \ldots, \boldsymbol{a}^{n-1}) \\ \boldsymbol{\pi}(B)' \succeq \boldsymbol{\nu}}} |\mathsf{M}^*(\boldsymbol{\pi}(B), \boldsymbol{\nu})|. \tag{5.32}$$

Proof. By Lemma 6, the left-hand side of the identity equals

$$\sum_{B \in \mathsf{M}(\boldsymbol{a}^1,\dots,\boldsymbol{a}^{n-1})} |\mathsf{M}^*(\boldsymbol{\Phi}(B),\boldsymbol{\nu})| . \tag{5.33}$$

But for any $B \in \mathsf{M}(\boldsymbol{a}^1,\dots,\boldsymbol{a}^{n-1})$, one has $|\mathsf{M}^*(\boldsymbol{\Phi}(B),\boldsymbol{\nu})| = |\mathsf{M}^*(\boldsymbol{\pi}(B),\boldsymbol{\nu})|$; and, by Theorem 9, $|\mathsf{M}^*(\boldsymbol{\pi}(B),\boldsymbol{\nu})| \neq 0$ if, and only if, $\boldsymbol{\pi}(B)' \succeq \boldsymbol{\nu}$. Then the claim follows. □

Proof (of Theorem 11). Let $X \in \mathsf{M}^*(\boldsymbol{a}^1,\dots,\boldsymbol{a}^{n-1},\boldsymbol{\nu})$ be a matrix of uniqueness. Lemma 7 implies that

$$\sum_{\substack{B \in \mathsf{M}(\boldsymbol{a}^1,\dots,\boldsymbol{a}^{n-1}) \\ \boldsymbol{\pi}(B)' \succeq \boldsymbol{\nu}}} |\mathsf{M}^*(\boldsymbol{\pi}(B),\boldsymbol{\nu})| = 1 . \tag{5.34}$$

Then there is a matrix $A \in \mathsf{M}(\boldsymbol{a}^1,\dots,\boldsymbol{a}^{n-1})$ such that $|\mathsf{M}^*(\boldsymbol{\pi}(A),\boldsymbol{\nu})| = 1$; therefore, by Theorem 8, $\boldsymbol{\pi}(A)' = \boldsymbol{\nu}$. Moreover, for any $B \in \mathsf{M}(\boldsymbol{a}^1,\dots,\boldsymbol{a}^{n-1})$, different from A, one has $|\mathsf{M}^*(\boldsymbol{\pi}(B),\boldsymbol{\nu})| = 0$. This implies that A is minimal and π-unique. Since $\mathsf{G}(A) \in \mathsf{M}^*(\boldsymbol{a}^1,\dots,\boldsymbol{a}^{n-1},\boldsymbol{\nu})$, our uniqueness assumption forces $X = \mathsf{G}(A)$.

Conversely, suppose X is the graph of a matrix $A \in \mathsf{M}(\boldsymbol{a}^1,\dots,\boldsymbol{a}^{n-1})$ that is minimal and π-unique. Let $\boldsymbol{\nu} = \boldsymbol{\pi}(A)'$. Since A is minimal and π-unique, Theorems 8 and 9 imply that Eq. (5.34) holds. Then, since $X \in \mathsf{M}^*(\boldsymbol{a}^1,\dots,\boldsymbol{a}^{n-1},\boldsymbol{\nu})$, Lemma 7 implies that X is a matrix of uniqueness. □

Proof (of Corollary 2). By Theorem 11, $\mathsf{G}(A)$ is a matrix of uniqueness whose 1-marginals are partitions. The claim follows from Theorem 6 and Lemma 5. □

Proof (of Theorem 12). It is immediate from Lemma 7. □

Proof (of Theorem 13). Suppose first that G is not bijective. Then there is a matrix $X \in \mathsf{M}^*(\boldsymbol{a}^1,\dots,\boldsymbol{a}^{n-1},\boldsymbol{\rho}')$ that is not in the image of G. Therefore, by Lemma 5, X is not a pyramid with respect to the nth direction, so there are $\boldsymbol{k}$, $\boldsymbol{l}$ such that $k_j = l_j$, for $1 \leq j < n$, $k_n < l_n$, $X(\boldsymbol{k}) = 0$, and $X(\boldsymbol{l}) = 1$. Let Y be obtained from X by switching the zero in position $\boldsymbol{k}$ and the one in position $\boldsymbol{l}$, that is, $Y(\boldsymbol{k}) = 1$, $Y(\boldsymbol{l}) = 0$ and $Y(\boldsymbol{m}) = X(\boldsymbol{m})$ for $\boldsymbol{m} \neq \boldsymbol{k}, \boldsymbol{l}$. Then Y has 1-marginals $\boldsymbol{a}^1,\dots,\boldsymbol{a}^{n-1}, \boldsymbol{b}$, where $b_{k_n} = \rho'_{k_n}+1$, $b_{l_n} = \rho'_{l_n}-1$, and $b_j = \rho'_j$ if $j \neq k_n, l_n$. The vector $\boldsymbol{b}$ might not be a partition, but $\boldsymbol{\pi}(\boldsymbol{b}) \succ \boldsymbol{\rho}'$ (this can be seen directly or by means of Lemma 1). Moreover, $\mathsf{Pr}(Y) \in \mathsf{M}(\boldsymbol{a}^1,\dots,\boldsymbol{a}^{n-1})$ and $\boldsymbol{\pi}(\mathsf{Pr}(Y))' \succeq \boldsymbol{\pi}(\boldsymbol{b}) \succ \boldsymbol{\rho}'$. Therefore, by (5.8), $\boldsymbol{\pi}(\mathsf{Pr}(Y)) \prec \boldsymbol{\rho} = \boldsymbol{\pi}(A)$. Thus, A is not minimal.

Conversely, suppose A is not minimal. Then there is a matrix B in $\mathsf{M}(\boldsymbol{a}^1,\dots,\boldsymbol{a}^{n-1})$ such that $\boldsymbol{\pi}(B) \prec \boldsymbol{\pi}(A) = \boldsymbol{\rho}$. Let $\boldsymbol{\lambda} = \boldsymbol{\pi}(B)$. Then $\mathsf{G}(B)$ is in $\mathsf{M}^*(\boldsymbol{a}^1,\dots,\boldsymbol{a}^{n-1},\boldsymbol{\lambda}')$. By (5.8), $\boldsymbol{\lambda}' \succ \boldsymbol{\rho}'$. We can, then, as in the proof of Theorem 9, apply Lemma 2 and shift ones *up* in $\mathsf{G}(B)$, along the nth direction, to obtain a matrix $Y \in \mathsf{M}^*(\boldsymbol{a}^1, \ldots, \boldsymbol{a}^{n-1}, \boldsymbol{\rho}')$. (We could also have used Lemma 6 and apply the idea in the proof of Theorem 9 to obtain a matrix Z in $\mathsf{M}^*(\boldsymbol{\Phi}(B), \boldsymbol{\rho}')$ from $\beta(\mathsf{G}(B))$ in $\mathsf{M}^*(\boldsymbol{\Phi}(B), \boldsymbol{\lambda}')$. Then Y would be $\beta^{-1}(Z)$.) The matrix Y is not a pyramid with respect to the nth direction. Then Lemma 5 implies that G is not a bijection. $\qquad\square$

5.6 Additivity for Integer Matrices

In this section we follow the same line of thought as in the last section and give a condition for an integer matrix A that is equivalent to $(0,1)$-additivity of its graph $\mathsf{G}(A)$. This new condition provides a more economic way of showing that a pyramid is $(0,1)$-additive. The results presented here are taken from [32].

We use the notation from Section 5.3. Let $\boldsymbol{a}^1, \ldots, \boldsymbol{a}^{n-1}, \boldsymbol{\nu}$ be as in Section 5.5. A matrix $A \in \mathsf{M}(\boldsymbol{a}^1, \ldots, \boldsymbol{a}^{n-1})$ is called *additive* if there are vectors $\boldsymbol{x}^i \in \mathbb{R}^{q_i}$, $i \in [n-1]$, such that for all $\overline{\boldsymbol{k}}, \overline{\boldsymbol{l}} \in \mathsf{B}(\overline{\boldsymbol{q}})$ the following condition holds:

$$A\left(\overline{\boldsymbol{k}}\right) > A\left(\overline{\boldsymbol{l}}\right) \implies \sum_{i=1}^{n-1} x^i_{k_i} > \sum_{i=1}^{n-1} x^i_{l_i} . \tag{5.35}$$

Theorem 14. *Let $X \in \mathsf{M}^*(\boldsymbol{a}^1, \ldots, \boldsymbol{a}^{n-1}, \boldsymbol{\nu})$. Then X is $(0,1)$-additive if, and only if, X is the graph $\mathsf{G}(A)$ of an additive matrix A in $\mathsf{M}(\boldsymbol{a}^1, \ldots, \boldsymbol{a}^{n-1})$.*

Example 10. The matrix C from Example 8 is additive: Let $\boldsymbol{x}^1 = (7,2,0)$ and $\boldsymbol{x}^2 = (6,3,0)$. Then the matrix of sums $(s_{i,j}) := (x^1_i + x^2_j)$ satisfies condition (5.35). Theorem 14 implies that the graph of C is $(0,1)$-additive, and Corollary 3 below implies that C is minimal and π-unique.

Example 11. The matrix D from Example 9 is not additive. This follows from Theorem 14, since its graph is not $(0,1)$-additive (see Example 5).

Proof (of Theorem 14). Suppose first that $X \in \mathsf{M}^*(\boldsymbol{a}^1, \ldots, \boldsymbol{a}^{n-1}, \boldsymbol{\nu})$ is $(0,1)$-additive. Then there are maps $f_i \colon [q_i] \longrightarrow \mathbb{R}$, $1 \le i \le n$, satisfying condition (5.11) in Section 5.3. Moreover, since $\boldsymbol{\nu}$ is a partition, we can use the same reasoning from the proof of Theorem 7 to conclude that X is a pyramid with respect to the nth direction, and therefore, by Lemma 5, X is the graph $\mathsf{G}(A)$ of some matrix $A \in \mathsf{M}(\boldsymbol{a}^1, \ldots, \boldsymbol{a}^{n-1})$. We will show that A is additive. Let $x^i_j = f_i(j)$ for $i \in [n-1]$ and $j \in [q_i]$. Let $\overline{\boldsymbol{k}}, \overline{\boldsymbol{l}} \in \mathsf{B}(\overline{\boldsymbol{q}})$ and suppose that $A\left(\overline{\boldsymbol{k}}\right) > A\left(\overline{\boldsymbol{l}}\right)$. Let $k_n = l_n = A(\overline{\boldsymbol{l}}) + 1$, $\boldsymbol{k} = (k_1, \ldots, k_n)$, and $\boldsymbol{l} = (l_1, \ldots, l_n)$. Then, since $X = \mathsf{G}(A)$, we have $X(\boldsymbol{k}) = 1$ and $X(\boldsymbol{l}) = 0$. Thus, by (5.11), $\sum_{i=1}^n f_i(k_i) \ge 0 > \sum_{i=1}^n f_i(l_i)$. Since $k_n = l_n$, condition (5.35) holds.

Conversely, if $X = \mathsf{G}(A)$, for some additive matrix $A \in \mathsf{M}(\boldsymbol{a}^1, \ldots, \boldsymbol{a}^{n-1})$. Then there are vectors $\boldsymbol{x}^i \in \mathbb{R}^{q_i}$ satisfying condition (5.35). For $i \in [n-1]$, let $f_i(j) = x^i_j$. The definition of f_n is more involved. Let $v_1, \ldots, v_m$ be the different values taken by the entries of A, arranged in decreasing order. Let $v_0 = q_n + 1 > v_1$ and $v_{m+1} = -1 < v_m$. For each $t \in [m]$, let

$$\varphi_t = \min \left\{ \sum_{i=1}^{n-1} x_{k_i}^i \ \Big| \ A\left(\overline{\boldsymbol{k}}\right) = v_t \right\} \tag{5.36}$$

and

$$\psi_t = \max \left\{ \sum_{i=1}^{n-1} x_{k_i}^i \ \Big| \ A\left(\overline{\boldsymbol{k}}\right) = v_t \right\} . \tag{5.37}$$

Let φ_0 and ψ_{m+1} be such that $\varphi_0 > \psi_1$ and $\psi_{m+1} < \varphi_m$. Then it follows from (5.35) that

$$\varphi_0 > \psi_1 \geq \varphi_1 > \psi_2 \geq \cdots \geq \varphi_{m-1} > \psi_m \geq \varphi_m > \psi_{m+1} . \tag{5.38}$$

Choose numbers d_t, $0 \leq t \leq m$ such that $\varphi_t > d_t > \psi_{t+1}$ (they could be rationals). Now, for any $j \in [q_n]$, there is a unique $0 \leq t(j) \leq m$ such that

$$v_{t(j)} \geq j > v_{t(j)+1} . \tag{5.39}$$

Let $f_n(j) = -d_{t(j)}$. Now we proceed to check condition (5.11). Let $\boldsymbol{k} \in \mathsf{B}(\boldsymbol{q})$. If $X(\boldsymbol{k}) = 1$, then $k_n \leq A\left(\overline{\boldsymbol{k}}\right) = v_s$ for some s. Then there is some $r \geq s$ such that $v_r \geq k_n > v_{r+1}$. Therefore,

$$\sum_{i=1}^{n} f_i(k_i) = \sum_{i=1}^{n-1} x_{k_i}^i - d_{t(k_n)}$$

$$\geq \varphi_s - d_r \geq \varphi_r - d_r > 0 . \tag{5.40}$$

Similarly, if $X(\boldsymbol{k}) = 0$, then $k_n > A\left(\overline{\boldsymbol{k}}\right) = v_s$ for some s. Then there is some $r < s$ such that $v_r \geq k_n > v_{r+1}$. Therefore,

$$\sum_{i=1}^{n} f_i(k_i) = \sum_{i=1}^{n-1} x_{k_i}^i - d_{t(k_n)}$$

$$\leq \psi_s - d_r \leq \psi_s - d_{s-1} < 0 . \tag{5.41}$$

Therefore, X is $(0,1)$-additive. $\square$

Corollary 3. *If A is an additive matrix, then A is minimal and π-unique. If, moreover, the 1-marginals of A are partitions, then A is a hyperpartition.*

Proof. Let A be an additive matrix. Then, by Theorem 14, $\mathsf{G}(A)$ is $(0,1)$-additive. Theorem 5 implies $\mathsf{G}(A)$ is a matrix of uniqueness. Finally, by Theorem 11, A is minimal and π-unique. The last claim follows from Corollary 2. $\square$

Example 12. Additivity can be more easily shown as $(0,1)$-additivity. For example, the graph of the $q \times q$ matrix

$$A = \begin{bmatrix} q & q-1 & q-2 & \cdots & \cdots & 2 & 1 \\ q-1 & q-2 & & \cdots & \cdots & 1 & 0 \\ q-2 & & \cdots & & \cdots & \cdots & 0 & 0 \\ \vdots & \vdots & \vdots & & \ddots & \vdots & \vdots \\ 2 & 1 & 0 & \cdots & & 0 & 0 \\ 1 & 0 & 0 & \cdots & & 0 & 0 \end{bmatrix} \tag{5.42}$$

is the matrix X in Example 4, which is $(0,1)$-additive. Additivity of A follows directly by taking $\boldsymbol{x}^1 = \boldsymbol{x}^2 = (q-1, q-2, \ldots, 1, 0)$. Then Theorem 14 provides a simpler proof of the $(0,1)$-additivity of X.

5.7 Uniqueness and $(0,1)$-Additivity in Dimension 3

In this section we present some results about three-dimensional $(0,1)$-matrices and two-dimensional integer matrices. We start by showing that pyramids are characterized by the absence of bad configurations of weight 2 [29, §3], [32, §3]. Then we prove (Theorem 15) a result analogous to Theorem 10 that shows the equivalence among being a pyramid, uniqueness, and $(0,1)$-additivity for matrices of size $2 \times q \times r$ [32]. For this we need to show that any plane partition of size $2 \times q$ is additive (Lemma 8). We present a new, shorter proof of this result than the one given in [32, §4]. We also mention the classification of bad configurations of weight 3 for pyramids from [29]. We conclude with several examples and some comments about the weight of bad configurations needed to determine if a pyramid is a matrix of uniqueness.

Let $\boldsymbol{\lambda}$, $\boldsymbol{\mu}$, $\boldsymbol{\nu}$ be partitions of some natural number N.

Proposition 1. *Let $X \in \mathsf{M}^*(\boldsymbol{\lambda}, \boldsymbol{\mu}, \boldsymbol{\nu})$. Then X is a pyramid if, and only if, X has no bad configurations of weight 2.*

Proof. One implication is Lemma 3. For the converse, suppose X has a bad configuration W of weight 2. Then W takes value 1 on two points, say $\boldsymbol{k}$, $\boldsymbol{l}$, and value -1 on two points, say $\boldsymbol{s}$, $\boldsymbol{t}$. If these four points lie on a plane parallel to a coordinate plane, then they must be the vertices of a rectangle; besides, $\boldsymbol{k}$ and $\boldsymbol{l}$ must be diagonally opposite. A simple case-by-case analysis shows that X is not a pyramid. If $\boldsymbol{k}$, $\boldsymbol{l}$, $\boldsymbol{s}$, $\boldsymbol{t}$ are not contained in a plane parallel to a coordinate plane, then $\boldsymbol{k}$ and $\boldsymbol{l}$ must be diagonally opposite vertices of a parallelepiped and $\boldsymbol{s}$, $\boldsymbol{t}$ must be a second pair of diagonally opposite vertices of the same parallelepiped. Again, a simple case-by-case analysis shows that X is not a pyramid. □

Lemma 8. *Every plane partition of size $2 \times q$ is additive.*

Proof. Let $A = (a_{ij})$ be a plane partition of size $2 \times q$ ($q \in \mathbb{N}$). Since there is a plane partition $B = (b_{ij})$ of size $2 \times q$ whose entries are all different and satisfies $a_{ij} > a_{kl} \Rightarrow b_{ij} > b_{kl}$, we can assume without loss of generality that A does not have two equal entries. Then we proceed by induction on q. The case $q = 1$ is trivial. Suppose then $q > 1$. The matrix $\overline{A}$ obtained from A by deleting the first column is a plane partition of size $2 \times (q - 1)$. By the induction hypothesis, $\overline{A}$ is additive. Then there exist real numbers x_1, x_2, $y_2, \ldots, y_q$ such that for all $i, k \in [2]$, $j, l \in \{2, \ldots, q\}$, the condition

$$a_{ij} > a_{kl} \Rightarrow x_i + y_j > x_k + y_l \qquad (5.43)$$

holds. We assume for simplicity that $x_2 = 0$ (this can always be done). Let $s = \max\{j \in [q] \mid a_{1j} > a_{21}\}$ (since $a_{11} > a_{21}$, s is well defined). If $s = 1$, then $a_{21} > a_{12}$, so we choose y_1 to be any number bigger than $x_1 + y_2$. If $1 < s < q$, then $a_{1s} > a_{21} > a_{1s+1}$, so we choose y_1 such that $x_1 + y_s > y_1 > \max\{x_1 + y_{s+1}, y_2\}$. If $s = q$, then $a_{1q} > a_{21}$, so we choose y_1 such that $x_1 + y_q > y_1 > y_2$. In the three cases, additivity follows easily from the induction hypothesis. □

Then by Corollary 3 we have

Corollary 4. *Every plane partition of size $2 \times q$ is minimal and π-unique.*

Theorem 15. *Let $X \in M^*(\lambda, \mu, \nu)$. If λ has length 2, the following are equivalent:*

(1) X is a pyramid;
(2) X has no bad configurations of weight 2;
(3) X is a matrix of uniqueness;
(4) X is $(0, 1)$-additive.

Proof. (1) $\Rightarrow$ (4). Let X be a pyramid. Then, by Lemma 5, there is a plane partition A of size $2 \times q$ (q is the length of μ) such that X is the graph of A. By Lemma 8, A is additive, and by Theorem 14, X is $(0, 1)$-additive. Finally, (4) $\Rightarrow$ (3) is Theorem 5, (3) $\Rightarrow$ (2) is Theorem 3, and (2) $\Rightarrow$ (1) is Lemma 3. □

Example 13. Theorem 15 is no longer true if λ has length greater than 2. Let X be the graph of matrix A in Example 8; then X is a pyramid that is not a matrix of uniqueness [29, §3]: Let $W : B(3, 3, 3) \longrightarrow \{-1, 0, 1\}$ be the matrix that takes value 1 on $(1, 2, 3)$, $(2, 3, 1)$, and $(3, 1, 2)$; value -1 on $(1, 3, 2)$, $(2, 1, 3)$, and $(3, 2, 1)$; and value 0 on the remaining points. Then W is a bad configuration for X of weight 3.

Bad configurations of weight 3 for pyramids have been classified. Any such bad configuration of weight 3 is essentially the bad configuration of Example 13 or its negative. The following theorem and its corollary are taken from [29, §5], where proofs can be found.

Theorem 16. *Let* $W\colon \mathsf{B}(p,q,r) \longrightarrow \{-1,0,1\}$ *be a bad configuration of weight 3 for some pyramid. Then there exist integers*

$$1 \le a < b < c \le p, \ 1 \le d < e < f \le q \text{ and } 1 \le g < h < i \le r \qquad (5.44)$$

such that W *or* $-W$ *takes value 1 on* (a,e,i), (b,f,g), (c,d,h), *value* -1 *on* (a,f,h), (b,d,i), (c,e,g), *and value 0 on the remaining points.*

Corollary 5. *Let* X *be the graph of a plane partition* A. *Then* X *has a bad configuration of weight 3 if, and only if, either* A *or its transpose contains a* 3×3 *submatrix* $B = (b_{ij})$ *satisfying*

$$b_{23} < b_{32} \le b_{31} < b_{13} \le b_{12} < b_{21} \,. \qquad (5.45)$$

Example 14. The graph $X = \mathsf{G}(E)$ of the matrix

$$E = \begin{bmatrix} 5\,5\,5\,4\,4 \\ 5\,5\,5\,3\,3 \\ 3\,3\,1\,1\,0 \\ 2\,1\,1\,1\,0 \\ 2\,1\,1\,1\,0 \\ 2\,1\,0\,0\,0 \end{bmatrix} \qquad (5.46)$$

has no bad configurations of weight 3 [29, §3]: Suppose X contains such a bad configuration. Then, by Corollary 5, E or its transpose contains a 3×3 submatrix $B = (b_{ij})$ satisfying (5.45). These inequalities imply that the three rows and the three columns of B are different. Then B or its transpose is a submatrix of matrix D in Example 9 (since D is obtained from E by deleting row 5). This is a contradiction because the graph of D is a set of uniqueness. However, E has a bad configuration of weight 6, namely W, where $W\colon \mathsf{B}(6,5,5) \longrightarrow \{-1,0,1\}$ is the matrix that takes value 1 on $(1,5,4)$, $(2,3,5)$, $(3,2,3)$, $(4,4,1)$, $(5,4,1)$, $(6,1,2)$, value -1 on $(1,4,5)$, $(2,4,4)$, $(3,5,1)$, $(4,2,2)$, $(5,1,3)$, $(6,3,1)$, and value 0 on the remaining points.

Remark 4. Example 14 shows how in dimension 3 bad configurations of weight 3 are not enough to determine whether a pyramid is a set of uniqueness. It is an open problem whether there is a finite upper bound (at least 4 by this example) on the weight of bad configurations that one need not go beyond to determine whether a pyramid of arbitrary size (number of ones) is a set of uniqueness; compare with [9, §5]. It seems likely that no finite upper bound exists. A similar result was proved in [17], where it was shown that when there is no upper bound on the weight of bad configurations, one needs to determine whether a 3-dimensional $(0,1)$-matrix is a matrix of uniqueness with respect to their *2-marginals* or *line sums*.

Remark 5. Not all minimal matrices are plane partitions. The simplest example of a minimal matrix that is not a plane partition is a permutation matrix.

A classification of all minimal matrices of size $2 \times q$ was achieved in [31]. A similar classification for minimal matrices or even for additive matrices of size $3 \times q$ seems much more difficult; compare, for example, the results in [7].

Remark 6. There are constructions for plane partitions analogous to the complement and rotation of a pyramid. A result similar to Lemma 4 can be stated for plane partitions. This is of interest in the applications to Kronecker products.

5.8 The Geometry of Real-Minimal Matrices

In this section we extend the notions for matrices with nonnegative integer entries given in Sections 5.5 and 5.6 to matrices with real entries. For a matrix A with real entries, we give characterizations involving the permutohedron determined by A, where A can be minimal, real-minimal, and/or π-unique. In particular, we obtain a new characterization for a binary matrix X to be a matrix of uniqueness (Corollary 10). We also show that minimal and real-minimal matrices appear as optimal solutions of quadratic transportation problems. In fact, the optimization problem from Proposition 3 has been used by H. Díaz-Leal, J. Martínez-Bernal, and D. Romero to compute the dimension of the variety of flags fixed by a nilpotent endomorphism [8]. The results presented here were obtained by S. Onn and the author for 2-dimensional matrices in [23]; their generalization to any dimension is easy, but needs some care.

We use the notation from Section 5.3. Let $\mathsf{M}(\boldsymbol{q})$ denote the set of all matrices with real entries of size $q_1 \times \cdots \times q_n$. As in Section 5.5, we associate to $A \in \mathsf{M}(\boldsymbol{q})$ two vectors in $\mathbb{R}^q$. The first uses the elements of $\mathsf{B}(\boldsymbol{q})$ arranged in lexicographic order $\boldsymbol{k}_1, \ldots, \boldsymbol{k}_q$ and is defined as

$$\boldsymbol{\Phi}(A) := (A(\boldsymbol{k}_1), \ldots, A(\boldsymbol{k}_q)) . \tag{5.47}$$

Then $\boldsymbol{\Phi} \colon \mathsf{M}(\boldsymbol{q}) \longrightarrow \mathbb{R}^q$ is a linear isomorphism. The second vector associated to A, called the π-sequence and denoted by $\boldsymbol{\pi}(A)$, is the vector formed by the entries of A arranged in weakly decreasing order. We proceed to extend, to matrices with real entries, the definitions given in previous sections for matrices with integer entries. Let $A \in \mathsf{F}(\boldsymbol{a}^1, \ldots, \boldsymbol{a}^n)$. Then A is called π-*unique* if there is no other $B \in \mathsf{F}(\boldsymbol{a}^1, \ldots, \boldsymbol{a}^n)$ such that $\boldsymbol{\pi}(B) = \boldsymbol{\pi}(A)$; A is called *real-minimal* if there is no other $B \in \mathsf{F}(\boldsymbol{a}^1, \ldots, \boldsymbol{a}^n)$ such that $\boldsymbol{\pi}(B) \prec \boldsymbol{\pi}(A)$; A is called *additive* if there are vectors $\boldsymbol{x}^i \in \mathbb{R}^{q_i}$, $1 \leq i \leq n$, such that for all $\boldsymbol{k}$, $\boldsymbol{l} \in \mathsf{B}(\boldsymbol{q})$, condition (5.35) in Section 5.6 holds; and A is called *hyperpartition* if for all $\boldsymbol{k}$, $\boldsymbol{l} \in \mathsf{B}(\boldsymbol{q})$ such that $k_i \leq l_i$, for all $1 \leq i \leq n$, one has $A(\boldsymbol{k}) \geq A(\boldsymbol{l})$. Clearly, any real-minimal matrix in $\mathsf{M}(\boldsymbol{a}^1, \ldots, \boldsymbol{a}^n)$ is minimal. The converse is false, as the following example shows.

Example 15. The matrix A from Example 8 is minimal, but not real-minimal. A matrix B with the same 1-marginals as A and such that $\boldsymbol{\pi}(B) \prec \boldsymbol{\pi}(A)$ can be constructed by taking a convex combination of A with its transpose, that is, $B = \varepsilon A + (1 - \varepsilon)A^{\mathsf{T}}$ for some $0 < \varepsilon < 1$.

It is important to note that if a matrix A is additive, then any other matrix B such that $B(\boldsymbol{k}) > B(\boldsymbol{l})$ if, and only if, $A(\boldsymbol{k}) > A(\boldsymbol{l})$ for all $\boldsymbol{k}, \boldsymbol{l}$, is additive. So, additivity for a matrix A (and by Theorem 19 also real-minimality) depends only on the connected region of the arrangement of hyperplanes

$$\{z_i - z_j = 0 \mid 1 \le i < j \le q\} \tag{5.48}$$

in $\mathbb{R}^q$ in which A lies.

Finally, the *permutohedron determined by* A is defined by

$$\mathsf{P}(A) := \mathsf{P}(\boldsymbol{\Phi}(A)) . \tag{5.49}$$

Note that $\boldsymbol{\pi}(A)$ is a vertex of $\mathsf{P}(A)$.

Theorem 17. *Let* $A \in \mathsf{F}(\boldsymbol{a}^1, \ldots, \boldsymbol{a}^n)$. *Then* A *is real-minimal if, and only if,*

$$\mathsf{P}(A) \cap \boldsymbol{\Phi}(\mathsf{F}(\boldsymbol{a}^1, \ldots, \boldsymbol{a}^n)) = \{\boldsymbol{\Phi}(A)\} . \tag{5.50}$$

Proof. Suppose first that there is some $B \in \mathsf{F}(\boldsymbol{a}^1, \ldots, \boldsymbol{a}^n)$, $B \ne A$, such that $\boldsymbol{\Phi}(B) \in \mathsf{P}(A)$. Then, by Theorem 2, $\boldsymbol{\pi}(B) \preceq \boldsymbol{\pi}(A)$. Since $A \ne B$, there is some $0 < \varepsilon < 1$ such that $\boldsymbol{\pi}(\varepsilon A + (1 - \varepsilon)B) \ne \boldsymbol{\pi}(A)$. Let $C = \varepsilon A + (1 - \varepsilon)B$; then, by convexity, $\boldsymbol{\Phi}(C)$ is in $\mathsf{P}(A) \cap \boldsymbol{\Phi}(\mathsf{F}(\boldsymbol{a}^1, \ldots, \boldsymbol{a}^n))$. Therefore, Theorem 2 implies that $\boldsymbol{\pi}(C) \prec \boldsymbol{\pi}(A)$; so, A is not real-minimal. Conversely, if A is not real-minimal, then there is some $B \in \mathsf{F}(\boldsymbol{a}^1, \ldots, \boldsymbol{a}^n)$ such that $\boldsymbol{\pi}(B) \prec \boldsymbol{\pi}(A)$. Thus, $B \ne A$, and by Theorem 2, $\boldsymbol{\Phi}(B)$ is in $\mathsf{P}(A) \cap \boldsymbol{\Phi}(\mathsf{F}(\boldsymbol{a}^1, \ldots, \boldsymbol{a}^n))$. □

Note that if $A \in \mathsf{T}(\boldsymbol{a}^1, \ldots, \boldsymbol{a}^n)$, then $\mathsf{P}(A)$ is in the first orthant. Therefore,

$$\mathsf{P}(A) \cap \boldsymbol{\Phi}(\mathsf{F}(\boldsymbol{a}^1, \ldots, \boldsymbol{a}^n)) = \mathsf{P}(A) \cap \boldsymbol{\Phi}(\mathsf{T}(\boldsymbol{a}^1, \ldots, \boldsymbol{a}^n)) . \tag{5.51}$$

Thus, in this case, we have

Corollary 6. *Let* $A \in \mathsf{T}(\boldsymbol{a}^1, \ldots, \boldsymbol{a}^n)$. *Then* A *is real-minimal if, and only if,*

$$\mathsf{P}(A) \cap \boldsymbol{\Phi}(\mathsf{T}(\boldsymbol{a}^1, \ldots, \boldsymbol{a}^n)) = \{\boldsymbol{\Phi}(A)\} . \tag{5.52}$$

Corollary 7. *Let* $A \in \mathsf{F}(\boldsymbol{a}^1, \ldots, \boldsymbol{a}^n)$. *Then* A *is real-minimal if, and only if, there is a hyperplane* $H \subset \mathbb{R}^q$ *that contains* $\boldsymbol{\Phi}(\mathsf{F}(\boldsymbol{a}^1, \ldots, \boldsymbol{a}^n))$ *and satisfies* $\mathsf{P}(A) \cap H = \{\boldsymbol{\Phi}(A)\}$.

Corollary 8. *If* $A \in \mathsf{F}(\boldsymbol{a}^1, \ldots, \boldsymbol{a}^n)$ *is real-minimal, then* A *is* $\boldsymbol{\pi}$-*unique.*

The following lemma is analogous to part (ii) of Theorem 1 in [28].

Lemma 9. *Suppose* $\boldsymbol{a}^1, \ldots, \boldsymbol{a}^n$ *are partitions. If* $A \in \mathsf{F}(\boldsymbol{a}^1, \ldots, \boldsymbol{a}^n)$ *is real-minimal, then* A *is a hyperpartition.*

Proof. Suppose A is not a hyperpartition. Then there are $\boldsymbol{k}$, $\boldsymbol{l} \in B(\boldsymbol{q})$ and $1 \leq i \leq n$, such that $k_i < l_i$, $k_j = l_j$, for $j \neq i$ and $A(\boldsymbol{k}) < A(\boldsymbol{l})$. Since $a^i_{k_i} \geq a^i_{l_i}$, there must exist $\boldsymbol{s}$, $\boldsymbol{t} \in B(\boldsymbol{q})$ such that $s_i = k_i$, $t_i = l_i$, $s_j = t_j$, for $j \neq i$ and $A(\boldsymbol{s}) > A(\boldsymbol{t})$. Choose $\varepsilon > 0$ such that $A(\boldsymbol{k}) + \varepsilon < A(\boldsymbol{l}) - \varepsilon$ and $A(\boldsymbol{s}) - \varepsilon > A(\boldsymbol{t}) + \varepsilon$. Let B be defined by $B(\boldsymbol{k}) = A(\boldsymbol{k}) + \varepsilon$, $B(\boldsymbol{l}) = A(\boldsymbol{l}) - \varepsilon$, $B(\boldsymbol{s}) = A(\boldsymbol{s}) - \varepsilon$, $B(\boldsymbol{t}) = A(\boldsymbol{t}) + \varepsilon$ and $B(\boldsymbol{m}) = A(\boldsymbol{m})$ for $\boldsymbol{m} \neq \boldsymbol{k}, \boldsymbol{l}, \boldsymbol{s}, \boldsymbol{t}$. Then, since $(A(\boldsymbol{l}), A(\boldsymbol{k})) \succ (A(\boldsymbol{l}) - \varepsilon, A(\boldsymbol{k}) + \varepsilon)$ and $(A(\boldsymbol{s}), A(\boldsymbol{t})) \succ (A(\boldsymbol{s}) - \varepsilon, A(\boldsymbol{t}) + \varepsilon)$, by Lemma 1, $\boldsymbol{\pi}(A) \succ \boldsymbol{\pi}(B)$. But $B \in \mathsf{F}(\boldsymbol{a}^1, \ldots, \boldsymbol{a}^n)$, then A is not real-minimal. $\qquad \square$

Theorem 18. *Let* $A \in \mathsf{M}(\boldsymbol{a}^1, \ldots, \boldsymbol{a}^n)$ *with π-sequence ρ. Then A is minimal if, and only if,*

$$\mathsf{P}(A) \cap \boldsymbol{\Phi}(\mathsf{T}(\boldsymbol{a}^1, \ldots, \boldsymbol{a}^n)) \cap \mathbb{Z}^q = \{ \boldsymbol{\Phi}(B) \mid B \in \mathsf{M}_\rho(\boldsymbol{a}^1, \ldots, \boldsymbol{a}^n) \} . \quad (5.53)$$

Proof. This is similar to the proof of Theorem 17. Note that the right-hand side is always contained in $\mathsf{P}(A) \cap \boldsymbol{\Phi}(\mathsf{T}(\boldsymbol{a}^1, \ldots, \boldsymbol{a}^n)) \cap \mathbb{Z}^q$. Suppose, first, that there is some $B \in \mathsf{M}(\boldsymbol{a}^1, \ldots, \boldsymbol{a}^n)$ with $\boldsymbol{\Phi}(B) \in \mathsf{P}(A)$ and $\boldsymbol{\pi}(B) \neq \boldsymbol{\pi}(A)$. Then, by Theorem 2; $\boldsymbol{\pi}(B) \prec \boldsymbol{\pi}(A)$, thus, A is not minimal. Conversely, if A is not minimal, there is some $B \in \mathsf{M}(\boldsymbol{a}^1, \ldots, \boldsymbol{a}^n)$ such that $\boldsymbol{\pi}(B) \prec \boldsymbol{\pi}(A)$; thus, $\boldsymbol{\Phi}(B) \in \mathsf{P}(A) \cap \boldsymbol{\Phi}(\mathsf{F}(\boldsymbol{a}^1, \ldots, \boldsymbol{a}^n)) \cap \mathbb{Z}^q$, and $\boldsymbol{\pi}(B) \neq \boldsymbol{\pi}(A)$. $\qquad \square$

Corollary 9. *Let* $A \in \mathsf{M}(\boldsymbol{a}^1, \ldots, \boldsymbol{a}^n)$. *Then A is minimal and π-unique if, and only if,*

$$\mathsf{P}(A) \cap \boldsymbol{\Phi}(\mathsf{T}(\boldsymbol{a}^1, \ldots, \boldsymbol{a}^n)) \cap \mathbb{Z}^q = \{ \boldsymbol{\Phi}(A) \} . \quad (5.54)$$

This corollary yields a new characterization, via Theorem 11, for a binary matrix X to be a matrix of uniqueness. Recall the definition of the projection of X after Theorem 13.

Corollary 10. *Let* X *be a pyramid with 1-marginals* $\boldsymbol{a}^1, \boldsymbol{a}^2, \ldots, \boldsymbol{a}^{n+1}$, *and let A be the projection of X. Then X is a matrix of uniqueness if, and only if,*

$$\mathsf{P}(A) \cap \boldsymbol{\Phi}(\mathsf{T}(\boldsymbol{a}^1, \ldots, \boldsymbol{a}^n)) \cap \mathbb{Z}^q = \{ \boldsymbol{\Phi}(A) \} . \quad (5.55)$$

Proposition 2. *Let* A^* *be the optimal solution to the problem*

$$\begin{aligned} &\min && \textstyle\sum_{\boldsymbol{k} \in B(\boldsymbol{q})} A(\boldsymbol{k})^2, \\ &\text{subject to} && A \in \mathsf{T}(\boldsymbol{a}^1, \ldots, \boldsymbol{a}^n) . \end{aligned} \quad (5.56)$$

Then A^* is real-minimal.

Proof. If A^* were not real-minimal, there would exist $B \in \mathsf{T}(\boldsymbol{a}^1, \ldots, \boldsymbol{a}^n)$ such that $\boldsymbol{\pi}(B) \prec \boldsymbol{\pi}(A^*)$. Then, by Rado's theorem, $B \in \mathsf{P}(A^*)$. Since the vertices of $\mathsf{P}(A^*)$ are all contained in the sphere S with center in the origin and radius $\sqrt{\sum_{\boldsymbol{k}} A^*(\boldsymbol{k})^2}$, and since B is not a vertex of $\mathsf{P}(A^*)$, B is in the interior of S, contradicting the optimality of A^*. $\qquad \square$

The same proof yields the following:

Proposition 3. *Let A^* be an optimal solution to the problem*

$$\min \qquad \sum_{k \in B(q)} A(k)^2,$$
$$\text{subject to} \quad A \in \mathsf{M}(a^1, \ldots, a^n).$$

(5.57)

Then A^* is minimal.

Remark 7. Propositions 2 and 3 still hold if $\sum_k A(k)^2$ is substituted by any strictly Schur-convex function defined on the first orthant. The proof is essentially the same as the one we gave above and follows from the very definition of Schur-convexity. See [20, Chapter 3] for many examples of Schur-convex functions and their applications.

Remark 8. A particular case of an algorithm due to M. Minoux [21] can be used to obtain, in polynomial time, an optimal solution to the optimization problem in Proposition 3. Therefore, there is a polynomial-time algorithm that produces a minimal matrix in $\mathsf{M}(a^1, \ldots, a^n)$ for any 1-marginals $a^1, \ldots, a^n$.

5.9 Real-Minimal and Additive Matrices

In this section we show the equivalence of real-minimality and additivity. This gives a description of additivity in terms of majorization, providing, in this way, a new approach to this notion. This also makes more transparent the relation between uniqueness and $(0, 1)$-additivity for a binary matrix and yields a new proof that $(0, 1)$-additivity is sufficient for uniqueness (Theorem 5). The results presented here were obtained by S. Onn and the author for 2-dimensional matrices in [23]; their generalization to any dimension is easy, but requires some care.

Proposition 4. *Let $A \in \mathsf{F}(a^1, \ldots, a^n)$, $a = \pi(A)$, and $a_\sigma = \Phi(A)$ for some permutation σ. Then A is real-minimal if, and only if, there is some vector $n \in \mathbb{R}^q$ such that*

(1) n is orthogonal to $\Phi(\mathsf{F}(a^1, \ldots, a^n))$.
(2) For any transposition τ adjacent relative to a, one has the inequality $\langle n, a_{\tau\sigma} - a_\sigma \rangle > 0$.

Proof. Suppose first that A is real-minimal. Then, by Corollary 7, there is a hyperplane H containing $\Phi(\mathsf{F}(a^1, \ldots, a^n))$ such that $\mathsf{P}(a_\sigma) \cap H = \{a_\sigma\}$. Therefore, there is a nonzero vector n, orthogonal to H, such that for all $x \in \mathsf{P}(a_\sigma)$, $x \neq a_\sigma$, one has $\langle n, x - a_\sigma \rangle > 0$. Then (1) and (2) hold. For the converse, suppose that there is some vector $n \in \mathbb{R}^q$ satisfying conditions (1) and (2). Let H be the hyperplane orthogonal to n containing a_σ. Since, by Theorem 1, the vertices of $\mathsf{P}(a_\sigma)$ adjacent to a_σ have the form $a_{\tau\sigma}$ for some transposition τ adjacent relative to a, condition (2) implies that $\langle n, x - a_\sigma \rangle > 0$ for all $x \in \mathsf{P}(a_\sigma)$ such that $x \neq a_\sigma$. Therefore, $\mathsf{P}(a_\sigma) \cap H = \{a_\sigma\}$. Condition (1) implies that $\mathbf{\Phi}(\mathsf{F}(a^1, \ldots, a^n)) \subseteq H$; therefore, $\mathsf{P}(A) \cap \mathbf{\Phi}(\mathsf{F}(a^1, \ldots, a^n)) = \{a_\sigma\}$. Then Theorem 17 implies that A is real-minimal. □

The set $\mathsf{F}(a^1, \ldots, a^n)$ is just the set of solutions of a system of linear equations. We describe below the matrix of coefficients of this system. In what follows we adopt the common convention that when a vector x with k coordinates is used in a matrix equation, x will denote the corresponding matrix of size $k \times 1$ and x^T will denote the corresponding matrix of size $1 \times k$. Let

$$m := (a_1^1, \ldots, a_{q_1}^1, a_1^2, \ldots, a_{q_2}^2, \ldots, a_1^n, \ldots, a_{q_n}^n), \tag{5.58}$$

and let $p = q_1 + \cdots + q_n$. We define a matrix T of size $p \times q$ as follows: Its rows will be indexed by the set of pairs (i, j) such that $1 \leq i \leq n$ and $1 \leq j \leq q_i$; they are arranged in lexicographic order. In practice, the pair (i, j) corresponds to the coordinate a_j^i of m. The columns of T will be indexed by the elements of $\mathsf{B}(q)$ arranged in lexicographic order. Then T is defined by

$$T((i, j), k) := \begin{cases} 1, & \text{if } k_i = j, \\ 0, & \text{otherwise.} \end{cases} \tag{5.59}$$

Then $\mathsf{F}(a^1, \ldots, a^n)$ equals the set of matrices A satisfying the equation

$$T\mathbf{\Phi}(A) = m . \tag{5.60}$$

For any vector $x = (x_1^1, \ldots, x_{q_1}^1, x_1^2, \ldots, x_{q_2}^2, \ldots, x_1^n, \ldots, x_{q_n}^n)$, we form a matrix $A_x : \mathsf{B}(q) \longrightarrow \mathbb{R}$ defined by $A_x(k) := \sum_{i=1}^n x_{k_i}^i$. The entries of A_x are just the numbers appearing in condition (5.35) in the definition of additivity. Then the following matrix equation holds for any x:

$$x^\mathsf{T} T = \mathbf{\Phi}(A_x) . \tag{5.61}$$

In particular, $x^\mathsf{T} T$ is orthogonal to $\mathbf{\Phi}(\mathsf{F}(a^1, \ldots, a^n))$.

Theorem 19. *Let $A \in \mathsf{F}(a^1, \ldots, a^n)$. Then A is real-minimal if, and only if, A is additive.*

Proof. Let $a = \pi(A)$. Then $\mathbf{\Phi}(A) = a_\sigma$ for some permutation σ. Suppose A is real-minimal; then by Proposition 4 there is a vector $n \in \mathbb{R}^q$ satisfying conditions (4.1) and (4.2). It follows from the proof of this proposition that $\langle n, x - a_\sigma \rangle > 0$ for all $x \in \mathsf{P}(a_\sigma)$, $x \neq a_\sigma$. Since n is orthogonal to $\mathbf{\Phi}(\mathsf{F}(a^1, \ldots, a^n))$, n is in the row space of T. Therefore, there is a vector x such that $-n = x^\mathsf{T} T$ or $n = -\mathbf{\Phi}(A_x)$. In order to prove that A is additive, we take $k, l \in \mathsf{B}(q)$ such that $A(k) > A(l)$. We have to show, by condition (5.35), that $A_x(k) = \sum_i x_{k_i}^i > \sum_i x_{l_i}^i = A_x(l)$. Suppose that, under the identity $a_\sigma = \mathbf{\Phi}(A)$, $A(k)$ corresponds to $a_{\sigma(s)}$ and $A(l)$ to $a_{\sigma(t)}$. Then

$n_s = -A_{\boldsymbol{x}}(\boldsymbol{k})$ and $n_t = -A_{\boldsymbol{x}}(\boldsymbol{l})$. Let $\tau = (\sigma(s)\ \sigma(t))$. Then $\langle \boldsymbol{n}, \boldsymbol{a}_{\tau\sigma} - \boldsymbol{a}_\sigma \rangle > 0$. But since

$$
\begin{aligned}
\langle \boldsymbol{n}, \boldsymbol{a}_{\tau\sigma} - \boldsymbol{a}_\sigma \rangle &= n_s(a_{\sigma(t)} - a_{\sigma(s)}) + n_t(a_{\sigma(s)} - a_{\sigma(t)}) \\
&= A_{\boldsymbol{x}}(\boldsymbol{k})[A(\boldsymbol{k}) - A(\boldsymbol{l})] - A_{\boldsymbol{x}}(\boldsymbol{l})[A(\boldsymbol{k}) - A(\boldsymbol{l})] ,
\end{aligned}
\tag{5.62}
$$

we conclude that $A_{\boldsymbol{x}}(\boldsymbol{k})[A(\boldsymbol{k}) - A(\boldsymbol{l})] > A_{\boldsymbol{x}}(\boldsymbol{l})[A(\boldsymbol{k}) - A(\boldsymbol{l})]$. But if $A(\boldsymbol{k}) > A(\boldsymbol{l})$, then $A_{\boldsymbol{x}}(\boldsymbol{k}) > A_{\boldsymbol{x}}(\boldsymbol{l})$. Therefore, A is additive.

The converse is similar. Assume that A is additive; then there are real vectors $\boldsymbol{x}^1, \ldots, \boldsymbol{x}^n$, satisfying condition (5.35). To prove that A is real-minimal, we use the equivalence given in Proposition 4. Let $\boldsymbol{x} = (x_j^i)$ and $\boldsymbol{n} = -\boldsymbol{x}^\mathsf{T} \cdot T$, then $\boldsymbol{n}$ is in the row space of T, so $\boldsymbol{n}$ is orthogonal to $\boldsymbol{\Phi}(\mathsf{F}(\boldsymbol{a}^1, \ldots, \boldsymbol{a}^n))$. Let τ be an transposition adjacent relative to $\boldsymbol{a}$. Let $\boldsymbol{k}, \boldsymbol{l} \in \mathsf{B}(\boldsymbol{q})$ be such that under the identity $\boldsymbol{\Phi}(A) = \boldsymbol{a}_\sigma$, entry $A(\boldsymbol{k})$ corresponds to $a_{\sigma(s)}$ and entry $A(\boldsymbol{l})$ corresponds to $a_{\sigma(t)}$. Without loss of generality, we assume that $A(\boldsymbol{k}) > A(\boldsymbol{l})$. Then, by condition (5.35), we have $A_{\boldsymbol{x}}(\boldsymbol{k}) > A_{\boldsymbol{x}}(\boldsymbol{l})$. Then identity (5.62) implies $\langle \boldsymbol{n}, \boldsymbol{a}_{\tau\sigma} - \boldsymbol{a}_\sigma \rangle > 0$. The claim follows.   □

Proof (of Theorem 5). Let X be a $(0,1)$-additive matrix. Assume, without loss of generality, that its 1-marginals are partitions. Then, by Theorem 14, X is the graph $\mathsf{G}(A)$ of an additive matrix A. Theorem 19 implies that A is real-minimal, therefore A is minimal, and, by Corollary 8, A is π-unique. Finally, Theorem 11 implies that X is a matrix of uniqueness.   □

Acknowledgments

Supported by DGAPA UNAM, Grant No. IN-111203, and by Consejo Nacional de Ciencia y Tecnología, Mexico, Grant No. 47086-F. I would also like to thank Pedro David Sánchez Salazar for providing the figures for this chapter.

References

1. Avella-Alaminos, D., Vallejo, E.: Kronecker products and RSK-correspondences for 3-dimensional matrices. In preparation.
2. Billera, L.J., Sarangarajan, A.: The combinatorics of permutation polytopes. In: Billera, L.J., Greene, C., Simion, R., Stanley R.P. (eds.), *Formal Power Series and Algebraic Combinatorics 1994*, DIMACS Series in Discrete Mathematics and Theoretical Computer Science, Vol. 24, AMS, Providence, RI, pp. 1–23 (1996).
3. Brylawsky, T.: The lattice of integer partitions. *Discr. Math.*, **6**, 201–219 (1973).
4. Brualdi, R.A.: Matrices of zeros and ones with fixed row and column sum vectors. *Lin. Algebra Appl.*, **33**, 159–231 (1980).
5. Brualdi, R.A.: Minimal nonnegative integral matrices and uniquely determined (0,1)-matrices. *Lin. Algebra Appl.*, **341**, 351–356 (2002).

6. Brunetti, S., Del Lungo, A., Gerard, Y.: On the computational complexity of reconstructing three-dimensional lattice sets from their two-dimensional X-rays. *Lin. Algebra Appl.*, **339**, 59–73 (2001).
7. De Loera, J., Onn, S.: The complexity of three-way statistical tables. *SIAM J. Comput.*, **33**, 819–836 (2004).
8. Díaz-Leal, H., Martínez-Bernal, J., Romero, D.: Dimension of the fixed point set of a nilpotent endomorphism on the flag variety. *Bol. Soc. Mat. Mexicana (3)*, **7**, 23–33 (2001).
9. Fishburn, P.C., Lagarias, J.C., Reeds, J.A., Shepp, L.A.: Sets uniquely determined by projections on axes II. Discrete case. *Discr. Math.*, **91**, 149–159 (1991).
10. Fishburn, P.C., Shepp, L.A.: Sets of uniqueness and additivity in integer lattices. In: Herman, G.T., Kuba, A. (eds.), *Discrete Tomography: Foundations, Algorithms, and Applications*, Birkhäuser, Boston, MA, pp. 35–58 (1999).
11. Gale, D.: A theorem of flows in networks. *Pacific J. of Math.*, **7**, 1073–1082 (1957).
12. Gritzmann, P., de Vries, S.: On the algorithmic inversion of the discrete Radon transform. *Theor. Comp. Science*, **281**, 455–469 (2001).
13. Gaiha, P., Gupta, S.K.: Adjacent vertices on a permutohedron. *SIAM J. Appl. Math.*, **32**, 323–327 (1977).
14. Grünbaum, B.: *Convex Polytopes*, 2nd edition. Springer, Berlin, Germany (2003).
15. Hardy, G., Littlewood, J.E., Pólya, G.: *Inequalities*, 2nd edition Cambridge Univ. Press, Cambridge, UK (1952).
16. Klee, V., Witzgall, C.: Facets and vertices of transportation polytopes. In: *Mathematics of Decision Sciences, Part I*. Amer. Math. Soc., Providence, RI, pp. 257–282 (1968).
17. Kong, T.Y., Herman, G.T.: On which grids can tomographic equivalence of binary pictures be characterized in terms of elementary switching operations? *Int. J. Imaging Syst. Technol.*, **9**, 118–125 (1998).
18. Kuba, A., Herman, G.T.: Discrete tomography: A historical overview. In: Herman, G.T., Kuba, A. (eds.), *Discrete Tomography. Foundations, Algorithms, and Applications*. Birkhäuser, Boston, MA, pp. 3–34 (1999).
19. Jurkat, W.B., Ryser H.J.: Extremal configurations and decomposition theorems I. *J. Algebra*, **8**, 194–222 (1968).
20. Marshall, A.W., Olkin, I.: *Inequalities: Theory of Majorization and Its Applications*. Academic Press, New York, NY (1979).
21. Minoux, M.: Solving integer minimum cost flows with separable convex cost objective polynomially. *Math. Programm. Stud.*, **26**, 237–239 (1986).
22. Muirhead, R.F.: Some methods applicable to identities and inequalities of symmetric algebraic functions of n letters. *Proc. Edinburgh Math. Soc.*, **21**, 144–157 (1903).
23. Onn, S., Vallejo, E.: Permutohedra and minimal matrices. *Lin. Algebra Appl.*, **412**, 471–489 (2006).
24. Rado, R.: An inequality. *J. London Math. Soc.*, **27**, 1–6 (1952).
25. Ryser, H.J.: Combinatorial properties of matrices of zeros and ones. *Canad. J. Math.*, **9**, 371–377 (1957).
26. Ryser, H.: *Combinatorial Mathematics*, Mathematical Association of America, Washington, DC (1963).
27. Snapper, E.: Group characters and nonnegative integral matrices. *J. Algebra*, **19**, 520–535 (1971).

28. Torres-Cházaro, A., Vallejo, E.: Sets of uniqueness and minimal matrices. *J. Algebra*, **208**, 444–451 (1998).
29. Vallejo, E.: Reductions of additive sets, sets of uniqueness and pyramids. *Discr. Math.*, **173**, 257–267 (1997).
30. Vallejo, E.: Plane partitions and characters of the symmetric group. *J. Algebraic Comb.*, **11**, 79–88 (2000).
31. Vallejo, E.: The classification of minimal matrices of size $2 \times q$. *Lin. Algebra Appl.*, **340**, 169–181 (2002).
32. Vallejo, E.: A characterization of additive sets. *Discr. Math.*, **259**, 201–210 (2002).
33. Vallejo, E.: Minimal matrices and discrete tomography. *Electr. Notes Discr. Math.*, **20**, 113–132 (2005).
34. Yemelichev, V.A., Kovalev, M.M., Kravtsov, M.K.: *Polytopes, Graphs and Optimisation*. Cambridge University Press, Cambridge, UK (1984).

6

Constructing $(0, 1)$-Matrices
with Given Line Sums and Certain Fixed Zeros

R.A. Brualdi and G. Dahl

Summary. Consider the class $\mathcal{A}_P(R, S)$ of $(0, 1)$-matrices with row sum vector R, column sum vector S, and zeros in all positions outside a certain set P. It is assumed that P satisfies a certain monotonicity property. We show the existence of a canonical matrix in this matrix class and give a simple algorithm for finding this matrix. Moreover, a classical interchange result of Ryser is generalized to the class $\mathcal{A}_P(R, S)$ and the uniqueness question for the class $\mathcal{A}_P(R, S)$ is discussed.

6.1 Introduction

Let m and n be positive integers and let $R = (r_1, r_2, \ldots, r_m)$ and $S = (s_1, s_2, \ldots, s_n)$ be nonnegative integral vectors satisfying $\sum_{i=1}^m r_i = \sum_{j=1}^n s_j$. We consider the class of $(0, 1)$-matrices with row sum vector R and column sum vector S, where ones are permitted only in a set P of positions. More precisely, let $\mathcal{A}_P(R, S)$ be the set of all $(0, 1)$-matrices $A = [a_{ij}]$ of size $m \times n$ that satisfy

$$\sum_{j=1}^n a_{ij} = r_i \quad (i \leq m),$$
$$\sum_{i=1}^m a_{ij} = s_j \quad (j \leq n),$$

and

$$a_{ij} = 0 \quad \text{for all } (i, j) \notin P. \tag{6.1}$$

Define the row index sets $P_j = \{i \leq m \mid (i, j) \in P\}$ $(j \leq n)$. We assume throughout the paper that the sets P_j $(j \leq n)$ satisfy the following condition:

$$\text{for each } i < j \text{ either } P_i \supseteq P_j \text{ or } P_i \cap P_j = \emptyset. \tag{6.2}$$

Thus, if a one is permitted in position (i, j), i.e., $i \in P_j$, then it is also permitted to place a one in all those positions (i, k) with $k < j$ for which $P_k \cap P_j \neq \emptyset$. The following matrix illustrates a possible pattern satisfying (6.2), where $m = 7$, $n = 13$, and positions in P are indicated by '$*$':

$$
\begin{bmatrix}
* & 0 & * & * & 0 & 0 & * & * & * & 0 & * & 0 & * \\
* & 0 & * & * & 0 & 0 & * & * & * & 0 & * & 0 & * \\
* & 0 & * & * & 0 & 0 & * & * & * & 0 & * & 0 & 0 \\
* & 0 & * & * & 0 & 0 & 0 & 0 & 0 & 0 & * & 0 & 0 \\
* & 0 & * & * & 0 & 0 & 0 & 0 & 0 & 0 & * & 0 & 0 \\
* & * & 0 & 0 & 0 & * & 0 & 0 & 0 & * & 0 & 0 & 0 \\
* & * & 0 & 0 & 0 & * & 0 & 0 & 0 & * & 0 & 0 & 0
\end{bmatrix} . \tag{6.3}
$$

We give some remarks related to assumption (6.2) on the sets P_j $(j \leq n)$.

(a) The following more general condition may be reduced to (6.2) after suitable reordering of the P_j's: $P_i \cap P_j = \emptyset$ or $P_i \subseteq P_j$ or $P_j \subseteq P_i$.

(b) It may also be of interest to consider matrices where certain entries are fixed to either zero or one. By replacing the fixed ones by zeros and updating row and column sums accordingly, one obtains an equivalent situation where certain entries are fixed to zero only. Thus, one obtains the situation treated in this paper provided that the remaining positions P_j satisfy condition (6.2).

(c) An interesting special case is when P is specified by a vector $K = (k_1, k_2, \ldots, k_n)$ satisfying $k_1 \geq k_2 \geq \cdots \geq k_n$ and for each $j \leq n$

$$
P_j = \{1, 2, \ldots, k_j\} . \tag{6.4}
$$

In this special case the position set P forms a Young diagram, so we say that P is a *Young-pattern* given by $K = (k_1, k_2, \ldots, k_n)$. Note that if $K = (m, m, \ldots, m)$, that is, $P = \{1, 2, \ldots, m\} \times \{1, 2, \ldots, n\}$, then $A_P(R, S)$ coincides with the well-known matrix class $A(R, S)$ of $(0, 1)$-matrices with row sum vector R and column sum vector S. We refer to [5] for a treatment of $A(R, S)$.

Note also that we do not require R or S to be monotone. Here, and later, we call a vector *monotone* if its components are nonincreasing.

The main contribution of this chapter is to generalize some results known for $A(R, S)$ to the class $A_P(R, S)$. These results include the existence of a canonical matrix in the class having certain properties and a simple extension of Ryser's algorithm for finding this canonical matrix. Moreover, an interchange result is generalized, and the uniqueness question for the class $A_P(R, S)$ is discussed.

A motivation for this work is in the area of discrete tomography, where $(0, 1)$-matrices with given line sums correspond to binary images with horizontal and vertical projections. If one knows that the image contains zeros in certain positions (satisfying (6.2)), one gets the problem discussed in this chapter. Moreover, this work extends some results in our previous paper [6], where we focused on the matrix class where P was a Young-pattern given by $K = (m, m, \ldots, m, k, k, \ldots, k)$ for some $k \leq m$. An introduction to discrete tomography can be found in [12]; see also the special issue of *Linear Algebra and Its Applications* [9]. For an extensive survey of the class $A(R, S)$, see [5].

The classical Gale–Ryser theorem says that the class $\mathcal{A}(R,S)$ is nonempty if, and only if, a simple majorization condition on R and S holds (S is majorized by the conjugate of R), see, e.g., the mentioned survey paper or the book [7].

Our work is related to paper [8], where Chen considered the class of integral matrices with given row and column sums and where each entry lies between a given lower and upper bound. This class includes our class $\mathcal{A}_P(R,S)$. The paper [8] contains an existence characterization of majorization type and studied an associated structure matrix. However, these results were shown under certain assumptions on the given vectors R and S and on the set P that do not include the situation considered in this chapter. A similar characterization in a restricted situation are found in [15]. In [3] a theorem was proved for a nonempty class $\mathcal{A}(R,S)$, where R and S are monotone and of the same size n. The theorem gives a simple necessary and sufficient condition for the class to contain a triangular matrix; in our notation this corresponds to a Young-pattern with $K=(n,n-1,\ldots,1)$. This condition is simply that $r_i \leq n-i+1$ and $s_i \leq n-i+1$ $(1 \leq i \leq n)$. Moreover, in [4] Anstee generalized the Gale–Ryser theorem to the situation where certain entries were fixed to 1 (but at most one such fixed 1 in each column). A related result was established in [11], where Fulkerson gave a characterization of the existence of $(0,1)$-matrices with given line sums and zero trace. More recently Kuba ([13]) discussed when $\mathcal{A}(R,S)$ contains a unique matrix with certain fixed zeros and ones. He characterized this situation in terms of certain sequences and also considered a reconstruction algorithm. Finally, we mention that the problem of constructing a matrix in $\mathcal{A}(R,S)$ with fixed ones and zeros in *any* set of positions may be solved efficiently as a maximum flow problem in a certain capacitated digraph (see the discussion of the feasible network flow problem in, e.g., [2] or [7]). Still, it is of interest to find theoretical results and simpler algorithms for more restricted situations, and the present chapter has this focus.

In this chapter, by the *class* of a matrix A we mean the class of $(0,1)$-matrices of the same size as A and having the same row and column sum vectors as A. For a matrix A and index sets I and J, we let $A(I,J)$ denote the submatrix of A consisting of the entries in rows indexed by I and columns indexed by J. Similarly, $A(:,J)$ is the submatrix of A containing (all rows and) columns indexed by J, and $A(:,j)$ is the jth column of A.

6.2 The Canonical Matrix

For the class $\mathcal{A}(R,S)$ the well-known Ryser's algorithm, introduced in [16], may be used to find a matrix in that class. The algorithm is simple (and efficient), and it actually constructs a canonical matrix in the class having certain properties; see [5]. We now follow a similar pattern for the more general class $\mathcal{A}_P(R,S)$ by performing the following steps:

1. Show the existence of a canonical matrix $\tilde{A}$ in the class $\mathcal{A}_P(R,S)$.

2. Use the special properties of this canonical matrix $\tilde{A}$ to set up an algorithm for finding $\tilde{A}$ column by column.

Before we start we remark, one may also use general network flow algorithms (see [2]) for finding a matrix in $\mathcal{A}_P(R, S)$, but our algorithm is much simpler (and faster).

As for the basic class $\mathcal{A}(R, S)$, the notion of an interchange is a central ingredient in our approach. An *interchange* applied to a $(0, 1)$-matrix A replaces a submatrix of order 2 of one of the forms

$$T_1 = \begin{bmatrix} 1 & 0 \\ 0 & 1 \end{bmatrix} \text{ and } T_2 = \begin{bmatrix} 0 & 1 \\ 1 & 0 \end{bmatrix} \tag{6.5}$$

by the other.

Ryser proved that given two matrices A and B in $\mathcal{A}(R, S)$, A can be transformed into B by a sequence of interchanges. Let $A \in \mathcal{A}_P(R, S)$ and assume that the 2×2 submatrix $A[\{i, j\}, \{k, l\}]$, where $i < j$ and $k < l$, is equal to T_1. This implies that $i \in P_k$ and $j \in P_l$. Assume, furthermore, that $i \in P_l$. Then $P_k \cap P_l \neq \emptyset$ (as $i \in P_k \cap P_l$), so by assumption (6.2) we must have $P_l \subseteq P_k$. Therefore, the matrix obtained from A by replacing the mentioned submatrix by T_2 will also lie in $\mathcal{A}_P(R, S)$. This operation will be called a $T_1 T_2$-*interchange*. The operation $T_2 T_1$-*interchange* is defined similarly.

Lemma 1. *Assume that $\mathcal{A}_P(R, S)$ is nonempty. Then $\mathcal{A}_P(R, S)$ contains a matrix $\widehat{A}$ where the 1's in column n appear in those rows in P_n in which r_i is largest, giving preference to the bottommost positions in case of ties.*

Proof. Let $A \in \mathcal{A}_P(R, S)$. Assume that $i, k \in P_n$ are such that $r_i > r_k$, $a_{in} = 0$, and $a_{kn} = 1$. Then (as $r_i > r_k$) there must be a $j < n$ such that $a_{ij} = 1$ and $a_{kj} = 0$. We then apply a ($T_1 T_2$- or $T_2 T_1$-) interchange to A (involving rows i, k and columns j, n) and thereby get a matrix that also lies in $\mathcal{A}_P(R, S)$ as $i, k \in P_n \subseteq P_j$. Note that here we used the chain assumption (6.2). Repeating this operation results in a matrix A^1 having the 1's in column n in those rows in P_n in which A has the largest row sums. Assume now that $i, k \in P_n$ are such that $i < k$, $r_i = r_k$, $a_{in} = 1$, and $a_{kn} = 0$. Then there must be a $j < n$ such that $a_{ij} = 0$ and $a_{kj} = 1$ so we apply an $T_2 T_1$-interchange involving rows i, k and columns j, n. The new matrix lies in $\mathcal{A}_P(R, S)$ as $i, k \in P_n \subseteq P_j$. By repeating this operation, we obtain a matrix $\widehat{A}$ with the desired properties. □

The matrix $\widehat{A}$ described in Lemma 1 may not be unique. But the last column is unique, and it is found directly from P_n, R, and s_n. We call any such matrix $\widehat{A}$ a *last-column canonical* matrix in the class $\mathcal{A}_P(R, S)$. Note that all matrices obtained from a last-column canonical matrix by deleting its last column must belong to the same matrix class (as the last column of $\widehat{A}$ is fixed).

We now apply the result in Lemma 1 recursively.

Theorem 1. *Assume that $\mathcal{A}_P(R,S)$ is nonempty. Then $\mathcal{A}_P(R,S)$ contains a unique matrix $\widetilde{A}$ such that for each $k \le n$ the submatrix $\widetilde{A}_k$ consisting of the first k columns of $\widetilde{A}$ is a last-column canonical matrix in its class.*

Proof. We shall construct $\widetilde{A}$ column by column. We may, using Lemma 1, find a last-column canonical matrix $\widehat{A}$ in $\mathcal{A}_P(R,S)$ and set $\check{A}(:,n) = \widehat{A}(:,n)$. Consider next the matrix $A' = \widehat{A}(:,\{1,2,\ldots,n-1\})$ and choose a last-column canonical matrix B in the class of A'. Let column $n-1$ of $\widetilde{A}$ be equal to the last column of B. Proceed like this and construct columns $n-2,\ldots,1$ of $\widetilde{A}$. Then $\widetilde{A}$ is the unique matrix with the desired properties stated in the theorem. $\square$

The matrix $\widetilde{A}$ described in Theorem 1 is called the *canonical matrix* in the class $\mathcal{A}_P(R,S)$. In the next section we discuss an algorithm for finding $\widetilde{A}$.

6.3 The Generalized Ryser Algorithm

The proof of Theorem 1 is constructive and it actually contains an algorithm for finding the canonical matrix. We call this procedure the generalized Ryser algorithm as it specializes into Ryser's algorithm when $P = \{1,2,\ldots,m\} \times \{1,2,\ldots,n\}$.

Generalized Ryser Algorithm

1. (Initialize) *Let $k = n$ and let $\hat{R} = R$.*
2. (Determine column k) *Find the indices in P_k corresponding to the s_k largest positive components of $\hat{R}$, where we prefer largest indices in case of ties. Let the kth column of $\widetilde{A}$ have ones in the s_k positions just found.*
3. (Update row sum) *Let $\hat{R} = R - \widetilde{A}(:,k)$ (the row sum vector after the last column has been deleted). If $k > 1$, reduce k by 1 and go to step 2.*

Due to Theorem 1, this algorithm will find the canonical matrix $\widetilde{A}$ provided the class is nonempty. If the class is empty, the procedure will break down at some stage. We see that this happens if, in an iteration k, the present row sum vector $\hat{R}$ has fewer than s_k ones in the positions corresponding to P_k. This may be seen as an algorithmic characterization of the nonemptyness of $\mathcal{A}_P(R,S)$.

The algorithm may alternatively be presented as follows. We start with the matrix $\overline{A}$, which is the $(0,1)$-matrix of size $m \times n$ whose ith row consists of r_i leading ones followed by $n - r_i$ zeros for $i \le m$. Then we shift ones to the right as in Ryser's algorithm, except that we use only the feasible positions P_k in each column k. Thus, the procedure is

Start with $A = \overline{A}$ and construct column n by shifting ones to the right so that ones occur in those rows of P_n where A has largest row sums, using the bottommost position in case of ties. Proceed to construct column k similarly by shifting in rows in P_k for $k = n-1, \ldots, 1$.

If the procedure breaks down at some point, the only reason can be that the matrix class $\mathcal{A}_P(R, S)$ is empty.

Example 1. Let $m = 5$, $n = 8$, $R = (5, 5, 4, 4, 3)$, $S = (3, 3, 3, 3, 3, 2, 2, 2)$, and let P correspond to the Young-pattern given by $K = (5, 5, 5, 5, 4, 4, 3, 3)$. The generalized Ryser algorithm proceeds as follows (where the forced zeros are shown in boldface):

$$
\begin{bmatrix}
1&1&1&1&1&0&0&0\\
1&1&1&1&1&0&0&0\\
1&1&1&1&0&0&0&0\\
1&1&1&1&0&0&0&\mathbf{0}\\
1&1&1&0&0&0&0&\mathbf{0}
\end{bmatrix}
\rightarrow
\begin{bmatrix}
1&1&1&1&0&0&0&1\\
1&1&1&1&0&0&0&1\\
1&1&1&1&0&0&0&0\\
1&1&1&1&0&0&0&\mathbf{0}\\
1&1&1&0&0&0&0&\mathbf{0}
\end{bmatrix}
\rightarrow
\begin{bmatrix}
1&1&1&1&0&0&0&1\\
1&1&1&0&0&0&1&1\\
1&1&1&0&0&0&1&0\\
1&1&1&1&0&0&0&\mathbf{0}\\
1&1&1&0&0&0&0&\mathbf{0}
\end{bmatrix}
\rightarrow
\begin{bmatrix}
1&1&1&0&0&1&0&1\\
1&1&1&0&0&0&1&1\\
1&1&1&0&0&0&1&0\\
1&1&1&0&0&1&0&\mathbf{0}\\
1&1&1&0&0&0&0&\mathbf{0}
\end{bmatrix}
\rightarrow
$$

$$
\begin{bmatrix}
1&1&1&0&0&1&0&1\\
1&1&0&0&1&0&1&1\\
1&1&0&0&1&0&1&0\\
1&1&0&0&1&1&0&\mathbf{0}\\
1&1&1&0&0&0&0&\mathbf{0}
\end{bmatrix}
\rightarrow
\begin{bmatrix}
1&1&0&1&0&1&0&1\\
1&1&0&0&1&0&1&1\\
1&1&0&0&1&0&1&0\\
1&0&0&1&1&1&0&\mathbf{0}\\
1&1&0&1&0&0&0&\mathbf{0}
\end{bmatrix}
\rightarrow
\begin{bmatrix}
1&1&0&1&0&1&0&1\\
1&0&1&0&1&0&1&1\\
1&0&1&0&1&0&1&0\\
1&0&0&1&1&1&0&\mathbf{0}\\
1&0&1&1&0&0&0&\mathbf{0}
\end{bmatrix}
\rightarrow
\begin{bmatrix}
1&1&0&1&0&1&0&1\\
1&0&1&0&1&0&1&1\\
1&0&1&0&1&0&1&0\\
0&1&0&1&1&1&0&\mathbf{0}\\
0&1&1&1&0&0&0&\mathbf{0}
\end{bmatrix}.
$$

6.4 Interchanges

A central result concerning the matrix class $\mathcal{A}(R, S)$ was proved by Ryser in [16]. It says that one can transform any given matrix in $\mathcal{A}(R, S)$ into another given matrix using a sequence of interchanges. It is natural to ask if a similar property holds for the more general class $\mathcal{A}_P(R, S)$, and the following theorem answers this question positively.

Theorem 2. *Let A and B be two given matrices in $\mathcal{A}_P(R, S)$. Then there is a sequence of interchanges that transforms A to B with every intermediate matrix in $\mathcal{A}_P(R, S)$.*

Proof. The proofs in our Lemma 1 and Theorem 1 show that any matrix in the class $\mathcal{A}_P(R, S)$ may be transformed using interchanges into the canonical matrix $\widetilde{A}$ in that class, and all intermediate matrices belong to the class. Therefore, both A and B may be transformed into $\widetilde{A}$, so by reversing the latter interchanges we get the desired sequence of interchanges that transforms A into B. Note here that all the interchanges involved here are "feasible," i.e., they don't put ones in forbidden positions. □

An interesting question is to find a more "direct" proof of this theorem which finds suitable interchanges without going via the canonical matrix $\widetilde{A}$. In the case of $\mathcal{A}(R, S)$, such an argument is known; actually the original proof of Ryser was along these lines.

6.5 Uniqueness and a Reconstruction Algorithm

From the point of view of discrete tomography, it is of particular interest to know when $\mathcal{A}_P(R, S)$ contains a unique matrix $A = [a_{ij}]$. Such a matrix A is then uniquely reconstructible given its row and column sum vectors R and S and its prescribed zeros as specified by the pattern P. Unique reconstructability of A is equivalent to the uniqueness of a solution of the system of equations

$$\sum_{j=1}^{n} a_{ij} = r_i \quad (1 \leq i \leq m),\tag{6.6}$$

$$\sum_{i=1}^{m} a_{ij} = s_j \quad (1 \leq j \leq n),\tag{6.7}$$

$$a_{ij} = 0 \text{ or } 1 \quad ((i, j) \in P),\tag{6.8}$$

$$a_{ij} = 0 \quad ((i, j) \notin P).\tag{6.9}$$

Such uniqueness questions have been studied in [1] in a more general context where certain entries are prescribed to be 0 as in (6.9) and certain other entries are prescribed to be 1. Also, uniqueness of particular entries is considered. It is to be observed that the coefficient matrix corresponding to the linear system (6.6) and (6.7) is totally unimodular (see, e.g., Lemma 3.1 of [1]), and this facilitates the analysis. From the general theory developed in [1], there follows the uniqueness characterization given in [10] in the case that no entries are prescribed. The relevant concept is that of *additivity*, where an m by n $(0, 1)$-matrix $A = [a_{ij}]$ is additive provided there are real vectors $(x_1, x_2, \ldots, x_m)$ and $(y_1, y_2, \ldots, y_n)$ such that $a_{ij} = 1$ if, and only if, $x_i + y_j \geq 0$. Uniqueness of A is equivalent to additivity of A.

We first discuss uniqueness for a special Young-pattern and then the same question is studied for a general pattern P. We call a $(0, 1)$-matrix Y a *Young matrix* if each row and column in Y consist of a sequence of 1's followed by a sequence of 0's, i.e., the ones in Y determine a Young-pattern.

Let P be a Young-pattern given by $K = (k_1, k_2, \ldots, k_n)$ for which the class $\mathcal{A}_P(R, S)$ is nonempty. First assume that $K = (m, m, \ldots, m)$. Then $\mathcal{A}_P(R, S) = \mathcal{A}(R, S)$, and without loss of generality we may assume that R and S are monotone nonincreasing. Then it is well known [5] that $\mathcal{A}(R, S)$ contains a unique matrix if, and only if, S equals the conjugate $R^* = (r_1^*, r_2^*, \ldots, r_n^*)$ of R, in which case the unique matrix is the Young matrix $\overline{A}$ with row sum vector R^* (its ith row consists of r_i^* ones followed by zeros).

We now consider the case studied in [6], where $K = (m, m, \ldots, m, k, k, \ldots, k)$ (p m's) for some positive integer $k \leq m$ and some positive integer $p \leq n$. Thus, every matrix in $\mathcal{A}_P(R, S)$ has an $(m - k)$-by-$(n - p)$ zero matrix in its lower right corner. Without loss of generality we may assume that $R' = (r_1, \ldots, r_k)$, $R'' = (r_{k+1}, \ldots, r_m)$, $S' = (s_1, \ldots, s_p)$, and

$S'' = (s_{p+1}, \ldots, s_n)$ are monotone nonincreasing. The following lemma explains, whenever $\mathcal{A}_P(R, S)$ contains a unique matrix, the structure of this matrix.

Lemma 2. *Assume that $\mathcal{A}_P(R, S)$ contains a unique matrix*

$$A = \begin{bmatrix} A_1 & A_2 \\ A_3 & O \end{bmatrix}, \tag{6.10}$$

where A_1 is a k by p matrix. Then A_1, A_2, and A_3 are all Young matrices.

Proof. From the uniqueness assumption, it follows that the submatrix $A' = [\,A_1\ A_2\,]$ is unique in its class. Let B' be obtained from A' by permuting columns so that B' has nonincreasing column sums. Since B' has monotone row and column sum vectors (the row sum vector of B' is R') and B' is unique in its class (as A' is), it follows that B' must be a Young matrix. Therefore, A' is obtained from a Young matrix by permuting columns and, moreover, its submatrix A_2 is itself a Young matrix. The last property follows from the fact that the column sum of A_2 is S'', which is monotone. A similar argument proves that A_3 is a Young matrix and that A_1 must be obtainable from a Young matrix by permuting its rows. Finally, we note that the properties established for A_1 imply that A_1 must be a Young matrix.   □

Consider a matrix A as in Lemma 2, where A_1, A_2, and A_3 are Young matrices. Assume that A has no row or column that contains only ones or only zeros. Then the last column of A_1 must be the zero vector and the entry in the upper right corner of A_3 must be a 1. Therefore, the first row of A_3 is an all-ones vector. Similarly, the first column of A_2 contains only ones. Thus, the following recursive procedure determines if a given matrix $A \in \mathcal{A}(R, S)$ is unique: Delete an all-zero or all-ones row or column, or delete a row where the corresponding row in A_3 contains only ones, or delete a column where the corresponding column in A_2 contains only ones. The initial matrix A is unique if, and only if, we end up with the empty matrix in this procedure.

We now generalize these ideas and discuss the uniqueness question for a general pattern P satisfying (6.2). To this end it is useful to discuss the problem in terms of certain graphs. To each matrix $A \in \mathcal{A}_P(R, S)$, we associate a directed graph G_A constructed as follows (a similar construction is used in [17]). G_A contains vertices $u_1, u_2, \ldots, u_m$ and $v_1, v_2, \ldots, v_n$. Moreover, for each $(i, j) \in P$, there is an arc in G_A: This arc is (u_i, v_j) if $a_{ij} = 1$ and it is (v_j, u_i) if $a_{ij} = 0$. Note that G_A represents A uniquely (different matrices correspond to different such graphs).

Theorem 3. *Let $A \in \mathcal{A}_P(R, S)$. Then the following statements are equivalent:*

(i) A is the unique matrix in $\mathcal{A}_P(R, S)$.
(ii) G_A is acyclic.
(iii) G_A contains no directed cycle of length 4.

(iv) Starting with A and recursively deleting rows and columns of all 0's in positions of P, or rows and columns of all 1's in positions in P, one eventually obtains the empty matrix.

Proof. A directed cycle in G_A corresponds to an even sequence of positions in P

$$(i_1, j_1), (i_2, j_1), (i_2, j_2), (i_3, j_2), \ldots, (i_t, j_t), (i_1, j_t) \tag{6.11}$$

such that the corresponding values a_{ij} is an alternating sequence of 0's and 1's. By interchanging 0's and 1's in this sequence, we obtain another matrix $A' \in \mathcal{A}_P(R, S)$ (as line sums are preserved and no positions lie outside P). In G_A this operation corresponds to reversing the direction on all arcs in the cycle. From this it is clear that (i) implies (ii). The converse implication also follows as if A, A' are two matrices in $\mathcal{A}_P(R, S)$, then the positions where $a_{ij} \neq a'_{ij}$ may be partitioned into disjoint sets corresponding to cycles as above (see [5] for details). Note that all these positions lie inside P as $a_{ij} = a'_{ij} = 0$ for all $(i, j) \notin P$. This proves that statements (i) and (ii) are equivalent.

The equivalence of statements (i) and (iii) follows from Theorem 2 as going from a matrix A to another matrix A' via an interchange corresponds to reversing the direction of a directed cycle of length 4 in the graph G_A.

Finally, statement (iv) is equivalent to statement (ii) since the recursive procedure is an algorithm for testing if the directed graph G_A is acyclic. It deletes vertices with indegree or outdegree zero as such vertices cannot belong to any cycle. If, eventually, all vertices are deleted, then there is no cycle. Otherwise, one finds a subgraph where each vertex has an ingoing arc and an outgoing arc, and this subgraph contains a directed cycle.   □

We remark that in this theorem the equivalence of statements (i), (ii), and (iv) holds for any pattern $P \subseteq \{1, 2, \ldots, m\} \times \{1, 2, \ldots, n\}$, while the equivalence to statement (ii) depends on our standard assumption (6.2) on P.

From Theorem 3 we may derive a simple reconstruction algorithm of interest in discrete tomography.

Reconstruction Algorithm

1. Initialize A by setting $a_{ij} = 0$ for all $(i, j) \notin P$.
2. Find a line in the matrix such that its line sum, together with the information provided by P and the previously determined entries in the algorithm, forces all remaining entries to be all one or all zero.
3. Set these entries accordingly, and return to step 2 until A is completely specified.

There are two possible outcomes of the algorithm: Either all entries are determined and then the constructed matrix is unique in the class, or the algorithm stops prematurely because of a "nonunique" line and then either the class is empty or it contains at least two matrices.

Corollary 1. *Assume that $\mathcal{A}_P(R, S)$ is nonempty. Then the reconstruction algorithm determines if the class $\mathcal{A}_P(R, S)$ contains a unique matrix and, if so, it finds this unique matrix.*

Proof. The correctness of the algorithm follows from statement (iv) in Theorem 3. The algorithm constructs the matrix in the reverse order compared to the deletion process described in statement (iv).   □

In the reconstruction setting of images in discrete tomography, an image is known to exist, and then the algorithm may be used for testing if the image is unique and finding this image if uniqueness holds.

As a concluding remark, we believe that it may be difficult to find simple conditions on R, S, and P that characterize the uniqueness in the class $\mathcal{A}_P(R, S)$. It would be of interest to find such a characterization although the simple algorithm above provides an algorithmic answer to this uniqueness question.

6.6 Conclusions and Summary

We have shown that some of the classical results known for $\mathcal{A}(R, S)$ generalize to the class $\mathcal{A}_P(R, S)$: (i) the existence of a canonical matrix; (ii) a simple algorithm for finding a matrix in the class; and (iii) the possibility of going between any pair of matrices in the class by using a sequence of interchanges. It is interesting that all these results hold although a nice and simple majorization characterization of the nonemptyness of $\mathcal{A}_P(R, S)$ is not present. Finally, we have given a simple reconstruction algorithm for the class $\mathcal{A}_P(R, S)$.

References

1. Aharoni, R., Herman, G.T., Kuba, A.: Binary vectors partially determined by linear equation systems. *Discr. Math.*, **171**, 1–16 (1997).
2. Ahuja, R.K., Magnanti, T.L., Orlin, J.B.: *Network Flows: Theory, Algorithms, and Applications.* Prentice-Hall, Englewood Cliffs, NJ (1993).
3. Anstee, R.P.: Triangular (0,1)-matrices with prescribed row and column sums. *Discr. Math.*, **40**, 1–10 (1982).
4. Anstee, R.P.: Properties of a class of (0, 1)-matrices covering a given matrix. *Can. J. Math.*, **34**, 438–453 (1982).
5. Brualdi, R.A.: Matrices of zeros and ones with fixed row and column sum vectors. *Lin. Algebra Appl.*, **33**, 159–231 (1980).
6. Brualdi, R.A., Dahl, G.: Matrices of zeros and ones with given line sums and a zero block. *Lin. Algebra Appl.*, **371**, 191–207 (2003).
7. Brualdi, R.A., Ryser, H.J.: *Combinatorial Matrix Theory.* Encyclopedia of Mathematics, Cambridge University Press, Cambridge, UK (1991).
8. Chen, W.Y.C.: Integral matrices with given row and column sums. *J. Combinatorial Theory, Series A*, **61**, 153–172 (1992).
9. Del Lungo, A. et al. (eds.). *Special Issue on Discrete Tomography. Lin. Algebra Appl.*, **339** (2001).
10. Fishburn, P.C., Lagarias, J.C., Reeds, J.A., Shepp, L.A.: Sets uniquely determined by projections on axes II. Discrete case. *Discr. Math.*, **91**, 153–172 (1991).

11. Fulkerson, D.R.: Zero-one matrices with zero trace. *Pacific J. Math.*, **10**, 831–836 (1960).
12. Herman, G.T., Kuba, A. (eds.): *Discrete Tomography. Foundations, Algorithms, and Applications*. Birkhäuser, Boston, MA (1999).
13. Kuba, A. Reconstruction of unique binary matrices with prescribed elements. *Acta Cybern.*, **12**, 57–70 (1995).
14. Marshall, A.W., Olkin, I.: *Inequalities: Theory of Majorization and Its Applications*. Academic Press, New York, NY (1979).
15. Nam, Y.: Integral matrices with given row and column sums. *Ars Combinatorica*, **52**, 141–151 (1999).
16. Ryser, H.J.: Combinatorial properties of matrices of zeros and ones. *Pacific J. Math.*, **7**, 1073–1082 (1957).
17. Sachnov, V.N., Tarakanov, V.E.: *Combinatorics of Nonnegative Matrices*. American Mathematical Society, Providence, RI (2002).

7

Reconstruction of Binary Matrices under Adjacency Constraints

S. Brunetti, M.C. Costa, A. Frosini, F. Jarray, and C. Picouleau

Summary. We are concerned with binary matrix reconstruction from their orthogonal projections. To the basic problem we add new kinds of constraints. In the first problems we study the ones of the matrix must be isolated: All the neighbors of a one must be a zero. Several types of neighborhoods are studied. In our second problem, every one has to be horizontally not isolated. Moreover, the number of successive zeros in a horizontal rank must be bounded by a fixed parameter. Complexity results and polynomial-time algorithms are given.

7.1 Introduction

Given a binary matrix, its horizontal and vertical projections are defined as the sum of its elements for each row and each column, respectively. The reconstruction of a binary matrix from its orthogonal projections has been studied by Ryser [22, 23]. One can refer to the book by Herman and Kuba [17] for further information on the theory, algorithms, and applications of this classical problem in discrete tomography. It is well-known that this basic problem, where the only constraints to verify are both projections, can be solved in polynomial time. Numerous studies deal with this problem when additional constraints have to be taken into account. Some examples of such constraints are different kind of convexity [6, 12, 16, 20], connectedness [4, 7, 24], periodicity [15, 19], and Gibbs priors [10]. In this chapter we study two other constraints for this problem. In a first part we take into account the "non-adjacency" constraint that depends on the definition of neighborhood: If a cell value is 1, then the values of each one of its neighbors must be 0. This problem arises especially in statistical physics to determine the microscopic properties (energy, density, entropy). In the model of hard square gas, two adjacent cells cannot be occupied simultaneously by particles because the energy of repulsion between them is very high (see, for instance, [5] or [9]). In this part several kinds of neighborhoods will be studied.

In the second part, we are concerned with a different constraint that imposes that in every row of the binary matrix no isolated cell with value 1 is permitted, and the maximum number of consecutive cells of value 0 is not greater than a prescribed integer k. Taking into account this constraint, the reconstruction of binary matrices has natural applications in timetabling and workforce scheduling. Indeed, given a company with a certain number of employees and a planning horizon of a certain number of days, 0's correspond to the working days of the employees and 1's corresponds to their days-off; the horizontal projections represent the total amount of days-off for the employees in the considered period, and the vertical projections give the number of employees at rest during the days. Hence, the social constraints state that a day-off cannot be isolated and an employee cannot have more than k successive working days. The reader can see, for instance, [2, 3, 8, 18] for some other days-off assignment problems.

7.2 Preliminaries

In this section we introduce notations and definitions that we use in the following sections.

Given an $m \times n$ binary matrix A, we denote its horizontal projection by $H = (h_1, \ldots, h_m)$, h_i being the number of 1's in row i, and its vertical projection by $V = (v_1, \ldots, v_n)$, v_j being the number of 1's in column j (see Fig. 7.1 for an example). The condition $\sum_{i=1}^{m} h_i = \sum_{j=1}^{n} v_j$, denoted by (C_0), is obviously necessary for the existence of a binary matrix respecting both projections in the problems we study in this chapter. Specially, we will consider the reconstruction problem from the horizontal and vertical projections for two classes of binary matrices obtained by imposing the nonadjacency constraint, and the timetabling constraint.

3	1	1	1	0	0
4	0	1	1	1	1
2	1	1	0	0	0
3	0	1	1	1	0
	2	4	3	2	1

Fig. 7.1. A binary matrix with projections $H = (3, 4, 2, 3)$ and $V = (2, 4, 3, 2, 1)$.

In order to define the nonadjacency constraint we recall several definitions of the neighborhood of a given cell $a_{i,j}$ of the matrix A. We speak of 2-*adjacency* if the two neighbors of $a_{i,j}$ are $a_{i,j+1}$ and $a_{i,j-1}$, i.e., its horizontal adjacent cells; 4-*adjacency* if the neighbors are $a_{i,j-1}, a_{i,j+1}, a_{i-1,j}$, and $a_{i+1,j}$, i.e., the horizontal and vertical adjacent cells; *6-adjacency* if, in addition to the previous ones, we add the neighbors on one diagonal: $a_{i-1,j-1}$ and $a_{i+1,j+1}$. Eventually, in the *8-adjacency* the neighbors of $a_{i,j}$ are its eight adjacent cells $a_{i,j-1}, a_{i,j+1}, a_{i-1,j}, a_{i+1,j}, a_{i-1,j-1}, a_{i-1,j+1}, a_{i+1,j-1}$, and $a_{i+1,j+1}$. We say that matrix A fulfills the *non p-adjacency constraint* if $a_{i,j} = 1$ implies that its p-adjacent cells have value 0. Figure 7.2 illustrates the non p-adjacency for $p = 2, p = 4, p = 6$, and $p = 8$ (from the left to the right). The class of binary matrices that fulfill non p-adjacency is denoted by $\mathcal{N}_p$, $p \in \{2, 4, 6, 8\}$.

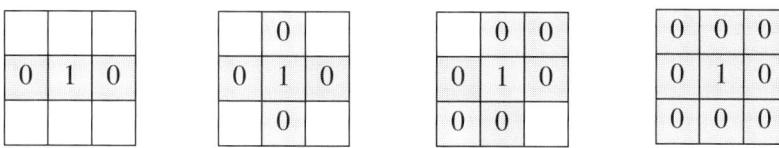

Fig. 7.2. Examples of the non $\{2, 4, 6, 8\}$-adjacency (from the left to the right).

We say that matrix A fulfills the *timetabling constraint* if $a_{i,j} = 1$ implies $a_{i,j-1} = 1$ or $a_{i,j+1} = 1$, and the number of successive 0's in each row of A is less than or equal to a given integer $k \geq 2$. Figure 7.3 shows a matrix that fulfills the timetabling constraint for $k = 3$. Given k, the class of binary matrices that fulfills timetabling constraint is denoted by $\mathcal{T}_k$.

1	1	1	0	0	0	1	1	1	0	0	0
0	1	1	1	1	0	0	1	1	0	1	1
1	1	0	0	0	1	1	0	1	1	0	0

Fig. 7.3. A matrix of $\mathcal{T}_3$.

7.3 Reconstructing Matrices under Nonadjacency Constraints

Let us consider the problem of reconstructing an $m \times n$ binary matrix of $\mathcal{N}_p$ from its horizontal $H = (h_1, \ldots, h_m)$ and vertical $V = (v_1, \ldots, v_n)$ projections, where $\mathcal{N}_p$ is the class of matrices that fulfill non p-adjacency constraints. We denote this problem by **Reconstruction**$_{\mathcal{N}_p}(\mathbf{m, n})$. In this section we deal with this problem and its modifications. In particular, we show how to solve **Reconstruction**$_{\mathcal{N}_2}$(**m, n**) in polynomial time. In Subsection 7.3.2, conditions for the existence of a solution to **Reconstruction**$_{\mathcal{N}_4}$(**m, n**) are given, and we solve it for matrices with two or three rows ($m = 2,3$). Finally, we prove that **Reconstruction**$_{\mathcal{N}_6}$(**m, n**) is NP-complete, and that **Reconstruction**$_{\mathcal{N}_8}$(**m, n**) is as difficult as the well-known open problem of reconstructing a three-colored matrix [13].

7.3.1 Binary Matrices under Non 2-Adjacency Constraint

We show that **Reconstruction**$_{\mathcal{N}_2}$(**m, n**), the problem of reconstructing a binary matrix under non 2-adjacency constraint from orthogonal projections, is equivalent to a particular packing reconstruction problem that can be solved in polynomial time.

In particular, we consider the horizontal domino packing problem. In this problem, every tile is a horizontally oriented domino, i.e., an array 1×2 or equivalently two consecutive cells in a row, and the packing consists in a placement of nonoverlapping horizontal oriented dominoes in a $m \times n$ array satisfying the orthogonal projections, i.e., a given number of distinct tiles in each row and column.

Lemma 1. Reconstruction$_{\mathcal{N}_2}$(**m, n**) *is equivalent to the horizontal domino packing problem.*

Proof. Consider an instance of **Reconstruction**$_{\mathcal{N}_2}$(**m, n**) defined by $H = (h_1, h_2, \ldots, h_m)$ and $V = (v_1, v_2, \ldots, v_n)$. Without loss of generality, we can suppose that $v_n = 0$.

The two problems are equivalent, since it is easy to see that the instance of the horizontal domino packing problem can be obtained by H, and V simply, and vice versa, and a solution for the horizontal domino packing problem corresponds to a solution of **Reconstruction**$_{\mathcal{N}_2}$(**m, n**) replacing every domino by two cells of values 1 (the leftmost) and 0 (the rightmost), and vice versa, two consecutive cells of **Reconstruction**$_{\mathcal{N}_2}$(**m, n**) with values 1 and 0 by a domino. Indeed, denoted by H', V', the orthogonal projections of the horizontal domino packing problem, $H = H'$ and $V = (v_1', v_2' - v_1', v_3' - (v_2' - v_1'), v_4' - (v_3' - (v_2' - v_1'))\ldots, v_n' - (v_{n-1}' - \ldots (v_2' - v_1')\ldots))$. This latter vector counts the number of horizontal dominoes starting in every column [21]. Since two consecutive dominoes in a row cannot start at consecutive columns, the first cells of each domino in a packing satisfying H' and V' also fulfill the nonadjacency constraint and satisfy H and V. □

Since there exists a polynomial-time algorithm for the horizontal domino packing problem [21], we can give the following theorem.

Theorem 1. Reconstruction$_{\mathcal{N}_2}$(**m, n**) *can be solved in polynomial time.*

7.3.2 Binary Matrices under Non 4-Adjacency Constraint

Reconstruction from One Projection

We are going to consider the problem of reconstructing a binary matrix under the non 4-adjacency constraint from one projection. Without loss of generality, we consider the horizontal projection. To solve **Reconstruction**$_{\mathcal{N}_4}(\mathbf{m})$, we shall use an "underlying" chessboard C of size $m \times n$ to provide forbidden positions (i.e., cells that cannot have value 1) and free positions (i.e., cells that can have either value 1 or value 0) for A. Notice that a chessboard verifies the non 4-adjacency constraint. In the chessboard, the cells $c_{i,j}$ such that $i + j$ is even (respectively, odd) have the same value as $c_{1,1}$ (respectively, $c_{2,1}$). Thus, there are two possible configurations of C depending on the value of $c_{1,1}$. Consider the configurations resulting from $c_{1,1} = 1$: If n is even, there are $n/2$ 1's in each row, and if n is odd, there are $(n+1)/2$ 1's in odd rows and $(n-1)/2$ 1's in even rows; such a chessboard is the most dense binary matrix respecting the non 4-adjacency constraint.

Now, we are going to give some necessary and sufficient conditions on H, depending on the parity of n, for the existence of an $m \times n$ matrix $A \in \mathcal{N}_4$ with horizontal projection H. We call **Consistency**$_{\mathcal{N}_4}(\mathbf{m})$ the corresponding decision problem. As a byproduct, we shall get a method to build A if it exists.

First, note that h_i 1's are required in each row i, and so at least $h_i - 1$ 0's: Thus, there is a solution only if, for all i, $h_i + h_i - 1 \le n$ or equivalently, for all i, $h_i \le (n+1)/2$. This condition, denoted by (C_1), is necessary whatever is the parity of n.

Proposition 1. *If n is even, then $h_i \le (n+1)/2$, for $i = 1, \ldots, m$, is a necessary and sufficient condition for* **Consistency**$_{\mathcal{N}_4}(\mathbf{m})$.

Proof. The necessity has been proved above. Let us prove the sufficiency. In each row i, n being even and h_i being integer, $h_i \le (n+1)/2 \Rightarrow h_i \le n/2$. Consider a chessboard: It has $\frac{n}{2}$ 1's per row; by choosing exactly h_i 1's per row and setting the other cells to 0, we get the solution.   □

Nevertheless, this condition is not sufficient in the case where n is odd: Just consider two adjacent rows with $h_i = h_{i+1} = (n+1)/2$; the condition (C_1) holds but there are 1's in vertically adjacent cells and the non 4-adjacency constraint is violated. When n is odd, we need to introduce more definitions. A row i is said to be *saturated* if $h_i = (n+1)/2$; that means that there must be a 1 in each odd column. We said that two saturated rows i_1 and i_2 are *consecutive* if there is no saturated *intermediate* row between them ($\forall i$ $i_1 < i < i_2$, row i is not saturated) (see Fig. 7.4). Let us denote by $A_{i_1 i_2}$ the submatrix of A restricted to rows i such that $i_1 \le i \le i_2$, and by **Consistency**$_{\mathcal{N}_4}([\mathbf{i_1}, \mathbf{i_2}])$ the corresponding subproblem. Obviously, **Consistency**$_{\mathcal{N}_4}(\mathbf{m})$ is satisfied only if for any consecutive saturated rows i_1 and i_2, **Consistency**$_{\mathcal{N}_4}([\mathbf{i_1}, \mathbf{i_2}])$ is satisfied.

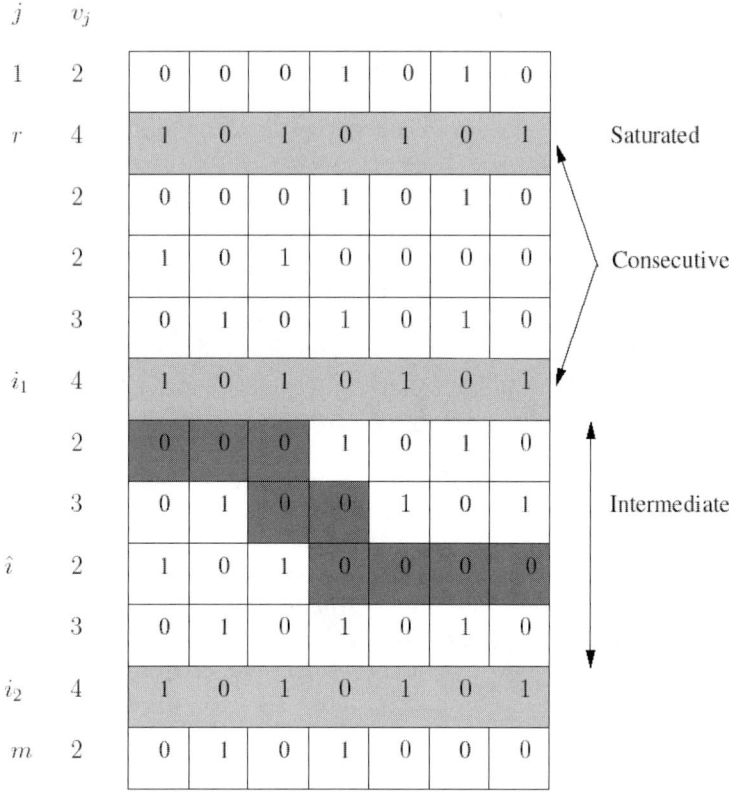

Fig. 7.4. A matrix of $\mathcal{N}_4$ with n odd.

Note that, as seen above, if two adjacent rows are saturated, then A cannot exist. Thus, from now we assume that $i_2 > i_1 + 1$.

Let $k = i_2 - i_1 - 1 \geq 1$ be the number of intermediate rows in $A_{i_1 i_2}$. The next three propositions give conditions on h_i's that ensure that **Consistency**$_{\mathcal{N}_4}([\mathbf{i_1}, \mathbf{i_2}])$ is true. These propositions are based on the parity of k. For an intermediate (unsaturated) row i, n being odd, we have $h_i \leq (n-1)/2$.

Proposition 2. *If n is odd and k is odd, then a necessary and sufficient condition for* **Consistency**$_{\mathcal{N}_4}([\mathbf{i_1}, \mathbf{i_2}])$ *is that $h_i \leq (n-1)/2$, for all i such that $i_1 < i < i_2,$.*

Proof. Just recall that a chessboard in $A_{i_1 i_2}$ has at least $(n-1)/2$ 1's per row i (but no more than $(n+1)/2$), $i_1 \leq i \leq i_2$. □

When n is odd and k is even, it is not possible to cover $A_{i_1 i_2}$ with a chessboard (see Fig. 7.4). In a first step we give a necessary condition for the existence of A. We call it (C_2); it is that $\sum_{i=i_1+1}^{i_2-1} h_i \leq kn/2 - (n+1)/2$.

Proposition 3. *If n is odd and k is even, then (C_2) is a necessary condition for* **Consistency**$_{N_4}([\mathbf{i_1}, \mathbf{i_2}])$.

Proof. Rows i_1 and i_2 are saturated. In the set of intermediate rows i, $i_1 < i < i_2$, there are at most $k/2$ 1's in an even column and $k/2 - 1$ 1's in an odd column. n being odd, there are $(n-1)/2$ even columns and $(n+1)/2$ odd columns. Hence the total number of 1's in the intermediate rows is at most $(n-1)/2 \times k/2 + (n+1)/2 \times (k/2 - 1) = kn/2 - (n+1)/2$; thus, (C_2) must be satisfied.   □

Now, let us show that when n is odd and k is even, (C_1) and (C_2) are sufficient for a solution to exist. Let f be the following integer function defined from $\{i = i_1, \ldots, i_2 - 1\}$ to $[1, \ldots, n]$ by

(a) $f(i_1) = 1$,
(b) $f(i_1 + 1) = n - 2h_{i_1+1}$,
(c) $f(i) = min(n, f(i-1) + n - 2h_i)$, for $i = i_1 + 2, \ldots, i_2 - 1$.

Without loss of generality, we assume now that i_1 is even. (If i_1 is odd, just exchange in the following on the one hand "odd" and "even" and on the other hand "have the same parity" and "have not the same parity.")
Let $\hat{i}$ be the smallest i such that $f(\hat{i}) = n$.

Property 1. $\hat{i}$ is such that $\hat{i} < i_2$.

Proof. Assume that $\hat{i} \geq i_2$, that is, $f(i_2 - 1) < n$. By induction, $f(i_2 - 1) = f(i_2 - 2) + n - 2h_{i_2-1} = \cdots = \sum_{i=i_1+1}^{i_2-1} n - 2h_i kn - 2\sum_{i=i_1+1}^{i_2-1} h_i$. Recall that (C_2) is $\sum_{i=i_1+1}^{i_2-1} h_i \leq kn/2 - (n+1)/2$; hence, we get $n + 1 \leq f(i_2 - 1) < n$, a contradiction.   □

Property 2. $f(i_1 + 1) \geq f(i_1)$ and f is increasing on $\{i_1 + 1, \ldots, \hat{i}\}$.

Proof. For $i_1 < i < i_2$, we have $h_i \leq (n-1)/2$, i.e., $n - 2h_i \geq 1$. Then $f(i_1 + 1) = n - 2h_{i_1+1} \geq f(i_1) = 1$ and $f(i) = f(i-1) + n - 2h_i > f(i-1)$, for $i = i_1 + 1, \ldots, \hat{i}$.   □

Property 3. For each i such that $i_1 < i < \hat{i}$, i and $f(i)$ have the same parity.

Proof. Recall that i_1 is even. Since n is odd, $f(i_1 + 1)$ is odd and the relation is satisfied for $i = i_1 + 1$. For $i > i_1 + 1$, $f(i) = f(i-1) + n - 2h_i$, then by induction i and $f(i)$ have the same parity.   □

Now, set to 0 all the cells in $\{(i,j) \mid i = i_1+1, \ldots, \hat{\imath}; j = f(i-1), \ldots, f(i)\}$. That defines "stairs" from column 1 to column n, splitting up the submatrix $A_{i_1 i_2}$ into two parts separated by these 0's (see Fig. 7.4). Let us cover the upper right part by a partial chessboard with $c_{i_1,1} = 1$, and the left lower part by another partial chessboard with $c_{i_2,1} = 1$. i_1 is even, $i_2 = i_1 + k + 1$, and k is even, thus i_2 is odd: The upper right partial chessboard has 1's in the cells (i,j) such that $i+j$ is odd, whereas the lower left partial chessboard has 1's in the cells such that $i+j$ is even. Clearly, the obtained binary matrix satisfies the non 4-adjacency constraint.

Property 4. For i, $i_1 < i < \hat{\imath}$, there are exactly h_i 1's in each row i.

Proof. Let us consider a row i with $i_1 < i < \hat{\imath}$. There is a stair of cells with 0 from column $f(i-1)$ to column $f(i)$. The cells $(i,1), (i,2), \ldots, (i, f(i-1)-1)$ are on the left of the stairs and belong to the lower left partial chessboard; note that for $i = i_1 + 1$, there are no cells on the left side. The cells $(i, f(i) + 1), (i, f(i) + 2), \ldots, (i, n)$ are on the right of the stair and belong to the upper right partial chessboard. The cell $(i, f(i-1) - 1)$ is adjacent to the stair by the left and from Property 3, $i + f(i-1) - 1$ is even and the cell $(i, f(i) + 1)$ is adjacent to the stair by the right and from Property 3, $i + f(i) + 1$ is odd: Thus, both cells have a 1. There are $\lceil (f(i-1) - 1)/2 \rceil$ 1's on the left of the stair, and $\lceil (n - f(i))/2 \rceil$ 1's on the right of the stair. Thus, the total number of 1's in row i is $\lceil (f(i-1) - 1)/2 \rceil + \lceil (n - f(i))/2 \rceil = \lceil (f(i-1) - 1)/2 \rceil + \lceil (2h_i - f(i-1))/2 \rceil = h_i + \lceil (f(i-1) - 1)/2 \rceil + \lceil -f(i-1)/2 \rceil = h_i$. □

Property 5. There are at least h_i 1's in each row $i, \hat{\imath} \leq i \leq i_2 - 1$.

Proof. First, consider the row $\hat{\imath}$. Since $\hat{\imath}$ and $f(\hat{\imath}-1) - 1$ have the same parity, there is a 1 in the cell $(\hat{\imath}, f(\hat{\imath}-1) - 1)$. So there are $\lceil (f(\hat{\imath}-1) - 1)/2 \rceil$ 1's on the left side of the stair in row $\hat{\imath}$. We have $f(\hat{\imath}) = n \leq f(\hat{\imath}-1) + n - 2h_i$; thus, $2h_i \leq f(\hat{\imath}-1) \Rightarrow h_i \leq \lfloor f(\hat{\imath}-1)/2 \rfloor = \lceil (f(\hat{\imath}-1) - 1)/2 \rceil$. Second, in each row i, $\hat{\imath} < i \leq i_2 - 1$, there are at least $(n-1)/2$ 1's. These rows being not saturated, we have $h_i \leq (n-1)/2$. □

We are ready to establish the following proposition:

Proposition 4. *If n is odd and k is even, then* **Consistency**$_{\mathcal{N}_4}([\mathbf{i_1, i_2}])$ *is satisfied if, and only if, (C_1) and (C_2) hold.*

Proof. (C_1) and (C_2) are necessary conditions. Now, if (C_1) and (C_2) are satisfied, to get a solution to **Reconstruction**$_{\mathcal{N}_4}([\mathbf{i_1, i_2}])$, we have to build the stairs of 0's as explained above. Then, from Property 4 and Property 5, each row i, $i_1 \leq i \leq i_2$, has at least h_i 1's; one can select exactly h_i 1's to get a solution to **Reconstruction**$_{\mathcal{N}_4}([\mathbf{i_1, i_2}])$. □

Now let the row r be the first saturated row of A and, if $r \neq 1$, consider the subproblem **Reconstruction**$_{\mathcal{N}_4}([\mathbf{1, r}])$ corresponding to the r first rows:

It has a solution if, and only if, the condition (C_1) is satisfied for $i = 1, \ldots, r$. The proof is the same as the proof given for Propositions 1 and 2. In addition, the subproblem **Reconstruction**$_{\mathcal{N}_4}([\mathbf{s}, \mathbf{m}])$, where $s < m$ is the last saturated row, can be solved as well.

Eventually, when n is odd, to solve **Reconstruction**$_{\mathcal{N}_4}(\mathbf{m})$ we have to solve each subproblem **Consistency**$_{\mathcal{N}_4}([\mathbf{i_1}, \mathbf{i_2}])$, where i_1 and i_2 are two consecutive saturated rows. If all these subproblems are satisfiable, putting together the solutions of the corresponding **Reconstruction**$_{\mathcal{N}_4}([\mathbf{i_1}, \mathbf{i_2}])$ provides a solution to **Reconstruction**$_{\mathcal{N}_4}(\mathbf{m})$; otherwise, **Consistency**$_{\mathcal{N}_4}(\mathbf{m})$ is not satisfiable. Now, we obtain the following result:

Theorem 2. Reconstruction$_{\mathcal{N}_4}(\mathbf{m})$ *has a solution if, and only if, (C_1) holds and either n is even or n is odd and (C_2) holds for each pair (i_1, i_2) of consecutive saturated rows such that $i_2 - i_1 - 1$ is even.*

Note that if **Reconstruction**$_{\mathcal{N}_4}(\mathbf{m})$ has a solution, then it can be obtained in a linear time using chessboards as indicated in the proofs above.

All the results obtained in this section can be settled symmetrically for the problem **Reconstruction**$_{\mathcal{N}_4}(\mathbf{n})$, where instead of a vector H of horizontal projections, we are given a vector V of vertical projections.

Reconstruction Satisfying the Orthogonal Projections

It seems that the complexity of **Reconstruction**$_{\mathcal{N}_4}(\mathbf{m}, \mathbf{n})$ is still an open problem. We first propose a sufficient and then a necessary condition for the existence of a solution to **Reconstruction**$_{\mathcal{N}_4}(\mathbf{m}, \mathbf{n})$, then we solve this problem in the special cases $m = 2$ and $m = 3$.

Sufficient Conditions for the Existence of a Solution to **Reconstruction**$_{\mathcal{N}_4}(\mathbf{m}, \mathbf{n})$

Let $H_O = (h_1, h_3, \ldots, h_{2p-1})$, $p = \lceil m/2 \rceil$, and $V_O = (v_1, v_3, \ldots, v_{2q-1})$, $q = \lceil n/2 \rceil$ (respectively, $H_E = (h_2, h_4, \ldots, h_{2p})$, $p = \lfloor m/2 \rfloor$, and $V_E = (v_2, v_4, \ldots, v_{2q})$, $q = \lfloor n/2 \rfloor$), be the projections of the odd (respectively, even) rows and columns. The existence of $\lceil m/2 \rceil \times \lceil n/2 \rceil$ binary matrices $A_O \in \mathcal{N}_4$ satisfying H_O and V_O and $A_E \in \mathcal{N}_4$ satisfying H_E and V_E implies that there is a solution to **Reconstruction**$_{\mathcal{N}_4}(\mathbf{m}, \mathbf{n})$. Indeed, this solution is obtained by aggregating the two binary matrices A_O and A_E: It obviously satisfies the projections and the non 4-adjacency constraint holds since the 1's are in cells $a_{i,j}$ such that $i + j$ is even.

In the same way, if the two subproblems restricted first to odd rows and even columns and second to even rows and odd columns both have a solution then **Reconstruction**$_{\mathcal{N}_4}(\mathbf{m}, \mathbf{n})$ has a solution: in that case, the 1's are in cells $a_{i,j}$ such that $i + j$ is odd.

However, these conditions are not necessary; just consider the instance $m = 3$, $n = 4$, $H = (2, 1, 2)$, and $V = (2, 1, 1, 1)$.

Necessary Conditions for the Existence of a Solution to
Reconstruction$_{\mathcal{N}_4}$(m, n)

Following the definitions of **Reconstruction$_{\mathcal{N}_4}$(m)**, **Reconstruction$_{\mathcal{N}_4}$(n)**, and **Reconstruction$_{\mathcal{N}_2}$(m, n)**, we have the obvious necessary condition: If a solution to **Reconstruction$_{\mathcal{N}_4}$(m, n)** exists, then there exists a solution to the corresponding instances of **Reconstruction$_{\mathcal{N}_4}$(m)**, **Reconstruction$_{\mathcal{N}_4}$(n)**, and **Reconstruction$_{\mathcal{N}_2}$(m, n)**. Nevertheless, these conditions are not sufficient as shown by the following instance: $m = n = 4$; $H = (2,1,2,1)$; and $V = (1,2,2,1)$. Now, we will focus on two particular cases: $m = 2$ and $m = 3$.

Solving **Reconstruction$_{\mathcal{N}_4}$(m, n)** *when $m = 2$*

In this case $v_j \in \{0,1\}$ for all j, for otherwise the non 4-adjacency constraint cannot be satisfied. From the columns such that $v_j = 1$, we make K blocks B^k, where each B^k is a maximal set of consecutive columns with unary vertical projection (see Fig. 7.5). Let l^k denote the number of columns in B^k, $k = 1, \ldots, K$. Since the columns j that are not in a block are such that $v_j = 0$, we have that $\sum_{k=1}^{K} l^k = \sum_{j=1}^{n} v_j$.

7	1	0	1	0	1	0	1	0	1	0	0	1	0	1	0	0
6	0	1	0	1	0	0	0	1	0	0	1	0	1	0	0	1
	1	2	3	4	5		1	2	3		1	2	3	4		1
			B^1					B^2				B^3				B^4

Fig. 7.5. A matrix of $\mathcal{N}_4$ with $m = 2$.

We can give the following proposition.

Proposition 5. *There exists a solution to* **Reconstruction$_{\mathcal{N}_4}$(m, n)** *for $m = 2$ if, and only if:*
  (C_0) $h_1 + h_2 = \sum_{j=1}^{n} v_j$;
  (C_1) $h_i \leq (n+1)/2$, *for* $i = 1, 2$;
  (C_2) $v_j \in \{0,1\}$, *for* $1 \leq j \leq n$;
  (C_3) $h_i \geq \sum_{k=1}^{K} \lfloor l^k/2 \rfloor$, *for* $i = 1, 2$.

Proof. (C_0) and (C_2) are obviously necessary as explained before. $h_i \leq (n+1)/2$ is the condition (C_1) necessary for **Reconstruction$_{\mathcal{N}_4}$(m)**: Any solution to **Reconstruction$_{\mathcal{N}_4}$(m, n)** is a solution to **Reconstruction$_{\mathcal{N}_4}$(m)**; thus, (C_1) is also necessary for **Reconstruction$_{\mathcal{N}_4}$(m, n)**. Eventually, for each block B_k there must be a 1 in each column; to respect the non 4-adjacency constraint, there must be at least $\lfloor l^k/2 \rfloor$ 1's in each row of each block B^k and (C_3) is necessary.

Now, assume that the conditions are all satisfied. (C_3) implies that $h_i - \sum_{k=1}^{K} \lfloor l^k/2 \rfloor \geq 0$; the number of blocks of odd length is equal to $\sum_{k=1}^{K} l^k - 2\sum_{k=1}^{K} \lfloor l^k/2 \rfloor = \sum_{j=1}^{n} v_j - 2\sum_{k=1}^{K} \lfloor l^k/2 \rfloor = h_1 + h_2 - 2\sum_{k=1}^{K} \lfloor l^k/2 \rfloor = \left(h_1 - \sum_{k=1}^{K} \lfloor l^k/2 \rfloor\right) + \left(h_2 - \sum_{k=1}^{K} \lfloor l^k/2 \rfloor\right) \geq 0$. Then we can obtain a solution to **Reconstruction**$_{\mathcal{N}_4}(\mathbf{m}, \mathbf{n})$ in the following way:

1. Renumber the columns of each block from 1 to l^k, $k = 1, \ldots, K$;
2. In the first row:
   a) "select" the first $h_1 - \sum_{k=1}^{K} \lfloor l^k/2 \rfloor$ blocks of odd length, then, for these selected blocks, $\lfloor l^k/2 \rfloor + 1$ cells lying in the odd columns are set to 1.
   b) for the non selected blocks, $\lfloor l^k/2 \rfloor$ cells lying in the even columns are set to 1.
3. in the second row: for each block B^k, the cells lying in the columns not having 1 in their first row (step 2) are set to 1.

Doing so, we get exactly a 1 in each column of each block, as required, and our solution satisfies the adjacency constraint. In addition, in the first row we get $\lfloor l^k/2 \rfloor$ 1's in each not selected block and $\lfloor l^k/2 \rfloor + 1$ 1's in the $h_1 - \sum_{k=1}^{K} \lfloor l^k/2 \rfloor$ selected blocks. That gives $\left(\sum_{k=1}^{K} \lfloor l^k/2 \rfloor\right) + \left(h_1 - \sum_{k=1}^{K} \lfloor l^k/2 \rfloor\right) = h_1$ 1's in the first row. Since the total number of blocks of odd length is $\left(h_1 - \sum_{k=1}^{K} \lfloor l^k/2 \rfloor\right) + \left(h_2 - \sum_{k=1}^{K} \lfloor l^k/2 \rfloor\right)$, there are $h_2 - \sum_{k=1}^{K} \lfloor l^k/2 \rfloor$ odd not selected blocks at step 2a. These not selected blocks are treated at step 2b and have 1's in the first row in even columns; from step 3, they get $\lfloor l^k/2 \rfloor + 1$ 1's in the second row in odd columns while the other blocks get $\sum_{k=1}^{K} \lfloor l^k/2 \rfloor$ 1's in the second row. Finally, we have $\sum_{k=1}^{K} \lfloor l^k/2 \rfloor + \left(h_2 - \sum_{k=1}^{K} \lfloor l^k/2 \rfloor\right) = h_2$ 1's in the second row. $\square$

Solving **Reconstruction**$_{\mathcal{N}_4}(\mathbf{m}, \mathbf{n})$ *when* $m = 3$

For a matrix $A \in \mathcal{N}_4$ with three rows, **Reconstruction**$_{\mathcal{N}_4}(\mathbf{m}, \mathbf{n})$ has a solution only if $v_j \in \{0, 1, 2\}$, for all j, since the non 4-adjacency constraint cannot be satisfied if $v_j = 3$ for some j. There is no 1 in columns j such that $v_j = 0$, and there must be a 1 in the first and third rows in column j such that $v_j = 2$. In order to satisfy the non 4-adjacency constraint, there is no column j such that $v_j = v_{j+1} = 2$, for $1 \leq j < n$. Thus, the condition (C_2') that follows must be satisfied: $v_j \in \{0, 1, 2\}$, $v_j + v_{j+1} < 4$, for $j = 1, \ldots, n-1$, and $v_n \in \{0, 1, 2\}$. In the sequel we suppose that (C_2') holds.

We have now to study columns with $v_j = 1$; they can be grouped in K blocks B^k of maximal length l^k as shown above in the case $m = 2$. Note that if there is a column j such that $v_j = 1$ and $(v_{j+1} = 2$ or $v_{j-1} = 2)$, the 1 of column j lies in the second row.

In a first step, let **Reconstruction**$_{\mathcal{N}_4}(\mathbf{m}, \mathbf{n})[\mathbf{B^k}]$ be the subproblem associated with a block B^k. We denote by $H^k = (h_1^k, h_2^k, h_3^k)$ its horizontal projections. Note that at this stage H^k is unknown. We are going to give some conditions on H^k for a solution to **Reconstruction**$_{\mathcal{N}_4}(\mathbf{m}, \mathbf{n})[\mathbf{B^k}]$ to exist. We consider three cases: a block B^k is adjacent to zero, to one, or to two columns with $v_j = 2$.

Proposition 6. *There exists a solution to* $\textbf{Reconstruction}_{\mathcal{N}_4}(\textbf{m}, \textbf{n})[\textbf{B}^k]$ *if, and only if,*
(C_0) $h_1^k + h_2^k + h_3^k = l^k$
and
Case 1: B^k is adjacent to two columns with $v_j = 0$, then
(C_4) $h_i^k \leq \lceil l^k/2 \rceil$, *for $i = 1, 2, 3$;*
Case 2: B^k is adjacent to a column with $v_j = 0$ and to a column with $v_j = 2$,
then
(C_5) $h_i^k \leq \lfloor l^k/2 \rfloor$, *$i = 1, 3$ and $1 \leq h_2^k \leq \lceil l^k/2 \rceil$;*
Case 3: B^k is adjacent to two columns with $v_j = 2$, then
(C_6) $l^k \neq 2$. *If $l^k = 1$, then $(h_1^k = h_3^k = 0$ and $h_2^k = 1)$ else*
$h_i^k \leq \lfloor (l^k - 1)/2 \rfloor$ *for $i = 1, 3$, and $2 \leq h_2^k \leq \lceil l^k/2 \rceil$.*

Proof. First let us prove the necessity of these conditions.

$h_1^k + h_2^k + h_3^k = \Sigma_{j=1}^n v_j = l^k$ is the necessary condition (C_0).

The non 4-adjacency implies (condition (C_1)) that $h_i^k \leq \lceil l^k/2 \rceil$, $i = 1, 2, 3$, must be satisfied for any case 1, 2, 3. Thus, for case 1, (C_4) is a necessary condition.

For case 2, without loss of generality, we assume that the column adjacent to the left of B^k has a vertical projection equal to two and that the column adjacent to the right of B^k has a vertical projection equal to zero. As noted above, there must be a 0 in the first and third rows and thus a 1 in the second row of the first column of B^k. Thus, the conditions of case 2 must be satisfied.

Eventually, in case 3, as noted above, there must be a 0 on the first and third rows and a 1 in the second row in the first and last columns of B^k. It follows that the non 4-adjacency cannot be satisfied if $l^k = 2$. If $l^k = 1$, the necessity of the condition (C_6) is trivial. If $l^k \geq 3$, then we must have $h_2^k \geq 2$ and for rows 1 and 3, the condition (C_1) is $h_i^k \leq \lceil (l^k - 2)/2 \rceil = \lfloor (l^k - 1)/2 \rfloor$. The conditions of case 3 must be satisfied.

Now, assume that these conditions are satisfied. Let us denote by j' and j'' the first and the last columns of B^k, respectively. The rows are numbered such that $h_i^k \geq h_{i'}^k \geq h_{i''}^k$.

We propose the following procedure to build a solution.

1. If $v_{j'-1} = 2$, then assign a 1 to the cell $(2, j')$ and do $v_{j'} = 0$ and update h_2^k to $h_2^k - 1$. If $v_{j''+1} = 2$, then assign a 1 to the cell $(2, j'')$ and do $v_{j''} = 0$ and update h_2^k to $h_2^k - 1$.
2. While $h_i^k \neq 0$, do the following: Let j be the leftmost column of B^k such that $v_j = 1$ and (i, j) is not 4-adjacent to a cell that contains a 1; assign 1 to (i, j) and do $v_j = 0$ and update h_i^k to $h_i^k - 1$ (row i is filled from the left).

3. While $h_{\hat{i}}^k \neq 0$, do the following: Let j be the rightmost column of B^k such that $v_j = 1$ and (i, j) is not 4-adjacent to a cell that contains a 1; assign a 1 to $(\hat{i}, j)$ and do $v_j = 0$ and $h_{\hat{i}}^k \leftarrow h_{\hat{i}}^k - 1$ (row $\hat{i}$ is filled from the right).
4. Assign a 1 to the cells (i', j) such that $v_j = 1$.

Let us prove the validity of our procedure: (C_5) and (C_6) ensure that we can perform step 1. The conditions (C_4), (C_5), and (C_6) ensure that we can perform step 2 whatever the row i is. Note that after this step there are no successive columns j and $j + 1$ with $v_j = v_{j+1} = 0$. Thus, step 3 can be performed. One notes that after step 3, the 1's cannot be non 4-adjacent. Now, from condition (C_0), step 4 can be executed. So it remains to show that the non 4-adjacency is always satisfied after this last step.

Since in step 4 the 1's are assigned to the cells (i', j) with $v_j = 1$, we have to prove that at the beginning of this step there are no columns j and $j + 1$ such that $v_j = v_{j+1} = 1$. In order to obtain a contradiction, let us suppose that there are such two columns. Let j_1, respectively j_2, be the last column where a 1 is assigned in row i (step 2), respectively row $\hat{i}$ (step 3). Following the manner in which steps 2 and 3 work, we have that $j \geq j_1 + 1$ and $j + 1 \leq j_2 - 1$. Thus, we have $h_{i'}^k \geq \lfloor h_i^k/2 \rfloor + \lfloor h_{\hat{i}}^k/2 \rfloor + 2 > (h_i^k + h_{\hat{i}}^k)/2$. Since $h_i^k \geq h_{\hat{i}}^k \geq h_{i'}^k$, we get a contradiction. $\square$

Now, in order to solve the whole problem, for each block B^k, we have to determine a projection H^k satisfying, first the conditions of Proposition 6, and second $\Sigma_{k=1}^K h_2^k = h_2$ and $\Sigma_{k=1}^K h_i^k - n_2 = h_i$ for $i = 1, 3$, where n_2 is the number of columns of A with $v_j = 2$. We propose to determine these H^k's by searching for a flow in a complete bipartite network $G = (X, Y, E)$ defined as follows (see Fig. 7.6): $X = \{R_1, R_2, R_3\}$, where the node R_i is associated to the row i; $Y = \{b^k, k = 1, \ldots, K\}$, where the node b^k is associated to the block B^k. We add a source node S and three arcs (S, R_i). The capacities of these arcs are set to h_2 for $i = 2$, and to $h_i - n_2$ for $i = 1, 3$. We add a sink node T and K arcs (b^k, T). These arcs have capacity l^k for $k = 1, \ldots, K$. Eventually, the capacities of the arcs (R_i, b^k) are as follows: If $i = 2$ or B^k is a block as in case 1 of Proposition 6, then the capacity is equal to $\lceil l^k/2 \rceil$; if $i = 1$ or $i = 3$ and B^k is as in case 2, then the capacity is equal to $\lfloor l^k/2 \rfloor$; finally, if $i = 1$ or $i = 3$ and B^k is as in case 3, then it is equal to $\lfloor (l^k - 1)/2 \rfloor$. We also have a lower bound for the arcs (R_2, b^k): If B^k is as in case 2, then the lower bound is 1; if B^k is as in case 3 and $l^k \neq 1$, then the lower bound is set to 2. The lower bound of every other arc is 0.

Theorem 3. *For $m = 3$, there exists a solution to* $\mathbf{Reconstruction}_{\mathcal{N}_4}(\mathbf{m}, \mathbf{n})$ *if, and only if, there exists a flow of total value $\Sigma_{k=1}^K l^k$ in the network G.*

Proof. If there exists such a flow in G, let h_i^k be equal to the flow on the arc (R_i, b^k). On the one hand, for each block B^k, the flow of the arcs (b^k, T) is l^k, for $k = 1, \ldots, K$, that means that $h_1^k + h_2^k + h_3^k = l^k$ (condition (C_0)) and as remarked above the other conditions of Proposition 6 are satisfied. Now using

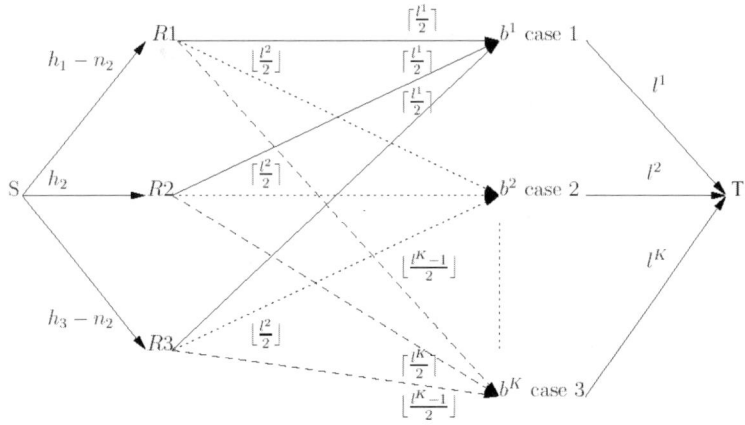

Fig. 7.6. The network associated with a matrix of $\mathcal{N}_4$ with $m = 3$.

the algorithm designed in the proof of Proposition 6, we know how to assign the 1's in each block B^k. On the other hand, since the value of the flow is $\Sigma_{k=1}^{K} l^k = h_1 + h_2 + h_3 - 2n_2$, the matrix A satisfies the horizontal projection and then A is a solution of **Reconstruction**$_{\mathcal{N}_4}(\mathbf{m}, \mathbf{n})$.

Conversely, if a solution of **Reconstruction**$_{\mathcal{N}_4}(\mathbf{m}, \mathbf{n})$ exists, $H^k = (h_1^k, h_2^k, h_3^k)$ is known for each block $B^k, k = 1, \ldots, K$. Thus, setting the value h_i^k for the flow of the arc (R_i, b^k), we obtain a feasible flow with value $\Sigma_{k=1}^{K} l^k$ in the network G.   □

Corollary 1. *For $m = 3$,* **Reconstruction**$_{\mathcal{N}_4}(\mathbf{m}, \mathbf{n})$ *can be solved in polynomial time.*

Proof. The computation of the flow in G can be done in polynomial time (see [1]). Clearly, the algorithm given in the proof of Proposition 6 is polynomial. Eventually, one can check the necessary conditions in polynomial time.   □

Binary Matrices under Non 6-Adjacency Constraint

We prove that **Consistency**$_{\mathcal{N}_6}(\mathbf{m}, \mathbf{n})$ is NP-complete. To do that, we show that a special case of **Consistency**$_{\mathcal{N}_6}(\mathbf{m}, \mathbf{n})$ is equivalent to an *L-tile packing problem* defined as follows: An *L-tile* is a polyomino with three cells as shown by Fig. 7.7. In addition, the lower left cell has a 1 and the two other cells have a 0. The projections are the number of 1's lying in each line (a cell not covered by an L-tile has a 0). The problem is to find L-tile packing with given projections $H = (h_1, \ldots, h_m)$ and $V = (v_1, \ldots, v_n)$.

Obviously, an L-tile packing exists only if $h_1 = v_n = 0$. Henceforth we are concerned with **Consistency**$_{\mathcal{N}_6}(\mathbf{m}, \mathbf{n} : \mathbf{h_1} = \mathbf{v_n} = \mathbf{0})$, the subproblem restricted to the instances with $h_1 = v_n = 0$.

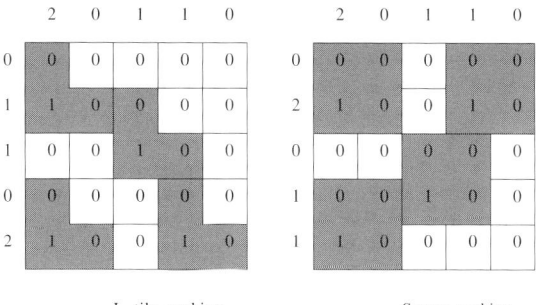

L–tile packing   Square packing

Fig. 7.7. A matrix of $\mathcal{N}_6$ (at left) and a matrix of $\mathcal{N}_8$ (at right) with their tile packings.

Lemma 2. Consistency$_{\mathcal{N}_6}$(m, n : h$_1$ = v$_n$ = 0) *is equivalent to the L-tile packing problem.*

Proof. Consider an instance $H = (0, h_2, \ldots, h_m)$ and $V = (v_1, \ldots, v_{n-1}, 0)$ common to both problems. Let S_1 be a solution to **Consistency$_{\mathcal{N}_6}$(m, n : h$_1$ = v$_n$ = 0)**. A solution S_2 to the L-tile packing problem can be obtained by assigning the 1's of S_1 to S_2. Indeed, since in S_1 two 1's are non 6-adjacent, two *L-tiles* cannot overlap in S_2. Conversely, a solution S_1 to **Consistency$_{\mathcal{N}_6}$(m, n : h$_1$ = v$_n$ = 0)** can be obtained from a solution S_2 to the L-tile packing problem, as well.   □

The L-tile packing problem is known to be NP-complete [11]. So we deduce the following theorem:

Theorem 4. Consistency$_{\mathcal{N}_6}$(m, n) *is NP-complete.*

Binary Matrices under Non 8-Adjacency Constraint

Here, we study **Consistency$_{\mathcal{N}_8}$(m, n)**. We first prove that a special case of **Consistency$_{\mathcal{N}_8}$(m, n)** is equivalent to the problem of 2×2 squares packing defined as follows: A 2×2 square is a polyomino with four cells as shown by Fig. 7.7. The lower left cell has a 1 and the other cells have a 0. The projections correspond to the number of 1's in each line (a cell not covered has a 0). The problem is to find a 2×2 square packing with given projections $H = (h_1, \ldots, h_m)$ and $V = (v_1, \ldots, v_n)$. Obviously, a 2×2 square packing is possible only if $h_1 = v_n = 0$.

Now, consider **Consistency$_{\mathcal{N}_8}$(m, n : h$_1$ = v$_n$ = 0)**, the subproblem restricted to instances with $h_1 = v_n = 0$.

Lemma 3. Consistency$_{\mathcal{N}_8}$(m, n : h$_1$ = v$_n$ = 0) *is equivalent to the 2×2 square packing problem.*

Proof. The proof uses the same arguments as proof of Lemma 2.   □

The 2×2 square packing problem has been proved to be as difficult as the three-colored image reconstruction problem, which is still an open problem [13]. We deduce the following theorem:

Theorem 5. Consistency$_{\mathcal{N}_8}(\mathbf{m}, \mathbf{n})$ *is as difficult as the three-colored image reconstruction problem.*

7.3.3 Conclusion

In this section we have studied problems **Reconstruction$_{\mathcal{N}_p}(\mathbf{m}, \mathbf{n})$** consisting of reconstructing a binary matrix that fulfills the non p-adjacency constraint from orthogonal projections. Polynomial-time algorithms are given to solve **Reconstruction$_{\mathcal{N}_2}(\mathbf{m}, \mathbf{n})$** and **Reconstruction$_{\mathcal{N}_4}(\mathbf{m}, \mathbf{n})$** in the special case where $m \leq 3$. We also give a polynomial-time algorithm for **Reconstruction$_{\mathcal{N}_4}(\mathbf{m})$**, the problem consisting of reconstructing a binary matrix that fulfills the non 4-adjacency constraint from only one projection. For **Reconstruction$_{\mathcal{N}_6}(\mathbf{m}, \mathbf{n})$**, we have proved the NP-completeness of **Consistency$_{\mathcal{N}_6}(\mathbf{m}, \mathbf{n})$**, its associated decision problem. The complexity status of both **Reconstruction$_{\mathcal{N}_4}(\mathbf{m}, \mathbf{n})$** and **Reconstruction$_{\mathcal{N}_8}(\mathbf{m}, \mathbf{n})$** remains an open question. However, we have shown that this last problem is harder than the three-colored image reconstruction problem, which is well known to be a major open problem in discrete tomography.

7.4 A Timetabling Constraint

We consider the problem of reconstructing an $m \times n$ binary matrix $A \in \mathcal{T}_k$ from its horizontal $H = (h_1, \ldots, h_m)$ and vertical $V = (v_1, \ldots, v_n)$ projections, where $\mathcal{T}_k$ is the class of binary matrices satisfying the timetabling constraint: If $a_{i,j} = 1$, then $a_{i,j-1} = 1$ or $a_{i,j+1} = 1$, and the number of successive 0's in each row of A is less than or equal to a given integer $k \geq 2$. We denote this problem by **Reconstruction$_{\mathcal{T}_k}(\mathbf{m}, \mathbf{n})$**.

This section is organized as follows. **Reconstruction$_{\mathcal{T}_k}(\mathbf{m}, \mathbf{n})$** is introduced, and we give necessary conditions for a solution to exist. Then we state some basic properties for **Reconstruction$_{\mathcal{T}_k}(\mathbf{m}, \mathbf{n} : \mathbf{m} = \mathbf{2})$**, the subproblem with $m = 2$. Finally, we use them to give a polynomial-time algorithm for **Reconstruction$_{\mathcal{T}_2}(\mathbf{m}, \mathbf{n} : \mathbf{m} = \mathbf{2})$**, the problem with $m = 2$ and $k = 2$.

7.4.1 The Basic Model

Formally, **Reconstruction$_{\mathcal{T}_k}(\mathbf{m}, \mathbf{n})$** is defined as follows: We are given two vectors $H = (h_1, \ldots, h_m)$ and $V = (v_1, \ldots, v_n)$ of nonnegative integers and an integer $k \geq 2$. From H and V we want to reconstruct an $m \times n$ binary matrix A such that, for $1 \leq i \leq m$ and $1 \leq j \leq n$,

$$\sum_{j=1}^{n} a_{i,j} = h_i, \tag{7.1}$$

$$\sum_{i=1}^{m} a_{i,j} = v_j, \tag{7.2}$$

if $a_{i,j} = 1$, then $a_{i,j} \times a_{i,j-1} + a_{i,j} \times a_{i,j+1} > 0$ $(a_{i,0} = a_{i,n+1} = 0)$, (7.3)

$$\sum_{l=0}^{k} a_{i,j'+l} > 0, \text{ with } 1 \leq j' \leq n - k + 1. \tag{7.4}$$

It is easy to see that (7.3) and (7.4) ensure that $A \in \mathcal{T}_k$ and (7.1) and (7.2) ensure that both projections are satisfied.

The following property gives necessary conditions for a solution to exist:

Property 6. If **Reconstruction**$_{\mathcal{T}_k}(\mathbf{m}, \mathbf{n})$ has a solution, then, for $1 \leq i \leq m$ and $1 \leq j \leq n$,

(a) $v_j \leq m$ and $n \geq h_i \geq \begin{cases} 2\lfloor n/(k+2) \rfloor, & \text{if } (n) mod_{k+2} \leq k, \\ 2\lfloor n/(k+2) \rfloor + 1, & \text{otherwise,} \end{cases}$

(b) $\sum_{i=1}^{m} h_i = \sum_{j=1}^{n} v_j$,
(c) $v_j \leq v_{j-1} + v_{j+1}, 1 \leq j \leq n$ (assuming $v_0 = v_{n+1} = 0$).

Proof. The inequalities $v_j \leq m$ and $n \geq h_i$ of (a) are trivial. From the definition of **Reconstruction**$_{\mathcal{T}_k}(\mathbf{m}, \mathbf{n})$, (7.3) and (7.4) imply that

- if $(n) mod_{k+2} \leq k$, then the sum of $k+2$ consecutive elements of a generic row of A has to be greater than 1, and thus $h_i \geq 2\lfloor n/(k+2) \rfloor$,
- if $(n) mod_{k+2} = k+1$, then the last $k+1$ elements of each row of A contain one entry 1 at least, so we have $h_i \geq 2\lfloor n/(k+2) \rfloor + 1$.

(b) and (c) follow from the definition of **Reconstruction**$_{\mathcal{T}_k}(\mathbf{m}, \mathbf{n})$. □

7.4.2 Necessary Conditions for Reconstruction$_{\mathcal{T}_k}(\mathbf{m}, \mathbf{n} : \mathbf{m} = 2)$

From now on, we concentrate our study on **Reconstruction**$_{\mathcal{T}_k}(\mathbf{m}, \mathbf{n} : \mathbf{m} = 2)$, giving further necessary conditions for a solution to exist.

The choice $m = 2$ allows the values of each vertical projection to belong to the set $\{0, 1, 2\}$. Furthermore, if a vertical projection, say v_j, has value 0 or 2, then the corresponding values of the jth column of A are fixed, i.e., $a_{1,j} = a_{2,j} = 0$ or $a_{1,j} = a_{2,j} = 1$, respectively. Thus, the nontrivial case is when $v_j = 1$, which implies $a_{1,j} + a_{2,j} = 1$.

Let us decompose the vector $V = (v_1, \ldots, v_n)$ of vertical projections into the subsequences $B_1^0, B_1^1, B_1^2, B_2^0, B_2^1, B_2^2, \ldots, B_p^0, B_p^1, B_p^2$, called blocks, such that the block B_i^0 is a maximal subsequence of successive 0's of length l_i^0, B_i^1 is a maximal subsequence of successive 1's of length l_i^1, and B_i^2 is a maximal subsequence of successive 2's of length l_i^2, with $1 \leq i \leq p$. We also allow a block B_i^j to be empty, i.e., $l_i^j = 0$. Obviously, the sum of the lengths of the blocks of consecutive 2's constitutes a lower bound to each horizontal projection.

For instance, if $V = (1, 1, 1, 0, 0, 2, 0, 0, 1, 2, 1)$, then its decomposition into blocks is

$$1, 1, 1, \qquad 0, 0, \qquad 2, \quad 0, 0, \quad 1, \quad 2, \qquad 1$$

$$\underbrace{}_{B_1^0} \underbrace{}_{B_1^1} \underbrace{}_{B_1^2} \underbrace{}_{B_2^0} \underbrace{}_{B_2^1} \underbrace{}_{B_2^2} \underbrace{}_{B_3^0} \underbrace{}_{B_3^1} \underbrace{}_{B_3^2} \underbrace{}_{B_4^0} \underbrace{}_{B_4^1} \underbrace{}_{B_4^2},$$

and the lengths of the blocks are

$$l_1^0 = l_1^2 = l_2^1 = l_4^0 = l_4^2 = 0, \quad l_2^2 = l_3^1 = l_3^2 = l_4^1 = 1, \quad l_2^0 = l_3^0 = 2, \text{ and } l_1^1 = 3.$$

It is straightforward that the length of every subsequence of any block depends on the length of the subsequences nearby. The following lemma provides necessary conditions for the existence of a solution.

Lemma 4. *If* **Reconstruction**$_{T_k}$(**m, n** : **m** = **2**) *has a solution, and the vector V is decomposed into p blocks, then, for $1 \leq i \leq p$,*

(a) $l_i^0 \leq k$,
(b) if $l_{i-1}^2 = 0$, then $l_i^0 \leq k - 1$,
(c) if $l_i^1 > 0$, then $l_i^0 \leq k - 1$,
(d) if $l_{i-1}^2 = 0$ and $(l_{i-1}^1 \geq 2$ or $l_i^1 \geq 2)$, then $l_i^0 \leq k - 2$.

Proof. If $l_i^0 = 0$, then the four statements are immediately satisfied. So, let B_i^0 be a nonempty block of consecutive 0's, and let q and r be the indices of its leftmost and rightmost positions in V, respectively. Now, (a) and (b) are immediate from (7.4). To show (c), we note that if $l_i^1 > 0$, then we have $a_{1,r+1} + a_{2,r+1} = 1$. Let us suppose, without loss of generality, that $a_{1,r+1} = 0$. If $l_i^0 > k-1$, then $\sum_{j=q}^{r+1} a_{1j} = 0$, which is inconsistent with (7.4). To show (d), we note that if $l_i^1 \geq 2$, then we have $a_{1,r+1} + a_{2,r+1} = 1$ and $a_{1,r+2} + a_{2,r+2} = 1$; without loss of generality, we suppose that $a_{1,r+1} = 0$. Since $a_{2,r} = 0$, (7.3) implies that $a_{2,r+2} = 1$, and, consequently, $a_{1,r+2} = 0$, which generates an inconsistency with (7.4). The case $l_{i-1}^1 \geq 2$ is analogous. □

7.4.3 A Polynomial Algorithm for Reconstruction$_{T_2}$(m, n : m = 2)

Let us consider an instance $I = (H, V)$ of **Reconstruction**$_{T_2}$(**m, n** : **m** = **2**). In the sequel, we furnish some operative lemmas that change I into an equivalent instance $\tilde{I} = (\tilde{H}, \tilde{V})$ with $\tilde{n} < n$, by reducing the lengths of some blocks of the decomposition of V. The equivalence of the two instances will directly follow from next lemmas.

Lemma 5. *Let $\tilde{I}$ be the instance I modified as follows: For each block B_i^2 in the decomposition of V such that $l_i^2 = q > 2$, let us set in $\tilde{I}$*

$$\tilde{l}_i^2 = 2, \quad \tilde{n} = n - q + 2, \quad \tilde{h}_1 = h_1 - q + 2, \quad \text{and} \quad \tilde{h}_2 = h_2 - q + 2, \quad (7.5)$$

and let us modify the vector $\tilde{V}$ in accordance with the new value of $\tilde{l}_i^2$. Then the instances I and $\tilde{I}$ are equivalent.

Proof. Let A be a binary matrix that is a solution of I. For each column j of A such that v_j belongs to the block B_i^2, it holds $a_{1,j} = a_{2,j} = 1$. Deleting $q - 2$ such columns, we obtain a binary matrix $\tilde{A}$, as can be easily checked to be a solution of $\tilde{I}$.

Conversely, let $\tilde{A}$ be a solution of $\tilde{I}$, and let the projection $\tilde{v}_j$ belong to $\tilde{B}_i^2$. If we add $q - 2$ columns after column j, and we set all their entries to the value 1, then we obtain the desired solution for I. $\square$

Lemma 6. *Let I be an instance of* **Reconstruction**$_{T_2}(\mathbf{m}, \mathbf{n} : \mathbf{m} = \mathbf{2})$. *There exists an instance $\tilde{I}$ equivalent to I, such that the vector $\tilde{V}$ has no elements equal to 0.*

Proof. Let the vector V of the instance I be divided into $3p$ blocks, and recall that from Lemma 4, we have $l_i^0 \leq 2$, with $1 \leq i \leq p$.

If $l_i^0 = 2$ (i.e., the block B_i^0 is composed of the vertical projections $(v_j, v_{j+1}) = (0,0)$), then from Lemma 4(b) and (c), we obtain that $l_{i-1}^2 > 0$ and $l_i^1 = 0$, and from Property 6(c), we have $l_{i-1}^2 \geq 2$ and $l_i^2 \geq 2$, i.e., $(v_{j-2}, \ldots v_{j+3}) = (2, 2, 0, 0, 2, 2)$.

Let $\tilde{A}$ be the matrix obtained from A by deleting columns j and $j + 1$. It is straightforward that A is a solution of I if, and only if, $\tilde{A}$ is a solution of the instance $\tilde{I}$ such that

$$H = \tilde{H} \quad \text{and} \quad \tilde{V} = (v_1, \ldots, v_{j-1}, v_{j+2}, \ldots, v_n). \tag{7.6}$$

We note that if $l_1^0 = 2$ or $l_p^0 = 2$ (i.e., $(0, 0, 2)$ is the initial subsequence of V or $(2, 0, 0)$ is the final subsequence of V), then the transformation still holds. Thus, we have that $I \equiv \tilde{I}$.

If $l_i^0 = 1$ (i.e., the block B_i^0 contains the single vertical projection $(v_j) = (0)$), then we analyze the following exhaustive series of subsequences of V.

(a) $(v_{j-2}, \ldots, v_{j+2}) = (2, 2, 0, 2, 2)$: If A is a solution of I, then acting similarly to the previous case, i.e., when $l_i^0 = 2$, we can construct a matrix $\tilde{A}$ that is a solution of the instance $\tilde{I}$ that is equivalent to I.

(b) $(v_{j-3}, \ldots, v_{j+3}) = (2, 2, 1, 0, 1, 2, 2)$: If A is a solutions of I, then there are only two possible submatrices corresponding to the seven columns $j - 3, \ldots j + 3$:

$$\begin{pmatrix} 1 1 1 0 0 1 1 \\ 1 1 0 0 1 1 1 \end{pmatrix} \quad \text{or} \quad \begin{pmatrix} 1 1 0 0 1 1 1 \\ 1 1 1 0 0 1 1 \end{pmatrix}. \tag{7.7}$$

Starting from A, we can construct the matrix $\tilde{A}$ by deleting its three columns $j - 1$, j, and $j + 1$, so that A is a solution of I if, and only if, $\tilde{A}$ is a solution of the instance $\tilde{I}$ such that

$$\tilde{H} = (h_1 - 1, h_2 - 1) \quad \text{and} \quad \tilde{V} = (v_1, \ldots, v_{j-2}, v_{j+2}, \ldots, v_n). \tag{7.8}$$

(c) $(v_{j-3}, \ldots, v_{j+3}) = (2, 2, 1, 0, 1, 2, 1)$: If A is a solution of I, then its only two possible submatrices corresponding to the seven columns $j-3, \ldots j+3$ are

$$\begin{pmatrix} 1 1 1 0 0 1 1 \\ 1 1 0 0 1 1 0 \end{pmatrix} \quad \text{or} \quad \begin{pmatrix} 1 1 0 0 1 1 0 \\ 1 1 1 0 0 1 1 \end{pmatrix}. \tag{7.9}$$

Starting from A, we can construct the matrix $\tilde{A}$ by deleting its four columns j, $j+1$, $j+2$, and $j+3$, so that $\tilde{A}$ is a solution of the instance $\tilde{I}$ such that

$$\tilde{H} = (h_1 - 2, h_2 - 2) \quad \text{and} \quad \tilde{V} = (v_1, \ldots, v_{j-1}, v_{j+4}, \ldots, v_n). \tag{7.10}$$

The equivalence of the instances I and $\tilde{I}$ can be easily deduced.

(d) $(v_{j-3}, \ldots, v_{j+3}) = (1, 2, 1, 0, 1, 2, 2)$: symmetrical to the previous case.
(e) $(v_{j-3}, \ldots, v_{j+3}) = (1, 2, 1, 0, 1, 2, 1)$: similar to the previous two cases.
(f) $(v_{j-1}, \ldots, v_{j+2}) = (2, 0, 1, 2)$: From Property 6, we have that $v_{j-2} = 2$. The matrix $\tilde{A}$ obtained after deleting column j from A is a solution of the instance $\tilde{I}$, where $\tilde{H} = H$, and $\tilde{V}$ is obtained from V after deleting the entry v_j. Obviously, I is equivalent to $\tilde{I}$.
(g) $(v_{j-1}, \ldots, v_{j+2}) = (2, 1, 0, 2)$: symmetrical to the previous case.
(h) $(v_1) = (0)$ (respectively, $(v_n) = (0)$): If A is a solution of I, then the matrix $\tilde{A}$ obtained from A after deleting its first (respectively, its last) column is obviously a solution of instance $\tilde{I}$ such that $\tilde{H} = H$, and $\tilde{V}$ is obtained from V after deleting the entry v_1 (respectively, v_n).

The given list of configurations of the entries of V surrounding column j when $B_i^0 = (v_j)$ is exhaustive, since Lemma 4 assures that the subsequences $(1, 1, 0)$ and $(0, 1, 1)$ cannot be subsequences of V.   □

Lemma 7. *Let I be an instance of* **Reconstruction**$_{T_2}(\mathbf{m}, \mathbf{n} : \mathbf{m} = \mathbf{2})$*. There exists an instance $\tilde{I}$, equivalent to I, such that the vector $\tilde{V}$ contains no subsequences of consecutive entries 1 having length greater than 4.*

Proof. Let the vector V of the instance I be divided into $3p$ blocks, and let us suppose that there exists a block $B_i^1 = (v_j, \ldots, v_{j+q}) = (1, \ldots, 1)$ such that $l_i^1 = q + 1 \geq 5$, with $1 \leq i \leq p$. If A is a solution of I, then the submatrix composed of its four columns j, $j+1$, $j+2$, and $j+3$ is one among

$$\begin{pmatrix} 1 1 0 0 \\ 0 0 1 1 \end{pmatrix}, \quad \begin{pmatrix} 0 0 1 1 \\ 1 1 0 0 \end{pmatrix}, \quad \begin{pmatrix} 1 0 0 1 \\ 0 1 1 0 \end{pmatrix}, \quad \text{and} \quad \begin{pmatrix} 0 1 1 0 \\ 1 0 0 1 \end{pmatrix}. \tag{7.11}$$

Moreover, for each of these four configurations, it is easy to check that the columns j and $j+4$ are identical, and so the matrix $\tilde{A}$ obtained from A by deleting its four columns j, $j+1$, $j+2$, and $j+3$ is a solution of the instance $\tilde{I}$, where

$$\tilde{H} = (h_1 - 2, h_2 - 2) \text{ and } \tilde{V} = (v_1, \ldots, v_{j-1}, v_{j+4}, \ldots, v_n). \tag{7.12}$$

The equivalence of I and $\tilde{I}$ is straightforward. Repeating the deletion of all the groups of four consecutive entries 1 from V, we obtain the lemma.   □

7.4.4 Graph Building

The three lemmas stated above allow us to solve **Reconstruction**$_{T_2}$(**m, n : m = 2**) by considering only its instances that satisfy the three constraints $l_i^0 = 0$, $l_i^1 \leq 4$, and $l_i^2 \leq 2$, with $1 \leq i \leq p$. Now, each one of such instances, say instance $I = (H, V)$ to keep the notation already introduced, is going to be reduced to an instance of a fast solvable problem concerning the search for paths inside a graph.

Let V be divided into $2p$ blocks $B_1^1, B_1^2, \ldots, B_p^1, B_p^2$. From the sequence of blocks, we construct a directed labelled graph $G = (X, A, lab)$.

The nodes of G, i.e., the elements of the set X, are associated to the blocks B_i^2 in the following way, for $1 \leq i \leq p$:

(a) if $l_i^2 = 2$, then we associate one node x_i to the block B_i^2;
(b) if $l_i^2 = 1$, then we associate two different nodes x_i^1 and x_i^2 to the block B_i^2.

We also add to X a source node x_0 and a sink node x_{p+1}.

The arcs of G, that is, the elements of A, connect the nodes associated to the blocks B_{i-1}^2, and B_i^2 and correspond to the blocks B_i^1. Since Lemma 6 allows us to get rid of the blocks composed of 0's, for each $1 \leq i \leq p$, we list all the possible configurations for the submatrix A_i^1 associated with the block B_i^1 (this permits us to reduce the number of arcs) as follows:

If $l_i^1 = 1$, then the submatrix A_i^1 can be one of the following:

$$\mu_1^1 = \begin{pmatrix} 1 \\ 0 \end{pmatrix} \quad \text{or} \quad \mu_2^1 = \begin{pmatrix} 0 \\ 1 \end{pmatrix};$$ (7.13)

if $l_i^1 = 2$, then A_i^1 can be one of the following:

$$\mu_1^2 = \begin{pmatrix} 11 \\ 00 \end{pmatrix}, \ \mu_2^2 = \begin{pmatrix} 00 \\ 11 \end{pmatrix}, \ \mu_3^2 = \begin{pmatrix} 10 \\ 01 \end{pmatrix} \quad \text{or} \quad \mu_4^2 = \begin{pmatrix} 01 \\ 10 \end{pmatrix};$$ (7.14)

if $l_i^1 = 3$, then A_i^1 can be one of the following:

$$\mu_1^3 = \begin{pmatrix} 110 \\ 001 \end{pmatrix}, \ \mu_2^3 = \begin{pmatrix} 001 \\ 110 \end{pmatrix}, \ \mu_3^3 = \begin{pmatrix} 100 \\ 011 \end{pmatrix} \quad \text{or} \quad \mu_4^3 = \begin{pmatrix} 011 \\ 100 \end{pmatrix};$$ (7.15)

finally, if $l_i^1 = 4$, then A_i^1 can be one of the following:

$$\mu_1^4 = \begin{pmatrix} 1100 \\ 0011 \end{pmatrix}, \ \mu_2^4 = \begin{pmatrix} 0011 \\ 1100 \end{pmatrix}, \ \mu_3^4 = \begin{pmatrix} 1001 \\ 0110 \end{pmatrix} \quad \text{or} \quad \mu_4^4 = \begin{pmatrix} 0110 \\ 1001 \end{pmatrix}.$$ (7.16)

Note that every possible configuration for A_i^1 satisfies (7.4) of the basic model, but not (7.3). So this last property is not local, but global. In other words, the "compatibility" of a specific configuration with the block B_i^1 strongly depends on the configurations associated to the blocks B_{i-1}^2 and B_i^2. As an "extreme" example, the submatrix μ_3^3 is not compatible with the block B_1^1 (assuming $l_1^1 = 3$), while it is compatible with the block B_p^1 when $l_p^1 = 3$

(assuming $l^2_{p-1} = 2$). Indeed, in order for this last property to be satisfied by the global solution, we need to express this constraint in terms of the arcs of the graph we are going to build.

We can now assign the arcs of the graph connecting the nodes associated to the block B^2_{i-1} with those associated to the B^2_i, as follows:

(a) If $l^2_{i-1} = l^2_i = 2$, then there is an arc (x_{i-1}, x_i);
(b) if $l^2_{i-1} = 2$ and $l^2_i = 1$, then there are two arcs (x_{i-1}, x^1_i) and (x_{i-1}, x^2_i);
(c) if $l^2_{i-1} = 1$ and $l^2_i = 2$, then there are two arcs (x^1_{i-1}, x_i) and (x^2_{i-1}, x_i);
(d) if $l^2_{i-1} = 1$ and $l^2_i = 1$, then
    a) if $l^1_i = 1$, then there are two arcs (x^1_{i-1}, x^2_i) and (x^2_{i-1}, x^1_i);
    b) if $l^1_i = 3$, then there are two arcs (x^1_{i-1}, x^1_i) and (x^2_{i-1}, x^2_i);
    c) if $l^1_i = 2$ or $l^1_i = 4$, then there are all four possible arcs (x^1_{i-1}, x^1_i), (x^1_{i-1}, x^2_i), (x^2_{i-1}, x^1_i), and (x^2_{i-1}, x^2_i).

Let us refer to y_i a generic node. The function *lab* associates to each arc (y_{i-1}, y_i) a set of integers (labels) in the interval $[0, 4]$, depending on the possible submatrices that are compatible with the blocks B^2_{i-1} and B^2_i in the final solution A.

More precisely, each label counts the number of 1's lying in the first row of each possible configuration μ^j_i of the block B^1_i which is compatible with the blocks B^2_{i-1} and B^2_i and is such that $l^1_i = j$. We remark that the word "compatible" is once again used with the meaning of satisfying the timetabling constraint.

A further assumption is needed: If an arc reaches the node x^1_i (respectively, x^2_i), then the configurations chosen for the assignment of its labels has to end with the column $(1, 0)^T$ (respectively, $(0, 1)^T$).

An example of such a graph is given by Fig. 7.8. The graph has seven nodes in addition to x_0 and x_5, since (1121112212111121) is composed of four blocks B^2_i, one of which, B^2_2 of length 2, gives rise to node x_2, and the others of lengths 1. Since B^1_1 has length 2 configurations, μ^2_1 and μ^2_2 are the only ones that satisfy property (7.3) of the basic model. Therefore, we assign label $\{2\}$ to (x_0, x^1_1) corresponding to configuration μ^2_1 and label $\{0\}$ to (x_0, x^2_1) corresponding to configuration μ^2_2. B^1_2 has length 3, and we assign label $\{1, 2\}$ to (x^1_1, x_2), since the compatible configurations are μ^3_2 and μ^3_4, and label $\{1, 2\}$ to (x^1_1, x_2), since the compatible configurations are μ^3_1 and μ^3_3. Then, B^1_3 has length 1, and since B^2_2 has length 2, all the configurations are compatible, and so we label (x_2, x^1_3) with $\{1\}$ (corresponding to μ^1_1), and (x_2, x^2_3) with 0 (corresponding to μ^1_2). B^1_4 has length 4, and the label $\{2\}$ to (x^1_3, x^1_4) corresponds to configuration μ^4_2, while the label to (x^1_3, x^2_4) corresponds to configuration μ^4_4. We do similarly for the arcs from x^2_3. Finally, (x^1_4, x_5) has label $\{1\}$, which corresponds to configuration μ^1_1, and (x^2_4, x_5) has label $\{0\}$, which corresponds to configuration μ^1_2.

To the path $\pi = (x_0, x^1_1, x_2, x^2_3, x^1_4, x_5)$ of Fig. 7.8, correspond the two matrices

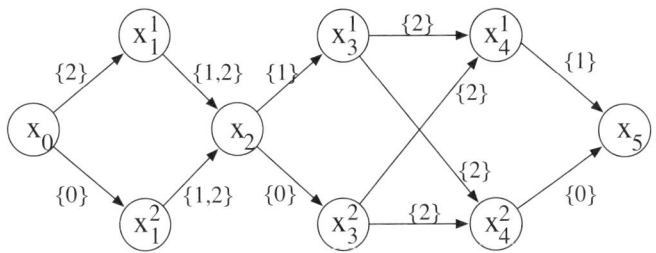

Fig. 7.8. The graph built from (1121112212111121).

$$M = \begin{pmatrix} 0011101101100110 \\ 1110011111011011 \end{pmatrix} \text{ and } M = \begin{pmatrix} 0011001101100110 \\ 1110111111011011 \end{pmatrix}. \quad (7.17)$$

The graph G has the following property:

Lemma 8. *There is a one-to-one correspondence between the paths of G and the matrices A satisfying (7.2), (7.3), and (7.4) of the basic model.*

Proof. Let $\pi = (x_0, y_1, \dots, y_p, x_{p+1})$ be a path of G. The matrices A corresponding to π are such that $M = A_1^1.A_1^2.A_2^1 \dots A_p^1.A_p^2$, where the submatrices A_i^2 are associated to the nodes y_i of π and the submatrices A_i^1 are associated to the arcs (y_{i-1}, y_i).

Consider any node y_i, $1 \le i \le p$: if $y_i = x_i$; then

$$A_i^2 = \begin{pmatrix} 11 \\ 11 \end{pmatrix}, \quad (7.18)$$

while if $y_i = x_i^1$ or $y_i = x_i^2$, then $A_i^2 = (1,1)^T$.

For an arc (x_{i-1}, x_i), $2 \le i \le p$, associated to the block B_i^1 of length $l_i^1 = j$, A_i^1 is a certain matrix μ_l^j.

In particular, for the first arc (x_0, y) of π, we have the following matrices A_1^1: If $j = 0$, then A_1^1 does not exist; if $y = x_1$, then we have $A_1^1 = \mu_1^1$ or $A_1^1 = \mu_2^1$ for $j = 1$, $A_1^1 = \mu_1^2$ or $A_1^1 = \mu_2^2$ for $j = 2$, $A_1^1 = \mu_1^3$ or $A_1^1 = \mu_2^3$ for $j = 3$, $A_1^1 = \mu_1^4$ or $A_1^1 = \mu_2^4$ for $j = 4$; if $y = x_1^1$, then we have $A_1^1 = \mu_1^1$ for $j = 1$, $A_1^1 = \mu_1^2$ for $j = 2$, $A_1^1 = \mu_2^3$ for $j = 3$, $A_1^1 = \mu_2^4$ for $j = 4$; and in the case $y = x_1^2$, we have $A_1^1 = \mu_2^1$ for $j = 1$, $A_1^1 = \mu_2^2$ for $j = 2$, $A_1^1 = \mu_1^3$ for $j = 3$, $A_1^1 = \mu_1^4$ for $j = 4$.

For the last arc (y, x_{p+1}), $y \ne x_p$, of π, we have the following matrices A_p^1: If $y = x_{p-1}$, then we have $A_p^1 = \mu_1^1$ or $A_p^1 = \mu_2^1$ for $j = 1$, $A_p^1 = \mu_1^2$ or $A_p^1 = \mu_2^2$ for $j = 2$, $A_3^1 = \mu_3^3$ or $A_p^1 = \mu_3^3$ for $j = 3$, $A_p^1 = \mu_1^4$ or $A_p^1 = \mu_1^4$ for $j = 4$; if $y = x_{p-1}^1$, then we have $A_p^1 = \mu_1^1$ for $j = 1$, $A_p^1 = \mu_2^2$ for $j = 2$, $A_p^1 = \mu_3^3$ for $j = 3$, $A_p^1 = \mu_2^4$ for $j = 4$; in the case where $y = x_{p-1}^2$, we have $A_p^1 = \mu_1^1$ for $j = 1$, $A_p^1 = \mu_1^2$ for $j = 2$, $A_p^1 = \mu_3^3$ for $j = 3$, $A_p^1 = \mu_1^4$ for $j = 4$.

For an arc (y, x_i^1), $2 \le i \le p$, A_i^1 is a matrix μ_l^j such that its last column is $(1,0)^T$, that is, $A_i^1 = \mu_1^1$ for the case $j = 1$, $A_i^1 = \mu_1^2$ or $A_i^1 = \mu_4^2$ in case of $j = 2$, $A_i^1 = \mu_2^3$ or $A_i^1 = \mu_4^3$ for the case $j = 3$, $A_i^1 = \mu_2^4$ or $A_i^1 = \mu_3^4$ for the case $j = 4$.

For an arc (y, x_i^2), $2 \le i \le p$, A_i^1 is a matrix μ_l^j such that the last column of μ_l^j is $(0,1)^T$, i.e., $A_i^1 = \mu_2^1$ for $j = 1$, $A_i^1 = \mu_2^2$ or $A_i^1 = \mu_3^2$ for $j = 2$, $A_i^1 = \mu_1^3$ or $A_i^1 = \mu_3^3$ for $j = 3$, $A_i^1 = \mu_1^4$ or $A_i^1 = \mu_4^4$ for $j = 4$.

In a same way, for an arc (x_{i-1}^1, y), $2 \le i \le p$, A_i^1 is a matrix μ_l^j having $(0,1)^T$ for last column, i.e., μ_2^1 for $j = 1$, μ_2^2 or μ_3^2 for $j = 2$, μ_1^3 or μ_3^3 for $j = 3$, μ_1^4 or μ_4^4 for $j = 4$.

Finally, for an arc (x_{i-1}^2, y), $2 \le i \le p$, A_i^1 is a matrix with last column $(1,0)^T$, i.e., μ_1^1 for $j = 1$, μ_1^2 or μ_4^2 for $j = 2$, μ_2^3 or μ_4^3 for $j = 3$, μ_2^4 or μ_3^4 for $j = 4$.

The matrices μ_l^j satisfy (7.2) and (7.4) of the basic model, and so the matrices A satisfy (7.2) and (7.4).

Trivially, the point (7.3) of the basic model is satisfied for the submatrix associated with a node x_i, $1 \le i \le p$, and for a matrix μ_l^j associated with an arc $(x_i - 1, x_i)$ of π. Now let us consider a node x_i^1: Following the choices made for the matrices μ_l^j associated with the arc (y, x_i^1) entering in x_i^1 and for the arc (x_i^1, y) leaving out x_i^1, (7.3) is satisfied. The same fact holds for the nodes x_i^2 of π.

Now let A be a matrix satisfying (7.2), (7.3), and (7.4) of the basic model. The nodes of $\mu = (x_0, \ldots, x_{p+1})$ are as follows: Let B_i^2 be a block such that $l_i^2 = 1$. We denote by A^j the column of A corresponding to B_i^2, and we denote by $\bar{A}^j$ the submatrix of A consisting of the three columns A^{j-1}, A^j, A^{j+1}. From (7.3), $\bar{A}^j$ is either

$$\bar{A}^j = \begin{pmatrix} 110 \\ 011 \end{pmatrix} \text{ or } \bar{A}^j = \begin{pmatrix} 011 \\ 110 \end{pmatrix}. \tag{7.19}$$

In the first case, μ passes through x_i^1, and in the second case, the path μ goes through the node x_i^2. If B_i^2 is a block such that $l_i^2 = 2$, then x_i^2 is a node of the path μ. Following the manner in which the arcs are set in G, we have that $\mu = (x_0, \ldots, x_{p+1})$ is a path of G. $\square$

Let μ be a path from x_0 to x_{p+1}. Denoting by $\lambda_i, 0 \le i \le p$, the set of integers making the label of the arc (y_i, y_{i+1}) of μ, the integer set $H(\mu)$ is defined as $H(\mu) = H(x_{p+1})$ with

$$H(y_i) = \begin{cases} \emptyset, & \text{if } i = 0, \\ \{a + b \mid a \in H(y_{i-1}), b \in \lambda_i\}, & \text{if } i > 0. \end{cases} \tag{7.20}$$

Using $\bar{h}_1 = |\{j \mid v_j = 1\}|$ (the number of columns with vertical projection equal to one), the next lemma gives a necessary and sufficient condition for a solution of **Reconstruction**$_{T_k}(\mathbf{m}, \mathbf{n} : \mathbf{m} = 2, \mathbf{k} = 2)$ to exist.

Lemma 9. *A solution of* **Reconstruction**$_{T_2}$(**m, n** : **m** = **2**) *exists if, and only if, there is a path* $\mu = (x_0, \ldots, x_{p+1})$ *of* G *such that* $\bar{h}_1 \in H(\mu)$.

Proof. From the previous lemma, it remains to prove that a matrix satisfying (7.1) of the basic model exists if, and only if, there exists a path μ of G such that $\bar{h}_1 \in H(\mu)$.

In G, the values making the label of an arc are the sums of the first row of the matrices μ_l^j associated with this arc (see the proof of the previous lemma). Thus, if A is a matrix with the first row sum equal to h_1, its corresponding path μ in G is such that $\bar{h}_1 \in H(\mu)$. Now, if there exists μ such that $\bar{h}_1 \in H(\mu)$, then there exists a matrix A with h_1 for the sum of its first row.   □

Hence, we are able to establish the following result.

Theorem 6. Reconstruction$_{T_2}$(**m, n** : **m** = **2**) *can be solved in time* $O(n^2)$.

Proof. G being a directed acyclic graph, we can use dynamic programming, i.e., the Ford algorithm (see [14], Section 24.2) to compute the values $H(x_i)$. Since a path from x_0 to x_{p+1} has length p and the label of an arc of G is such that $\lambda \subset \{0, 1, 2\}$, we have that $H(x_i) \in \{0, \ldots, 2p\}$, $0 \leq i \leq p+1$. Each node of G has at most two ancestors, so $H(x_i)$ can be computed with time $O(p)$. So we can compute the values $H(x)$ in time $O(p^2)$.   □

7.4.5 Conclusion

In this section we have studied **Reconstruction**$_{T_k}$(**m, n**), the problem of constructing a binary matrix that fulfills a particular timetabling constraint from orthogonal projections. We have designed a polynomial-time algorithm for the special subproblem **Reconstruction**$_{T_2}$(**m, n** : **m** = **2**), where $m = 2$ and $k = 2$. Using similar but more combinatorial and sophisticated arguments, we can design a polynomial-time algorithm for **Reconstruction**$_{T_k}$(**m, n** : **m** = **2**). The complexity status of **Reconstruction**$_{T_k}$(**m, n**) is still open even for its subproblem in which $m = 3$ and $k = 2$.

References

1. Ahuja, R.K., Magnanti, T.L., and Orlin, J.B.: *Network Flows.* Prentice Hall, Englewood Cliffs, NJ (1993).
2. Alfares, H.K.: Four day workweek scheduling with two or three consecutive days off. *J. Math. Modeling Algorithms*, **2**, 67–80 (2003).
3. Alfares, H.K.: Survey, categorization, and comparison of recent tour scheduling literature. *Annals of Operations Research*, **127**, 147–177 (2004).
4. Barcucci, E., Del Lungo, A, Nivat, M., Pinzani, R.: Reconstructing convex polyominoes from horizontal and vertical projections. *Theor. Comp. Sci.*, **155**, 321–347 (1996).

5. Baxter, R.J.: Planar lattice gases with nearest-neighbour exclusion. *Annals of Combinatorics*, **3**, 191–203 (1999).
6. Brunetti, S., Daurat, A.: An algorithm reconstructing convex lattice sets. *Theor. Comp. Sci.*, **304**, 35–57 (2003).
7. Brunetti, S., Del Lungo, A., Del Ristoro, F., Kuba, A., Maurice, N.: Reconstruction of 4- and 8-connected convex discrete sets from row and column projections. *Lin. Algebra Appl.*, **339**, 37–57 (2001).
8. Burns, R.N., Narasimhan, R., Smith, L.D.: A set processing algorithm for scheduling staff on 4-day or 3-day work weeks. *Naval Research Logistics*, **45**, 839–853 (1998).
9. Calkin, N.J., Wilf, H.S.: The number of independent sets in a grid graph. *SIAM J. Discr. Math.*, **11**, 54–60 (1998).
10. Chan, M.T., Herman, G.T., Levitan, E.: Bayesian image reconstruction using image-modeling Gibbs priors. *Int. J. Imaging Systems Techn.*, **9**, 85–98 (1998).
11. Chrobak, M., Couperus, P., Dürr, C., Woeginger, G.: A note on tiling under tomographic constraints. *Theor. Comp. Sci.*, **290**, 2125–2136 (2003).
12. Chrobak, M., Dürr, C.: Reconstructing hv-convex polyominoes from orthogonal projections. *Inform. Process. Lett.*, **69**, 283–289 (1999).
13. Chrobak, M., Dürr, C.: Reconstructing polyatomic structures from X-rays: NP-completeness proof for three atoms. *Theor. Comp. Sci.*, **259**, 81–98 (2001).
14. Cormen, T., Leiserson, C., Rivest, R., Stein, C.: *Introduction to Algorithms.* 2nd edition, MIT Press, Cambridge, MA (2001).
15. Del Lungo, A., Frosini, A., Nivat, M., Vuillon, L.: Reconstruction under periodicity constraints. In: Widmayer, P., Triguero, F., Morales, R., Hennessy, M., Eidenbenz, S., Conejo, R. (eds.), *Automata, Languages and Programming*, Springer, Berlin, Germany, pp. 38–56 (2002).
16. Del Lungo, A., Nivat, M.: Reconstruction of connected sets from two projections. In Herman, G.T., Kuba, A. (eds.), *Discrete Tomography: Foundations, Algorithms, and Applications*, Birkhäuser, Boston, MA, pp. 163–188 (1999).
17. Herman, G.T., Kuba, A. (eds.): *Discrete Tomography: Foundations, Algorithms, and Applications.* Birkhäuser, Boston, MA (1999).
18. Hung, R.: Single-shift off-day scheduling of a hierarchical workforce with variable demands. *European J. Operational Research*, **78**, 49–57 (1994).
19. Jarray F.: *Résolution de problèmes de tomographie discrète. Applications à la planification de personnel.* Ph.D. Thesis, CNAM, Paris, France (2004).
20. Kuba, A., Balogh, E.: Reconstruction of convex 2D discrete sets in polynomial time. *Theor. Comput. Sci.*, **283**, 223–242 (2000).
21. Picouleau, C.: Reconstruction of domino tiling from its two orthogonal projections. *Theor. Comp. Sci.*, **255**, 437–447 (2001).
22. Ryser, H.J.: Combinatorial properties of matrices of zeros and ones. *Canad. J. Math.*, **9**, 371–377 (1957).
23. Ryser, H.: *Combinatorial Mathematics*, Mathematical Association of America, Washington, DC (1963).
24. Woeginger, G.J.: The reconstruction of polyominoes from their orthogonal projections. *Info. Process. Lett.*, **77**, 225–229 (2001).

Part II

Discrete Tomography Reconstruction
Algorithms

Decomposition Algorithms for Reconstructing Discrete Sets with Disjoint Components

P. Balázs

Summary. The reconstruction of discrete sets from their projections is a frequently studied field in discrete tomography with applications in electron microscopy, image processing, radiology, and so on. Several efficient reconstruction algorithms have been developed for certain classes of discrete sets having some good geometrical properties. On the other hand, it has been shown that the reconstruction under certain circumstances can be very time-consuming, even NP-hard. In this chapter we show how prior information that the set to be reconstructed consists of several components can be exploited in order to facilitate the reconstruction. We present some general techniques to decompose a discrete set into components knowing only its projections and thus reduce the reconstruction of a general discrete set to the reconstruction of single components, which is usually a simpler task.

8.1 Introduction

The reconstruction of two-dimensional discrete sets from few (usually up to four) projections is a frequently studied field of discrete tomography. Reconstruction algorithms have a wide area of applications, e.g., in electron microscopy, image processing, nondestructive testing, radiology, statistical data security, and so on (see the final chapters of this book and [14] for some of the applications).

The main challenge in designing reconstruction algorithms is that the reconstruction problem is usually underdetermined; therefore, the number of solutions for a given reconstruction task can be very large. Moreover, the reconstruction under certain circumstances can be NP-hard [10, 12, 18]. Since applications require fast algorithms that give unambiguous solutions, scientists of this field began to study the possibility of keeping the reconstruction process tractable and to reduce the number of solutions. A commonly used technique that can lead to efficient reconstruction is to suppose some prior information on the set to be reconstructed. The most frequently used properties are connectedness, directedness, and some kind of discrete versions of the convexity. A lot of work has been done in designing efficient reconstruction algorithms for different classes of discrete sets satisfying some of the above properties [4, 5, 6, 7, 8, 11, 15, 16, 17]. While the reconstruction from two projections in the class of hv-convex sets is in general NP-hard [18], it turned out that the additional prior knowledge that the set has only one component (i.e., it is 4-connected) leads to a polynomial-time reconstruction algorithm [6]. Later, this algorithm was generalized for the class of 8-connected hv-convex sets [4]. Surprisingly, in [3] the authors showed that in this class the prior information that the set to be reconstructed consists of more than one component (i.e., if the set is not 4-connected) leads to a more efficient reconstruction algorithm than the general one developed in [4]. The above results show that prior knowledge about the number of components can have an effect on the reconstruction task.

The aim of this chapter is to present what we know about reconstruction complexity in several classes when the additional information that the set consists of several disjoint components is also given. The chapter is structured as follows: After introducing the necessary definitions and notations (Section 8.2), we investigate the problem of reconstructing discrete sets with disjoint components from two projections in Section 8.3. In Section 8.4, we describe a general technique for reconstructing decomposable discrete sets from four projections. Section 8.5 is about the correctness and complexity of the algorithms presented in the previous two sections. Finally, in Section 8.6, we conclude our results.

8.2 Preliminaries

A *discrete set* F is a finite subset of $\mathbb{Z}^2$ and can be represented as a set of pixels or by a binary matrix $\hat{F}$ (see Fig. 8.1). The elements of a discrete set are called *points* or *positions*. The smallest containing discrete rectangle (SCDR) of F is denoted by $R(F)$. For any discrete set F, we define the vectors $\mathcal{H}(F) = H = (h_1, \ldots, h_m)$, $\mathcal{V}(F) = V = (v_1, \ldots, v_n)$, $\mathcal{D}(F) = D = (d_1, \ldots, d_{m+n-1})$, and $\mathcal{A}(F) = A = (a_1, \ldots, a_{m+n-1})$, where

$$h_i = \sum_{j=1}^{n} \hat{f}_{ij}, \qquad i = 1, \ldots, m , \tag{8.1}$$

$$v_j = \sum_{i=1}^{m} \hat{f}_{ij}, \qquad j = 1, \ldots, n , \tag{8.2}$$

$$d_k = \sum_{i+(n-j)=k} \hat{f}_{ij}, \qquad a_k = \sum_{i+j=k+1} \hat{f}_{ij}, \qquad k = 1, \ldots, m+n-1. \tag{8.3}$$

The vectors H, V, D, and A are called the *horizontal*, *vertical*, *diagonal*, and *antidiagonal projections* of F, respectively. The *cumulated vectors* of F are denoted by $\widetilde{H} = (\widetilde{h}_1, \ldots, \widetilde{h}_m)$, $\widetilde{V} = (\widetilde{v}_1, \ldots, \widetilde{v}_n)$, $\widetilde{D} = (\widetilde{d}_1, \ldots, \widetilde{d}_{m+n-1})$, and $\widetilde{A} = (\widetilde{a}_1, \ldots, \widetilde{a}_{m+n-1})$ and defined by the following formulas:

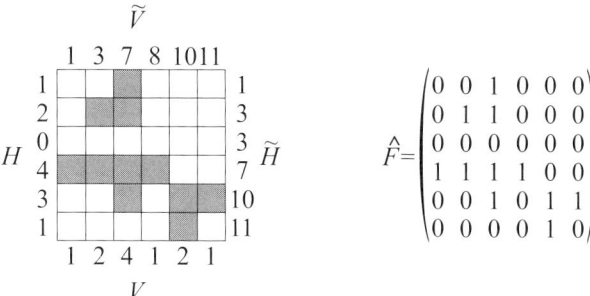

Fig. 8.1. A discrete set F represented by gray unitary squares and the corresponding binary matrix $\hat{F}$. The projections of F are H, V, $D = (0, 0, 0, 1, 2, 3, 2, 2, 1, 0, 0)$, and $A = (0, 0, 2, 2, 1, 1, 2, 0, 1, 2, 0)$. The cumulated vectors of F are $\tilde{H}$, $\tilde{V}$, $\tilde{D} = (0, 0, 0, 1, 3, 6, 8, 10, 11, 11, 11)$, and $\tilde{A} = (0, 0, 2, 4, 5, 6, 8, 8, 9, 11, 11)$.

$$\tilde{h}_i = \sum_{l=1}^{i} h_l, \qquad i = 1, \ldots, m \; ; \tag{8.4}$$

$$\tilde{v}_j = \sum_{l=1}^{j} v_l, \qquad j = 1, \ldots, n \; ; \tag{8.5}$$

$$\tilde{d}_k = \sum_{l=1}^{k} d_l, \qquad \tilde{a}_k = \sum_{l=1}^{k} a_l, \qquad k = 1, \ldots, m+n-1 \; . \tag{8.6}$$

Given an arbitrary class $\mathcal{G}$ of discrete sets, we say that the discrete set $F \in \mathcal{G}$ is *unique in the class* $\mathcal{G}$ (with respect to some projections) if there is no other discrete set $F' \in \mathcal{G}$ with the same projections.

In this chapter, we study the reconstruction problem from two and four projections in several classes, whose tasks for a given class $\mathcal{G} \subseteq \mathcal{F}$ can be formulated as follows:

2-RECONSTRUCTION($\mathcal{G}$)

Instance: Two nonnegative vectors $H \in \mathbb{N}_0^m$ and $V \in \mathbb{N}_0^n$.

Task: Construct a discrete set $F \in \mathcal{G}$ such that $\mathcal{H}(F) = H$ and $\mathcal{V}(F) = V$.

4-RECONSTRUCTION($\mathcal{G}$)

Instance: Four nonnegative vectors $H \in \mathbb{N}_0^m$, $V \in \mathbb{N}_0^n$, $D \in \mathbb{N}_0^{m+n-1}$, and $A \in \mathbb{N}_0^{m+n-1}$.

Task: Construct a discrete set $F \in \mathcal{G}$ such that $\mathcal{H}(F) = H$, $\mathcal{V}(F) = V$, $\mathcal{D}(F) = D$, and $\mathcal{A}(F) = A$.

In order to keep the reconstruction process tractable and to reduce the number of solutions of a given reconstruction problem, it is often supposed that the set to be reconstructed has some special geometrical features. In the following, we briefly describe the ones used most frequently.

Connectedness and Convexity

Two points $P = (p_1, p_2)$ and $Q = (q_1, q_2)$ in a discrete set F are said to be *4-adjacent* if $|p_1 - q_1| + |p_2 - q_2| = 1$. The points P and Q are said to be *8-adjacent* if they are 4-adjacent or ($|p_1 - q_1| = 1$ and $|p_2 - q_2| = 1$). The sequence of distinct points $P_0, \ldots, P_k$ is a *4/8-path* from point P_0 to point P_k in a discrete set F if each point of the sequence is in F and P_l is 4/8-adjacent, respectively, to P_{l-1} for each $l = 1, \ldots, k$. A discrete set F is *4/8-connected* if for any two points of F there is a 4/8-path, respectively, in F between them. The 4-connected set is also called as *polyomino* [13]. Clearly, every 4-connected set is also 8-connected, but the converse is not true [see, e.g., Fig. 8.2(b)]. The discrete set F is *horizontally convex/vertically convex* (or shortly, *h-convex/v-convex*) if its rows/columns are 4-connected, respectively. The *h-* and *v-*convex sets are called *hv-convex* [see Figs. 8.2(b) and (d)].

For any point $P = (p_1, p_2)$, we define the four quadrants around P by

$$R_0(P) = \{Q = (q_1, q_2) \mid q_1 \leq p_1 \text{ and } q_2 \leq p_2\},$$
$$R_1(P) = \{Q = (q_1, q_2) \mid q_1 \geq p_1 \text{ and } q_2 \leq p_2\},$$
$$R_2(P) = \{Q = (q_1, q_2) \mid q_1 \geq p_1 \text{ and } q_2 \geq p_2\},$$
$$R_3(P) = \{Q = (q_1, q_2) \mid q_1 \leq p_1 \text{ and } q_2 \geq p_2\}. \tag{8.7}$$

A discrete set F is *Q-convex* if $R_k(P) \cap F \neq \emptyset$ for all $k \in \{0, 1, 2, 3\}$ implies $P \in F$ [see, e.g., Fig. 8.2(c)].

Remark 1. More precisely, the above definition corresponds to Q-convexity along the horizontal and vertical directions as Q-convexity can be defined in a more general manner [7]. However, for the sake of simplicity, we will use this abbreviated form.

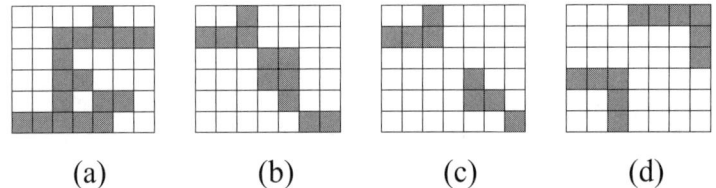

(a)   (b)   (c)   (d)

Fig. 8.2. (a) A NE-directed polyomino. (b) An *hv-*convex 8- but not 4-connected discrete set. (c) A Q-convex but not 8-connected discrete set. (d) An *hv-*convex decomposable but not Q-convex discrete set.

Directedness

A 4-path in a discrete set F is a *northeast path* (or shortly, NE-path) from point P_0 to point P_t if each point P_l of the path is in north or east of P_{l-1}

for each $l = 1, \ldots, t$. SW-, SE-, NW-paths are defined similarly. The discrete set F is *NE-directed* if there is a particular point of F, called the *source*, such that there is an NE-path in F from the source to any other point of F. It follows from the definition that the source of a NE-directed set is necessarily the point $(m, 1)$ [see Fig. 8.2(a)]. Similar definitions can be given for SW-, SE-, and NW-directedness. We simply say that the discrete set is *directed* if it is NE-, SW-, SE-, or NW-directed.

Decomposability

A maximal 4-connected subset of a discrete set F is called a *component* of F. We say that that two components F_1 and F_2 of F are *disjoint* if both the sets of the row indices and the sets of the column indices of F_1 and F_2 are disjoint. For example, the discrete set in Fig. 8.1 has three components: $F_1 = \{(1,3), (2,2), (2,3)\}$; $F_2 = \{(4,1), (4,2), (4,3), (4,4), (5,3)\}$; and $F_3 = \{(5,5), (5,6), (6,5)\}$, where F_1 and F_3 are disjoint.

Given two discrete sets C and D represented by the binary matrices $\hat{C} = (\hat{c}_{ij})_{m_1 \times n_1}$ and $\hat{D} = (\hat{d}_{ij})_{m_2 \times n_2}$, respectively, we say that we get the discrete set F represented by the binary matrix $\hat{F} = (\hat{f}_{ij})_{m_3 \times n_3}$ by a *northwest-gluing* (or shortly, NW-gluing) from C and D if

$$\hat{F} = \begin{pmatrix} \hat{C} & \mathbf{0} \\ \mathbf{0} & \hat{D} \end{pmatrix} \text{ such that } m_3 \geq m_1 + m_2 \text{ and } n_3 \geq n_1 + n_2 . \tag{8.8}$$

We stress the importance of the fact that in the resulting set F there can be empty rows or/and columns between the subsets C and D (namely, if $m_3 > m_1 + m_2$ or/and $n_3 > n_1 + n_2$). If C is a single component, then we say that C is the *NW-component* of F. NE-, SE-, SW-gluings and -components are defined similarly. We say that a discrete set F consisting of k ($k \geq 2$) components is *decomposable* if

(α) the components are uniquely reconstructible from their horizontal and vertical projections in polynomial time, and
(β) the components are pairwise disjoint, and
(γ) if $k > 2$, then we get F by gluing a single component to a decomposable discrete set consisting of $k - 1$ components using one of the four gluing operators.

As a straightforward consequence of this definition, we obtain that every discrete set consisting of one component is nondecomposable and every discrete set consisting of two or three components and satisfying properties (α) and (β) is decomposable. Figure 8.3 shows some decomposable and nondecomposable configurations if the set satisfies property (β) and consists of four components.

If omitting empty rows and columns the SCDRs of the components of a decomposable discrete set F are connected to each other with their bottom

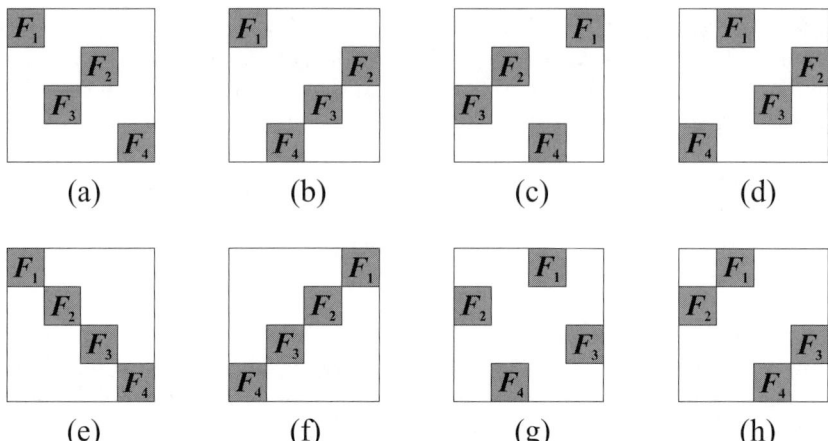

Fig. 8.3. Some decomposable (**a**)–(**f**) and nondecomposable (**g**)–(**h**) configurations of the components F_1, F_2, F_3, and F_4. The SCDRs of the components are marked with gray squares. The possible empty rows and columns are not indicated.

right and upper left (bottom left and upper right) corners, then we say that F is of *type 1/2*, respectively [see Figs. 8.3(e) and (f) in the case of four components].

Throughout this chapter we will use the following notations for classes of discrete sets.

(a) $\mathcal{S}_8'$ for the class of 8- but not 4-connected hv-convex sets.
(b) $\mathcal{Q}'$ for the class of non-4-connected Q-convex discrete sets.
(c) $\mathcal{DEC}$ for the class of decomposable discrete sets.
(d) $\mathcal{S}^*, \mathcal{S}^{**}$ for the class of discrete sets of type 1/2, respectively.

8.3 Reconstruction from Two Projections

The reconstruction from horizontal and vertical projections in classes of discrete sets having some convexity and connectedness properties has been frequently studied by mathematicians and computer scientists. In [10] a survey is given for the reconstruction complexity in classes of discrete sets having properties h-convexity, v-convexity, or 4-connectedness. Discrete sets satisfying none of the above properties can be reconstructed in O(mn) time by an early result from Ryser [17]. In [10] it is shown that if a set satisfies only one or two of the above properties, then its reconstruction is NP-complete. In the same time, if all three properties are satisfied, i.e., in the class of hv-convex polyominoes, the reconstruction can be solved in polynomial time. Several methods have been presented for reconstructing hv-convex polyominoes and, later on, they have been improved to reconstruct also 8-connected hv-convex discrete sets in polynomial time (see [4] for the comparison of the algorithms' complexities). In both classes of hv-convex 8- and 4-connected sets, the worst-case time complexity of the fastest algorithm for solving the reconstruction problem is of $O(mn \cdot \min\{m^2, n^2\})$. Surprisingly, in [3] the authors showed that the additional knowledge that the hv-convex 8-connected set is not 4-connected (i.e., it is in $\mathcal{S}'_8$) leads to a reconstruction algorithm with worst-case time complexity of $O(mn \cdot \min\{m, n\})$. The aim of this section is to describe a generalized version of the algorithm given in [3] for reconstructing discrete sets of $\mathcal{Q}'$ from its horizontal and vertical projections.

8.3.1 Q-Convex Sets with Disjoint Components

Consider that we want to reconstruct a Q-convex discrete set from its horizontal and vertical projections having the prior information that the set has at least two components. That is, we want to solve problem 2-RECONSTRUCTION($\mathcal{Q}'$). We first summarize some results from [9] and [16] concerning directed discrete sets, which will be important in designing the reconstruction algorithm.

Theorem 1. *Every hv-convex directed discrete set can be reconstructed from its source and its horizontal and vertical projections uniquely in $O(mn)$ time.*

Following from the definitions directly, we can check the directedness of an hv-convex polyomino by investigating a single position.

Proposition 1. *Let G be an hv-convex polyomino with $R(G) = \{i', \ldots, i''\} \times \{j', \ldots, j''\}$.*

1. *G is SE-directed if, and only if, $\hat{g}_{i',j'} = 1$.*
2. *G is NW-directed if, and only if, $\hat{g}_{i'',j''} = 1$.*
3. *G is SW-directed if, and only if, $\hat{g}_{i',j''} = 1$.*
4. *G is NE-directed if, and only if, $\hat{g}_{i'',j'} = 1$.*

Our algorithm will reconstruct the Q-convex discrete set component by component. This can be done with the aid of the following theorem, which describes the relation between decomposable and Q-convex discrete sets.

Theorem 2. $\mathcal{Q}' \subseteq \mathcal{S}^* \cup \mathcal{S}^{**}$.

Proof. (Sketch.) Let $F \in \mathcal{Q}'$ having components $F_1, \ldots, F_k$ with $R(F_l) = \{i'_l, \ldots, i''_l\} \times \{j'_l, \ldots, j''_l\}$ ($l = 1, \ldots, k$). Since F is non-4-connected, it has at least two components, i.e., $k \geq 2$. Every Q-convex set is hv-convex, too, therefore, any two arbitrary components of F are disjoint; thus, property (β) is satisfied. Without loss of generality, we can assume that

$$1 \leq i'_1 \leq i''_1 < i'_2 \leq i''_2 < \cdots \leq i''_k = m . \tag{8.9}$$

Then, exactly one of the following cases is possible:

$$1 \leq j'_1 \leq j''_1 < j'_2 \leq j''_2 < \cdots \leq j''_k = n, \text{ or} \tag{8.10}$$

$$n = j'_1 \geq j''_1 > j'_2 \geq j''_2 > \cdots \geq j''_k \geq 1 . \tag{8.11}$$

If for F (8.10)/(8.11) holds, then $F_1, \ldots, F_{k-1}$ are NW/NE-directed and $F_2, \ldots, F_k$ are SE/SW-directed, respectively. Since in both cases all the components are directed, therefore, by Theorem 1, property (α) is satisfied, too. Finally, if (8.10) holds, then $F \in \mathcal{S}^*$; otherwise (if (8.11) holds), $F \in \mathcal{S}^{**}$. Certainly, property (γ) is satisfied, too. $\square$

Remark 2. For further details of the proof, see [2].

Now, we can show how to represent a set of $\mathcal{Q}'$.

Corollary 1. *Let $F \in \mathcal{Q}'$ having components $F_1, \ldots, F_k$. Then there are uniquely determined row indices $0 < i_1 < \cdots < i_k \le m$ and column indices $0 < j_1 < \cdots < j_k \le n$ such that for each $l = 1, \ldots, k$ $(k \ge 2)$, (i_l, j_l) is the bottom right position of $R(F_l)$ if $F \in \mathcal{S}^*$ and (i_l, j_{k-l+1}) is the bottom left position of $R(F_l)$ if $F \in \mathcal{S}^{**}$.*

Depending on the type of F, let us define

$$
C_F = \begin{cases} \{(i_l, j_l) \mid l = 1, \ldots, k-1\} & \text{if } F \in \mathcal{S}^*, \\ \{(i_l, j_{k-l+1}) \mid l = 1, \ldots, k-1\} & \text{if } F \in \mathcal{S}^{**}, \end{cases} \tag{8.12}
$$

where $i_1, \ldots, i_k$ and $j_1, \ldots, j_k$ denote the uniquely determined indices mentioned in Corollary 1. That is, on the basis of Proposition 1, C_F consists of the source points of the NW-/NE-directed components $F_1, \ldots, F_{k-1}$ if F has type $1/2$, respectively (see Fig. 8.4). The knowledge of any element of C_F is useful in the reconstruction of an $F \in \mathcal{Q}'$, as we can see on the basis of the following theorem.

Theorem 3. *Any $F \in \mathcal{Q}'$ is uniquely determined by its horizontal and vertical projections, its type, and an arbitrary element of C_F.*

Proof. Let us suppose that $F \in \mathcal{S}^*$ and $(i_l, j_l) \in C_F$ is given for some $l \in \{1, \ldots, k-1\}$. Then (i_l, j_l) is the source of the NW-directed component F_l, which can be reconstructed uniquely on the basis of Theorem 1. Suppose that $R(F_l) = \{i', \ldots, i_l\} \times \{j', \ldots, j_l\}$. Then, the source (i^*_{l+1}, j^*_{l+1}) of the

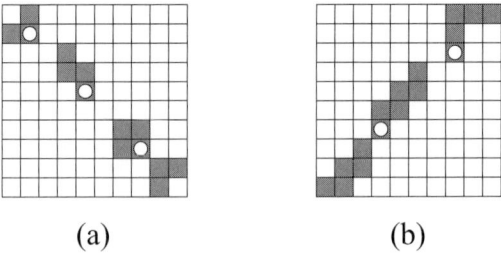

(a)   (b)

Fig. 8.4. (a) A discrete set $F \in \mathcal{Q}'$ of type 1 and (b) a discrete set $F' \in \mathcal{Q}'$ of type 2. The elements of C_F and $C_{F'}$ are marked with white dots.

SE-directed component F_{l+1} and the source (i_{l-1}, j_{l-1}) of the NW-directed component F_{l-1} are uniquely determined. Namely,

$$i^*_{l+1} = \min\{i \mid i > i_l \text{ and } h_i \neq 0\} , \tag{8.13}$$

$$j^*_{l+1} = \min\{j \mid j > j_l \text{ and } v_j \neq 0\} , \tag{8.14}$$

$$i_{l-1} = \max\{i \mid i < i' \text{ and } h_i \neq 0\} , \tag{8.15}$$

$$j_{l-1} = \max\{j \mid j < j' \text{ and } v_j \neq 0\} . \tag{8.16}$$

Again, by Theorem 1, F_{l+1} and F_{l-1} can be reconstructed uniquely. Then the sources of F_{l+2} and F_{l-2} are determined. The method can be continued until F_1 and F_k are reconstructed. The proof is similar if $F \in \mathcal{S}^{**}$.   □

As a direct consequence, we see from Theorem 3 that different solutions of 2-RECONSTRUCTION$(\mathcal{Q}')$ with the same type must have different source points.

Corollary 2. *If $F, F' \in \mathcal{Q}'$ are different solutions of the same reconstruction problem and they have the same type, then $C_F \cap C_{F'} = \emptyset$.*

8.3.2 Equality Positions

Let $\widetilde{H}$ and $\widetilde{V}$ be the cumulated vectors of $F \in \mathcal{Q}'$. We say that $(i,j) \in \{1,\dots,m-1\} \times \{1,\dots,n-1\}$ is an *equality position of type 1* of F if $\widetilde{h}_i = \widetilde{v}_j$. We say that $(i,j) \in \{1,\dots,m\} \times \{2,\dots,n+1\}$ is an *equality position of type 2* of F if $\widetilde{h}_i = \widetilde{v}_n - \widetilde{v}_{j-1}$. Equality positions (i,j) for which $h_i = 0$ and/or $v_j = 0$ are not interesting for this study and are omitted. We denote the set of equality positions of type 1/2 by L^1_F/L^2_F, respectively. Equality positions are useful for finding the elements of C_F.

Lemma 1. *Let $F \in \mathcal{Q}'$. Then $C_F \subseteq L^1_F$ if $F \in \mathcal{S}^*$ and $C_F \subseteq L^2_F$ if $F \in \mathcal{S}^{**}$.*

Proof. Let us suppose that $F \in \mathcal{S}^*$ and define a set E as follows:

$$E = (\{1,\dots,i\} \times \{j+1,\dots,n\}) \cup (\{i+1,\dots,m\} \times \{1,\dots,j\}) . \tag{8.17}$$

If $(i,j) \in C_F$, then $F \cap E = \emptyset$, and so $C_F \subseteq L^1_F$ since

$$\widetilde{h}_i = \sum_{t=1}^{i} h_t = |F \cap \{1,\dots,i\} \times \{1,\dots,n\}| = |F \cap \{1,\dots,i\} \times \{1,\dots,j\}|$$

$$= |F \cap \{1,\dots,m\} \times \{1,\dots,j\}| = \sum_{t=1}^{j} v_t = \widetilde{v}_j . \tag{8.18}$$

If $F \in \mathcal{S}^{**}$, then define E' as follows:

$$E' = (\{1,\dots,i\} \times \{1,\dots,j-1\}) \cup (\{i+1,\dots,m\} \times \{j,\dots,n\}) . \tag{8.19}$$

If $(i, j) \in C_F$, then $F \cap E' = \emptyset$, and so $C_F \subseteq L_F^2$ since

$$\widetilde{h}_i = \sum_{t=1}^{i} h_t = |F \cap \{1, \ldots, i\} \times \{1, \ldots, n\}| = |F \cap \{1, \ldots, i\} \times \{j, \ldots, n\}|$$

$$= |F \cap \{1, \ldots, m\} \times \{j, \ldots, n\}| = \sum_{t=j}^{n} v_t = \widetilde{v}_n - \widetilde{v}_{j-1} . \qquad \square \qquad (8.20)$$

8.3.3 The Reconstruction Algorithm

The algorithm for reconstructing sets of $\mathcal{Q}'$ from their horizontal and vertical projections can now be outlined as follows.

Algorithm 1
1. *Identify the sets L_F^1 and L_F^2;*
2. **while** $L_F^1 \neq \emptyset$ **do**
   $F = \emptyset; l := 1;$
   take an arbitrary element $(i, j) \in L_F^1$ and let $L_F^1 = L_F^1 \setminus \{(i, j)\};$
   try to reconstruct the NW-directed component F_1 from source (i, j)
   with $\mathcal{H}(F_1) = (h_1, \ldots, h_i)$ and $\mathcal{V}(F_1) = (v_1, \ldots, v_j);$
   repeat
       if F_l *is not reconstructed* **then break;**
       $F := F \cup F_l; l := l + 1;$
       identify the source (i_l^*, j_l^*) of F_l and try to reconstruct the
       SE-directed component F_l from source (i_l^*, j_l^*) with the
       corresponding projections;
       if F_l *is reconstructed* **then**
           if F_l *is the last component* **then** *output $F \cup F_l$;*
               else if F_l *is NW-directed* **then** $L_F^1 = L_F^1 \setminus \{(i_l, j_l)\};$
       until F_l *is the last component* **or** F_l *is not NW-directed;*
3. *Repeat step 2 with NE- and SW-directed components using set L_F^2;*

This algorithm works as follows. We first assume that the set $F \in \mathcal{Q}'$ to be reconstructed has type 1. On the basis of Theorem 3, it is sufficient to find an arbitrary element of C_F to reconstruct F from its horizontal and vertical projections uniquely. The elements of C_F are equality positions of type 1 on the basis of Lemma 1. So, in order to find all solutions of the reconstruction problem, we check for every element of L_F^1 whether it is an element of C_F. Without losing any solution, we can assume that if an investigated equality position $(i, j) \in L_F^1$ is in C_F, then it is the source of the first component F_1. From the proof of Theorem 2, we know that this component is NW-directed. Now, in order to decide if (i, j) is the source of F_1, we try to reconstruct an hv-convex NW-directed polyomino G with source (i, j) such that $\mathcal{H}(G) = (h_1, \ldots, h_i)$ and $\mathcal{V}(G) = (v_1, \ldots, v_j)$. If there is no such polyomino, then, clearly, (i, j) cannot be the source of F_1 and we continue with the investigation of the next equality position from L_F^1. Otherwise, we can assume that $F_1 = G$ and we try to reconstruct the remaining components iteratively. The lth component F_l $(l = 2, \dots)$ is SE-directed, so we try to reconstruct an hv-convex SE-directed polyomino G such that the number of its points in each row and column are equal to the corresponding elements of H and V, respectively. The source of F_l must be the position (i_{l+1}^*, j_{l+1}^*), where i_{l+1}^* and j_{l+1}^* are defined by (8.13) and (8.14), respectively. If it is not possible to reconstruct the SE-directed polyomino, then, clearly, (i_{l+1}^*, j_{l+1}^*) cannot be the source of F_l, which contradicts the assumption that (i, j) is the source of F_1, and we continue with the investigation of the next equality position from L_F^1. Otherwise, we check whether the reconstructed component was the last one. This can be done by checking the bottom right position (i'', j'') of G. If $(i'', j'') \neq (m, n)$, then G cannot be the last component. Then, G must be NW-directed on the basis of the proof of Theorem 2. This can be investigated by Proposition 1. If $\hat{g}_{i'',j''} \neq 1$, then G is not NW-directed and, clearly, $F_l \neq G$, which contradicts the assumption that (i, j) is the source of F_1. We continue with the investigation of the next equality position from L_F^1. Otherwise, that is, when $\hat{g}_{i'',j''} = 1$, we can assume that $F_l = G$. On the basis of Corollary 2, G cannot be the first component of any other solution of the same type; therefore, (i'', j'') can be eliminated from L_F^1 and we continue with the next iteration. If $(i'', j'') = (m, n)$, then $F_l = G$ and $F = F_1 \cup \dots \cup F_l$. We found a solution and we continue with the investigation of the next equality position from L_F^1 in order to find another solutions. Step 3 of the algorithm is similar. We assume that F has type 2 and try to build NE- and SW-directed components from the corresponding sources. If no solutions are found after investigating all equality positions of both types, then the assumption that $F \in \mathcal{Q}'$ is not met, i.e., there is no discrete set with the given projections which is Q-convex and consists of at least two components. However, in some cases there can be several solutions (see Fig. 8.5).

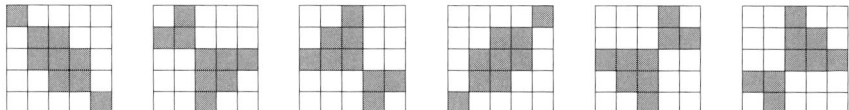

Fig. 8.5. Six sets of $\mathcal{Q}'$ with the same horizontal and vertical projections.

Example 1. Suppose that we wish reconstruct the Q-convex discrete set F in Fig. 8.6(a) from the vectors H and V. In this case, $L_F^1 = \{(1, 1), (2, 3), (3, 4)\}$, $L_F^2 = \{(4, 2)\}$, and $C_F = \{(2, 3)\}$. First we assume that the set to be reconstructed is of type 1. Supposing that $(1, 1)$ is the source of the NW-directed component F_1 [Fig. 8.6(b)], the algorithm fails after reconstructing the SE-directed second component [Fig. 8.6(c)] because there is no room for F_3. Then the position $(3, 4)$ can be deleted from L_F^1. Assuming that $(2, 3)$ is the source of F_1 [Fig. 8.6(d)] the algorithm gives a solution of type 1 [Fig. 8.6(e)]. Finally, assuming that the set to be reconstructed is of type 2, we suppose that $(4, 2)$ is the source of F_1. Since there is no room for F_1, the algorithm ends (there is no solution of type 2).

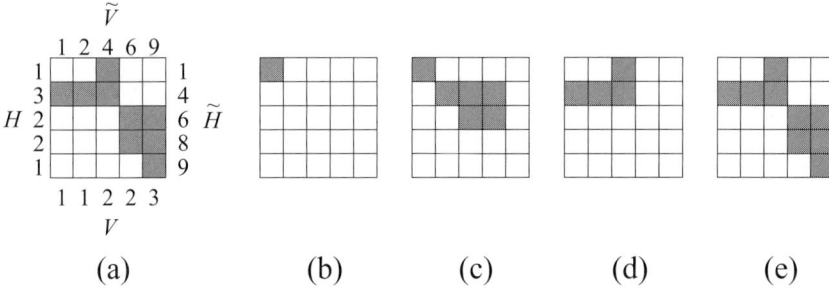

Fig. 8.6. An illustration of how Algorithm 1 works.

8.4 Reconstruction from Four Projections

The aim of this section is to present a general decomposition technique for reconstructing discrete sets from four projections. The algorithm uses similar ideas as the one of the previous section. Although this method works in more general classes of discrete sets, the price we pay is that we need four projections and some more technical lemmas. Due to space considerations, the technical proofs of the theoretical results in this chapter are omitted. The interested reader can find them in [1].

8.4.1 The Center of a Decomposable Discrete Set

We can give a description of decomposability as follows:

Lemma 2. *A discrete set F is decomposable if, and only if, it satisfies property (α) and there exists a sequence of discrete sets $F^{(1)}, \ldots, F^{(k)}$ ($k \geq 2$) such that $F^{(1)}$ consists of one component, $F^{(k)} = F$, and for each $l = 1, \ldots, k-1$, we get $F^{(l+1)}$ by gluing a component to $F^{(l)}$ using a gluing operator.*

For a given discrete set $F \in \mathcal{DEC}$, the sequence described in Lemma 2 is not uniquely determined. We will refer to any sequence satisfying the properties of Lemma 2 as a *gluing sequence* of F. For example, the sequences $F^{(1)} = \{(1, 1)\}$, $F^{(2)} = \{(1, 1), (2, 2)\}$, $G^{(1)} = \{(2, 2)\}$, and $G^{(2)} = \{(1, 1), (2, 2)\}$ are both gluing sequences of the same discrete set $F = \{(1, 1), (2, 2)\}$. Clearly, every gluing sequence of a given decomposable discrete set must be of the same length (namely, the length is always equal to the number of the components of the discrete set). If the discrete set $F \in \mathcal{DEC}$ consists of two components, then, clearly, either $F \in \mathcal{S}^*$ or $F \in \mathcal{S}^{**}$. Moreover, from property (γ) it follows that if $F^{(1)}, \ldots, F^{(k)}$ is a gluing sequence of $F \in \mathcal{DEC} \setminus (\mathcal{S}^* \cup \mathcal{S}^{**})$, then there exists a unique integer $1 < j < k$ such that $F^{(j)} \in \mathcal{S}^* \cup \mathcal{S}^{**}$ and $F^{(j+1)} \notin \mathcal{S}^* \cup \mathcal{S}^{**}$. The following lemma shows the relation between two arbitrary gluing sequences of a same discrete set.

Lemma 3. *Let $F^{(1)}, \ldots, F^{(k)}$ and $G^{(1)}, \ldots, G^{(k)}$ be two different gluing sequences of the same discrete set $F \in \mathcal{DEC} \setminus (\mathcal{S}^* \cup \mathcal{S}^{**})$. Moreover, let $1 < j, j' < k$ such that $F^{(j)}, G^{(j')} \in \mathcal{S}^* \cup \mathcal{S}^{**}$, and $F^{(j+1)}, G^{(j'+1)} \notin \mathcal{S}^* \cup \mathcal{S}^{**}$. Then $j = j'$ and $F^{(j)} = G^{(j')}$.*

Based on this lemma we can say that, for every set $F \in \mathcal{DEC}$, there exists an integer j such that, in every gluing sequence $F^{(1)}, \ldots, F^{(k)} = F$, $F^{(j)}$ is the same, $F^{(j)} \in \mathcal{S}^* \cup \mathcal{S}^{**}$, and $F^{(j+1)} \notin \mathcal{S}^* \cup \mathcal{S}^{**}$ (if $F \in \mathcal{S}^* \cup \mathcal{S}^{**}$, then $j = k$ and this latter relation is not important). The uniquely determined set $F^{(j)}$ is called the *center* of F and is denoted by $C(F)$. For example, if the configuration of the components of the set F is given as in Fig. 8.3(a), then $C(F) = F_2 \cup F_3$, while in the case given in Fig. 8.3(b), $C(F) = F_2 \cup F_3 \cup F_4$.

8.4.2 Finding a Component

Before giving any further details, we must mention one important fact according to property (α). In fact, to satisfy this property, we usually need to have some a priori information about the components. For example, one can assume that the components are NW-directed and hv-convex since in this case property (α) is fulfilled (see Theorem 1). In the following, where it is important to emphasize this in order to avoid confusion, we will write $\mathcal{DEC}_{\mathcal{C}}$ for the class of decomposable discrete sets whose components are from a certain class $\mathcal{C}$ where property (α) holds. On the basis of properties (α) and (β) in the reconstruction of a decomposable discrete set, it is sufficient to identify the SCDRs of the components. In this subsection we only deal with NW-components. However, the results given in the following can easily be modified to find NE-, SE-, or SW-components, too. In order to find the SCDR of a NW-component, we first give a necessary condition that is quite similar to Lemma 1.

Lemma 4. *Let $F \in \mathcal{DEC}$. If (i, j) is the bottom right position of the SCDR of the NW-component of F, then i is the smallest integer for which there exists an integer j with $\tilde{h}_i = \tilde{v}_j = \tilde{a}_{i+j-1} > 0$ and $a_{i+j} = 0$.*

Unfortunately, this lemma does not give a sufficient condition for identifying the SCDR of a component of F. For example, if the discrete set is $F = \{(1, 3), (2, 2), (5, 1)\}$, then for the position $(2, 2)$ the conditions of Lemma 4 hold (since $\tilde{h}_2 = \tilde{v}_2 = \tilde{a}_3 = 2$ and $a_4 = 0$) but F has no NW-component.

With the aid of the following theorem, it is possible to test whether the decomposable discrete set has a NW- or SE-component.

Theorem 4. *Let $F \in \mathcal{DEC}_\mathcal{C}$, $\mathcal{H}(F) = (h_1, \ldots, h_m)$, $\mathcal{V}(F) = (v_1, \ldots, v_n)$, and $\mathcal{A}(F) = (a_1, \ldots, a_{m+n-1})$. If (i, j) is a position satisfying the necessary conditions of Lemma 4 such that a polyomino $P \in \mathcal{C}$ exists with $\mathcal{H}(P) = (h_1, \ldots, h_i)$, $\mathcal{V}(P) = (v_1, \ldots, v_j)$, and $\mathcal{A}(P) = (a_1, \ldots, a_{i+j-1})$, then P is the NW-component of F or/and F has a SE-component. If no such position exists, then F has no NW-component.*

Note that if the conditions of the above theorem hold, then in some cases the discrete set can have both NW- and SE-components; for example, if the discrete set is in $\mathcal{S}^*$. However, Theorem 4 does not state that the discrete set necessarily has a NW-component (see, e.g., Fig. 8.7).

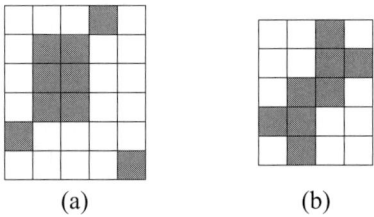

(a)   (b)

Fig. 8.7. (a) A decomposable discrete set that has no NW-component although the position $(5, 4)$ satisfies the conditions of Theorem 4 with the polyomino in (b).

Remark 3. The polyomino in Fig. 8.7(b) is not uniquely determined by its horizontal and vertical projections. Its symmetrical pair has the same projections. However, using the prior information that the set to be reconstructed can consist of rectangle-shaped components or polyominoes shown in Fig. 8.7(b), property (α) can be satisfied.

If the set is of $\mathcal{S}^*/\mathcal{S}^{**}$, then with the aid of the NW/NE-version of Theorem 4, it is possible to find the SCDR of the NW/NE-component of F, respectively. This means that once we have decomposed all the components around the center of F, Theorem 4 gives an effective tool to reconstruct the center itself. On the basis of the following theorem, one can find the NW-component of F (if it exists) if $F \in \mathcal{DEC} \setminus (\mathcal{S}^* \cup \mathcal{S}^{**})$.

Theorem 5. *Assume that $F \in \mathcal{DEC} \setminus (\mathcal{S}^* \cup \mathcal{S}^{**})$ and (i, j) satisfies the conditions of Theorem 4 with a polyomino P. Moreover, let $R(C(F)) = \{i_1, \ldots, i_2\} \times \{j_1, \ldots, j_2\}$. Then P is the NW-component of F if, and only if, there exists $i' \in \{i_1, \ldots, i_2\}$ such that $i < i'$ or there exists $j' \in \{j_1, \ldots, j_2\}$ such that $j < j'$.*

An observation similar to Corollary 2 will speed up the reconstruction.

Corollary 3. *If $F, F' \in \mathcal{DEC}$ are different solutions of the same reconstruction problem, then $R(C(F))$ and $R(C(F'))$ are disjoint.*

8.4.3 The Reconstruction Algorithm

Now, an algorithm can be outlined for reconstructing decomposable discrete sets with given horizontal, vertical, diagonal, and antidiagonal projections. We first describe a procedure for decomposing a NW-component knowing that it belongs to a given class $\mathcal{C}$ where property (α) holds.

Procedure 1 DecomposeNW

1. *Find the position (i, j) for which $\widetilde{h}_i = \widetilde{v}_j = \widetilde{a}_{i+j-1} > 0$ and $a_{i+j} = 0$;*
   if *no such position exists* **then return**(*no component*);
2. **if** $j \geq l$ **then return**(*no component*);
3. *Construct a polyomino $P \in \mathcal{C}$ with $\mathcal{H}(P) = (h_1, \ldots, h_i)$,*
   $\mathcal{V}(P) = (v_1, \ldots, v_j)$*, and $\mathcal{A}(P) = (a_1, \ldots, a_{i+j-1})$;*
   if *no such polyomino exists* **then return**(*no component*);
4. $F := F \cup P$;
5. *Update H, V, D, and A according to the projections of P;*
6. **return**;

The procedures for decomposing components from the other three directions can be outlined similarly. The main algorithm for reconstructing decomposable discrete sets produces four vectors $H \in \mathbb{N}_0^m$, $V \in \mathbb{N}_0^n$, $D \in \mathbb{N}_0^{m+n-1}$, and $A \in \mathbb{N}_0^{m+n-1}$ as input, and outputs the set S containing all the decomposable discrete sets with the projections H, V, D, and A such that the components are from a given class $\mathcal{C}$ where property (α) holds. This algorithm reconstructs the solutions component by component, calling the procedures for decomposition. The algorithm can be outlined as follows:

Algorithm 2
1. $C := \{1, \ldots, n\} \setminus \{j \mid v_j = 0\}$; $S := \emptyset$;
2. $F := \emptyset$; $l := \min C$; *restore H, V, D, and A;*
3. **repeat**
       call DecomposeNW;
       if *(no component)* **then** *call DecomposeNE;*
       if *(no component)* **then** *call DecomposeSE;*
       if *(no component)* **then** *call DecomposeSW;*
     until *(no component)*;
4. *Try to reconstruct the last component;*
5. **if** $D = 0$ **and** $A = 0$ **then** $\{$ $S := S \cup \{F\}$;
                               $C := C \setminus \{columns\ of\ C(F)\}$; $\}$
6. **if** $C = \emptyset$ **then return** S **else goto** *Step 2;*

This algorithm works as follows. First, the set of solutions is $S = \emptyset$, and the set C contains the possible columns of a solution's center (step 1). Then in step 2, we set $F = \emptyset$, we restore the vectors H, V, D, and A to their original values, and we try to find a solution such that the leftmost column of its center is $l = \min C$. In step 3, we first try to decompose a NW-component. This is done by Procedure 1, which seeks the SCDR of the NW-component of F by trying to find the uniquely determined position that satisfies the conditions of Theorems 4 and 5 with a polyomino P (steps 1–3 of Procedure 1). If no such position exists, then either the assumption that the set to be reconstructed has a NW-component was false or the lth column cannot be a column of the center. In both cases, the procedure simply returns. Otherwise, the polyomino P is assumed to be the NW-component of F; we simulate the effect of this component on the projections of F (steps 4 and 5 of Procedure 1) and we return to the main algorithm. If we were not able to find a NW-component, then we try to decompose a NE-, SE-, and SW-component, similarly, in this order. Note that Theorem 5 cannot be applied on sets of $F \in \mathcal{S}^* \cup \mathcal{S}^{**}$, but this does not lead to failing our algorithm since in this case instead of a NW/NE-component we will decompose a SE/SW-component if the set is of type 1/2, respectively. If we found a component (which can be any of the four kinds), then we go on and try to decompose further components from the remaining set. We repeat this until we cannot decompose a component. In this case, the remaining set is nondecomposable; therefore, it must consist of a single component. We try to reconstruct this last component in step 4. Then in step 5 we check whether the reconstructed set F has the given projections; if so, then we set $S := S \cup \{F\}$. On the basis of Corollary 3, columns of $C(F)$ cannot be the columns of any other solution; therefore, we eliminate the columns of $C(F)$ from C and we go on to step 2 in order to find possible further solutions with other centers. Algorithm 2 investigates in each iteration whether a solution with a certain center exists by assuming that a given column is a column of the center, too. On the basis of Theorem 5, this strategy can also be applied to the rows of the center. If $m < n$, then we will choose the latter version of our strategy.

Example 2. Suppose that we wish to reconstruct discrete sets of $\mathcal{DEC}_\mathcal{C}$ (where $\mathcal{C}$ is the same class as mentioned in Remark 3) from the vectors

$$H = (1, 2, 2, 2, 1, 1, 2, 2, 2, 1, 1),$$
$$V = (1, 3, 3, 1, 0, 1, 3, 3, 1, 1),$$
$$D = (0, 0, 0, 0, 0, 0, 1, 2, 2, 3, 4, 2, 2, 1, 0, 0, 0, 0, 0, 0),$$
$$A = (0, 0, 1, 3, 3, 1, 0, 0, 0, 0, 0, 0, 1, 3, 3, 1, 0, 0, 0, 1). \tag{8.21}$$

First, it is assumed that the first column is a column of the center; therefore, the position (i, j) that satisfies $\tilde{h}_i = \tilde{v}_j = \tilde{a}_{i+j-1} > 0$ and $a_{i+j} = 0$ violates Theorem 5 [Fig. 8.8(a)]. Then the algorithm reconstructs SW-components in two iterations [Figs. 8.8(b) and 8.8(c)]. After that, in the next two iterations, the algorithm decomposes two NE-components in the remaining part

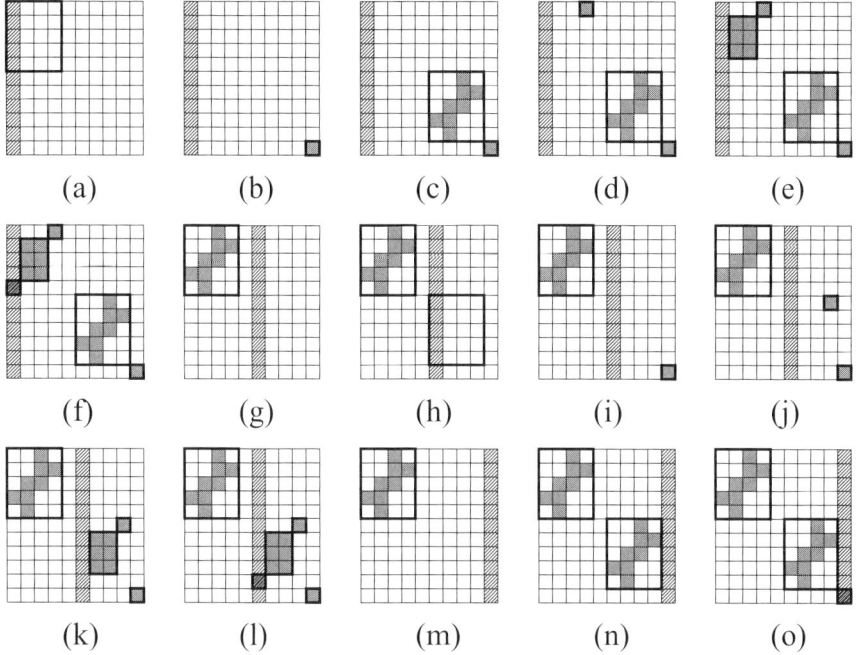

Fig. 8.8. An example how Algorithm 2 works. The identified discrete rectangles which must contain the next component are marked with bold squares. The column assumed to be a column of $C(F)$ is filled with slanted lines.

of the discrete set [Figs. 8.8(d) and (e)]. Finally, the algorithm reconstructs the last component and finds a solution F [Fig. 8.8(f)]. After eliminating the columns of $C(F)$ from C, we go on by assuming that the sixth column is a column of a possible other solution's center. With this assumption, we decompose a NW-component [Fig. 8.8(g)]. Then, again, a NW-component cannot be decomposed in the remaining part as its SCDR violates Theorem 5 [(Fig. 8.8(h)]. In the following, we decompose a SE-, a NE- and, again, a NE-component [Fig. 8.8(i),(j), and (k), respectively]. Reconstructing the last component [Fig. 8.8(l)], we find another solution F'. Finally, assuming that the last column is the center, we decompose two NW-components [Figs. 8.8(m) and (n)] and reconstruct the last component [Fig. 8.8(o)]. However, the reconstructed set does not have the given diagonal projection; therefore, the algorithm ends and the number of solutions is two.

8.5 Correctness and Complexity

In this section we prove the correctness and state the complexity of the algorithms of the previous two sections. First, we study the complexity of the reconstruction using only two projections.

Theorem 6. *Algorithm 1 solves problem* 2-RECONSTRUCTION$(\mathcal{Q}')$ *in* $O(mn \cdot \min\{m, n\})$ *time. The algorithm finds all sets of* $\mathcal{Q}'$ *with the given projections.*

Proof. Every row and column index can be in an equality position of both types at most once. This means that we have at most $\min\{m, n\}$ equality positions of type 1 and at most $\min\{m, n\}$ equality positions of type 2. Moreover, equality positions can be found in time $O(m + n)$ by the comparison of the cumulated horizontal and vertical vectors. Building the components of F assuming that an equality position (i, j) is in C_F takes $O(mn)$ time (see Theorem 1). We have to examine every equality position if it is in C_F, so we get the execution time $O(mn \cdot \min\{m, n\})$ in the worst case.

On the basis of Theorems 2 and 3, the reconstructed sets are Q-convex and have the given projections H and V. On the basis of Theorem 3, any element of C_F together with the projections and the knowledge of the type of F is sufficient to reconstruct F uniquely. Elements of C_F are equality positions, too, on the basis of Lemma 1. Algorithm 1 examines every equality position whether it is in C_F, and so the second part of the theorem follows. □

Sets of $\mathcal{S}'_8$ have the same properties as sets of $\mathcal{Q}'$ (see [3] for further details). The only difference is that the SCDRs of the components in the class $\mathcal{Q}'$ might be separated (i.e., there can be empty rows and/or columns between two consecutive components) while in the class $\mathcal{S}'_8$ they are always 8-connected [see also Fig. 8.2(c) for an example]. This observation immediately implies that 2-RECONSTRUCTION$(\mathcal{S}'_8)$ can also be solved in $O(mn \cdot \min\{m, n\})$ time. However, there is an interesting improvement in the complexity of the reconstruction if the set of $\mathcal{Q}'$ to be reconstructed is not 8-connected.

Theorem 7. 2-RECONSTRUCTION$(\mathcal{Q}' \backslash \mathcal{S}'_8)$ *can be solved in* $O(mn)$ *time. The number of solutions is at most two.*

Proof. Let $F \in \mathcal{Q}' \backslash \mathcal{S}'_8$. Since F is not 8-connected, there exists at least one empty row in $R(F)$ (say the ith) such that $\widetilde{h}_i \neq 0$ or an empty column in $R(F)$ (say the jth) such that $\widetilde{v}_j \neq 0$. Assume that the ith row of $R(F)$ is empty and $\widetilde{h}_i \neq 0$. Let $i^* = \max\{i' \mid \widetilde{h}_{i'} = \widetilde{h}_i \text{ and } h_{i'} \neq 0\}$ and

$$j^* = \begin{cases} \min\{j' \mid \widetilde{v}_{j'} = \widetilde{h}_i\} & \text{if } F \in \mathcal{S}^*, \\ \max\{j' \mid \widetilde{v}_n - \widetilde{v}_{j'-1} = \widetilde{h}_i\} & \text{if } F \in \mathcal{S}^{**}. \end{cases} \qquad (8.22)$$

Note that (i^*, j^*) can be found in $O(m + n)$ time. Since F is Q-convex, the position (i^*, j^*) must be the source of a NW/NE-directed component if F is of type 1/2, respectively (see Fig. 8.9). Therefore $(i^*, j^*) \in C_F$ and the solution is uniquely determined on the basis of Theorem 3. Consequently, there can be ambiguity only in the type of F, i.e., the number of solutions is at most two. In some cases, there exist solutions of both types (see Fig. 8.9). The proof can be given analogously if the SCDR of the discrete sets $F \in \mathcal{S}^* \cup \mathcal{S}^{**}$ has an empty column.   □

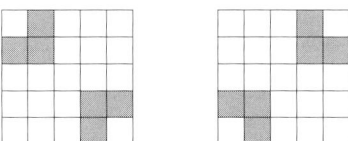

Fig. 8.9. Two sets of $\mathcal{Q}'$ with an empty row and column and the same horizontal and vertical projections.

Now we prove the correctness of the algorithm that uses four projections.

Theorem 8. *Let $\mathcal{C}$ be an arbitrary class of polyominoes that can be reconstructed in this class uniquely from their horizontal and vertical projections in polynomial time (say in $O(f(m, n))$ time). Then Algorithm 2 solves 4-*RECONSTRUCTION$(\mathcal{DEC}_{\mathcal{C}})$ *in $O(\min\{m, n\} \cdot f(m, n))$ time. The algorithm finds all sets of $\mathcal{DEC}_{\mathcal{C}}$ with the given projections.*

Proof. Let F be an arbitrary set of S. From Theorems 4 and 5, it follows that F is decomposable. Due to step 3 of Procedure 1, the horizontal and vertical projections of F are equal to the given vectors H and V, respectively. Moreover, step 5 of Algorithm 2 guarantees that the diagonal and antidiagonal projections of F are also equal to the vectors D and A, respectively. Assuming that the lth ($l = 1, \dots, k$) component to be reconstructed is a NW-component, it takes $O(m + n)$ time to find the (uniquely determined) position that satisfies the necessary conditions of Lemma 4. We do it simply by scanning the vectors $\widetilde{H}$, $\widetilde{V}$, and $\widetilde{A}$. In order to test whether this position is the bottom right position of the SCDR of the NW-component, we try to reconstruct this component based on Theorem 4, which takes $O(f_l)$ time. The same is true if the lth component is a NE-, SE- or SW-component. In the worst case, the component is a SW-component, i.e., we try to reconstruct the lth component at most four times, and so the time complexity of reconstructing all the components (steps 3 and 4 of Algorithm 2) is of $O(f(m, n))$, which is polynomial on the basis of property (α). In the worst case, we iterate steps 3 and 4 of Algorithm 2 by assuming that the first, second, ..., nth columns of G are also columns of $C(G)$ (if $n < m$) or by assuming that the first, second, ..., mth rows of G are also rows of $C(G)$ (if $m \leq n$). This means that steps 3 and 4 of Algorithm 2 must be repeated at most $\min\{m, n\}$ times. So we get that the total execution time of Algorithm 2 is of $O(\min\{m, n\} \cdot f(m, n))$.

Since we check every possible column (row) of F whether it is a column (row) of $C(F)$, it follows that the algorithm reconstructs all sets of $\mathcal{DEC}$ with the given projections. Consequently, if the algorithm returns $S = \emptyset$, then there is no solution of 4-RECONSTRUCTION($\mathcal{DEC}$).   □

If a discrete set is of type 1/2, then, following from Corollary 3, the solution is uniquely determined. With the aid of Theorem 4, this solution can be found with a single iteration of steps 3 and 4 of Algorithm 2. Knowing that $\mathcal{S}'_8 \subseteq \mathcal{Q}' \subseteq \mathcal{S}^* \cup \mathcal{S}^{**}$, this observation leads to the following corollaries.

Corollary 4. 4-RECONSTRUCTION($\mathcal{Q}'$) *can be solved in $O(mn)$ time. The solution is uniquely determined.*

Corollary 5. 4-RECONSTRUCTION($\mathcal{S}'_8$) *can be solved in $O(mn)$ time. The solution is uniquely determined.*

Remark 4. (a) If a discrete set is of type 1, then the horizontal, vertical, and antidiagonal projections are sufficient for the reconstruction. Similarly, for reconstructing a set of type 2, it is sufficient to know its horizontal, vertical, and diagonal projections. That is, knowing the type of the discrete set, the reconstruction can be solved even from three projections uniquely.
(b) The class of decomposable discrete sets for which the NW/NE/SE/SW-version of Theorem 4 gives both necessary and sufficient conditions for the existence of a NW/NE/SE/SW-component, respectively, is somewhat broader than $\mathcal{S}^* \cup \mathcal{S}^{**}$. This class of sets is called strongly decomposable and was studied in [2].
(c) Although the reconstruction of hv-convex discrete sets is, in general, an NP-hard problem [18], the decomposition technique described in this section can be applied to a subclass of hv-convex discrete sets yielding a polynomial-time reconstruction algorithm [1].

8.6 Conclusions and Discussion

In this chapter we studied the reconstruction complexity in some well-known classes of discrete sets using the additional knowledge that the discrete set consists of several (disjoint) components. We learned that in two important classes, namely in the class of hv-convex 8-connected discrete sets and in the class of Q-convex discrete sets, using the extra information that the set consists of at least two components (i.e., it is in $\mathcal{S}'_8$, and $\mathcal{Q}'$, respectively), the reconstruction problems can be solved from two projections quite effectively. Moreover, we got the interesting result that the reconstruction from two projections in the class of non-8-connected Q-convexes can be even faster. In the case of four projections, we investigated the general class of decomposables and presented a polynomial-time algorithm for reconstructing discrete sets of this class from four projections. All presented algorithms are able to find all the solutions for a given reconstruction problem. The complexity of reconstructing decomposable discrete sets from two projections is an open question. What we do know is that in some cases there can be exponentially large numbers of decomposable discrete sets with the same horizontal and vertical projections. Therefore, if an algorithm that reconstructs all the solutions of such a reconstruction task exists, then for some instances the time complexity of the algorithm is exponential. However, it might be possible that finding only one solution can be done in polynomial time.

References

1. Balázs, P.: A decomposition technique for reconstructing discrete sets from four projections. *Image and Vision Computing*, submitted.
2. Balázs, P.: Reconstruction of discrete sets from four projections: Strong decomposability. *Electr. Notes Discr. Math.*, **20**, 329–345 (2005).
3. Balázs, P., Balogh, E., Kuba, A.: Reconstruction of 8-connected but not 4-connected *hv*-convex discrete sets. *Discr. Appl. Math.*, **147**, 149–168 (2005).
4. Balogh, E., Kuba, A., Dévényi, C., Del Lungo, A.: Comparison of algorithms for reconstructing *hv*-convex discrete sets. *Lin. Algebra Appl.* **339**, 23–35 (2001).
5. Barcucci, E., Del Lungo, A., Nivat, M., Pinzani, R.: Reconstructing convex polyominoes from horizontal and vertical projections. *Theor. Comput. Sci.*, **155**, 321–347 (1996).
6. Barcucci, E., Del Lungo, A., Nivat, M., Pinzani, R.: Medians of polyominoes: A property for the reconstruction. *Int. J. Imaging Systems Techn.*, **9**, 69–77 (1998).
7. Brunetti, S., Daurat, A.: An algorithm reconstructing convex lattice sets. *Theor. Comput. Sci.*, **304**, 35–57 (2003).
8. Chrobak, M., Dürr, C.: Reconstructing *hv*-convex polyominoes from orthogonal projections. *Inform. Process. Lett.*, **69**, 283–289 (1999).
9. Del Lungo, A.: Polyominoes defined by two vectors. *Theor. Comput. Sci.*, **127**, 187–198 (1994).
10. Del Lungo, A., Nivat, M.: Reconstruction of connected sets from two projections. In [14], pp. 163–188 (1999).
11. Del Lungo, A., Nivat, M., Pinzani, R.: The number of convex polyominoes reconstructible from their orthogonal projections. *Discr. Math.*, **157**, 65–78 (1996).
12. Gardner, R.J., Gritzmann, P.: Uniqueness and complexity in discrete tomography. In [14], pp. 85–113 (1999).
13. Golomb, S.W.: *Polyominoes*. Scribner, New York, NY (1965).
14. Herman, G.T., Kuba, A. (eds.), *Discrete Tomography: Foundations, Algorithms, and Applications*. Birkhäuser, Boston, MA (1999).
15. Kuba, A.: The reconstruction of two-directionally connected binary patterns from their two orthogonal projections. *Comp. Vision, Graphics, Image Proc.*, **27**, 249–265 (1984).
16. Kuba, A., Balogh, E.: Reconstruction of convex 2D discrete sets in polynomial time. *Theor. Comput. Sci.*, **283**, 223–242 (2002).
17. Ryser, H.J.: Combinatorial properties of matrices of zeros and ones. *Canad. J. Math.*, **9**, 371–377 (1957).
18. Woeginger, G.W.: The reconstruction of polyominoes from their orthogonal projections. *Inform. Process. Lett.*, **77**, 225–229 (2001).

9

Network Flow Algorithms for Discrete Tomography

K.J. Batenburg

Summary. There exists an elegant correspondence between the problem of reconstructing a 0–1 lattice image from two of its projections and the problem of finding a maximum flow in a certain graph. In this chapter we describe how network flow algorithms can be used to solve a variety of problems from discrete tomography. First, we describe the network flow approach for two projections and several of its generalizations. Subsequently, we present an algorithm for reconstructing 0–1 images from more than two projections. The approach is extended to the reconstruction of 3D images and images that do not have an intrinsic lattice structure.

9.1 Introduction

The problem of reconstructing a 0–1 image from a small number of its projections has been studied extensively by many authors. Most results deal with images that are defined on a lattice, usually a subset of $\mathbb{Z}^2$. Already in 1957, Ryser studied the problem of reconstructing an $m \times n$ 0–1-matrix from its row and column sums [19, 20]. He also provided an algorithm for finding a reconstruction if it exists. Ryser's algorithm is extremely efficient. In fact, it can be implemented in linear time, $O(m + n)$, by using a compact representation for the output image [5].

The problem of reconstructing a 0–1 matrix from its row and column sums can also be modeled elegantly as a *network flow problem*. In 1957, Gale was the first to describe the two-projection reconstruction problem in the context of flows in networks, providing a completely different view from Ryser's approach [7]. In the latter work, there was no reference to the algorithmic techniques for solving network flow problems. In 1956, Ford and Fulkerson published their seminal paper on an algorithm for computing a maximum flow in a network [6], which can be used to solve the two-projection reconstruction problem. Using the network flow model, Anstee derived several mathematical properties of the reconstruction problem [2].

The reconstruction problem from two projections is usually severely underdetermined. The number of solutions can be exponential in the size of the image. In practice, the goal of tomography is usually to obtain a reconstruction of an *unknown original image*, not just to find any solution that has the given projections. If only two projections are available, additional prior knowledge must be used. Certain types of prior knowledge can be incorporated efficiently into the network flow approach, by using the concept of *min cost flows*.

A drawback of the network flow approach is that it cannot be generalized to the case of more than two projections. The reconstruction problem is NP-hard for any set of more than two projections [8]. Recently, an iterative approach for reconstructing 0–1 images from more than two projections was proposed by Batenburg [3]. In each iteration a reconstruction is computed from only two projections, using the network flow approach. The reconstruction from the previous iteration, which was computed using a different pair of projections, is used as prior knowledge such that the new reconstruction resembles the previous one.

In this chapter the network flow approach will be described, starting with the basic two-projection case. Section 9.2 describes the basic network flow formulation. In Section 9.3, the model is extended to incorporate prior knowledge in the reconstruction procedure. Section 9.4 deals with how the network flow approach can be made tolerant to noise and other errors. The implementation of network flow algorithms for discrete tomography is discussed in Section 9.5. Several highly efficient implementations of network flow algorithms are available. This section also addresses the time complexity of the relevant network flow algorithms. The basic iterative algorithm for reconstructing from more than two projections is described in Section 9.6. This algorithm can be generalized to 3D reconstruction very efficiently, which is discussed in Section 9.7. So far, all sections deal with *lattice images*. In Section 9.8, we discuss how the algorithms from the previous sections can be adapted to the problem of reconstructing binary images that do not have a lattice structure.

9.2 Network Flow Formulation for Two Projections

The reconstruction problems of this paper can be posed in several different forms. We mainly consider the reconstruction of a *subset* F of $\mathbb{Z}^2$ from its projections, but one can also formulate this problem in the context of reconstructing *binary matrices* or *black-and-white images*. In the case of binary matrices, the set F is represented by the set of matrix entries that have a value of 1. If we want to display a set $F \subseteq \mathbb{Z}^2$ and F is contained in a large rectangle $A \subseteq \mathbb{Z}^2$ (e.g., 256^2 elements), it is convenient to represent F as a *black-and-white* image. The white pixels correspond to the elements of F; the black pixels correspond to the remaining elements of A. *Continuous tomography algorithms*, such as the algebraic reconstruction technique (see, e.g., Chapter 7 of [17]), represent the reconstruction as a *gray-level image*. At several points in this chapter, we discuss how to utilize algorithms for continuous tomography for solving the discrete reconstruction problems. In these cases we use the black-and-white image representation of F, as this representation can easily be connected with the gray-level images from continuous tomography. Depending on the representation of the set F, points in A may also be called *entries* (in the context of binary matrices) or *pixels* (in the context of black-and-white images).

In this section we consider the problem of reconstructing a subset F of the lattice $\mathbb{Z}^2$ from its projections in *two* lattice directions, $v^{(1)}$ and $v^{(2)}$. This is a generalization of the problem of reconstructing a binary matrix from its row and column sums.

We assume that a *finite* set $A \subseteq \mathbb{Z}^2$ is given such that $F \subseteq A$. We call the set A the *reconstruction lattice*. As an illustration of the concept of the reconstruction lattice, consider the representation of F as a black-and-white image. The set A defines the *boundaries* of the image: All white pixels are known to be within these boundaries.

We denote the cardinality of any finite set F by $|F|$. Define $\mathbb{N}_0 = \{x \in \mathbb{Z} \mid x \geq 0\}$. Let $v^{(1)}, v^{(2)} \in \mathbb{Z}^2$. A *lattice line* is a line in $\mathbb{Z}^2$ parallel to either $v^{(1)}$ or $v^{(2)}$ that passes through at least one point in $\mathbb{Z}^2$. Any lattice line parallel to $v^{(k)}$ ($k = 1, 2$) is a *set* of the form $\{nv^{(k)} + t \mid n \in \mathbb{Z}\}$ for $t \in \mathbb{Z}^2$. The sets $\mathcal{L}^{(1)}$ and $\mathcal{L}^{(2)}$ denote the sets of lattice lines for directions $v^{(1)}$ and $v^{(2)}$ respectively. For $k = 1, 2$, put $L^{(k)} = \{\ell \in \mathcal{L}^{(k)} \mid \ell \cap A \neq \emptyset\}$. Note that $L^{(1)}$ and $L^{(2)}$ are finite sets. We denote the elements of $L^{(k)}$ by $\ell_{k,i}$ for $i = 1, \ldots, |L^{(k)}|$. As an example, Fig. 9.1 shows the reconstruction lattice for $A = \{1, 2, 3\} \times \{1, 2, 3\}$, $v^{(1)} = (1, 0)$, and $v^{(2)} = (1, 1)$. For this example, the sets $L^{(1)}$ and $L^{(2)}$ contain three and five lattice lines, respectively.

For any lattice set $F \subseteq \mathbb{Z}^2$, its projection $P_F^{(k)} : L^{(k)} \to \mathbb{N}_0$ in direction $v^{(k)}$ is defined as

$$P_F^{(k)}(\ell) = |F \cap \ell| = \sum_{x \in \ell} f(x), \tag{9.1}$$

where f denotes the characteristic function of F. The reconstruction problem can now be formulated as follows:

Problem 1. Let $v^{(1)}$, $v^{(2)}$ be given distinct lattice directions, and let $A \subseteq \mathbb{Z}^2$ be a given lattice set. Let $p^{(1)} : L^{(1)} \to \mathbb{N}_0$ and $p^{(2)} : L^{(2)} \to \mathbb{N}_0$ be given functions. Construct a set $F \subseteq A$ such that $P_F^{(1)} = p^{(1)}$ and $P_F^{(2)} = p^{(2)}$.

Define $S^{(k)} = \sum_{\ell \in L^{(k)}} p^{(k)}(\ell)$. We call $S^{(k)}$ the *projection sum for direction* $v^{(k)}$. Note that if F is a solution of Problem 1, we have $S^{(k)} - |F|$ for $k = 1, 2$. In Section 9.4, a generalization of Problem 1 will be described for which the prescribed projections $p^{(1)}$ and $p^{(2)}$ may contain errors. In that case the projection sum for direction $v^{(1)}$ may be different from the projection sum for direction $v^{(2)}$.

With the triple $(A, v^{(1)}, v^{(2)})$, we associate a *directed* graph $G = (V, E)$, where V is the set of nodes and E is the set of edges. We call G the *associated graph* of $(A, v^{(1)}, v^{(2)})$.

The set V contains a node s (the *source*), a node t (the *sink*), one node for each $\ell \in L^{(1)}$, and one node for each $\ell \in L^{(2)}$. The node that corresponds to $\ell_{k,i}$ has label $n_{k,i}$. We call the nodes $n_{k,i}$ *line nodes*.

Nodes $n_{1,i}$ and $n_{2,j}$ are connected by a (directed) edge $(n_{1,i}, n_{2,j})$ if, and only if, $\ell_{1,i}$ and $\ell_{2,j}$ intersect in A. We call these edges *point edges* and denote the set of all point edges by $E_p \subseteq E$. There is a bijective mapping $\Phi : E_p \to A$ that maps $(n_{1,i}, n_{2,j}) \in E_p$ to the intersection point of $\ell_{1,i}$ and $\ell_{2,j}$. We call Φ the *edge-to-point mapping* of G. For $e \in E_p$, we call $\Phi(e)$ the *corresponding point* of e and for $x \in A$, we call $\Phi^{-1}(x)$ the *corresponding edge* of x.

Besides the point edges, the set E contains the subsets $E_1 = \{(s, n_{1,i}) \mid i = 1, \ldots, |L^{(1)}|\}$ and $E_2 = \{(n_{2,j}, t) \mid j = 1, \ldots, |L^{(2)}|\}$ of directed edges. We call the elements of E_1 and E_2 the *line edges* of G. The complete set of edges of G is given by $E = E_p \cup E_1 \cup E_2$. Figure 9.2 shows the associated graph for the triple $(A, v^{(1)}, v^{(2)})$ of Fig. 9.1.

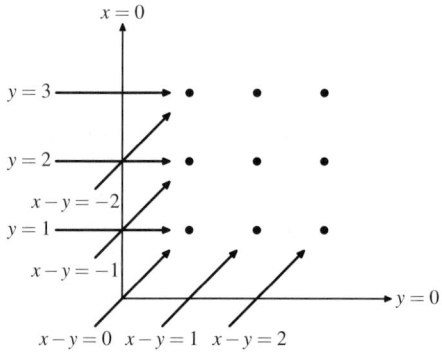

Fig. 9.1. Example lattice: $A = \{1, 2, 3\} \times \{1, 2, 3\}$, $v^{(1)} = (1, 0)$, $v^{(2)} = (1, 1)$.

Note that the structure of the associated graph is independent of the projections $p^{(1)}$ and $p^{(2)}$. To use the associated graph G for solving a particular instance of the reconstruction problem, we assign *capacities* to the edges of G. A *capacity function for G* is a mapping $E \to \mathbb{N}_0$. We use the following capacity function U:

$$\text{for } i = 1, \ldots, |L^{(1)}|; \ j = 1, \ldots, |L^{(2)}|; \tag{9.2}$$
$$U((n_{1,i}, n_{2,j})) = 1 ; \tag{9.3}$$
$$U((s, n_{1,i})) = p^{(1)}(\ell_{1,i}) ; \tag{9.4}$$
$$U((n_{2,j}, t)) = p^{(2)}(\ell_{2,j}) . \tag{9.5}$$

A *flow* in G is a mapping $Y : E \to \mathbb{R}_{\geq 0}$ such that $Y(e) \leq U(e)$ for all $e \in E$ and such that for all $v \in V \setminus \{s, t\}$,

$$\sum_{w: (w,v) \in E} Y((w, v)) = \sum_{w: (v,w) \in E} Y((v, w)) . \tag{9.6}$$

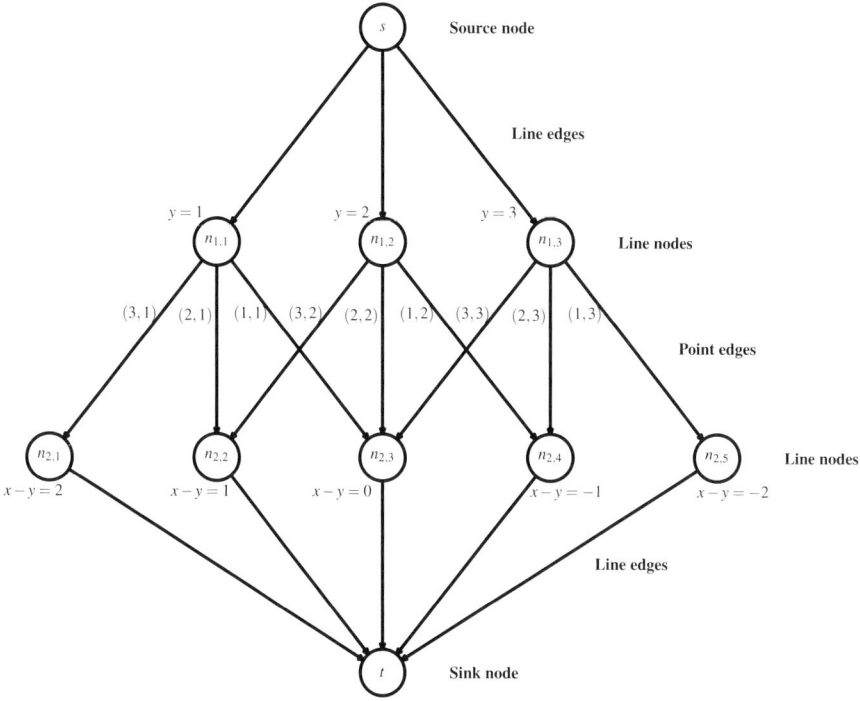

Fig. 9.2. Associated graph G for the triple $(A, v^{(1)}, v^{(2)})$ from Fig. 9.1.

The latter constraint is called the *flow conservation constraint*. Flows in graphs are also known as *network flows* in the literature. Let $\mathcal{Y}$ be the set of all flows in G. For a given flow $Y \in \mathcal{Y}$, the *size* $T(Y)$ of Y is given by $T(Y) = \sum_{(s,v)\in E} Y((s,v))$. If we consider G as a network of pipelines, carrying flow from s to t, the size of a flow is the net amount of flow that passes through the network. Due to the flow conservation constraint, we also have $T(Y) = \sum_{(v,t)\in E} Y((v,t))$. The associated graph G has a layered structure: All flow that leaves the source s must pass through the point edges. This yields the equality $T(Y) = \sum_{e\in E_p} Y(e)$. If $Y(e) \in \mathbb{N}_0$ for all $e \in E$, we call Y an *integral flow*. Note that for any integral flow Y in the associated graph G, we have $Y(e) \in \{0, 1\}$ for all $e \in E_p$, as the capacity of all point edges is 1.

There is an elegant correspondence between the solutions of the reconstruction problem and the integral flows of maximal size (*max flows*) in the associated graph G:

Theorem 1. *Suppose that $S^{(1)} = S^{(2)} =: \bar{T}$. Problem 1 has a solution if, and only if, there exists an integral flow in G of size $\bar{T}$. Moreover, there is a 1-1* *correspondence between the solutions of Problem 1 and the integral flows of size $\bar{T}$ in G.*

Proof. We show first that any integral flow in G of size $\bar{T}$ corresponds to a unique solution of Problem 1. Let Y be a flow in G of size $\bar{T}$. For each $e \in E_p$, we have $Y(e) \in \{0, 1\}$. Put $F_Y = \{\Phi(e) \mid e \in E_p \text{ and } Y(e) = 1\}$, where Φ is the edge-to-point mapping of G. The set F_Y contains all lattice points for which the corresponding point edge in G carries a flow of 1. We call F_Y the *corresponding point set of* Y. We claim that F_Y is a solution of Problem 1. We show that $P_{F_Y}^{(1)} = p^{(1)}$; the proof for direction $v^{(2)}$ is completely analogous.

From the capacity constraints on the line edges of G and the fact that $T(Y) = S^{(1)}$, it follows that all line edges of G must be filled completely by Y. Therefore, we have $Y((s, n_{1,i})) = p^{(1)}(\ell_{1,i})$ for all $i = 1, \ldots, |L^{(1)}|$. Because of the flow conservation constraint at the line nodes of G, we have

$$\sum_{j=1}^{|L^{(2)}|} Y((n_{1,i}, n_{2,j})) = p^{(1)}(\ell_{1,i}) \quad \text{for } i = 1, \ldots, |L^{(1)}| \tag{9.7}$$

and, therefore,

$$|\{\Phi((n_{1,i}, n_{2,j})) \mid Y((n_{1,i}, n_{2,j})) = 1\}| = p^{(1)}(\ell_{1,i}) \quad \text{for } i = 1, \ldots, |L^{(1)}| . \tag{9.8}$$

From the structure of G, it follows that

$$F_Y \cap \ell_{1,i} = \{\Phi((n_{1,i}, n_{2,j})) \mid Y((n_{1,i}, n_{2,j})) = 1\} , \tag{9.9}$$

which yields $P_{F_Y}^{(1)}(\ell_{1,i}) = p^{(1)}(\ell_{1,i})$ for $i = 1, \ldots, |L^{(1)}|$. To prove that every flow Y of size $\bar{T}$ in G corresponds to a *unique solution* of Problem 1, we note that Y is completely determined by its values on the point edges of G. Therefore, a flow $Y' \neq Y$ of size $\bar{T}$ must be different from Y at at least one of the point edges; hence, $F_{Y'} \neq F_Y$.

We will now show that the mapping from flows of size $\bar{T}$ in G to solutions of Problem 1 is surjective. For any solution F of Problem 1, define the *corresponding flow* Y_F:

$$Y_F((n_{1,i}, n_{2,j})) = \begin{cases} 1 & \text{if } \Phi((n_{1,i}, n_{2,j})) \in F , \\ 0 & \text{otherwise} . \end{cases} \tag{9.10}$$

Specifying Y_F on the point edges completely determines the flow through the remaining edges by the conservation of flow constraint. We call Y_F the *corresponding flow of* F. It is easy to verify that Y_F satisfies all edge capacity constraints. By definition, F is the corresponding point set of Y_F. We have $T(Y_F) = \sum_{(v,w) \in E_p} Y((v, w)) = |F|$, so Y_F is a flow of size $|F| = S^{(1)} = \bar{T}$. This shows that the mapping $Y \rightarrow F_Y$ is a bijection. $\square$

The proof of Theorem 1 shows that we can find a solution of Problem 1 by finding an integral flow of size $\bar{T} = S^{(1)} = S^{(2)}$ in the associated graph. This flow is a *maximum flow* in G, because all line edges are completely saturated. Finding a maximum integral flow in a graph is an important problem in operations research, and efficient algorithms have been developed to solve this problem; see Section 9.5.

The equivalence between the reconstruction problem for two projections and the problem of finding a maximum flow in the associated graph was already described by Gale in 1957 [7] in the context of reconstructing binary matrices from their row and column sums. Theorem 1 generalizes this result to the case of any reconstruction lattice A and any pair of lattice directions $(v^{(1)}, v^{(2)})$.

In the next sections we will see that the network flow approach can be extended to solve more complex variants of the reconstruction problem and that it can be used as a building block for algorithms that compute a reconstruction from more than two projections.

9.3 Weighted Reconstruction

Problem 1 is usually severely underdetermined: The number of solutions can be exponential in the size of the reconstruction lattice A. In practical applications of tomography, the projection data are usually obtained by measuring the projections of an unknown object (the *original object*), and it is important that the reconstruction closely resembles this object. One way to achieve this is to use *prior knowledge* of the original object in the reconstruction algorithm. One of the first attempts to incorporate prior knowledge in the network flow approach was described in [22], in the context of medical image reconstruction.

In this section we consider a weighted version of Problem 1:

Problem 2. Let A, $v^{(1)}$, $v^{(2)}$, $p^{(1)}$, $p^{(2)}$ be given as in Problem 1. Let $W : A \to \mathbb{R}$ be a given mapping, the *weight map*. Construct a set $F \subseteq A$ such that $P_F^{(1)} = p^{(1)}$ and $P_F^{(2)} = p^{(2)}$ and the *total weight* $\sum_{x \in F} W(x)$ is maximal.

As a shorthand notation, we refer to the total weight of F as $W(F)$. Problem 2 is a generalization of Problem 1. Through the weight map, one can express a preference for a particular solution if the reconstruction problem has more than one solution. This preference is specified independently for each $x \in A$. The higher the weight $W(x)$, the stronger is the preference to include x in the reconstruction F. Note that a preference for image features that involve several pixels cannot be specified directly through the weight map.

The associated graph G can also be used to solve the weighted version of the reconstruction problem. Define the mapping $C : E \to \mathbb{R}$ as follows:

$$C(e) = \begin{cases} -W(\Phi(e)), & \text{for } e \in E_p \,, \\ 0, & \text{otherwise} \,. \end{cases} \qquad (9.11)$$

The *cost* $C(Y)$ of a flow Y in G is defined as $\sum_{e \in E} C(e)Y(e)$. The *min cost flow problem* in G deals with finding an integral flow Y of a prescribed size $\bar{T}$ in G such that the cost $C(Y)$ is minimal. If we choose $\bar{T} = S^{(1)} = S^{(2)}$, any integral flow Y of size $\bar{T}$ is a maximum flow in G and corresponds to a solution of Problem 1. The total weight of the solution that corresponds to a flow Y equals $-C(Y) = W(F_Y)$. Therefore, solving the integral min cost flow problem in G yields a solution of the reconstruction problem of maximum weight, solving Problem 2.

Just as for the max flow problem, efficient algorithms are available for solving the (integral) min cost flow problem. However, most such algorithms assume that the edge costs are integer values. If the edge costs are all in $\mathbb{Q}$, we can simply multiply all edge costs by the smallest common multiple of the denominators to obtain integer costs. If the edge costs are not in $\mathbb{Q}$, the solution of Problem 2 can be approximated by multiplying all edge costs with a large integer and rounding the resulting costs.

In [22] Slump and Gerbrands described an application of Problem 2 to the reconstruction of the left ventricle of the heart from two orthogonal angiographic projections. They used a min cost flow approach to solve a specific instance of Problem 2.

Having the ability to solve Problem 2 can be very helpful in solving a variety of reconstruction problems. We will describe two such problems. These problems deal with the reconstruction of *binary images*, i.e., images for which all pixels are either black or white. Each pixel in the image corresponds to a lattice point. A binary image corresponds to the lattice set $F \subseteq A$, where F contains the lattice points of all white pixels in the image.

Example 1. As an application of Problem 2, consider an industrial production line, where a large amount of similar objects has to be produced. Suppose that a *blueprint* is available, which specifies what the objects should look like. Occasionally, flaws occur in the production process, resulting in objects that don't match the blueprint. To check for errors, the factory uses a tomographic scanner that scans the objects in two directions: horizontal and vertical. To obtain a meaningful reconstruction from only two projections, the blueprint is used as a *model image*. For each object on the factory line, the reconstruction is computed that matches the blueprint in as many points as possible.

This problem can be formulated in the context of Problem 2. Suppose we want to reconstruct an $n \times n$ image. Put $A = \{1, \ldots, n\} \times \{1, \ldots, n\}$, $v^{(1)} = (1, 0)$, and $v^{(2)} = (0, 1)$. Let F_M be the lattice set that corresponds to the blueprint. We want to compute the solution F of Problem 1 such that

$$|(F \cap F_M) \cup (A \backslash F \cap A \backslash F_M)| = |A| - |F \bigtriangleup F_M| \qquad (9.12)$$

is maximal, where $\bigtriangleup$ denotes the symmetric set difference. The term $F \cap F_M$ represents the white pixels shared by F and F_M; the term $A \backslash F \cap A \backslash F_M$

represents the shared black pixels. To formulate this problem as an instance of Problem 2, put

$$W(x) = \begin{cases} 1 & \text{if } x \in F_M , \\ 0 & \text{otherwise} . \end{cases} \qquad (9.13)$$

The solution of Problem 2 for this weight map maximizes $|F \cap F_M|$, the number of common elements of F and F_M, subject to the constraints $P_F^{(1)} = p^{(1)}$ and $P_F^{(2)} = p^{(2)}$.

For the symmetric difference $F \triangle F_M$, the following equality holds:

$$|F \triangle F_M| = (|F| - |F \cap F_M|) + (|F_M| - |F \cap F_M|) . \qquad (9.14)$$

Noting that $|F| = S^{(1)}$ is constant for all solutions of Problem 1 yields

$$|(F \cap F_M) \cup (A \backslash F \cap A \backslash F_M)| \qquad (9.15)$$
$$= |A| - (S^{(1)} - |F \cap F_M|) - (|F_M| - |F \cap F_M|) \qquad (9.16)$$
$$= 2|F \cap F_M| + (|A| - |F_M| - S^{(1)}) . \qquad (9.17)$$

The term $(|A| - |F_M| - S^{(1)})$ is constant, which shows that maximizing $|(F \cap F_M) \cup (A \backslash F \cap A \backslash F_M)|$ is equivalent to maximizing $|F \cap F_M|$. We conclude that the given weight map indeed computes the reconstruction that corresponds to the blueprint in as many pixels as possible.

Figure 9.3(a) shows a blueprint image that represents a semiconductor part. The white pixels correspond to the wiring; the black pixels correspond to the background. Suppose that the object shown in Fig. 9.3(b) passes the scanner. The object clearly contains a gap that is not present in the blueprint and should be detected. Figure 9.3(c) shows a reconstruction computed from the horizontal and vertical projection data of the faulty object, using the blueprint image of Fig. 9.3(a). It has the same projections as the image in Fig. 9.3(b) and corresponds to the blueprint in as many pixels as possible. Although the reconstruction is not perfect, the gap is clearly visible and the object can be easily identified as faulty. For comparison, consider the image in Fig. 9.3(d), which also has the same projections as the images in Fig. 9.3(b) and (c). This time, the reconstruction corresponds to the blueprint in as *few* pixels as possible. Comparing this reconstruction to the original image of the faulty part shows how severely underdetermined the reconstruction problem is when only two projections are available. Of course, using a blueprint image does not guarantee that the reconstruction resembles the scanned object, but it is likely that the reconstruction will be much better than if no prior knowledge is used at all.

Example 2. Another practical problem that can be formulated in the framework of Problem 2 is how to obtain a 0–1 reconstruction from an already computed real-valued reconstruction. Computing a 0–1 reconstruction from

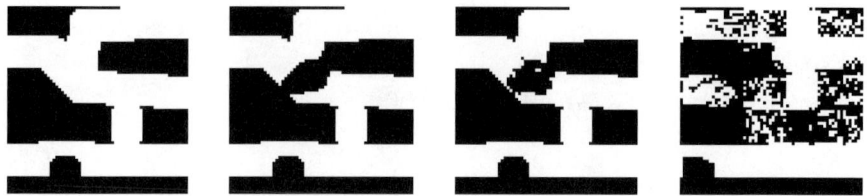

Fig. 9.3. (**a**) Blueprint image of a semiconductor part. (**b**) Test image, containing a gap in one of the wires. (**c**) Reconstruction of the test image from the horizontal and vertical projections, using the image from (a) as a model image. (**d**) Reconstruction using an inverted version of the blueprint image as a model image.

more than two projections is a computationally hard problem, but for computing a real-valued reconstruction several algorithms are available, such as the algebraic reconstruction technique (ART, see Chapter 7 of [17]). These algorithms typically require many projections to compute an accurate reconstruction. Figure 9.4(a) shows an ART reconstruction of the image in Fig. 9.3(b) from six projections. If we want the reconstruction to be binary, this reconstruction can be "rounded," such that all pixel values less than 1/2 become 0 and all pixel values of 1/2 or more become 1. The result is shown in Fig. 9.4(b). A different way to obtain a binary reconstruction is to solve Problem 2 using the pixel values of the original image as the weight map: the higher the gray value of a pixel in the continuous reconstruction, the higher the preference for this pixel to be assigned a value of 1 in the binary reconstruction. In this way the reconstruction will perfectly satisfy two of the projections, while "resembling" the continuous reconstruction. Figure 9.4(c) and (d) show two such reconstructions. The reconstruction in Fig. 9.4(c) was obtained using $v^{(1)} = (1, 0)$, $v^{(2)} = (0, 1)$. For the second reconstruction, the lattice directions $v^{(1)} = (0, 1)$, $v^{(2)} = (1, 1)$ were used. Both reconstructions are better than the one in Fig. 9.4(b) at some features, but it is not clear how to detect automatically which one is better, or how the two solutions can be combined into one superior solution. In Section 9.6, we describe how the reconstructions for different pairs of lattice directions can be combined to compute a single, more accurate reconstruction (see Fig. 9.9).

9.4 Reconstruction from Noisy Projections

The network model from Sections 9.2 and 9.3 is only suitable for computing reconstructions from *perfect* projection data. In simulation experiments, it is easy to compute perfect projections of a given image, but data that are obtained by physical measurements are usually polluted by noise. As an example of what happens in the network of Section 9.2, when the projection data contain errors, consider the possibility that $S^{(1)} \neq S^{(2)}$. In this case, it

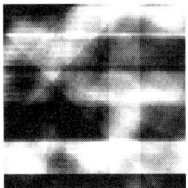 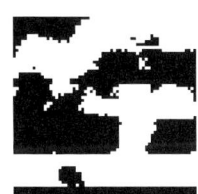 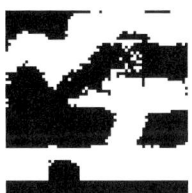 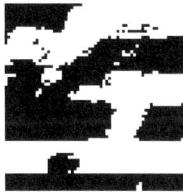

Fig. 9.4. (a) ART reconstruction of the image in Fig. 9.3(b) from six projections. (b) Rounded ART reconstruction. (c) Solution of Problem 2, using the ART reconstruction as the weight map, for lattice directions $(1,0)$ and $(0,1)$. (d) Solution of Problem 2 using lattice directions $(0,1)$ and $(1,1)$.

is clear that no perfect solution of the reconstruction problem exists. One can still compute a maximum flow in the associated graph G. Due to the line arc capacity constraints, such a flow will always have size at most $\min(S^{(1)}, S^{(2)})$. If the measured projection for a line ℓ is lower than the number of points on that line in the original object, that line will always contain too few points in the reconstruction, regardless of the measured line projections in the other direction, because of the capacity constraint on the corresponding line edge of ℓ.

In this section we consider a modification of the associated graph which can be used to compute a reconstruction F for which the norm of the residue, i.e., the difference between the projections of F and the two prescribed projections is minimal. This network does not have the drawbacks that we described above of the network from Section 9.2.

Let $F \subseteq A$. For $k = 1, 2$, the projections $P_F^{(k)}$ of F have finite domains, so we can regard $P_F^{(k)}$ as a vector of $|L^{(k)}|$ elements. We denote the sum-norm of this vector by $|P_F^{(k)}|_1$. For a given prescribed projection $p^{(k)}$, the norm

$$|P_F^{(k)} - p^{(k)}|_1 = \sum_{\ell \in L^{(k)}} |P_F^{(k)}(\ell) - p^{(k)}(\ell)| \tag{9.18}$$

equals the total summed projection difference over all lines in $L^{(k)}$. Another norm that is often used in tomography is the Euclidean norm $|\cdot|_2$. The sum-norm is better suited for incorporation in the network flow approach. We now define a generalization of Problem 1 that allows for errors in the prescribed projections.

Problem 3. Let A, $v^{(1)}$, $v^{(2)}$, $p^{(1)}$, $p^{(2)}$ be given as in Problem 1. Let $\bar{T} \in \mathbb{N}_0$. Construct a set $F \subseteq A$ with $|F| = \bar{T}$ such that $|P_F^{(1)} - p^{(1)}|_1 + |P_F^{(2)} - p^{(2)}|_1$ is minimal.

Problem 3 asks for a set F that has a prescribed number of $\bar{T}$ elements such that F corresponds as well as possible to the two prescribed projections, according to the sum-norm. If Problem 1 has a solution, we can find all solutions by putting $\bar{T} = S^{(1)}$ and solving Problem 3. We will show that Problem 3 can be solved within the network flow model. For any n-dimensional vector $p \in \mathbb{R}^n$, define

$$|p|^+ = \sum_{i=1}^{n} \max(p_i, 0) . \tag{9.19}$$

To solve Problem 3, we need to make some modifications to the associated graph. Before introducing the modified graph, we prove the following lemma.

Lemma 1. *Let $F \subseteq A$, $|F| = \bar{T}$. Then, for $k = 1, 2$,*

$$|P_F^{(k)} - p^{(k)}|_1 = 2|P_F^{(k)} - p^{(k)}|^+ + S^{(k)} - \bar{T} . \tag{9.20}$$

Proof. Let $k \in \{1, 2\}$. By definition, we have

$$|P_F^{(k)} - p^{(k)}|_1 = |P_F^{(k)} - p^{(k)}|^+ + |p^{(k)} - P_F^{(k)}|^+ . \tag{9.21}$$

For each line $\ell \in L^{(k)}$, we have

$$P_F^{(k)}(\ell) = p^{(k)} + \max(P_F^{(k)}(\ell) - p^{(k)}(\ell), 0) - \max(p^{(k)}(\ell) - P_F^{(k)}(\ell), 0) . \tag{9.22}$$

Summing this equation over all lines $\ell \in L^{(k)}$, it follows that

$$\bar{T} = S^{(k)} + |P_F^{(k)} - p^{(k)}|^+ - |p^{(k)} - P_F^{(k)}|^+ ; \tag{9.23}$$

hence,

$$|P_F^{(k)} - p^{(k)}|_1 = 2|P_F^{(k)} - p^{(k)}|^+ + S^{(k)} - \bar{T} . \tag{9.24}$$

$\square$

Lemma 1 shows that solving Problem 3 is equivalent to finding a set F with $|F| = \bar{T}$ for which

$$|P_F^{(1)} - p^{(1)}|^+ + |P_F^{(2)} - p^{(2)}|^+ \tag{9.25}$$

is minimal, since $S^{(1)}$, $S^{(2)}$, and $\bar{T}$ are constant.

We will now describe how the associated graph can be modified for solving Problem 3. The network from Section 9.2 forms the basis for the new network. From this point on we refer to the line edges of the network from Section 9.2 as *primary line edges*. As before, we denote the sets of all primary line edges for directions $v^{(1)}$ and $v^{(2)}$ by E_1 and E_2, respectively. Let $\ell \in L^{(k)}$ be any lattice line for direction $v^{(k)}$, and let $e \in E_k$ its corresponding primary line edge. The capacity of e imposes a hard upper bound on the number of points on ℓ in the network flow reconstruction. To relax this hard constraint, we add a second edge for each lattice line, the *excess edge*. The excess edges are parallel to their corresponding primary line edges and have the same orientation. We denote the set of excess edges for directions $v^{(1)}$ and $v^{(2)}$ by E_1' and E_2', respectively.

The resulting graph G' is shown in Fig. 9.5. The capacities of the primary line edges remain unchanged. The excess edges have unbounded capacities. Effectively, this means that the total flow through a primary line edge and its corresponding excess edge — both belonging to a line $\ell \in L^{(k)}$ — is bounded by $|A \cap \ell|$, as all outgoing flow from the line edges must pass through $|A \cap \ell|$ point edges where each has capacity 1. Therefore, it is still possible to assign finite capacities to the excess edges.

The primary line edges of the new graph are still assigned a cost of 0, as in the original network. The excess edges are assigned a cost of K, where K is a positive constant. In this way it is possible to allow more points on a line ℓ than $p^{(k)}(\ell)$, but only at the expense of a cost increase.

Now consider the problem of finding a min cost flow in G' of size $\bar{T}$. Without computing such a flow, we can already be sure that any excess edge will only carry flow if its corresponding primary line edge is saturated up to its capacity. Otherwise, the cost could be decreased by transferring flow from the excess edge to the primary edge.

Suppose that $Y : E \rightarrow \mathbb{Z}$ is a min cost flow in G' of size $\bar{T}$. The total cost of Y, given by

$$C(Y) = K \Big(\sum_{e \in E_1'} Y(e) + \sum_{e \in E_2'} Y(e) \Big). \tag{9.26}$$

Let F_Y be the set of points for which the corresponding point edges in Y carry a positive flow, as in the Proof of Theorem 1. For any line $\ell \in L^{(k)}$, the total flow through the primary and excess edges of ℓ must equal $P_{F_Y}^{(k)}(\ell)$, because of the flow conservation constraints. Therefore, we have

$$\sum_{e \in E_k'} Y(e) = |P_{F_Y}^{(k)} - p^{(k)}|^+ ; \tag{9.27}$$

hence,

$$C(Y) = K(|P_{F_Y}^{(1)} - p^{(1)}|^+ + |P_{F_Y}^{(2)} - p^{(2)}|^+). \tag{9.28}$$

Applying Lemma 1, we conclude that a min cost flow in G' of size $\bar{T}$ yields a solution of Problem 3.

The new network can also be used to solve an extended version of Problem 2.

Problem 4. Let A, $v^{(1)}$, $v^{(2)}$, $p^{(1)}$, $p^{(2)}$ be as given in Problem 2. Let $\bar{T} \in \mathbb{N}_0$, $\alpha \in \mathbb{R}_{>0}$. Construct a set $F \subseteq A$ with $|F| = \bar{T}$ such that

$$\alpha(|P_F^{(1)} - p^{(1)}|_1 + |P_F^{(2)} - p^{(2)}|_1) - \sum_{x \in F} W(x) \tag{9.29}$$

is minimal.

Similar to the procedure for solving Problem 2, we set $C(e) = -W(\Phi(e))$ for all $e \in E_p$. Assuming that an excess edge only carries flow if its corresponding primary line edge is completely full, the total cost of an integral flow $Y \in \mathcal{Y}$ now becomes

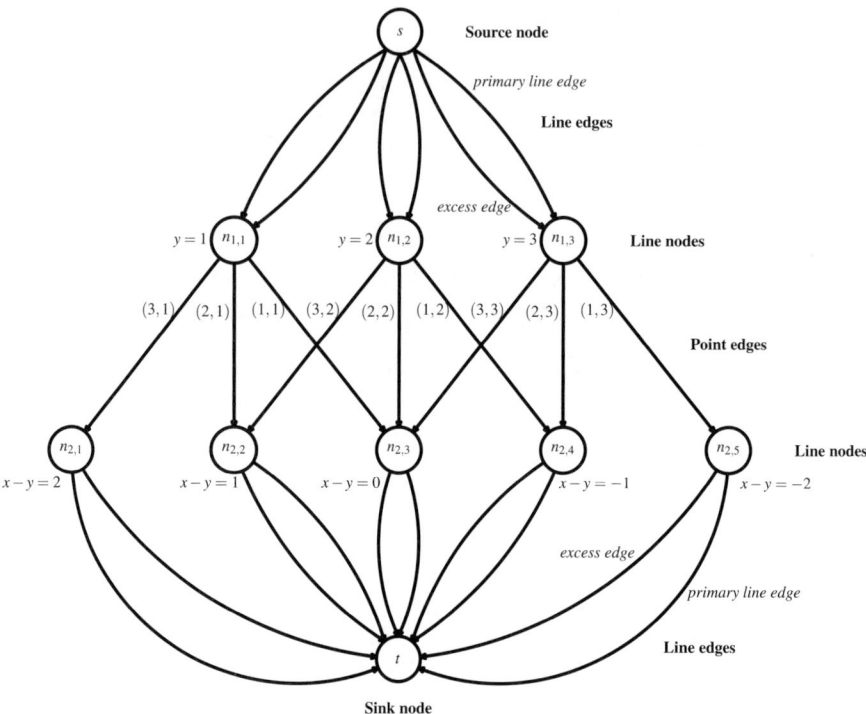

Fig. 9.5. Modified associated graph G' for the triple $(A, v^{(1)}, v^{(2)})$ from Fig. 9.1.

$$C(Y) = K(|P_{F_Y}^{(1)} - p^{(1)}|^+ + |P_{F_Y}^{(2)} - p^{(2)}|^+) - \sum_{x \in F_Y} W(x) \, . \qquad (9.30)$$

Setting $K = 2\alpha$ and using Eq. (9.24) yield

$$C(Y) = \alpha(|P_{F_Y}^{(1)} - p^{(1)}|_1 + |P_{F_Y}^{(2)} - p^{(2)}|_1) - \sum_{x \in F_Y} W(x) - C_0 \, , \qquad (9.31)$$

where C_0 is a constant. We conclude that if Y is an integral min cost flow of size $\bar{T}$ in G', then F_Y is a solution to Problem 4.

9.5 Algorithms and Implementation

As described in the previous sections, Problem 1, 2, 3, and 4 can all be solved as instances of network flow problems. Both the max flow problem and the min cost flow problem have been studied extensively. The book [1] provides an overview of available algorithms. A survey of the time complexities of various network flow algorithms can be found in [21] (max flow: Chapter 10; min cost flow: Chapter 12).

We now assume that the reconstruction lattice A is a square of size $N \times N$, and we fix a pair $(v^{(1)}, v^{(2)})$ of lattice directions. It is clear that the number of points in A on each lattice line parallel to $v^{(1)}$ or $v^{(2)}$ is $O(N)$. It is also clear that the number of lattice lines parallel to $v^{(1)}$ or $v^{(2)}$ that have a nonempty intersection with A is $O(N)$.

Problem 1 can be solved as an instance of the max flow problem in the associated graph. In [10], Goldberg and Rao describe an algorithm to compute a maximum flow in a graph with n nodes, m edges, and maximum edge capacity c in $O(n^{2/3} m \log(n^2/m) \log c)$ time. The associated graph of the triple $(A, v^{(1)}, v^{(2)})$ has $n = O(N)$ nodes, $m = O(N^2)$ edges, and a maximum edge capacity of $c = O(N)$. Therefore, Problem 1 can be solved in $O(N^{8/3} \log N)$ time.

Problems 2 and 3 can both be solved as instances of the min cost flow problem, i.e., the problem of finding a flow of fixed size that has minimal cost. The min cost flow problem can be reformulated as a minimum-cost circulation problem by adding an edge from the sink node t to the source node s; see Section 12.1 of [21]. In [11], Goldberg and Tarjan describe an algorithm to compute a minimum-cost circulation in a graph with n nodes, m edges, and maximum (integral) edge cost K in $O(nm \log(n^2/m) \log(nK))$ time. For the associated graph from Section 9.3, as well as for the modified associated graph from Section 9.4, this yields a time complexity of $O(N^3 \log(NK))$ for solving the min cost flow problem.

The problem of finding a maximum flow in the associated graph is known in the literature as *simple b-matching*. A flow that saturates all line edges is called a *perfect simple b-matching*, and the weighted variant of finding a perfect b-matching is known as *perfect weighted b-matching*; see Chapter 21 of [21]. For these particular network flow problems, special algorithms have been developed that are sometimes faster than general network flow algorithms.

Implementing fast network flow algorithms is a difficult and time-consuming task. The fastest way to use such algorithms is to use an existing implementation. Several network flow program libraries are available, some commercially and some for free. The ILOG CPLEX solver [15] performs very well for a wide range of network flow problems. The CS2 library from Goldberg [9] performs well and is free for noncommercial use. The same holds for the RelaxIV library from Bertsekas [4].

9.6 Extension to More Than Two Projections

As shown in the previous sections, the reconstruction problem from two projections is well understood and can be solved efficiently. We now move to the case where more than two projections are available.

Problem 5. Let $n > 2$ and let $v^{(1)}, \ldots, v^{(n)}$ be given distinct lattice directions. Let $A \subseteq \mathbb{Z}^2$ be a given lattice set. For $k = 1, \ldots, n$, let $p^{(k)} : L^{(k)} \to \mathbb{N}_0$ be given functions. Construct a set $F \subseteq A$ such that $P_F^{(k)} = p^{(k)}$ for $k = 1, \ldots, n$.

When more projections are available, the reconstruction problem is less underdetermined and we would like to be able to use the additional projections to increase the reconstruction quality. However, the reconstruction problem for more than two projections is NP-hard. Therefore, we have to resort to approximation algorithms. In this section we will describe an iterative algorithm that uses only two projections in each iteration. Within an iteration, a new pair of projections is first selected. Subsequently, an instance of Problem 2 is solved to obtain a reconstruction that satisfies the current two projections. The reconstruction from the previous iteration, which was computed using a different pair of projections, is used to construct the weight map of Problem 2 in such a way that the new reconstruction will resemble the previous one. In this way the other projections are incorporated in the reconstruction procedure in an implicit way.

Compute the start solution F^0;

$i := 0$;

while (stop criterion is not met) **do**
begin

    $i := i + 1$;

    Select a new pair of directions v_a and v_b $(1 \leq a < b \leq n)$;

    Compute a new weight map W^i from the previous solution F^{i-1};

    Compute a new solution F^i by solving Problem 2 for
    directions v_a and v_b, using the weight map W^i;

end

Fig. 9.6. Basic steps of the algorithm.

Figure 9.6 describes the basic structure of the algorithm. In the next subsections each of the steps will be described. The algorithm relies heavily on the methods for solving two-projection subproblems, which we described in the previous sections.

9.6.1 Computing the Start Solution

At the start of the algorithm, there is no "previous reconstruction"; a start solution has to be computed for the iterative algorithm. Ideally, the start solution should satisfy two criteria:

(a) **Accuracy**. The start solution should correspond well to the prescribed projection data.

(b) **Speed**. The start solution should be computed fast (compared with the running time of the rest of the algorithm).

These are conflicting goals. Computing a highly accurate binary reconstruction will certainly take too much time, as the reconstruction problem is NP-hard.

There are several options for computing the start solutions, each having a different tradeoff between speed and accuracy. The first option is to choose the empty set $F^0 = \emptyset$ as a start solution, i.e., an image that is completely black.

A better alternative is to use a very fast approximate reconstruction algorithm, such as one of the greedy algorithms described in [12]. The running time of these algorithms is comparable to the time it takes to solve a single network flow problem in the body of the main loop of our algorithm.

A third possibility is to start with a continuous reconstruction. A binary start solution can then be computed from the continuous reconstruction, as described in Example 2 of Section 9.3. One class of reconstruction algorithms that can be used consists of the *algebraic reconstruction algorithms* (see Chapter 7 of [17]). The basic idea of these algorithms is to describe Problem 5 as a system of linear equations:

$$Mx = b. \qquad (9.32)$$

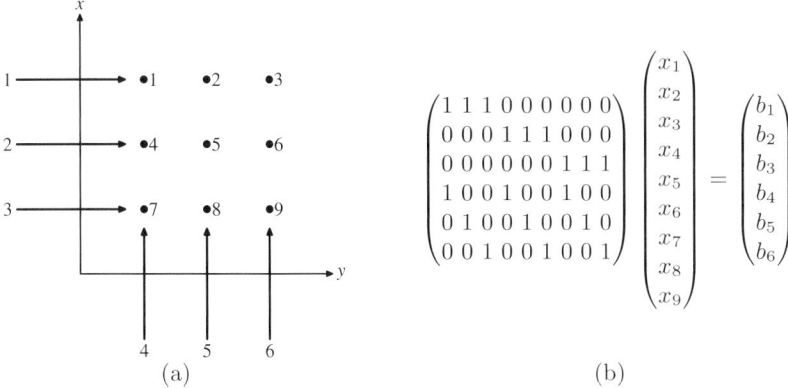

Fig. 9.7. (a) Numbering scheme for the lattice points and the lattice lines in a rectangular reconstruction lattice. (b) System of equations corresponding to the numbering in (a).

Figure 9.7 shows an example 3×3 grid with the corresponding system of equations for two directions, $v^{(1)} = (1,0)$ and $v^{(2)} = (0,1)$. Each entry of the vector x represents an element of A. The entries of the vector b correspond to the line projections for lattice directions $v^{(1)}, \ldots, v^{(n)}$. Each row of the binary matrix M represents a lattice line. The entry M_{ij} is 1 if, and only if, its corresponding lattice line i passes through point j.

The system (9.32) is usually underdetermined. The shortest solution of the system with respect to the Euclidean norm $| \cdot |_2$, which we denote as x^*, is a good choice for a start solution in discrete tomography. It can be shown that if Problem 5 has several solutions, then the Euclidean distance of x^* to any of these solutions is the same, so x^* is "centered" between the solutions. In addition, if the system (9.32) has binary solutions, any of these solutions has minimal norm among all integral solutions. Therefore, a short solution is likely to be a good start solution. We refer to [13] for the details of these arguments. The shortest solution of (9.32) can be computed efficiently by iterative methods, as described in [23]. After this solution has been computed, a pair $(v^{(a)}, v^{(b)})$ of lattice directions has to be selected for computing the binary start solution. The start solution is computed by solving Problem 2, using the pixel values in x^* as the weight map.

9.6.2 Computing the Weight Map

In each iteration of the main loop an instance of Problem 2 is solved. The weight map for this reconstruction problem is computed from the reconstruction of the previous iteration; it does not depend on the selected pair of lattice directions.

The weight map should be chosen in such a way that the new reconstruction resembles the reconstruction from the previous iteration. In the new instance of Problem 2, only two of the projections are used. If the new reconstruction is similar to the previous reconstruction, which was computed using a different pair of projections, the new image will also approximately adhere to the prescribed two projections from the previous iteration. Repeating this intuitive argument, we would hope that the new image also satisfies the projections from the iteration before the previous one, from the iteration before that one, etc.

The most straightforward way to make the new reconstruction resemble the previous one is to follow the approach from Example 1 in Section 9.3. If we put

$$W^i((x,y)) = \begin{cases} 1 & \text{if } (x,y) \in F^{i-1} , \\ 0 & \text{otherwise} , \end{cases} \qquad (9.33)$$

the new reconstructed image F^i will have the same pixel value as F^{i-1} in as many pixels as possible. Unfortunately, this choice usually does not lead to good results. Typically, the main loop of the algorithm does not converge, making it difficult to decide when the algorithm should be terminated. This behavior is by no means surprising. The reconstruction problem from a small number of projections is severely underdetermined. If no additional prior knowledge is used, a small number of projections (e.g., four or five) may not even be nearly enough data to uniquely determine a reconstruction.

To deal with this problem, we focus on the reconstruction of images that satisfy additional properties. *Smoothness* is a property that can often be observed in practical images: Images consist of large areas that are completely black or completely white, instead of exhibiting completely random pixel patterns. A nice property of the smoothness concept is that it can be measured *locally*. We say that an image F is *perfectly smooth* at pixel $x \in A$ if all neighboring points of x have the same value as x. Of course, this notion requires the definition of a *neighborhood* of x, which we will describe below.

From this point on, we assume that the reconstruction lattice A is rectangular. If this assumption is not satisfied, we can use any square reconstruction lattice A' for which $A \subseteq A'$, as increasing the size of the reconstruction lattice does not affect the projections.

Let F^{i-1} be the reconstructed image from the previous iteration. As a neighborhood of the point $p = (x_p, y_p) \in A$, we choose a square centered in (x_p, y_p). The reason for preferring a square neighborhood over alternatives is that the required computations can be performed very efficiently in this case. Let $p = (x_p, y_p) \in A$. Let r be a positive integer, the *neighborhood radius*. Put

$$N_p = \{ (x,y) \in A \mid x_p - r \le x \le x_p + r,\ y_p - r \le y \le y_p + r \} . \quad (9.34)$$

N_p contains all pixels in the neighborhood of p, including p. In case p is near the boundary of A, the set N_p may contain fewer than $(2r + 1)^2$ pixels. Let s_p be the number of pixels $q \in N_p$ for which $F(p) = F(q)$. Define

$$f_p = \frac{s_p}{|N_p|} . \quad (9.35)$$

We call f_p the *similarity fraction* of p. A high similarity fraction corresponds to a smooth neighborhood of p.

Let $g : [0,1] \to \mathbb{R}_{>0}$ be a nondecreasing function, the *local weight function*. This function determines the preference for locally smooth regions. We compute the pixel weight $W(p)$ of p as follows:

$$W(p) = 2(F(p) - \frac{1}{2})g(f_p) . \quad (9.36)$$

Note that $2(F(p) - \frac{1}{2})$ is either -1 or $+1$.

When we take $g(f) = 1$ for all $f \in [0,1]$, there is no preference for local smoothness. To express the preference, we make the local weight function g an increasing function of f_p. Now a pixel having a value of 1 that is surrounded by other pixels having the same value will obtain a higher weight than such a pixel that is surrounded by 0-valued pixels. A higher weight expresses a preference to retain the value of 1 in the next reconstruction. The same reasoning holds for pixels having a value of 0, except that in this case the pixel weights are negative. Three possible choices for the local weight function are

(a) $g(f_p) = f_p$,
(b) $g(f_p) = \sqrt{f_p}$,
(c) $g(f_p) = f_p^2$.

The last choice results in a strong preference for pixels that are (almost) perfectly smooth. Of course, many other local weight functions are possible. In [3], extensive results are reported for the local weight function

$$g(f_p) = \begin{cases} 1 & (f_p \leq 0.65) , \\ 4f & (0.65 < f_p < 1) , \\ 9 & (f_p = 1) . \end{cases} \tag{9.37}$$

The choice for this particular function is somewhat arbitrary. In each case, a preference is expressed for retaining the pixel value of p in the next reconstruction, instead of changing it. In the case that the whole neighborhood of p has the same value as p, this preference is very strong. If the neighborhood contains a few pixels having a different value, the preference is less. If there are many pixels in the neighborhood that have a different value, the preference is even smaller.

So far we have not discussed how the neighborhood radius should be chosen. If the start solution is already a good approximation of the final reconstruction, using a fixed value of $r = 1$ works well. For this neighborhood radius, the differences between consecutive reconstructions F^i are typically small. It is usually better to start with a larger neighborhood radius, e.g., $r = 5$ or $r = 8$. This typically results in large changes between consecutive reconstructions. Only very large regions of pixels that have the same value obtain a strong preference to keep this value. Regions that are less smooth can easily change. A choice that works well for the range of images studied in [3] is to start the algorithm with $r = 8$ and to set $r = 1$ after 50 iterations.

9.6.3 Choosing the Pair of Directions

In each iteration of the main loop of the algorithm, a new pair of lattice directions is selected. There is no selection scheme that is "obviously best" in all cases. Yet there are several ways for choosing the direction pairs that perform well in practice.

A good choice for the new direction pair is to choose the lattice directions $v^{(a)}$, $v^{(b)}$, for which the total projection error

$$|P_F^{(a)} - p^{(a)}|_1 + |P_F^{(b)} - p^{(b)}|_1 \tag{9.38}$$

is largest. After solving the new instance of Problem 2, the total projection error for these two lattice directions will be zero, assuming perfect projection data. This also guarantees that if at least two projections have a positive projection error after the previous iteration, both new lattice directions will be different from the ones used in the previous iteration.

If the number of projections is very small (e.g., four or five) the projection error is not a good criterion for selecting the new projection pair. For the case of four projections, this scheme leads to cycling behavior between two pair of projections. The other projection pairs are not used at all. To avoid this behavior, it is better to use a fixed order of direction pairs, in which all pairs occur equally often. Such schemes, for four and five projections, are shown in Table 9.1.

Table 9.1. (left) Lattice Direction Scheme for Four Projections (Each projection pair is used equally often. No projection pair is used in two consecutive iterations.) (right) Lattice Direction Scheme for Five Projections

Iteration	1 2 3 4 5 6
1st dir.	1 3 1 2 1 2
2nd dir.	2 4 3 4 4 3

Iteration	1 2 3 4 5 6 7 8 9 10
1st dir.	1 3 5 2 4 1 2 3 4 5
2nd dir.	2 4 1 3 5 3 4 5 1 2

9.6.4 Stop Criterion

In general, it is not easy to determine when the iterative algorithm from Fig. 9.6 should terminate, because there is no guaranteed convergence. Yet, the experiments from [3] show that if enough projections are available, the algorithm often converges to the exact solution of Problem 5. Detecting that an exact solution has been found is easy, and the algorithm always terminates in that case.

To measure the quality of the current reconstruction F, the *total projection difference*

$$D(F) = \sum_{k=1}^{n} |P_F^{(k)} - p^{(k)}|_1 \tag{9.39}$$

can be used. This distance is 0 for any perfect solution of Problem 5 and greater than 0 otherwise. The total projection difference can be used for defining termination conditions. If no new minimal value is found for the total projection distance during the last T iterations, where T is a positive integer, the algorithm terminates. We used $T = 100$ for all experiments in the next subsection.

9.6.5 Some Results

We will now show some experimental results obtained by the iterative algorithm from Fig. 9.6. The performance of the algorithm, as for any other general discrete tomography algorithm, depends heavily on the type of image that is being reconstructed and the number of available projections. In order to give extensive statistical results about the reconstruction quality, a *class of images* has to be defined first. All images in this class should have similar characteristics. The performance of the algorithm can then be measured for this particular image class. In [3], reconstruction results were reported for several different image classes. The results in this section show a varied set of test images with their reconstructions, rather than providing extensive quantitative results. Figure 9.8 shows six test images, each having different characteristics, and their reconstructions. The number n of projections that was used is shown in the figure captions. The reconstructions of the first five images (a–e) are all *perfect reconstructions*, obtained using the weight function in Eq.(9.37) from Section 9.6.2. For the first four images (a–d), the linear local weight function also works very well, even faster than the function in Eq.(9.37). The image in Fig. 9.8(e) contains many fine lines of only a single pixel's thickness. In this case, the local weight function $g(f_p) = \sqrt{f_p}$ works well. Which local weight function is best for a certain class of image depends strongly on characteristics of the particular class. This is also true for the *number of projections* required to reconstruct an image.

For reconstructing the image in Fig. 9.8(a), four projections suffice. The structure of the object boundary is fairly complex, but the object contains no "holes." The iterative algorithm reconstructed the image perfectly from four projections (horizontal, vertical, diagonal, and antidiagonal).

Figure 9.8(b) shows a much more complicated example. The object contains many cavities of various sizes and has a very complex boundary. Some of the black holes inside the white region are only a single pixel in size. In this case, our algorithm requires six projections to compute an accurate reconstruction. Some of the fine details in this image are not smooth at all. Still, the fine details are reconstructed with great accuracy. The image from Fig. 9.8(c) is even more complex. It requires eight projections to be reconstructed perfectly.

The image in Fig. 9.8(d) has a lot of local smoothness in the black areas, but it contains no large white areas. Still, the image is smooth enough to be reconstructed perfectly from only five projections. This example also illustrates that very fine, nonsmooth details can be reconstructed by the algorithm, as long as the entire image is sufficiently smooth.

Figure 9.8(e) shows a vascular system containing several very thin vessels. The iterative algorithm can reconstruct the original image perfectly from 12 projections. This is quite surprising, since the very thin vessels have a width of only one pixel, so they are not smooth. Still, the smoothness of the thicker vessels and the background area provides the algorithm with enough guidance to reconstruct the original image.

When the image contains no structure at all, the algorithm performs very badly. Figure 9.8(f) shows an image of random noise. The reconstruction from 12 projections shows that our algorithm has a preference for connected areas of white and black pixels. In this case, however, the smoothness assumption is obviously not satisfied by the original image. The distance between the projections of the image found by our algorithm and the prescribed projections is very small, however.

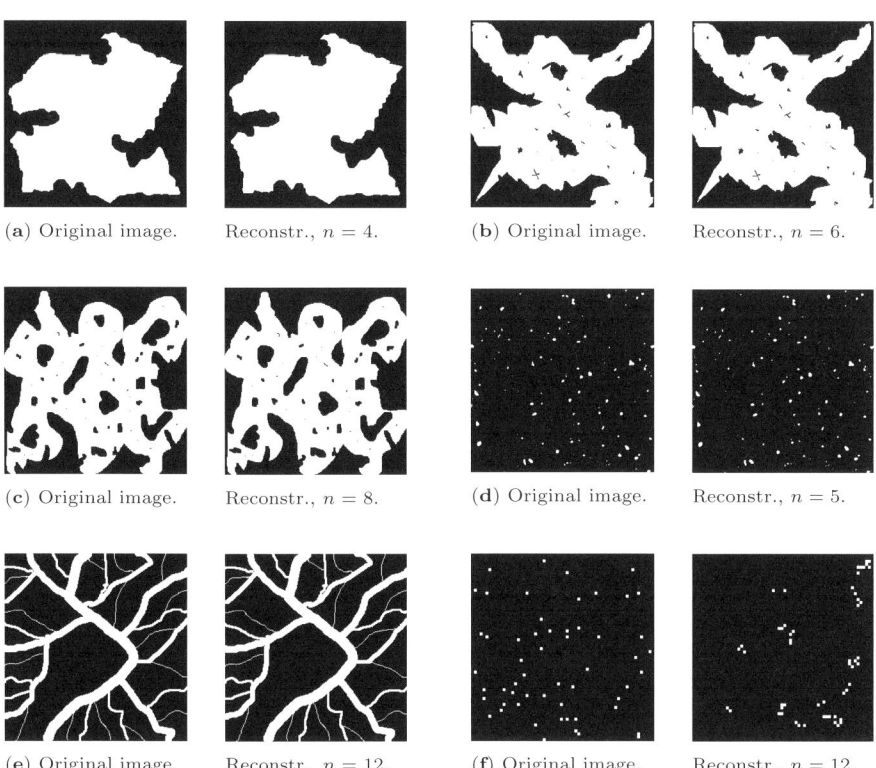

(a) Original image.   Reconstr., $n = 4$.   (b) Original image.   Reconstr., $n = 6$.

(c) Original image.   Reconstr., $n = 8$.   (d) Original image.   Reconstr., $n = 5$.

(e) Original image.   Reconstr., $n = 12$.   (f) Original image.   Reconstr., $n = 12$.

Fig. 9.8. Six original images and their reconstructions. The number n of projections is shown in the figure caption. [The images in Fig. 9.8(f) show a zoomed portion of the center of the actual images, to make the details clearly visible.]

For reconstructing the images in Fig. 9.8, a sufficiently large set of projections was used. Figures 9.9 and 9.10 demonstrate the result of using the algorithm if too few projections are available.

Figure 9.9 shows the results of reconstructing the semiconductor image of Fig. 9.3(b) from three and four projections, respectively. When we use only three projections, a reconstruction is found that has exactly the prescribed projections, but the reconstruction is very different from the original image.

If we use too few projections, the algorithm may also get stuck in a local minimum of the projection distance, which is shown in Fig. 9.10. The original image can be reconstructed perfectly from five projections, but when only four projections are used, the algorithm fails to find a good reconstruction. The projections of the reconstructed image are significantly different from the four prescribed projections, yet the algorithm is unable to find a better reconstruction.

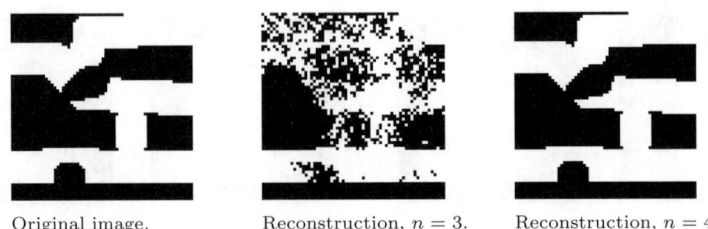

Original image.   Reconstruction, $n = 3$.   Reconstruction, $n = 4$.

Fig. 9.9. (a) Original image. (b) Reconstruction from three projections (horizontal, vertical, diagonal) that has exactly the prescribed projections. (c) Perfect reconstruction of the original image from four projections (horizontal, vertical, diagonal, antidiagonal).

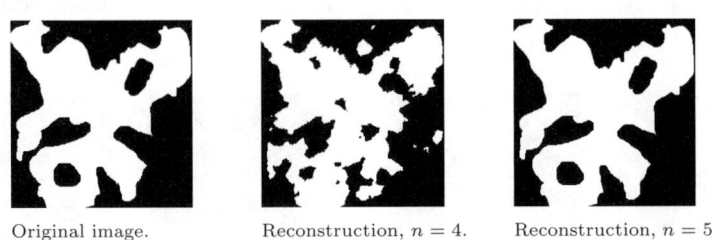

Original image.   Reconstruction, $n = 4$.   Reconstruction, $n = 5$.

Fig. 9.10. (a) Original image. (b) Reconstruction from four projections, which does not have the prescribed projections. The horizontal and vertical projections are identical to those of the first image. The diagonal and antidiagonal projections have a total projection difference (sum of absolute values) of 184 and 126, respectively. (c) Perfect reconstruction of the original image from five projections.

9.7 Reconstructing 3D Volumes

So far our approach has been concerned with the reconstruction of two-dimensional images. In many practical applications of tomography, it is important to obtain 3D reconstructions. Computing 3D reconstructions is usually a computationally very demanding task, as large amounts of data are involved. There is a slight difference in terminology between 2D and 3D reconstructions. *Pixels* in 2D images are usually called *voxels* in the context of 3D images, where they represent a unit cube in the 3D volume.

If there exists a plane H in $\mathbb{Z}^3$ such that all projection directions lie in H, all algorithms for 2D reconstruction can be used directly for 3D reconstruction as well, reconstructing the volume as a series of slices. All slices can be reconstructed in parallel, which allows for a large speedup if several processors are used. A disadvantage of reconstructing all slices independently is that certain types of prior knowledge cannot be exploited. For example, if we generalize the preference for local smoothness from Section 9.6 to 3D, voxels from adjacent slices are required to compute the neighborhood density of a certain voxel. Therefore, the reconstruction computations of the slices are no longer independent.

If the projection directions are not coplanar, reconstructing the volume as a series of slices is not possible. This situation occurs, for example, in the application of atomic resolution electron microscopy. The crystal sample is tilted in two directions to obtain as many useful projections as possible.

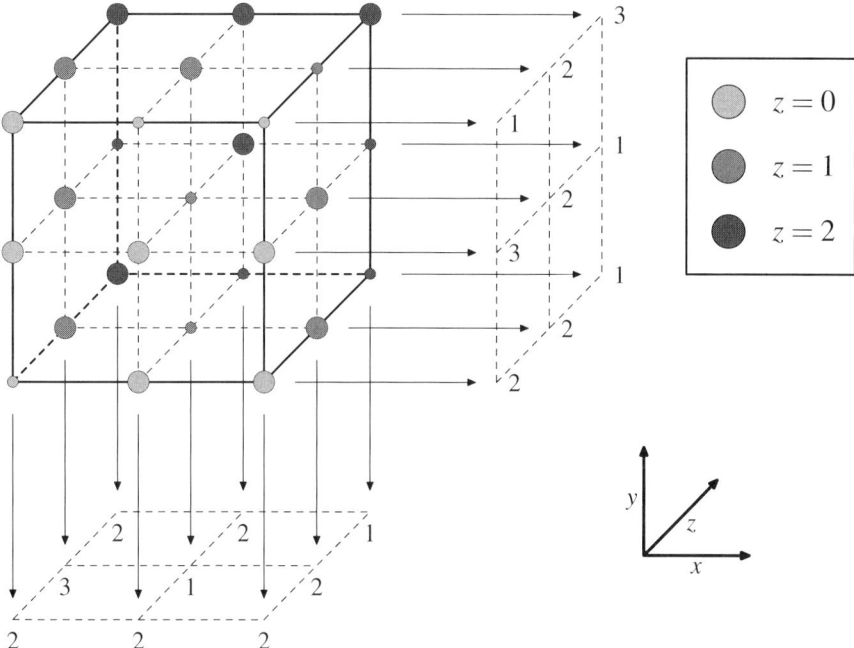

Fig. 9.11. $3 \times 3 \times 3$ binary volume with its projections in directions $v^{(1)} = (1, 0, 0)$ and $v^{(2)} = (0, 1, 0)$. A large circle indicates a value of 1; a small circle indicates a value of 0.

We will now show how the algorithm for 2D reconstruction from the previous section can be generalized to the 3D case. Figure 9.11 shows an example of a $3 \times 3 \times 3$ volume A with its projections parallel to the lattice directions

$v^{(1)} = (1,0,0)$ and $v^{(2)} = (0,1,0)$. Lattice points that have a value of 1 (i.e., lattice points included in the set F) are indicated by large dots. Similar to the associated network from Section 9.2, each two-projection problem in 3D also has an associated graph. The associated graph for the volume in Fig. 9.11 is shown in Fig. 9.12. Just as in the 2D case, the associated graph contains a line edge for every projected lattice line. The middle layer of edges contains one edge for every voxel, connecting the two line nodes for which the corresponding lines intersect with that voxel.

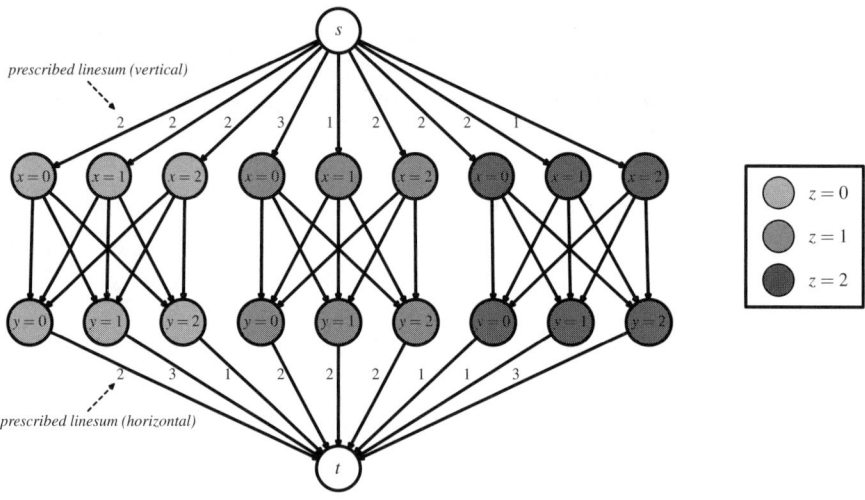

Fig. 9.12. Network corresponding to the two-projection reconstruction problem in Fig. 9.11.

Figure 9.12 shows a nice property of the two-projection reconstruction problem. For any point edge $(n_{1,i}, n_{2,j}) \in E_p$ in the associated graph, the lines $\ell_{1,i}$ and $\ell_{2,j}$ have a nonempty intersection in A, so there is a plane in $\mathbb{Z}^3$ that contains both $\ell_{1,i}$ and $\ell_{2,j}$. Since $\ell_{1,i}$ and $\ell_{2,j}$ are translates of $v^{(1)}$ and $v^{(2)}$, respectively, this plane will always be a translate of the plane spanned by $v^{(1)}$ and $v^{(2)}$. If two lines $\ell_{1,i}$ and $\ell_{2,i}$ lie in different translates of this plane, there will be no voxel edge connecting the corresponding line nodes. Therefore, the max flow problem can be solved for each translate of the plane independently. In the example network of Fig. 9.12, the subproblems for each of the planes $z = 0$, $z = 1$, and $z = 2$ can be solved independently. This property holds for any pair $(v^{(a)}, v^{(b)})$ of lattice directions, although the sizes of the subproblems depend on the direction pair. The number of point edges in each subproblem is bounded by the maximal number of voxels in A that lie in a single plane.

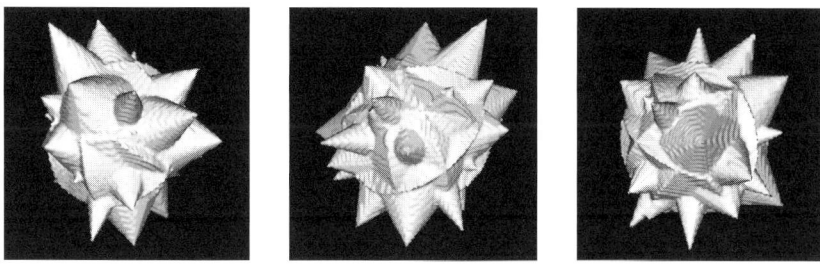

(**a**) Cones pointing out, 128×128×128: perfect reconstruction from 4 projections.

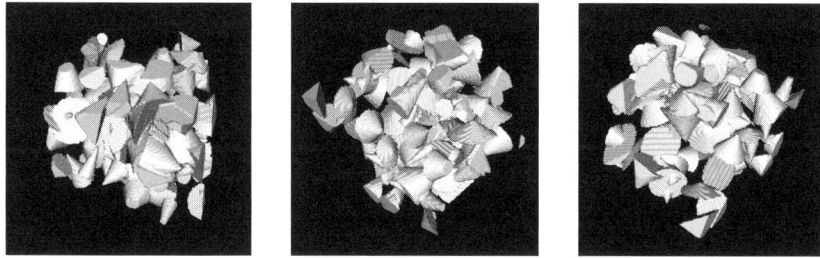

(**b**) Random cones, 128×128×128: perfect reconstruction from 6 projections.

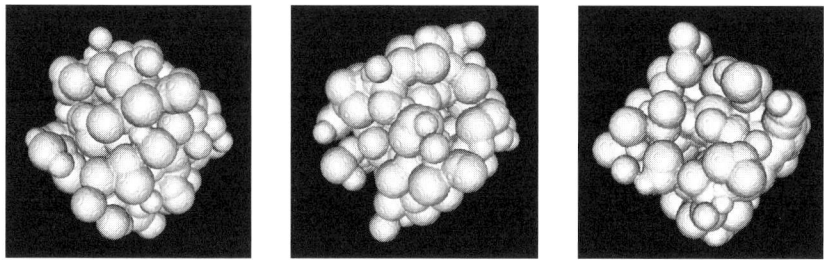

(**c**) 100 spheres, 169×169×169: perfect reconstruction from 6 projections.

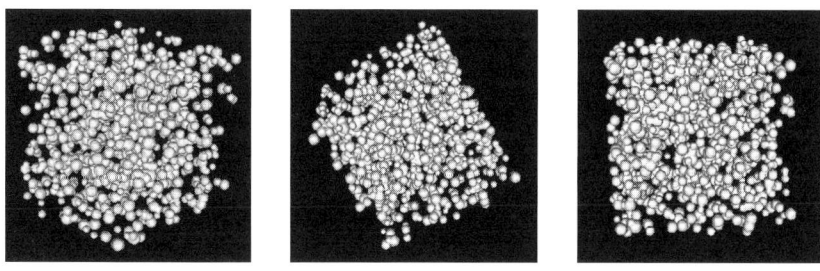

(**d**) 1000 small spheres, 139×139×139: perfect reconstruction from 6 projections.

Fig. 9.13. Reconstruction results for four 3D volumes.

Figure 9.13 shows four different test volumes, each displayed from three different viewing directions. The directions were selected to provide a clear view of the volume; they are not parallel to any of the projection directions. The iterative network flow algorithm can reconstruct each of these images from projections along the six lattice directions $(1,0,0), (0,1,0), (0,0,1), (1,1,0)$, $(1,0,1)$, and $(0,1,1)$. The image dimensions are shown in the figure. For the test image in Fig. 9.13(a), a perfect reconstruction is already found if only the first four projections are used. The test volumes are surrounded by a black background, which is not counted in the image dimensions. For all four test volumes, the algorithm computed the 3D reconstruction within 7 minutes on a standard 2.4GHz Pentium IV PC.

9.8 Extension to Plane Sets

So far we have considered the reconstruction of lattice sets in 2D and 3D. This model is well suited for the application of nanocrystal reconstruction at atomic resolution in electron microscopy [16]: Atoms in a crystalline solid are arranged regularly in a lattice structure. In many other applications of tomography there is no "intrinsic lattice." In this section, we consider the reconstruction of subsets of $\mathbb{R}^2$ from its projections in a small number of directions. We will also refer to such subsets as *planar black-and-white images*. In this new context, the projection along a line is no longer a sum over a discrete set; rather it is a *line integral* or *strip integral* of a function $\mathbb{R}^2 \to \{0,1\}$, which yields a real value.

Binary tomography problems without an intrinsic lattice structure occur often in practice, for example, in medical imaging [14]. Besides using a pixel representation for the reconstructed image, other representations have also been proposed. If the object of interests can be approximated well by a polygon, for example, one can use a polygonal, representation in the reconstruction algorithm (see [18]).

The iterative network flow algorithm can be adapted in such a way that it can be used for the reconstruction of planar black-and-white images. We will only give a high-level overview of the algorithm. The details will be described in a future publication.

Figure 9.14 shows an example of a planar black-and-white image along with two of its projections. If strip projections are used, the total amount of "white" (or black) in a set of consecutive strips parallel to the projection direction is measured. As it is impossible to represent all planar images in a computer program, they are approximated by representing the images on a pixel grid. Each of the pixels can have a value of either 1 (white) or 0 (black).

The weighted reconstruction problem for two projections (i.e., Problem 2 in the context of lattice sets) can also be solved efficiently in the case of planar subsets. However, a specifically chosen pixel grid must be used, which depends on the two projection directions. Figure 9.15 shows how the grid is

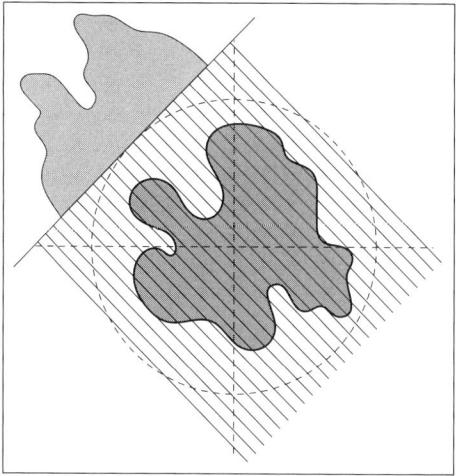

Fig. 9.14. A planar black-and-white image with one of its projections. If strip projections are used, the total amount of "black" in a set of consecutive strips parallel to the projection direction is measured.

formed from two projections. Every pixel on the grid is the intersection of a strip in the first direction with a strip in the second direction. The network flow approach can be used for this pixel grid, to compute a 0–1 reconstruction from the given two projections.

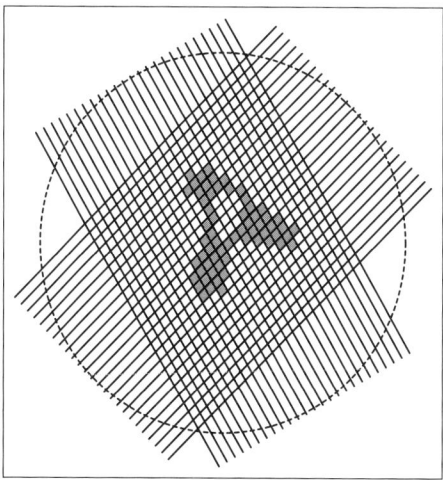

Fig. 9.15. Two parallel beams span a pixel grid. On this pixel grid, network flow methods can be used to solve the two-projection 0–1 reconstruction problem.

In every iteration of the iterative network flow algorithm, a new pair of projections is selected. Therefore, the pixel grid on which the new solution is computed is different in each iteration. To compute the weight map for the new pixel grid, the image from the previous iteration (defined on a different pixel grid) is first converted to a grayscale image on the pixel grid by interpolation. Recall that the computation of the *similarity fraction* for a pixel p does not require that neighboring pixels of p are *binary*. Therefore, the new weight map can be computed in a straightforward way. An overview of the adapted version of the iterative algorithm is shown in Fig. 9.16.

Compute the start solution F^0 on the standard pixel grid;

$i := 0$;

while (stop criterion is not met) **do**
begin

$\quad i := i + 1$;

$\quad$ Select a new pair of directions $v^{(a)}$ and $v^{(b)}$ $(1 \leq a < b \leq n)$;

$\quad$ Convert the previous solution F^{i-1} to an image $\hat{F}^{i-1}$ that is defined on the pixel grid spanned by directions $v^{(a)}$ and $v^{(b)}$;

$\quad$ Compute a new weight map W^i from the image $\hat{F}^{i-1}$;

$\quad$ Compute a new solution F^i on the grid spanned by $v^{(a)}$ and $v^{(b)}$ by solving a variant of Problem 4, using the weight map W^i.

end

Fig. 9.16. Basic steps of the algorithm for plane sets.

Just as for lattice images, the iterative network flow algorithm for plane sets is capable of computing very accurate reconstructions if a sufficient number of projections is available. However, if the original image does not have an intrinsic lattice structure, we cannot expect a reconstruction that perfectly matches the projection data, as it is unlikely that the original image can be represented as a binary image on the pixel grid used by the algorithm.

Acknowledgments

The author would like to thank Robert Tijdeman, Herman te Riele, and Willem, Jan Palenstijn for their valuable comments and suggestions.

References

1. Ahuja, R.K., Magnanti, T.L., Orlin, J.B.: *Network Flows: Theory, Algorithms and Applications.* Prentice-Hall, Englewood Cliffs, NJ (1993).

2. Anstee, R.P.: The network flows approach for matrices with given row and column sums. *Discr. Math.*, **44**, 125–138 (1983).

3. Batenburg, K.J.: Reconstructing binary images from discrete X-rays. *Tech. Rep. PNA-E0418*, CWI, Amsterdam, The Netherlands (2004).

4. Bertsekas, D.P., Tseng, P.: RELAX-IV: A faster version of the RELAX code for solving minimum cost flow problems. *LIDS Technical Report LIDS-P-2276*, MIT, Cambridge, MA (1994).

5. Dürr, C.: Ryser's algorithm can be implemented in linear time. http://www.lix.polytechnique.fr/~durr/Xray/Ryser/.

6. Ford, L.R., Fulkerson, D.R.: Maximal flow through a network. *Can. J. Math.*, **8**, 399–404 (1956).

7. Gale, D.: A theorem on flows in networks. *Pac. J. Math.*, **7**, 1073–1082 (1957).

8. Gardner, R.J., Gritzmann, P., Prangenberg, D.: On the computational complexity of reconstructing lattice sets from their X-rays. *Discr. Math.*, **202**, 45–71 (1999).

9. Goldberg, A.V.: An efficient implementation of a scaling minimum-cost flow algorithm. *J. Algebra*, **22**, 1–29 (1997).

10. Goldberg, A.V., Rao, S.: Beyond the flow decomposition barrier. *J. ACM*, **45**, 783–797 (1998).

11. Goldberg, A.V., Tarjan, R.E.: Finding minimum-cost circulations by successive approximation. *Math. Oper. Res.*, **15**, 430–466 (1990).

12. Gritzmann, P., de Vries, S., Wiegelmann, M.: Approximating binary images from discrete X-rays. *SIAM J. Opt.*, **11**, 522–546, (2000).

13. Hajdu, L., Tijdeman, R.: Algebraic aspects of discrete tomography. *J. Reine Angew. Math.*, **534**, 119–128 (2001).

14. Herman, G.T.,Kuba, A.: Discrete tomography in medical imaging. *Proc. IEEE*, **91**, 380–385 (2003).

15. *ILOG CPLEX*, http://www.ilog.com/products/cplex/.

16. Jinschek, J.R., Calderon, H.A., Batenburg, K.J., Radmilovic, V., Kisielowski, C.: Discrete tomography of Ga and InGa particles from HREM image simulation and exit wave reconstruction. *Mat. Res. Soc. Symp. Proc.*, **839**, 4.5.1–4.5.6 (2004).

17. Kak, A.C., Slaney, M.: *Principles of Computerized Tomographic Imaging.* SIAM, Philadelphia, PA (2001).

18. Mohammad-Djafari, A.: Binary polygonal shape image reconstruction from a small number of projections. *ELEKTRIK*, **5**, 127–139 (1997).

19. Ryser, H.J.: Combinatorial properties of matrices of zeros and ones. *Can. J. Math.*, **9**, 371–377 (1957).

20. Ryser, H.: *Combinatorial Mathematics*, Mathematical Association of America, Washington, DC (1963).

21. Schrijver, A.: *Combinatorial Optimization: Polyhedra and Efficiency.* Springer, Heidelberg, Germany (2003).

22. Slump, C.H., Gerbrands, J.J.: A network flow approach to reconstruction of the left ventricle from two projections. *Comp. Graph. Image Proc.*, **18**, 18–36 (1982).

23. Tanabe, K.: Projection method for solving a singular system. *Num. Math.*, **17**, 203–214 (1971).

10

A Convex Programming Algorithm for Noisy Discrete Tomography

T.D. Capricelli and P.L. Combettes

Summary. A convex programming approach to discrete tomographic image reconstruction in noisy environments is proposed. Conventional constraints are mixed with noise-based constraints on the sinogram and a binariness-promoting total variation constraint. The noise-based constraints are modeled as confidence regions that are constructed under a Poisson noise assumption. A convex objective is then minimized over the resulting feasibility set via a parallel block-iterative method. Applications to binary tomographic reconstruction are demonstrated.

10.1 Introduction

The tomographic reconstruction problem is to estimate a multidimensional signal $\overline{x}$ in a Hilbert space $\mathcal{H}$ from lower-dimensional measurements of its line integrals. In computerized tomography, the signals are discretized over a bounded domain and $\mathcal{H}$ is the usual Euclidean space $\mathbb{R}^N$ (using standard lexicographic ordering, an N-voxel signal is represented as an N-dimensional vector). A popular approach for solving this problem is to pose it as a convex feasibility problem of the form

$$\text{find } \overline{x} \in \bigcap_{i=1}^{m} S_i \, , \tag{10.1}$$

where $(S_i)_{1 \leq i \leq m}$ are closed convex sets in $\mathbb{R}^N$ arising from prior knowledge (bounds, support information, spectral information, information about the noise corrupting the measurements, etc.) and the discrete line integral (line sum) measurements [4, 6, 21, 31]. This set theoretic approach to tomographic image reconstruction goes back to [18]; further developments can be found in [24, 25, 30, 32, 35]. In some instances it may be justified on physical grounds to seek a feasible image that is optimal in some sense. The problem then assumes the form

$$\text{find } \overline{x} \in S = \bigcap_{i=1}^{m} S_i \text{ such that } \varphi(\overline{x}) = \inf \varphi(S), \tag{10.2}$$

where $\varphi \colon \mathbb{R}^N \to (-\infty, +\infty]$ is a convex function. The advantage of this convex programming formulation is that it allows the incorporation of a wide range of prior information in the reconstruction process, and, at the same time, it benefits from the availability of powerful algorithms; see [1, 4, 7, 8, 9] and the references therein.

In discrete tomography, the range of the signal $\overline{x}$ to be reconstructed is known to be a finite set, for instance, the set $\{0, 1\}$ in binary tomography. This additional information is of paramount importance and has profound consequences on the theoretical and practical aspects of the reconstruction problem [22]. As underlined in [22], classical computer tomography algorithms do not perform well in the presence of few (say 10 or less) views (we do not employ the standard term "projection," as it will be reserved to describe the best metric approximation from a convex set). Consequently, they are not directly applicable in discrete tomography, where such low numbers of views are common. Furthermore, classical algorithms do not exploit nor enforce the discrete nature of the original signal.

In this chapter, we propose a convex programming approach to the discrete tomography problem in noisy environments. In recent years, many papers have been devoted to the theoretical and numerical investigations of discrete reconstruction problems; see [15, 17, 19, 22, 23, 29, 34] and the references therein. The novelty of our work is to propose a convex programming formulation of this problem that explicitly takes into account the presence of noise in the measured data, and to provide a numerical method to solve it. Our formulation is of the form (10.2), and our algorithm is based on the block-iterative methods recently developed in [8, 9]. While our approach is applicable to general discrete problems, we shall focus on the case of binary images for simplicity. Since the set of binary images is nonconvex, our first task will be to find pertinent convex constraints that will promote the binary nature of the image: Total variation will be used for this purpose. Thus, the image produced by the algorithm will be relatively close to being binary, which will minimize the number of errors incurred by the final binarization step. Other constraints will exploit standard information (bounds, support) as well as information about the data model and the noise.

The remainder of the chapter is organized as follows. In Section 10.2, we review the parallel block-iterative algorithm that will be employed to solve the convex program (10.2). In Section 10.3, we address the construction of constraints for noisy binary tomography. The new constraints are confidence regions that are based on statistical attributes of the noise perturbing the sinogram, and a total variation constraint aimed at promoting the binary nature of the reconstructed image. A Poisson noise model is assumed in our statistical analysis of the confidence regions. In Section 10.4, we describe several applications of this convex programming framework to binary image reconstruction in the presence of noisy measurements. A few remarks conclude the chapter in Section 10.5.

10.2 Proposed Algorithm

Throughout the chapter, the signal space containing the original image $\bar{x}$ is the standard Euclidean space $\mathbb{R}^N$, with scalar product $\langle \cdot \mid \cdot \rangle$, norm $\| \cdot \|$, and distance d. The distance to a nonempty set $C \subset \mathbb{R}^N$ is $d_C(x) = \inf \|x - C\|$. If $C \subset \mathbb{R}^N$ is nonempty, closed, and convex, then, for every $x \in \mathbb{R}^N$, there is a unique point $P_C x \in C$ such that $\|x - P_C x\| = d_C(x)$; $P_C x$ is called the *projection* of x onto C.

To solve (10.2), we use the parallel block-iterative algorithm described in [9], where the framework of [8] was adapted to problems with quadratic objective functions. Although more general strictly convex objectives φ can be used [8], we restrict our attention to quadratic functions in this chapter, as they lead to particularly simple implementations.

Let

$$\varphi \colon \mathbb{R}^N \to \mathbb{R} \colon x \mapsto \langle R(x - r) \mid x - r \rangle, \tag{10.3}$$

where $r \in \mathbb{R}^N$ and $R \in \mathbb{R}^{N \times N}$ is a positive definite symmetric matrix. In addition, we suppose (without loss of generality) that the closed convex constraint sets $(S_i)_{1 \le i \le m}$ in (10.2) assume the form

$$(\forall i \in \{1, \ldots, m\}) \quad S_i = \{x \in \mathbb{R}^N \mid f_i(x) \le \delta_i\}, \tag{10.4}$$

where $(f_i)_{1 \le i \le m}$ are convex functions from $\mathbb{R}^N$ to $\mathbb{R}$ and $(\delta_i)_{1 \le i \le m}$ are real numbers such that $S = \bigcap_{i=1}^m S_i \ne \emptyset$. Recall that, under these assumptions, for every $x \in \mathbb{R}^N$, each f_i admits at least one *subgradient* at x, i.e., a point $g_i \in \mathbb{R}^N$ such that [27]

$$(\forall y \in \mathbb{R}^N) \quad \langle y - x \mid g_i \rangle + f_i(x) \le f_i(y). \tag{10.5}$$

For instance, if C is a nonempty closed convex subset of $\mathbb{R}^N$ and $x \in \mathbb{R}^N \setminus C$, then

$$\partial d_C(x) \ni (x - P_C x)/d_C(x). \tag{10.6}$$

The set of all subgradients of f_i at x is the *subdifferential* of f_i at x and is denoted by $\partial f_i(x)$; if f_i is differentiable at x, then $\partial f_i(x) = \{\nabla f_i(x)\}$. Moreover, the *subgradient projection* $G_i x$ of x onto S_i is obtained by selecting an arbitrary $g_i \in \partial f_i(x)$ and setting [7]

$$G_i x = \begin{cases} x + \dfrac{\delta_i - f_i(x)}{\|g_i\|^2} g_i & \text{if } f_i(x) > \delta_i, \\ x & \text{if } f_i(x) \le \delta_i. \end{cases} \tag{10.7}$$

The algorithm proposed in [9] to solve (10.2)–(10.3) constructs a sequence $(x_n)_{n \in \mathbb{N}}$ of approximate solutions as follows:

1. Fix $\varepsilon \in (0, 1/m)$. Set $x_0 = r$ and $n = 0$.
2. Take a nonempty index set $I_n \subset \{1, \ldots, m\}$.

3. Set $z_n = x_n - \lambda_n R^{-1} u_n$, where:
   (a) for every $i \in I_n$, $p_{i,n} = G_i x_n$;
   (b) the weights $(\omega_{i,n})_{i \in I_n}$ lie in $[\varepsilon, 1]$ and $\sum_{i \in I_n} \omega_{i,n} = 1$;
   (c) $u_n = x_n - \sum_{i \in I_n} \omega_{i,n} p_{i,n}$;
   (d) $\lambda_n \in [\varepsilon L_n, L_n]$, where

$$
L_n = \begin{cases} \dfrac{\displaystyle\sum_{i \in I_n} \omega_{i,n} \|p_{i,n} - x_n\|^2}{\langle R^{-1} u_n \mid u_n \rangle} & \text{if } \max_{i \in I_n} \left(f_i(x_n) - \delta_i \right) > 0, \\[2ex] 1/\|R^{-1}\| & \text{otherwise.} \end{cases}
$$

4. Set $\pi_n = \langle R(x_0 - x_n) \mid x_n - z_n \rangle$, $\mu_n = \langle R(x_0 - x_n) \mid x_0 - x_n \rangle$, $\nu_n = \langle R(x_n - z_n) \mid x_n - z_n \rangle$, and $\rho_n = \mu_n \nu_n - \pi_n^2$.
5. Set

$$
x_{n+1} = \begin{cases} z_n & \text{if } \rho_n = 0 \,, \ \pi_n \geq 0, \\[2ex] x_0 + \left(1 + \dfrac{\pi_n}{\nu_n}\right)(z_n - x_n) & \text{if } \rho_n > 0, \ \pi_n \nu_n \geq \rho_n, \\[2ex] x_n + \dfrac{\nu_n}{\rho_n}\left(\pi_n(x_0 - x_n) + \mu_n(z_n - x_n)\right) & \text{if } \rho_n > 0, \ \pi_n \nu_n < \rho_n. \end{cases}
$$

6. Set $n = n + 1$ and go to step 2.

The following convergence result is an application of [9, Theorem 16].

Theorem 1. *Suppose that there exists a strictly positive integer J such that*

$$
(\forall n \in \mathbb{N}) \quad \bigcup_{k=n}^{n+J-1} I_k = \{1, \ldots, m\}. \tag{10.8}
$$

Then every sequence $(x_n)_{n \in \mathbb{N}}$ generated by the above algorithm converges to the unique solution to (10.2)–(10.3).

Some comments about this result and the algorithm are in order.

(a) Condition (10.8) is satisfied in particular when $I_n = \{1, \ldots, m\}$, i.e., when all the sets are activated at each iteration. In general, (10.8) allows for variable blocks of sets to be used, which provides great flexibility in terms of parallel implementation (see [7] for examples). More details on the importance of block-processing for task scheduling on parallel architectures can be found in [4]. Further flexibility is provided by the fact that the relaxations and the weights can vary at each iteration.
(b) The algorithm activates the constraints by means of subgradient projections rather than exact projections. The former are significantly easier to implement than the latter, as they require only the computation of

subgradients (gradients in the differentiable case). Analytically complex constraints can therefore be incorporated in the recovery algorithm and processed at low cost.

(c) The parameter L_n is always at least equal to $1/\|R^{-1}\|$ [9, Proposition 12], and it can attain large values. Choosing λ_n large (e.g., equal to L_n) usually yields faster convergence.

In [9], it was shown that in order to reduce the computational load of the method, an iteration of the algorithm could be implemented as follows (only one application of the matrices R and R^{-1} is required):

1. For every $i \in I_n$, set $a_i = -f_i(x_n)g_i/\|g_i\|^2$, where $g_i \in \partial f_i(x_n)$, if $f_i(x_n) > \delta_i$; $a_i = 0$ otherwise.
2. Choose weights $(\omega_i)_{i \in I_n}$ in $[\varepsilon, 1]$ adding up to 1. Set $v = \sum_{i \in I_n} \omega_i a_i$ and $L = \sum_{i \in I_n} \omega_i \|a_i\|^2$.
3. If $L = 0$, set $x_{n+1} = x_n$, and exit iteration. Otherwise, set $b = x_0 - x_n$, $c = Rb$, $d = R^{-1}v$, and $L = L/\langle d \mid v \rangle$.
4. Choose $\lambda \in [\varepsilon L, L]$ and set $d = \lambda d$.
5. Set $\pi = -\langle c \mid d \rangle$, $\mu = \langle b \mid c \rangle$, $\nu = \lambda \langle d \mid v \rangle$, and $\rho = \mu\nu - \pi^2$.
6. Set $x_{n+1} = \begin{cases} x_n + d & \text{if } \rho = 0 \text{ and } \pi \geq 0, \\ x_0 + (1 + \pi/\nu)d & \text{if } \rho > 0 \text{ and } \pi\nu \geq \rho, \\ x_n + \dfrac{\nu}{\rho}(\pi b + \mu d) & \text{if } \rho > 0 \text{ and } \pi\nu < \rho. \end{cases}$

Remark 1. If the projector P_i onto S_i is easy to implement, one can set $f_i = d_{S_i}$ since S_i can certainly be described as the level set

$$S_i = \{x \in \mathbb{R}^N \mid d_{S_i}(x) \leq 0\}. \tag{10.9}$$

In this case, it follows at once from (10.6) and (10.7) that $G_i = P_i$ (the subgradient projector reduces to the usual projector) and, moreover, that $a_i = P_i x_n - x_n$ at step 1 of the algorithm.

10.3 Construction of Closed Convex Constraint Sets

10.3.1 Data Model

The sinogram is the image under the Radon transform of the original image $\bar{x}$. The portion of the sinogram corresponding to a given observation angle θ will be referred to as a *view*. The observed data consist of q noisy views $(z_i)_{1 \leq i \leq q}$ at angles $(\theta_i)_{1 \leq i \leq q}$. For every $i \in \{1, \ldots, q\}$, we let L_i be the restriction of the Radon transform for a fixed angle θ_i. In other words, the ith measurement is

$$z_i = L_i \bar{x} + w_i, \tag{10.10}$$

where w_i is the noise vector corrupting the observation. Each view z_i is a one-dimensional signal of M points and will be represented by a vector $z_i = [\zeta_{i,k}]_{1 \leq k \leq M}^T$ in $\mathbb{R}^M$; L_i is therefore a matrix in $\mathbb{R}^{M \times N}$. Finally, we denote by $\underline{1}$ the vector $[1, \ldots, 1]^T$ in $\mathbb{R}^N$ or $\mathbb{R}^M$.

10.3.2 Standard Constraints

Further details on standard constraint sets can be found in [6, 31].

Range

The first standard constraint arises from the fact that pixel values are nonnegative and have known maximal value. After normalization, the corresponding set is

$$[0,1]^N. \tag{10.11}$$

In the context of binary tomography, this is simply the convex hull of the set $\{0,1\}^N$.

Support

A second common piece of a priori information in tomography is the knowledge of the support K of the body under investigation. The associated set is

$$\{x \in \mathbb{R}^N \mid x1_K = x\}, \tag{10.12}$$

where 1_K is the characteristic function of K and where the product $x1_K$ is taken componentwise. The projector onto this set is $x \mapsto x1_K$ [6].

Pixel Sum

Let μ be the sum of the pixel values in the original image, i.e.,

$$\mu = \langle \overline{x} \mid \underline{1} \rangle. \tag{10.13}$$

The knowledge of μ leads to the set

$$\{x \in \mathbb{R}^N \mid \langle x \mid \underline{1} \rangle = \mu\}. \tag{10.14}$$

Since μ is never known exactly, this set should be relaxed into the hyperslab

$$\{x \in \mathbb{R}^N \mid \mu^- \leq \langle x \mid \underline{1} \rangle \leq \mu^+\}, \tag{10.15}$$

where $[\mu^-, \mu^+]$ is a confidence interval. The projector onto this set is [6]

$$x \mapsto \begin{cases} x + \dfrac{\mu^- - \langle x \mid \underline{1} \rangle}{N}\underline{1} & \text{if } \langle x \mid \underline{1} \rangle < \mu^-, \\[2ex] x + \dfrac{\mu^+ - \langle x \mid \underline{1} \rangle}{N}\underline{1} & \text{if } \langle x \mid \underline{1} \rangle > \mu^+, \\[2ex] x & \text{otherwise.} \end{cases} \tag{10.16}$$

The values of μ^- and μ^+ depend on prior information about the experimental setup and about the noise. An example is provided in Subsection 10.3.5.

10.3.3 Binariness-Promoting Constraint

The constrained image recovery method presented in Section 10.2 is limited to problems with convex constraints. As a result, since the set of binary images is nonconvex, the binariness constraint cannot be enforced directly in such a framework. Furthermore, the convex set (10.11) will not properly enforce binariness, and we must find a more effective means to promote binariness through a convex constraint.

In recent years, total variation has emerged as an effective tool to recover piecewise-smooth images in variational methods. This approach was initiated in [28] in the context of denoising problems and has since been used in various image recovery problems. Recently, it has also been applied in certain variational computerized tomography problems [2, 36]. In all of these approaches, total variation appears in the objective of a minimization problem. Such nondifferentiable problems are not easy to solve, and they offer very limited potential in terms of incorporating constraints [5, 11].

In [12], it was observed that, in many problems, the total variation $\mathrm{tv}(\overline{x})$ of the original image, which measures the amount of oscillations, does not exceed some known bound τ. This constraint, which is associated with the set

$$\left\{ x \in \mathbb{R}^N \mid \mathrm{tv}(x) \leq \tau \right\}, \tag{10.17}$$

appears to be particularly relevant in binary (and more generally in discrete) tomography, as it attenuates the oscillating components in the image, thereby forcing the creation of flat areas and promoting binariness. An important issue is, of course, the availability of the parameter τ in (10.17). In this respect, binary tomography places us on favorable grounds. Indeed, since the total variation of a binary image is related to the length of its contours (i.e., the sum of the perimeters of the elementary shapes), it can be estimated with good accuracy in certain typical problems from prior experiments or by sampling databases [12].

Numerically, the total variation of a discrete image $x = [\xi_{i,j}] \in \mathbb{R}^{\sqrt{N} \times \sqrt{N}}$ is computed as

$$
\begin{aligned}
\mathrm{tv}(x) = \sum_{i=1}^{\sqrt{N}-1} \sum_{j=1}^{\sqrt{N}-1} & \sqrt{|\xi_{i+1,j} - \xi_{i,j}|^2 + |\xi_{i,j+1} - \xi_{i,j}|^2} \\
+ \sum_{i=1}^{\sqrt{N}-1} & |\xi_{i+1,\sqrt{N}} - \xi_{i,\sqrt{N}}| + \sum_{j=1}^{\sqrt{N}-1} |\xi_{\sqrt{N},j+1} - \xi_{\sqrt{N},j}| .
\end{aligned} \tag{10.18}
$$

The subgradient projector onto the set (10.17) can be found in [12].

10.3.4 Constraints on the Residual Views

Using an approach developed in [13] and [33], we can form a wide range of statistical constraints modeled by closed convex sets for each of the q views.

Indeed, (10.10) gives

$$z_i - L_i \overline{x} = w_i. \tag{10.19}$$

Hence, the residual signal $z_i - L_i x$ associated with an estimate x of $\overline{x}$ should be constrained to be statistically consistent with every known attribute (e.g., moment, periodogram, etc.) of the noise. Consistency is usually enforced via some statistical confidence bound (see [10] for an analysis of the global confidence level in terms of confidence levels of each set). We now provide examples of such constraint sets.

Amplitude

Let us denote by $(e_k)_{1 \le k \le M}$ the canonical basis of $\mathbb{R}^M$ (recall that M is the length of each view z_i). If no noise were present, (10.10) would confine $\overline{x}$ to the intersection of the Mq hyperplanes

$$\left\{ x \in \mathbb{R}^N \mid \langle L_i x \mid e_k \rangle = \langle z_i \mid e_k \rangle \right\}. \tag{10.20}$$

These sets were used in the early ART reconstruction technique [18]. In the presence of noise, the hyperplanes must be replaced by hyperslabs of the form [20]

$$\left\{ x \in \mathbb{R}^N \mid |\langle L_i x - z_i \mid e_k \rangle| \le \alpha_{i,k} \right\}. \tag{10.21}$$

The confidence interval $[-\alpha_{i,k}, \alpha_{i,k}]$ can be determined from the distribution of the random variable $\langle w_i \mid e_k \rangle$. Such distributions can be available in certain problems, e.g., [6, 14, 33]. However, in the present problem, the noise is best modeled by a signal-dependent process that makes it impossible to obtain reliable bounds. We shall therefore not use these sets in our experiments.

ℓ^p Norms

Let $p \in [1, +\infty)$ and $i \in \{1, \ldots, q\}$. Suppose that an estimate $\delta_{i,p}^{1/p}$ of the ℓ^p norm of the noise vector w_i is available from physical considerations or past experience with tomographic reconstructions of similar objects. Then one can construct the set [13]

$$\left\{ x \in \mathbb{R}^N \mid \|L_i x - z_i\|_p^p \le \delta_{i,p} \right\}. \tag{10.22}$$

The projector onto this set has no simple closed form, but the subgradient projector can be obtained as follows. Let us denote by $(L_{i,k})_{1 \le k \le M}$ the M rows of L_i and by $L_{i,k,l}$ an entry of the matrix L_i, i.e.,

$$L_i = \left[L_{i,k,l} \right]_{\substack{1 \le k \le M \\ 1 \le l \le N}}. \tag{10.23}$$

Then, by elementary subdifferential calculus [27],

$$\partial \| L_i x - z_i \|_p^p = \sum_{k=1}^{M} \partial |\langle L_{i,k} \mid x \rangle - \zeta_{i,k}|^p . \tag{10.24}$$

Hence, if $p > 1$, the unique subgradient of $x \mapsto \| L_i x - z_i \|_p^p$ is

$$g = p \left(\sum_{k=1}^{M} L_{i,k,l} |\langle L_{i,k} \mid x \rangle - \zeta_{i,k}|^{p-1} \operatorname{sign}(\langle L_{i,k} \mid x \rangle - \zeta_{i,k}) \right)_{1 \leq l \leq N} . \tag{10.25}$$

Now suppose that $p = 1$. Recall that

$$\operatorname{sign} \colon \xi \mapsto \begin{cases} -1 & \text{if } \xi < 0, \\ 0 & \text{if } \xi = 0, \\ +1 & \text{if } \xi > 0, \end{cases} \tag{10.26}$$

is a selection of the subdifferential of $\xi \mapsto |\xi|$, which is given by

$$(\forall \xi \in \mathbb{R}) \quad \partial |\xi| = \begin{cases} \{-1\} & \text{if } \xi < 0, \\ [-1,1] & \text{if } \xi = 0, \\ \{+1\} & \text{if } \xi > 0. \end{cases} \tag{10.27}$$

Therefore, a subgradient of $x \mapsto \| L_i x - z_i \|_1$ is

$$g = \left(\sum_{k=1}^{M} L_{i,k,l} \operatorname{sign}(\langle L_{i,k} \mid x \rangle - \zeta_{i,k}) \right)_{1 \leq l \leq N} . \tag{10.28}$$

One can compute the subgradient projection (10.7) via (10.25) and (10.28).

Energy

The case $p = 2$ corresponds to the set

$$\{ x \in \mathbb{R}^N \mid \| L_i x - z_i \|^2 \leq \delta_{i,2} \}. \tag{10.29}$$

In this case, (10.25) reduces to $g = 2 L_i^T (L_i x - z_i)$. As discussed in [7, 33], the projection of an image x onto this set requires an iterative procedure, while the subgradient projector is given explicitly by (10.7) as

$$x \mapsto \begin{cases} x + \dfrac{\delta_{i,2} - \| L_i x - z_i \|^2}{2 \| L_i^T (L_i x - z_i) \|^2} L_i^T (L_i x - z_i) & \text{if } \| L_i x - z_i \|^2 > \delta_{i,2}, \\ x & \text{if } \| L_i x - z_i \|^2 \leq \delta_{i,2}. \end{cases} \tag{10.30}$$

10.3.5 Bound Estimation in the Case of Poisson Noise

In this subsection, we address the problem of computing the parameters μ^- and μ^+ in (10.15) and $\delta_{i,2}$ in (10.29).

Noise modeling in computerized tomography is a research topic in its own right, and it is beyond the scope of the present chapter to attempt to provide a precise model for the various complex underlying physical phenomena. In [3], a simple additive Gaussian noise model is considered. Since many data collection processes in discrete tomography are counting processes (e.g., counting the number of atoms in a structure along a certain direction), we adopt here a Poisson noise model. More specifically, we assume that the observation z_i in (10.10) is a realization of a random vector

$$Z_i = \left[Z_{i,k} \right]^T_{1 \leq k \leq M}, \tag{10.31}$$

the components of which are independent Poisson variables with means $(\lambda_{i,k})_{1 \leq k \leq M}$. It is also assumed that the random vectors $(Z_i)_{1 \leq i \leq q}$ are independent. Now, let Λ_i be the mean of Z_i. Then

$$\Lambda_i = \mathsf{E} Z_i = [\lambda_{i,k}]^T_{1 \leq k \leq M} = L_i \overline{x}. \tag{10.32}$$

Bound on the View Sums

Our purpose here is to determine the parameters μ^- and μ^+ in (10.15). A property of the discrete Radon transform is that it preserves pixel sums in the sense that

$$(\forall i \in \{1, \ldots, q\}) \quad \mu = \langle \overline{x} \mid \underline{1} \rangle = \langle L_i \overline{x} \mid \underline{1} \rangle. \tag{10.33}$$

Since $\langle Z_i \mid \underline{1} \rangle$ is the sum of M independent Poisson variables, it is also a Poisson variable, with mean $\langle \Lambda_i \mid \underline{1} \rangle = \mu$ and variance $\mathsf{var} \langle Z_i \mid \underline{1} \rangle = \mu$. The parameter μ can be approximated by the sample mean of the q views, i.e.,

$$\gamma = \frac{1}{q} \sum_{i=1}^{q} \langle z_i \mid \underline{1} \rangle. \tag{10.34}$$

The associated statistical estimator is

$$\Gamma = \frac{1}{q} \sum_{i=1}^{q} \langle Z_i \mid \underline{1} \rangle, \tag{10.35}$$

with mean

$$\mathsf{E} \Gamma = \frac{1}{q} \sum_{i=1}^{q} \mathsf{E} \langle Z_i \mid \underline{1} \rangle = \mu \tag{10.36}$$

and variance

$$\text{var}\,\Gamma = \frac{1}{q^2} \sum_{i=1}^{q} \text{var}\,\langle Z_i \mid \underline{1} \rangle = \frac{\mu}{q}. \tag{10.37}$$

We look for a confidence interval of the form

$$\left[\, \mathsf{E}\Gamma - \beta_1 \sqrt{\text{var}\,\Gamma},\ \mathsf{E}\Gamma + \beta_1 \sqrt{\text{var}\,\Gamma}\,\right] = \left[\,\mu - \beta_1\sqrt{\mu/q},\ \mu + \beta_1\sqrt{\mu/q}\,\right], \tag{10.38}$$

for some $\beta_1 > 0$. Upon approximating μ by the observed sample mean γ, the confidence interval becomes $\left[\,\gamma - \beta_1\sqrt{\gamma/q},\ \gamma + \beta_1\sqrt{\gamma/q}\,\right]$. Monte Carlo experiments show that $\beta_1 = 2.3$ gives 98% of the realizations within this interval. Thus, with a confidence level of $c_1 = 98\%$, we can use the values

$$\mu^- = \gamma - 2.3\sqrt{\gamma/q} \quad \text{and} \quad \mu^+ = \gamma + 2.3\sqrt{\gamma/q} \tag{10.39}$$

in (10.15).

Bound on the Residual Energy

Let $i \in \{1,\dots,q\}$. Our purpose is to determine the parameter $\delta_{i,2}$ in (10.29). The mean square residual error is

$$\mathsf{E}\|Z_i - L_i\overline{x}\|^2 = \mathsf{E}\|Z_i - \Lambda_i\|^2 = \sum_{k=1}^{M} \text{var}\,Z_{i,k} = \sum_{k=1}^{M} \lambda_{i,k} = \|\Lambda_i\|_1. \tag{10.40}$$

To compute $\mathsf{E}\|Z_i - L_i\overline{x}\|^4$, we need the moments of $Z_{i,k}$ up to order 4. We have

$$\mathsf{E}|Z_{i,k}|^3 = \lambda_{i,k}^3 + 3\lambda_{i,k}^2 + \lambda_{i,k} \tag{10.41}$$

and

$$\mathsf{E}|Z_{i,k}|^4 = \lambda_{i,k}^4 + 6\lambda_{i,k}^3 + 7\lambda_{i,k}^2 + \lambda_{i,k}. \tag{10.42}$$

The fourth central moment is therefore

$$\begin{aligned}
\mathsf{E}|Z_{i,k} - \lambda_{i,k}|^4 &= \mathsf{E}|Z_{i,k}|^4 - 4\lambda_{i,k}\mathsf{E}|Z_{i,k}|^3 + 6\lambda_{i,k}^2\mathsf{E}|Z_{i,k}|^2 - 4\lambda_{i,k}^3\mathsf{E}Z_{i,k} + \lambda_{i,k}^4 \\
&= 3\lambda_{i,k}^2 + \lambda_{i,k}.
\end{aligned} \tag{10.43}$$

We can now compute the second-order moment of the residual energy as

$$\begin{aligned}
\mathsf{E}\|Z_i - L_i\overline{x}\|^4 &= \mathsf{E}\|Z_i - \Lambda_i\|^4 \\
&= \mathsf{E}\left| \sum_{k=1}^{M} |Z_{i,k} - \lambda_{i,k}|^2 \right|^2 \\
&= \sum_{k=1}^{M} \mathsf{E}|Z_{i,k} - \lambda_{i,k}|^4 + 2\sum_{1 \le k < j \le M} \mathsf{E}|Z_{i,j} - \lambda_{i,j}|^2 \mathsf{E}|Z_{i,k} - \lambda_{i,k}|^2 \\
&= \sum_{k=1}^{M} (3\lambda_{i,k}^2 + \lambda_{i,k}) + 2\sum_{1 \le k < j \le M} \lambda_{i,j}\lambda_{i,k} \\
&= 2\|\Lambda_i\|^2 + \|\Lambda_i\|_1 + \|\Lambda_i\|_1^2,
\end{aligned} \tag{10.44}$$

and its variance as

$$\text{var}\|Z_i - L_i\overline{x}\|^2 = \mathsf{E}\|Z_i - \Lambda_i\|^4 - \mathsf{E}^2\|Z_i - \Lambda_i\|^2 = 2\|\Lambda_i\|^2 + \|\Lambda_i\|_1. \quad (10.45)$$

An upper bound on its standard deviation is

$$\sigma = \sqrt{2\|\Lambda_i\|_1^2 + \|\Lambda_i\|_1} \geq \sqrt{2\|\Lambda_i\|^2 + \|\Lambda_i\|_1} = \sqrt{\text{var}\|Z_i - L_i\overline{x}\|^2}. \quad (10.46)$$

We look for a confidence interval of the form $[0, \mu + \beta_2\sigma]$ for some $\beta_2 > 0$. As seen above, $\mu = \|\Lambda_i\|_1$ can be approximated by the sample mean γ of (10.34) and, therefore, σ can be approximated by $\sqrt{2\gamma^2 + \gamma}$. In turn, the confidence interval becomes $[0, \gamma + \beta_2\sqrt{2\gamma^2 + \gamma}]$. Monte Carlo experiments show that $\beta_2 = 0.51$ gives 98% of the realizations within this interval. Thus, with a confidence level of $c_2 = 98\%$, we can use the bound

$$\delta_{i,2} = \gamma + 0.51\sqrt{2\gamma^2 + \gamma} \quad (10.47)$$

in (10.29).

Global Confidence Analysis

There are $q + 1$ sets that are confidence regions. In the previous discussion, the bounds on the sets (10.15) and (10.29) were determined so as to obtain individual confidence levels of $c_1 = c_2 = 98\%$. Using the analysis of [10], the global confidence level c on the feasibility set $S = \bigcap_{i=1}^{m} S_i$ satisfies

$$c \geq 1 - (1 - c_1) - q(1 - c_2). \quad (10.48)$$

In our experiments, which will involve $q = 4$ or $q = 3$ views, we shall thus obtain global confidence levels of $c \geq 90\%$ or $c \geq 92\%$, respectively.

10.4 Numerical Simulations

Most theoretical results in discrete tomography impose conditions on the shape of the objects to be reconstructed. Thus, experiments are usually performed on connected, convex, or even hv-convex objects [22]. Our algorithm does not require such stringent assumptions, and we shall use an original 32×32 binary image $\overline{x}$ displayed in Fig. 10.1. This image features two disconnected components, one of which is nonconvex. As in most of the experiments presented in [22], few views will be used, namely $q = 4$ or $q = 3$ views.

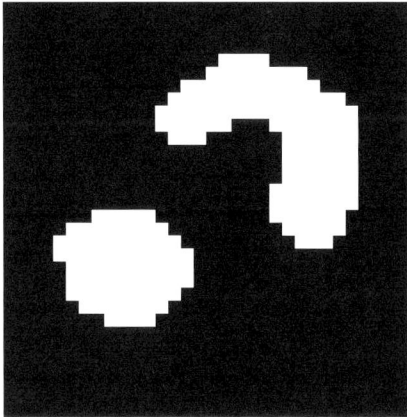

Fig. 10.1. Original image in the last experiment.

10.4.1 Noise Simulation

As discussed above, the noise corrupting the views in (10.10) is assumed to be Poisson-distributed. The pointwise variance of such a noise is directly related to the amplitude of the signal. On the other hand, the data acquisition process typically induces a multiplicative factor between the actual line sums and the measured views, due, for instance, to exposure time. In order to obtain a reasonable noise level, we set this multiplicative factor to 255.

We now describe the methodology used for creating the noisy views. First, for each $i \in \{1, \ldots, q\}$, the exact line sum is computed and then multiplied by the proportionality factor 255 in order to generate the noiseless view $L_i \overline{x}$. Then, each point $\langle L_i \overline{x} \mid e_k \rangle$ of the ith view is replaced by a realization of a Poisson variable with mean $\langle L_i \overline{x} \mid e_k \rangle$ (see [16, 26] for the numerical simulation of Poisson noise).

A typical noisy sinogram view is shown in Fig. 10.2. The SNR (signal-to-noise ratio) on the views varies from 31 dB to 33 dB.

10.4.2 Binarization

The binarization process consists of mapping an image in $[0, 1]^N$ into an image in $\{0, 1\}^N$. The scheme we adopt here is straightforward: Since the algorithm produces an image in the set (10.11), each pixel value is rounded to 0 if the original value is less than 0.5, and to 1 otherwise. It is clear that binarization could be performed in a more sophisticated fashion, especially in the light of additional a priori information on the original image.

10.4.3 Experimental Setup

The algorithm described in Section 10.2 is implemented with $\varphi \colon x \mapsto \|x\|^2$ in (10.3) (hence R is the identity matrix and r is the zero image). In other words,

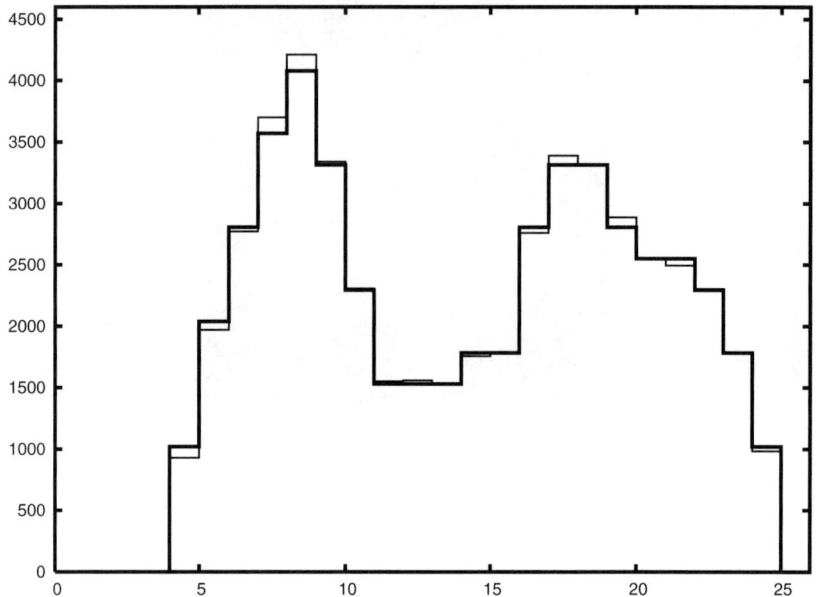

Fig. 10.2. Example of a sinogram view: noiseless view (bold lines) and view with Poisson noise (thin lines).

we seek the image with minimum energy in the feasibility set $S = \bigcap_{i=1}^{m} S_i$. The $m = q + 4$ constraint sets to be used are

(a) S_1: pixel range; see (10.11).
(b) S_2: image support; see (10.12) and Fig. 10.3.

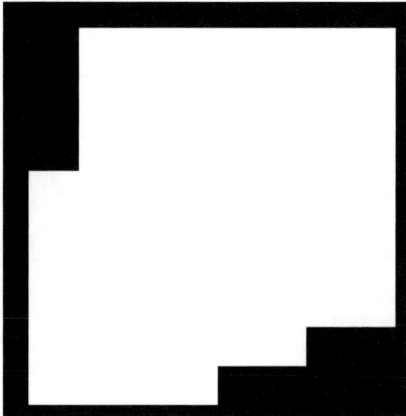

Fig. 10.3. Support K used in (10.12) in the experiments.

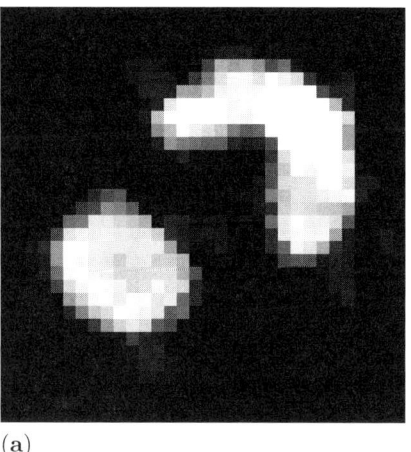
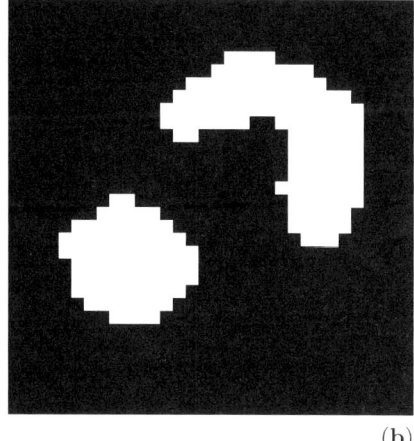

(a)   (b)

Fig. 10.4. No noise, $q = 4$ views, without the total variation constraint. Before (**a**) and after (**b**) binarization (error: 6 pixels).

(c) S_3: sum of pixel values; see (10.15) and (10.39).
(d) $(S_{i+3})_{1\leq i\leq q}$: residual energy of the views; see (10.29) and (10.47).
(e) $S_{q+4} = S_m$: total variation; see (10.17).

   To illustrate the benefit of using the total variation set S_m, experiments with the sets $(S_i)_{1\leq i\leq m-1}$ and $(S_i)_{1\leq i\leq m}$ will be performed. Since they are easily computable in closed form, exact projections onto the sets S_1, S_2, and S_3 are used. On the other hand, subgradient projections are used for the sets $(S_i)_{4\leq i\leq m}$.

10.4.4 Numerical Results

We first use $q = 4$ views at observation angles 0, $\pi/4$, $\pi/2$, and $3\pi/4$. In the case of noiseless views, the algorithm produces the image shown in Fig. 10.4.
   We now turn to the case of noise-corrupted views. Figures 10.5 and 10.6 show two typical reconstructions produced by the algorithm, for two arbitrary realizations of the noise. To illustrate the impact of the total variation constraint, we display the images obtained with and without this constraint.
   In order to test the variability of our results, several hundreds of tests were performed, using different realizations of the noise and various types of images. These experiments reveal that, for a given image, the number of wrong pixels does not vary significantly. This variability is quantified in Fig. 10.7 in the case of the original image of Fig. 10.1.
   Finally, we show how the algorithm behaves on a standard image from the binary tomography literature. This image, shown in Fig. 10.8, can be reconstructed uniquely from its exact (noiseless) horizontal and vertical views [22]. This theoretical result is, of course, no longer true in a noisy environment.

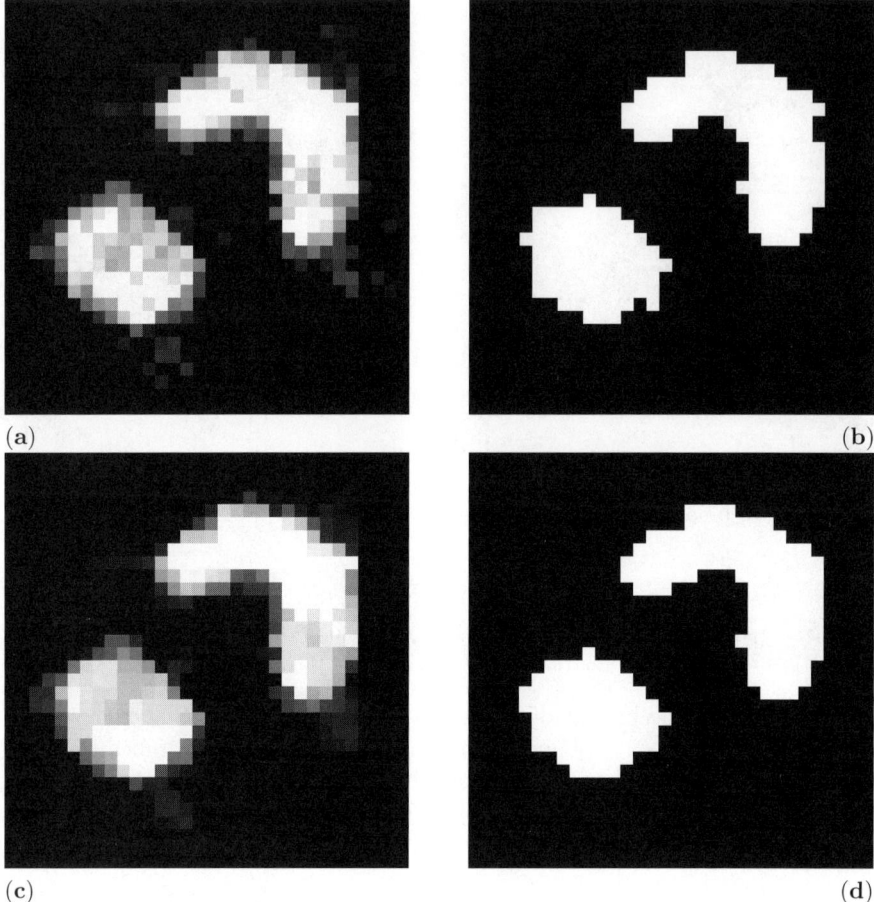

Fig. 10.5. Poisson noise, $q = 4$ views. Reconstruction without the total variation constraint: before (**a**) and after (**b**) binarization (error: 16 pixels). Reconstruction with the total variation constraint: before (**c**) and after (**d**) binarization (error: 8 pixels).

However, our algorithm reconstructs the image almost perfectly in the presence of $q = 3$ noise-corrupted views at angles 0, $\pi/4$, and $\pi/2$ (see Fig. 10.9) with the 6 sets:

(a) S_1: pixel range; see (10.11).
(b) S_2: sum of pixel values; see (10.15) and (10.39).
(c) $(S_{i+2})_{1 \leq i \leq 3}$: residual energy of the views; see (10.29) and (10.47).
(d) S_6: total variation; see (10.17).

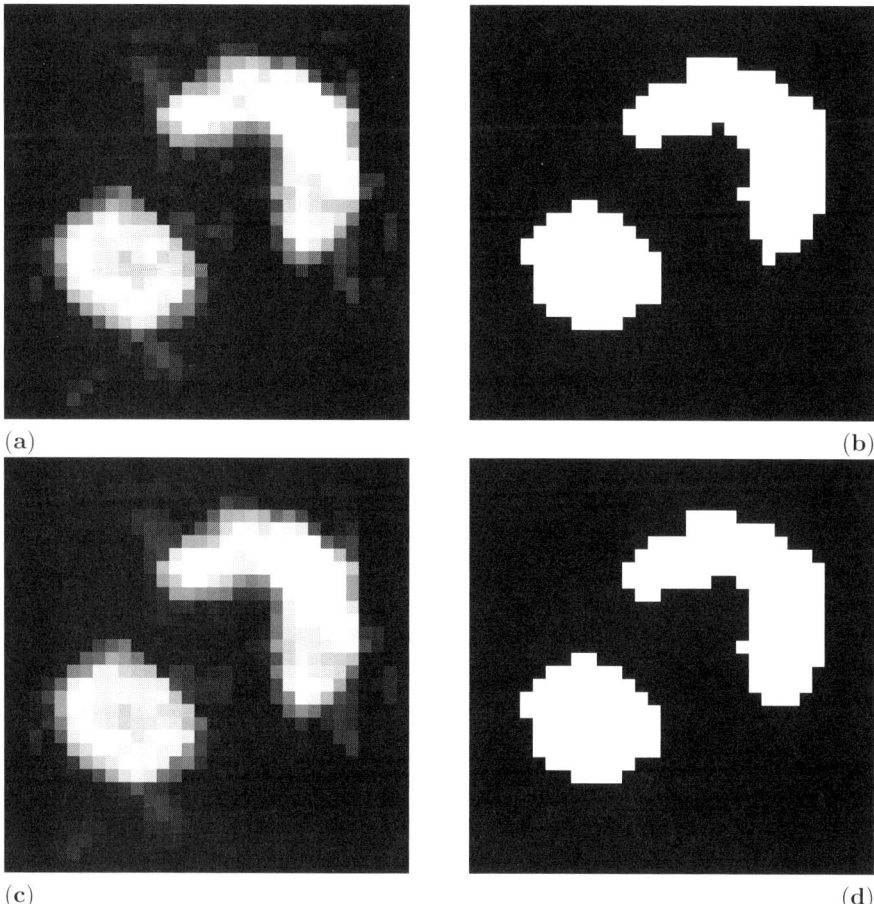

(a)   (b)

(c)   (d)

Fig. 10.6. Same experiments as in Fig. 10.5 with a different realization of the noise. Reconstruction without the total variation constraint: before (**a**) and after (**b**) binarization (error: 12 pixels). Reconstruction with the total variation constraint: before (**c**) and after (**d**) binarization (error: 9 pixels).

10.5 Concluding Remarks

We have proposed a convex programming approach to the discrete tomographic image reconstruction problem. Promising results have been obtained with a limited number of constraints and a quadratic objective function. The proposed algorithm can also handle a wide range of additional constraints as well as more general objective functions. The exploration of such extensions is left for future work. In particular, additional constraints could be derived from a better understanding of the noise process. Likewise, while total variation appears to give good results, soft enforcement of binariness should be possible through alternative convex functionals.

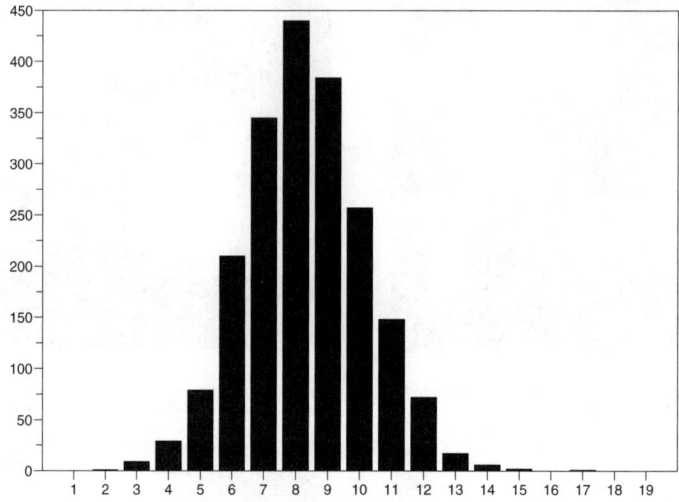

Fig. 10.7. Experiments of Figs. 10.5 and 10.6: histogram of the number of wrong pixels based on 2000 realizations of the noise.

Fig. 10.8. Original image.

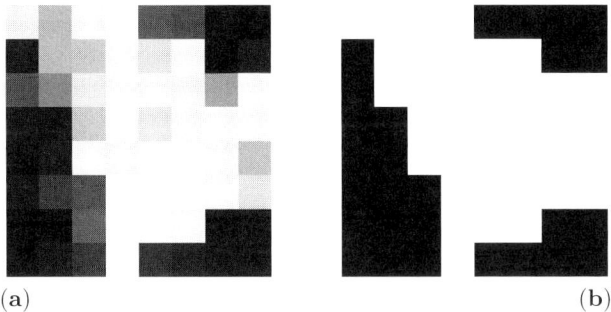

(a)   (b)

Fig. 10.9. Poisson noise, $q = 3$ views. Reconstruction before (**a**) and after (**b**) binarization (error: 1 pixel).

References

1. Bauschke, H., Borwein, J.M.: On projection algorithms for solving convex feasibility problems. *SIAM Rev.*, **38**, 367–426 (1996).
2. Bronstein, M., Bronstein, A.M., Zibulevsky, M., Azhari, H.: Reconstruction in diffraction ultrasound tomography using nonuniform FFT. *IEEE Trans. Medical Imaging*, **21**, 1395–1401 (2002).
3. Capricelli, T.D., Combettes, P.L.: Parallel block-iterative reconstruction algorithms for binary tomography. *Elect. Notes Discr. Math.*, **20**, 263–280 (2005).
4. Censor, Y., Zenios, S.A.: *Parallel Optimization — Theory, Algorithms and Applications.* Oxford University Press, New York, NY (1997).
5. Chambolle, A.: An algorithm for total variation minimization and applications. *J. Math. Imaging Vision*, **20**, 89–97 (2004).
6. Combettes, P.L.: The convex feasibility problem in image recovery. In: Hawkes, P.W. (ed.), *Advances in Imaging and Electron Physics*, Academic Press, New York, NY, pp. 155–270 (1996).
7. Combettes, P.L.: Convex set theoretic image recovery by extrapolated iterations of parallel subgradient projections. *IEEE Trans. Image Processing*, **6**, 493–506 (1997).
8. Combettes, P.L.: Strong convergence of block-iterative outer approximation methods for convex optimization. *SIAM J. Control Optim.*, **38**, 538–565 (2000).
9. Combettes, P.L.: A block-iterative surrogate constraint splitting method for quadratic signal recovery. *IEEE Trans. Signal Processing*, **51**, 1771–1782 (2003).
10. Combettes, P.L., Chaussalet, T.J.: Combining statistical information in set theoretic estimation. *IEEE Signal Process. Lett.*, **3**, 61–62 (1996).
11. Combettes, P.L., Luo, J.: An adaptive level set method for nondifferentiable constrained image recovery. *IEEE Trans. Image Processing*, **11**, 1295–1304 (2002).
12. Combettes, P.L., Pesquet, J.C.: Image restoration subject to a total variation constraint. *IEEE Trans. Image Processing*, **13**, 1213–1222 (2004).
13. Combettes, P.L., Trussell, H.J.: The use of noise properties in set theoretic estimation. *IEEE Trans. Signal Processing*, **39**, 1630–1641 (1991).
14. Combettes, P.L., Trussell, H.J.: Deconvolution with bounded uncertainty. *Int. J. Adapt. Control Signal Processing*, **9**, 3–17 (1995).
15. Del Lungo, A., Gronchi, P., Herman, G.T.: Special issue on discrete tomography. *Lin. Algebra Appl.*, **339**, 1–2 (2001).

16. Devroye, L.: *Non-Uniform Random Variate Generation*. Springer, New York, NY (1986).
17. Gardner, R.J.: *Geometric Tomography*. Cambridge University Press, Cambridge, UK (1995).
18. Gordon, R., Bender, R., Herman, G.T.: Algebraic reconstruction techniques (ART) for three-dimensional electron microscopy and X-ray photography. *J. Theoret. Biology*, **29**, 471–481 (1970).
19. Gritzmann, P., de Vries, S., Wiegelmann, M.: Approximating binary images from discrete X-rays. *SIAM J. Optim.*, **11**, 522–546 (2000).
20. Herman, G.T.: A relaxation method for reconstructing objects from noisy X-rays. *Math. Program.*, **8**, 1–19 (1975).
21. Herman, G.T.: *Image Reconstruction from Projections, the Fundamentals of Computerized Tomography*. Academic Press, New York, NY (1980).
22. Herman, G.T., Kuba, A. (eds.): *Discrete Tomography: Foundations, Algorithms, and Applications*. Birkhäuser, Boston, MA (1999).
23. Herman, G.T., Kuba, A. Eds.: Proc. Workshop on Discrete Tomography and Its Applications. *Electr. Notes Discr. Math.*, **20**, 1–622 (2005).
24. Kudo, H., Saito, T.: Sinogram recovery with the method of convex projections for limited-data reconstruction in computed tomography. *J. Opt. Soc. Amer. A*, **8**, 1148–1160 (1991).
25. Oskoui-Fard, P., Stark, H.: Tomographic image reconstruction using the theory of convex projections. *IEEE Trans. Medical Imaging*, **7**, 45–58 (1988).
26. Press, W.H., Flannery, B.P., Teukolsky, S.A., Vetterling, W.T.: *Numerical Recipes in C Example Book: The Art of Scientific Computing*, 2nd ed. Cambridge University Press, Cambridge, UK (1992).
27. Rockafellar, R.T.: *Convex Analysis*. Princeton University Press, Princeton, NJ. (1970).
28. Rudin, L.I., Osher, S., Fatemi, E.: Nonlinear total variation based noise removal algorithms. *Physica D*, **60**, 259–268 (1992).
29. Schapira, P.: Tomography of constructible functions. In: Cohen, G., Giusti, M., Mora, T. (eds.), *Algebraic Algorithms and Error–Correcting Codes*, Springer, Berlin, Germany, pp. 427–435 (1995).
30. Sezan, M.I., Stark, H.: Tomographic image reconstruction from incomplete view data by convex projections and direct Fourier inversion. *IEEE Trans. Medical Imaging*, **3**, 91–98 (1984).
31. Stark, H., Ed.: *Image Recovery: Theory and Applications*. Academic Press, San Diego, CA (1987).
32. Stark, H., Yang, Y: *Vector Space Projections: A Numerical Approach to Signal and Image Processing, Neural Nets, and Optics*. Wiley, New York, NY (1998).
33. Trussell, H.J., Civanlar, M.R.: The feasible solution in signal restoration. *IEEE Trans. Acoust., Speech, Signal Processing*, **32**, 201–212 (1984).
34. Weber, S., Schüle, T., Hornegger, J., Schnörr, C.: Binary tomography by iterating linear programs from noisy projections. In: Klette, R, Zunic, J.D. (eds.), *Combinatorial Image Analysis*, Springer, Berlin, Germany, pp. 38–51 (2004).
35. Wernick, M.N., Chen, C.T.: Superresolved tomography by convex projections and detector motion. *J. Opt. Soc. Amer. A*, **9**, 1547–1553 (1992).
36. Zhang, X.-Q., Froment, J.: Constrained total variation minimization and application in computerized tomography. In: Rangarajan, A., Vemuri, B.C., Yuille, A.L. (eds.), *Energy Minimization Methods in Computer Vision and Pattern Recognition*, Springer, Berlin, Germany, pp. 456–472 (2005).

11

Variational Reconstruction with DC-Programming

C. Schnörr, T. Schüle, and S. Weber

Summary. We present an approach to binary tomography by variational reconstruction and difference-of-convex-functions (DC) programming. Because we use a standard functional comprising a reconstruction error and a smoothness prior, the integer conditions are relaxed to convex box constraints. Complementing the functional with a concave penalty term allows a gradual enforcement of binary solutions. A DC-programming approach leads to an iterative reconstruction algorithm that is also applicable to large-scale problems. We show that hidden parameters, which model uncertainties of the imaging process, can be estimated as part of the variational reconstruction. Besides presenting a concise overview over recent results, we also include novel results concerning the optimization performance of our approach.

11.1 Introduction

We consider the reconstruction problem of transmission tomography for binary objects. As explained in Fig. 11.1, the imaging process is represented by the algebraic system of equations

$$\mathsf{A}\mathbf{x} = \mathbf{b}, \tag{11.1}$$

where $\mathsf{A} \in \mathbb{R}^{m \times n}$ and $\mathbf{b} \in \mathbb{R}^m$ are given, and where the binary indicator vector $\mathbf{x} \in \{0,1\}^n$ represents some unknown object to be reconstructed. This scenario arises in numerous application areas [14, 15].

Problem (11.1) is difficult for two reasons. First, the linear system is often underdetermined because, for instance, only a few projection directions are taken. In the absence of the binary constraint $\mathbf{x} \in \{0,1\}^n$, and for a large number of variables, this problem is often dealt with by iteratively determining a least-squares solution to (11.1) [5, 11, 17, 21], based on the convex feasibility problem [2] defined by the m equations (11.1). Another natural approach is to regularize the problem by picking out a particular feasible solution having an additional desired property. A typical example of such a property that is useful in many applications is to require a certain amount of spatial homogeneity of reconstructed objects, as measured, for instance, by

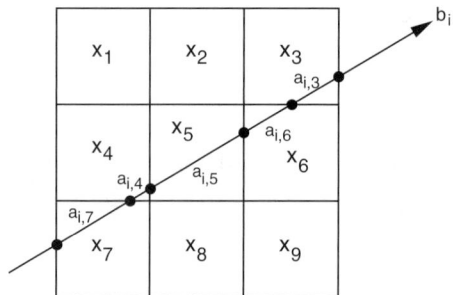

Fig. 11.1. Discretization model for binary transmission tomography. The measured projection data are given in terms of a vector $\mathbf{b} \in \mathbb{R}^m$. Each component b_i corresponds to a projection ray measuring the absorption along the ray through the volume, which is discretized into cells. The absorption $a_{i,j}$ in each cell is assumed to be proportional to the density of the unknown object. $x_1, x_2, \ldots$ are binary variables indicating whether the corresponding cells belong to the object ($x_k = 1$) or not ($x_k = 0$). Assembling all projection rays into a linear system gives $\mathbf{Ax} = \mathbf{b}$, $\mathbf{x} \in \{0,1\}^n$, from which the unknown binary object, represented by $\mathbf{x}$, has to be determined.

$$\sum_{ij \in E} (x_i - x_j)^2 =: \langle \mathbf{x}, \mathsf{L}\mathbf{x} \rangle. \tag{11.2}$$

Here, E denote the edges of a regular grid graph, corresponding to a uniform discretization of the spatial domain (cf. Fig. 11.1), with nodes $i \in \{1, \ldots, n\}$ indexing the components x_i, $i = 1, \ldots, n$, of $\mathbf{x}$. Note that (11.2) defines a quadratic form with positive semidefinite matrix L. A prototypical approach to restoring underdetermined images or objects, based on (11.1) and (11.2), is to compute them as minimum of the functional

$$G(\mathbf{x}) := \frac{1}{2} \Big(\|\mathbf{Ax} - \mathbf{b}\|^2 + \alpha \langle \mathbf{x}, \mathsf{L}\mathbf{x} \rangle \Big), \qquad \mathbb{R} \ni \alpha > 0, \tag{11.3}$$

yielding a regularized least-squares solution to (11.1) [1, 6, 7]. The weighting parameter α allows us to control the smoothness of reconstructions.

A second source of difficulties related to (11.1) is that we require $\mathbf{x}$ to be binary. On the one hand, this is motivated by the considerably reduced degrees of freedom that have to be determined from (11.1) (as opposed to an unconstrained vector $\mathbf{x} \in \mathbb{R}^n$). On the other hand, the feasible set $\{0,1\}^n$ gives rise to the combinatorial integer programming problem

$$G(\mathbf{x}^*) = \inf_{\mathbf{x} \in \{0,1\}^n} G(\mathbf{x}), \tag{11.4}$$

which, in general, cannot be solved in polynomial time. Rather, we have to confine ourselves to efficiently compute a good local optimum close to $\mathbf{x}^*$. Still, this is a challenging task for large-scale problems as they arise in 3D tomography.

The objective of this chapter is to give a concise account of our recent work based on a relaxation of problem (11.4), concave minimization, and DC-programming, where "DC" stands for "difference of convex functions." While DC-programming usually refers to algorithms for global optimization of a certain class of nonconvex functions [16], which is feasible for small problem sizes only, our focus here is on local optimization of large-scale problems. Besides summarizing results from previous work [23, 24, 26], we also include novel results and experiments with respect to the optimization performance of our approach.

Section 11.2 describes the relaxation and concave minimization part of our approach. In Section 11.3, we state conditions for local and global optimality. The DC-programming part of our approach is detailed in Section 11.4. Our framework is sufficiently general to allow for various extensions. Of particular interest is the ability to take into account uncertainty with respect to the model of the imaging process. Two examples in Section 11.5 show how corresponding parameters can be estimated by extending our approach accordingly. Section 11.6 reports experimental results obtained by applying our approach to discrete tomography and quantitative information about optimization performance. Although this work has been motivated by binary tomography, we believe that our results are also of interest for other scientific problems involving large-scale quadratic optimization problems with binary variables. We conclude with corresponding remarks in Section 11.7.

Our notation will be as follows:

$\|\mathbf{x}\|$	Euclidean norm $\left(\sum_{i=1} x_i^2\right)^{1/2}$ of vector $\mathbf{x}$
$\langle \mathbf{x}, \mathbf{y} \rangle$	inner product $\sum_{i=1}^{n} x_i y_i$ of vectors $\mathbf{x}$ and $\mathbf{y}$
$\mathbb{B}$	convex set ("box") $[0,1]^n$: $\mathbf{x} \in \mathbb{B}$ if $0 \leq x_i \leq 1$, for all i
$I_{\mathbb{B}}(\mathbf{x})$	indicator function of the set $\mathbb{B}$: $I_{\mathbb{B}}(\mathbf{x}) = 0$ if $\mathbf{x} \in \mathbb{B}$, and $I_{\mathbb{B}}(\mathbf{x}) = +\infty$ if $\mathbf{x} \notin \mathbb{B}$
$\lambda_{\min}(\mathsf{M}), \lambda_{\max}(\mathsf{M})$	smallest and largest eigenvalue of matrix M
$\mathrm{Diag}(\mathsf{M})$	diagonal matrix with the diagonal of matrix M
$\mathrm{Diag}(\mathbf{x})$	diagonal matrix with vector $\mathbf{x}$ on its diagonal
$\mathbf{e}$	vector $(1,1,\ldots,1)^T \in \mathbb{R}^n$
I	$\mathrm{Diag}(\mathbf{e})$ (the $n \times n$ unit matrix)
$\mathbf{x}^*$	global optimum of Problem (11.4)
$\mathbf{x}_\mu$	local optimum of Problem (11.6)

11.2 Variational Approach

Our approach to (11.4) is to relax the binary constraint $\mathbf{x} \in \{0,1\}^n$ to the convex constraint $\mathbf{x} \in \mathbb{B}$, and to minimize the family of functionals

$$J_\mu(\mathbf{x}_\mu) = \inf_{\mathbf{x} \in \mathbb{B}} J_\mu(\mathbf{x}), \tag{11.5}$$

where

$$0 \leq \mu \in \mathbb{R}, \quad J_\mu(\mathbf{x}) := G(\mathbf{x}) - \mu H(\mathbf{x}), \tag{11.6}$$

G is defined in (11.3), and

$$H(\mathbf{x}) := \frac{1}{2} \langle \mathbf{x}, \mathbf{x} - \mathbf{e} \rangle. \tag{11.7}$$

The following theorem explains the connection of problem (11.5) with the original problem (11.4).

Theorem 1. *[9, 16] Suppose that G is twice continuously differentiable on $\mathbb{B}$. Then there exists $\mu_c \in \mathbb{R}$ such that, for all $\mu > \mu_c$,*

(i) Problem (11.4) and the minimization of J_μ are equivalent:

$$J_\mu(\mathbf{x}^*) = \inf_{\mathbf{x} \in \mathbb{B}} J_\mu(\mathbf{x}). \tag{11.8}$$

(ii) J_μ is concave on $[0, 1]^n$.

Theorem 1 asserts that for a sufficiently large value of the parameter μ in (11.5), the global optima of (11.6) and (11.4) coincide. Assertion (ii), on the other hand, implies that not only does the global optimum satisfy the binary constraint in (11.4), but any local optimum too (all vertices of $\mathbb{B}$ are local minima). This means that for such a large value μ, problem (11.5) is as difficult as problem (11.4).

For $\mu = 0$, however, minimization of the functional $J_0 \equiv G$ over $\mathbb{B}$ is a convex optimization problem. Thus, the global optimum $\mathbf{x}_0$ can be easily computed. This suggests the one-parameter family of optimization problems (11.6) for an increasing sequence of values $0 = \mu^0 < \mu^1 < \cdots < \mu^K$, $\mu^K > \mu_c$, and the computation of a corresponding sequence of local optima $\{\mathbf{x}_{\mu^k}\}$. Because we start with a global optimum $\mathbf{x}_0$ and use as starting value $\mathbf{x}_\mu^{k-1}$ in order to determine $\mathbf{x}_\mu^k$, there is some hope to determine a final local optimum x_μ^K that is close, if not identical, to the global optimum $\mathbf{x}^*$ in (11.4). This approach, akin to numerical continuation or homotopy methods for studying general nonlinear systems, is the subject of the present chapter.

We introduce some further notation in connection with (11.1), (11.3), and (11.6), which will be convenient later on:

$$J_\mu(\mathbf{x}) = \frac{1}{2} \langle \mathbf{x}, Q_\mu \mathbf{x} \rangle - \langle \mathbf{q}_\mu, \mathbf{x} \rangle + const.; \tag{11.9a}$$

$$Q_\mu := A^T A + \alpha L - \mu I; \tag{11.9b}$$

$$\mathbf{q}_\mu := A^T \mathbf{b} - \frac{\mu}{2} \mathbf{e}. \tag{11.9c}$$

Assumption. Throughout this chapter, we assume the symmetric matrix Q_0 to be positive definite.

This assumption is natural because the matrix $A^T A$ is symmetric and positive semidefinite. Moreover, as the nullspace of L in (11.2) contains constant grid functions only, its intersection with the nullspace of $A^T A$ is typically empty.

Corollary 1. *The value μ_c of the parameter μ in Theorem 1 is*

$$\mu_c = \lambda_{\max}(Q_0). \tag{11.10}$$

11.3 Optimality

Problem (11.5) belongs to the class of quadratic optimization problems [8]. While the objective function is nonconvex for $\mu > \lambda_{\min}(Q_0)$, the constraints $\mathbf{x} \in \mathbb{B}$ are convex and therefore simple.

In Subsection 11.3.1, we state conditions for local optimality. These are important for the design of optimization algorithms, because they have to be satisfied after convergence. In Subsection 11.3.2, we briefly address the much more difficult problem of global optimality. We confine ourselves to reporting from the literature necessary and sufficient conditions that can easily be checked in practice. They provide the basis for corresponding experimental results discussed in Subsection 11.6.2.

11.3.1 Local Optimality

Minimizing the functional (11.6) over the convex set $\mathbb{B}$ leads to the first-order necessary conditions for a local optimum $\mathbf{x}_\mu$.

$$-\nabla J_\mu(\mathbf{x}_\mu) \in N_\mathbb{B}(\mathbf{x}_\mu), \tag{11.11}$$

where $N_\mathbb{B}(\mathbf{x}_\mu)$ is the normal cone to $\mathbb{B}$ at $\mathbf{x}_\mu$ [22]. Due to the simple structure of $\mathbb{B} = [0,1]^n$, condition (11.11) reads more explicitly:

$$\left(\nabla J_\mu(\mathbf{x}_\mu)\right)_i \begin{cases} \leq 0 & \text{if } (\mathbf{x}_\mu)_i = 1, \\ \geq 0 & \text{if } (\mathbf{x}_\mu)_i = 0, \\ = 0 & \text{if } (\mathbf{x}_\mu)_i \in (0,1). \end{cases} \tag{11.12}$$

This condition is sufficient in the convex case $\mu \leq \lambda_{\min}(Q_0)$, and also in the nonconvex case if $\mathbf{x}_\mu$ is nondegenerate [8]. The latter means that no component of the gradient $\left(\nabla J_\mu(\mathbf{x}_\mu)\right)_i$ vanishes if a corresponding constraint is active: $x_i \in \{0,1\}$.

11.3.2 Global Optimality

The following conditions, to be read elementwise, can be numerically checked in practice:

Theorem 2. *[3] If $\mathbf{x}_\mu \in \{0,1\}^n$ and*

$$\frac{1}{4}\lambda_{\min}(Q_\mu)\mathbf{e} \geq \left(\mathrm{Diag}(\mathbf{x}_\mu) - \frac{1}{2}\mathrm{I}\right)(Q_\mu\mathbf{x}_\mu - \mathbf{q}_\mu), \tag{11.13}$$

then $\mathbf{x}_\mu = \mathbf{x}^*$. *Conversely, let* $\mathbf{x}_\mu = \mathbf{x}^*$. *Then*

$$\frac{1}{4}\mathrm{Diag}(\mathbf{Q}_\mu)\mathbf{e} \geq \left(\mathrm{Diag}(\mathbf{x}_\mu) - \frac{1}{2}\mathsf{I}\right)(\mathbf{Q}_\mu\mathbf{x}_\mu - \mathbf{q}_\mu). \tag{11.14}$$

Condition (11.13) is sufficient for $\mathbf{x}_\mu$ to be globally optimal. It can be used to check a posteriori whether a local minimum $\mathbf{x}_\mu$ is also a global minimum. Conversely, (11.14) is a necessary condition for global optimality. Thus, if $\mathbf{x}_\mu$ violates (11.14), then it cannot be the global optimum.

11.4 DC-Programming

In this section, a series of algorithms is developed for solving (11.8) and (11.4). Each algorithm utilizes the family of optimization problems (11.5) together with a particular decomposition of the functional (11.6).

Subsection 11.4.1 describes the overall iterative algorithm based on (11.5). At each iteration, a quadratic functional is locally optimized by DC-programming. Subsection 11.4.2 describes the DC-framework and two particular instances related to (11.6). Results of a numerical evaluation of these two approaches are reported in Section 11.6.

11.4.1 Overall Algorithm

The following algorithm computes a locally optimal solution to (11.8).

Algorithm 1 Compute a local optimum to (11.8).

Require: $0 \leq \mu < \lambda_{\min}(\mathbf{Q}_0)$
Require: $\delta_\mu > 0$ {μ-increment}
Require: $\varepsilon > 0$ {termination criterion: $\mathbf{x}$ is approximately binary}
 1: $\mathbf{x} \Leftarrow$ global minimum of $J_\mu \equiv G$ in $\mathbb{B}$ {see (11.3), (11.6)}
 2: **repeat**
 3:     $\mu \Leftarrow \mu + \delta_\mu$
 4:     $\mathbf{x} \Leftarrow$ local minimum of J_μ in $\mathbb{B}$ {see (11.6)}
 5: **until** $x_i \notin [\varepsilon, 1 - \varepsilon]$, for all $i = 1, \ldots, n$
 6: **return x**

Note that the first computation of $\mathbf{x}$ is done by computing the global minimum of a convex quadratic functional. For increasing values of μ, however, the optimization problem in line 1 becomes nonconvex. Algorithms for solving this problem are described in Subsection 11.4.2. Algorithm 1 terminates according to Theorem 1.

In Subsection 11.6.2, we numerically assess the optimization performance of Algorithm 1. If it returns the global optimum, then this is also the solution $\mathbf{x}^*$ of (11.4).

To determine a starting value of μ, we compute $\lambda_{\min}(\mathbf{Q}_0)$. Because $\mathbf{Q}_0$ is positive definite and the computation can be done offline, we apply the power iteration [10] to the matrix $\mathbf{Q}_0^{-1}$. The inverse does not have to be computed explicitly. Just a stable linear system with $\mathbf{Q}_0$ as matrix has to be solved in each step. For large-scale problems, this also can be done iteratively [12].

Determination of a value for δ_μ is based on the following consideration. Having computed the global optimum of J_μ in line 1 of Algorithm 1, the components x_i of $\mathbf{x}$ lying in the interior of $\mathbb{B}$ are assumed to be most critical for computing a good local minimum as μ varies. Consequently, we determine δ_μ so as to bound the initial "speed" of these values.

To simplify the analysis, we consider the situation in which $\mathbf{x}$ is in the interior of $\mathbb{B}$, and that $\mu = 0$ in line 1. Then (11.11) reduces to $\nabla J_0(\mathbf{x}) = 0$. Because $\mathbf{Q}_0$ is positive definite, we have

$$\mathbf{x} = \mathbf{Q}_0^{-1}\mathbf{q}_0. \tag{11.15}$$

Let $\mathbf{x}' = \mathbf{x} + \delta\mathbf{x}$ be the first local minimum, computed in line 1, corresponding to the parameter with $\mu' = 0 + \delta_\mu = \delta_\mu$. Our objective is to bound the shift $\delta\mathbf{x}$. To this end, we ignore again the constraints $\mathbb{B}$ and assume $\mathbf{Q}_{\mu'}$ to be invertible as well:

$$\mathbf{x}' = \mathbf{Q}_{\mu'}^{-1}\mathbf{q}_{\mu'}. \tag{11.16}$$

Using the first-order expansion in δ_μ (see the Appendix), we obtain

$$\|\delta\mathbf{x}\| \leq \delta_\mu \|\mathbf{Q}_0^{-1}\| \left\|\mathbf{x} - \frac{1}{2}\mathbf{e}\right\|. \tag{11.17}$$

We propose choosing δ_μ such that $|\delta x_i| \leq \varepsilon$, on average. This yields

$$\delta_\mu \leq \frac{\varepsilon n^{1/2}\lambda_{\min}(\mathbf{Q}_0)}{\left\|\mathbf{x} - \frac{1}{2}\mathbf{e}\right\|}. \tag{11.18}$$

This result is consistent with the above assumption that $\mathbf{Q}_{\mu'} = \mathbf{Q}_{\delta_\mu}$ is invertible provided $\delta_\mu < \lambda_{\min}(\mathbf{Q}_0)$. As a rule, this is true in real applications, in which $\mathbf{x}$ sufficiently deviates from $\mathbf{e}$. The analysis does not apply for arbitrary values of μ, however, because $\mathbf{Q}_\mu$ becomes singular if μ is equal to some eigenvalue of $\mathbf{Q}_0$. Still, the result is plausible because the actual computation corresponding to line 1 — see Subsection 11.4.2 — avoids any singularities and is based on convex optimization of functionals with quadratic forms in $\mathbf{Q}_0$, independent of the value of μ.

11.4.2 DC-Optimization

In view of functional (11.6) and problem (11.8), we consider the family of optimization problems

$$\inf_{\mathbf{x} \in \mathbb{B}} \{g(\mathbf{x}) - h(\mathbf{x})\}, \tag{11.19}$$

where both g and h are convex and continuously differentiable. The following proposition follows from general results described in [20, 23].

Proposition 1. *The sequence* $\{\mathbf{x}^k\}$ *of global optima of the convex optimization problems defined by*

$$\mathbf{x}^{k+1} \in \operatorname*{argmin}_{\mathbf{x} \in \mathbb{B}} \left\{ g(\mathbf{x}) - \langle \nabla h(\mathbf{x}^k), \mathbf{x} \rangle \right\} \tag{11.20}$$

is decreasing and converges to a point $\overline{\mathbf{x}}$ *satisfying the necessary conditions for a local minimum of (11.19):*

$$\nabla h(\overline{\mathbf{x}}) \in \nabla g(\overline{\mathbf{x}}) + N_{\mathbb{B}}(\overline{\mathbf{x}}). \tag{11.21}$$

Consequently, Algorithm 1 gives rise to the following:

Algorithm 2 Compute a local optimum to (11.8).

Require: $0 \leq \mu < \lambda_{\min}(\mathbf{Q}_0)$
Require: $\delta_\mu > 0$ {μ-increment}
Require: $\varepsilon_1 > 0$ {termination criterion: $\mathbf{x}$ is approximately binary}
Require: $\varepsilon_2 > 0$ {termination criterion of the DC-iteration}
 1: $\mathbf{x} \Leftarrow$ global minimum of $J_\mu \equiv G$ in $\mathbb{B}$ {see (11.3), (11.6)}
 2: **repeat**
 3:     $\mu \Leftarrow \mu + \delta_\mu$
 4:     **repeat**
 5:         $\mathbf{x}' \Leftarrow \mathbf{x}$
 6:         $\mathbf{x} \Leftarrow$ global minimum of $g(\mathbf{x}) - \langle \nabla h(\mathbf{x}'), \mathbf{x} \rangle$ in $\mathbb{B}$ {see (11.20)}
 7:     **until** $\left(g(\mathbf{x}') - h(\mathbf{x}') \right) - \left(g(\mathbf{x}) - h(\mathbf{x}) \right) \leq \varepsilon_2$
 8: **until** $x_i \notin [\varepsilon_1, 1 - \varepsilon_1]$, for all $i = 1, \ldots, n$
 9: **return** $\mathbf{x}$

Depending on the decomposition of (11.6), Algorithm 2 can be applied to (11.8) in different ways. We consider the following two alternatives.

I. Choose $\mathbb{R} \ni \lambda > \lambda_{\max}(Q_\mu)$ and

$$g(\mathbf{x}) := \frac{\lambda}{2} \|\mathbf{x}\|^2, \quad h(\mathbf{x}) := \frac{\lambda}{2} \|\mathbf{x}\|^2 - J_\mu(\mathbf{x}). \tag{11.22}$$

Based on this definition, (11.20) corresponds to the sequence of convex programs

$$\mathbf{x}^{k+1} \in \operatorname*{argmin}_{\mathbf{x} \in \mathbb{B}} \left\{ \frac{1}{2} \lambda \|\mathbf{x}\|^2 - \langle \lambda \mathbf{x}^k - \nabla J_\mu(\mathbf{x}^k), \mathbf{x} \rangle \right\}. \tag{11.23}$$

II. Choose [cf. (11.6)]

$$g(\mathbf{x}) := G(\mathbf{x}), \quad h(\mathbf{x}) := \mu H(\mathbf{x}). \tag{11.24}$$

In this case, (11.20) corresponds to

$$\mathbf{x}^{k+1} \in \operatorname*{argmin}_{\mathbf{x} \in \mathbb{B}} \left\{ G(\mathbf{x}) - \mu \langle \nabla H(\mathbf{x}^k), \mathbf{x} \rangle \right\}. \tag{11.25}$$

After convergence, either version satisfies (11.21), which then corresponds to (11.11).

Decomposition (11.22) leads to a straightforward optimization algorithm based on sparse matrix-vector products and thresholding [23], but with slower convergence. Decomposition (11.24), on the other hand, leads to more involved iterative steps (11.25) that are still efficiently solvable [4], and with faster convergence. Other decompositions are conceivable but have not been investigated so far.

11.5 Extensions

In real applications, the mathematical model (11.1) of the imaging process is often not precisely known. As such uncertainties may considerably affect the reconstructions, they have to be taken into account whenever possible. This can be done if a parametric model of the uncertainties is known.

An example is given by [24]

$$\nu_1 A\mathbf{x} + \nu_0 A(\mathbf{e} - \mathbf{x}) = \mathbf{b}, \tag{11.26}$$

which generalizes (11.1) to include two unknown absorption coefficients. Other examples are [26]

$$AG_\sigma \mathbf{x} = \mathbf{b}, \tag{11.27}$$

and

$$G_\sigma A\mathbf{x} = \mathbf{b}, \tag{11.28}$$

which take into account that projections were taken from blurred objects or that the projection data themselves were blurred, respectively. Here, G_σ denotes a block-circulant matrix representing the blurring operation with a Gaussian and unknown scale parameter σ.

In either case, Algorithm 2 can be extended so as to incorporate parameter estimation, during reconstruction, by means of the well-known expectation-maximization (EM) approach [18]. While the actual computations for setting up the respective extension are application-dependent [24, 26], the general principle is the same: Function $g(\mathbf{x})$ in (11.20) is modified through integration over the space of unknown parameters (i.e., marginalization in the language of probabilistic inference), to become a convex function $g(\mathbf{x}; \hat{\mathbf{x}})$ (E-step). Here, $\hat{\mathbf{x}}$ denotes the reconstruction based on the current parameter estimate. Both parameters and reconstruction are iteratively updated, as part of the DC-loop (M-step). Algorithm 3 provides these steps in detail.

11.6 Experimental Results

In Subsection 11.6.1, we illustrate our approach by applying it to binary discrete tomography. Performance from the viewpoint of optimization is assessed

---

Algorithm 3 Locally optimize (11.8), estimate unknown parameters.

Require: $0 \leq \mu < \lambda_{\min}(\mathbf{Q}_0)$
Require: $\delta_\mu > 0$ {μ-increment}
Require: $\varepsilon_1 > 0$ {termination criterion: $\mathbf{x}$ is approximately binary}
Require: $\varepsilon_2 > 0$ {termination criterion of the DC-iteration}
Require: $\varepsilon_3 > 0$ {termination criterion of the EM-iteration}
 1: $\mathbf{x} \Leftarrow$ global minimum of $J_\mu \equiv G$ in $\mathbb{B}$ {see (11.3), (11.6)}
 2: **repeat**
 3:     $\mu \Leftarrow \mu + \delta_\mu$
 4:     **repeat**
 5:         $\mathbf{x}' \Leftarrow \mathbf{x}$
 6:         **repeat**
 7:             $\hat{\mathbf{x}} \Leftarrow \mathbf{x}$
 8:             $\mathbf{x} \Leftarrow$ global minimum of $g(\mathbf{x}; \hat{\mathbf{x}}) - \langle \nabla h(\mathbf{x}'), \mathbf{x} \rangle$ in $\mathbb{B}$ {EM-update}
 9:         **until** $\|\mathbf{x} - \hat{\mathbf{x}}\| \leq \varepsilon_3$
10:     **until** $\big(g(\mathbf{x}') - h(\mathbf{x}')\big) - \big(g(\mathbf{x}) - h(\mathbf{x})\big) \leq \varepsilon_2$
11: **until** $x_i \notin [\varepsilon_1, 1 - \varepsilon_1]$, for all $i = 1, \ldots, n$
12: **return** $\mathbf{x}$

---

in Subsection 11.6.2. Finally, we illustrate in Subsection 11.6.3 the extensions described in Section 11.5.

11.6.1 Discrete Tomography

To illustrate Algorithm 2 with Decomposition I (11.22), Fig. 11.2(a) shows a 2D image from which three projections within 90 degrees were taken. The other images in Fig. 11.2 show intermediate results of the iteration and how the binary constraint is gradually enforced. The final binary result [Fig. 11.2(f)] shows that although the initial solution of the convex problem for $\mu = 0$ is far from the original image, the algorithm is able to reconstruct the original image without error.

To illustrate the application of our approach to a sizable 3D reconstruction problem, we used a binarized medical data set of size 256^3. This volume was calculated as the difference of two volumes based on a standard computer tomography reconstruction. The first volume was the reconstruction of a human head without, and the other volume with a contrast agent. As a result, the binarized difference volume shows the tree structure of a vessel system inside a human head.

For this binary volume, we simulated 5 projections with angles $31.5°$, $48°$, $66°$, $84°$, and $103.5°$. The reconstruction was calculated with Decomposition II (11.24). The parameter α was set to 1, and the increment δ_μ was computed according to Eq. (11.18) with $\varepsilon = 1$. We eliminated beforehand from the optimization procedure all redundant voxels with projection value equal to zero by setting them to the fixed value zero. The remaining number of unknowns was $279,074$, and the number of projection constraints was $485,791$ [Fig. 11.3(a)].

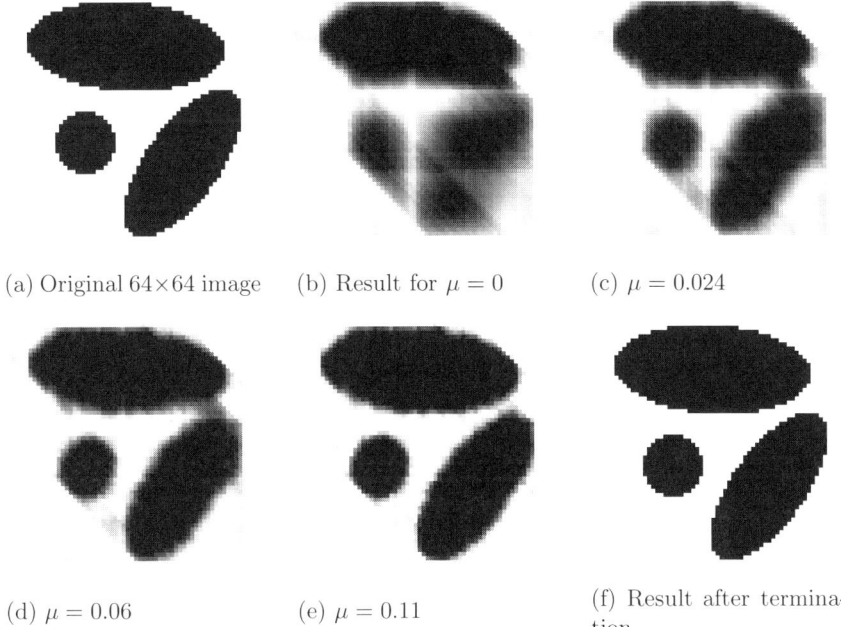

(a) Original 64×64 image   (b) Result for $\mu = 0$ (c) $\mu = 0.024$

(d) $\mu = 0.06$ (e) $\mu = 0.11$ (f) Result after termination

Fig. 11.2. (a) Original image (64×64). (b)-(f) Reconstructions from three projections ($0°$, $45°$, $90°$). Each image shows the reconstruction result after termination of the DC-iteration (cf. Algorithm 2, lines 4–7) for a corresponding value of μ.

While this relationship of unknowns/constraints seems to indicate that the reconstruction problem is easy, this is essentially not the case. Even standard tomographic reconstruction employs regularization (filtered backprojection) while using much more constraints — 133 projections over $200°$ in the present example. Consequently, regularization is all the more crucial when taking five projections only. This is effectively done by our approach by reducing the degrees of freedom of the reconstruction to those of binary volume functions.

The algorithm was able to reconstruct the ground truth volume [Fig. 11.3 (b)] within a run time of about 1900 sec on a dual 2.4GHz AMD Opteron system.

11.6.2 Optimization Performance

We assessed the optimization performance of our approach using a 64×64 image shown in Fig. 11.4, from which three projections were taken at $0°$, $45°$, and $90°$. We denote the corresponding vector with $\mathbf{x}^*$, and the final reconstruction $\mathbf{x}_{\mu_{\max}}$ with $\mathbf{x} = \mathbf{x}_{\mu_{\max}}$. The regularization parameter α was set to 0.5. The μ-increment δ_μ was computed using Eq. (11.18) with $\varepsilon = 1$.

Note that in this subsection, we use the symbol $\mathbf{x}^*$ to denote the *ground truth* depicted in Fig. 11.4. We do not know, of course, whether this also

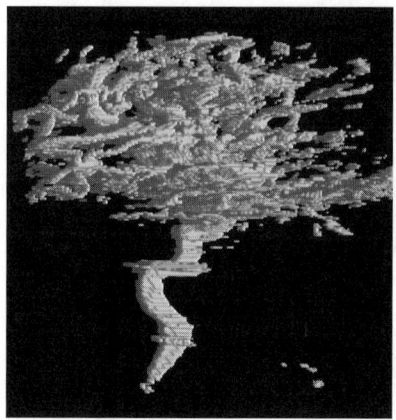 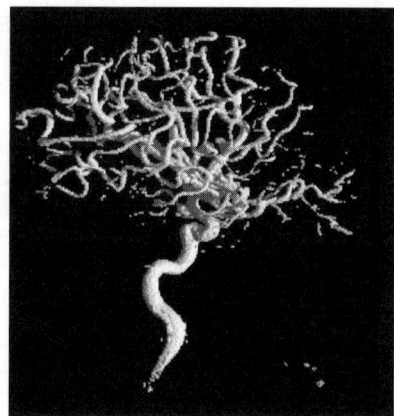

(a) Peel volume   (b) Reconstructed vessel system

Fig. 11.3. Variational binary reconstruction of a vessel system in a discretized volume of size 256^3. (a) Locations of unknown variables corresponding to nonzero projection constraints. (b) The reconstructed vessel system.

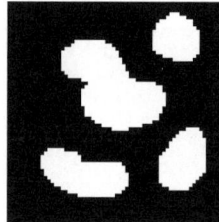

Fig. 11.4. Ground truth of a 64×64 reconstruction problem with three projections within $90°$.

corresponds to the *global* optimum. It is reasonable to assume, however, that it is quite close to it. Our results shown below confirm this and thus yield useful quantitative insights into the optimization performance of our approach. We preferred this way over experiments of very small size, for which the global optimum can be computed as a reference by exhaustive search.

Figure 11.5 displays the error $\|Ax - b\|_2$, and Fig. 11.6 shows the corresponding run times, as a function of a factor $s > 1$ specifying various coarser schedules in terms of a μ-increment $s\delta_\mu$ that was larger than specified by Eq. (11.18), and that was fixed for each schedule. Both decompositions were able to reconstruct x^* for fine schedules. This also confirms the validity of the estimate (11.18), which seems to be a bit conservative but safe. For coarser schedules the run time decreases, of course, but the error increases as well. Moreover, Decomposition II converges faster, that is, a smaller number of iterations necessary to converge compensates by far the additional costs in each step, in comparison to Decomposition I.

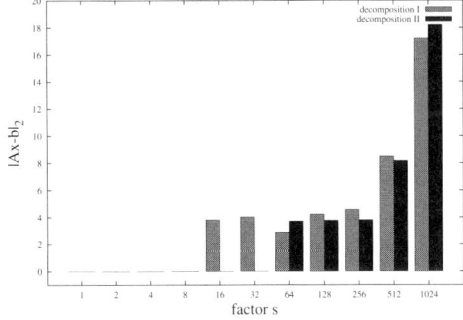

Fig. 11.5. Error $\|\mathbf{Ax} - \mathbf{b}\|_2$ for different schedules.

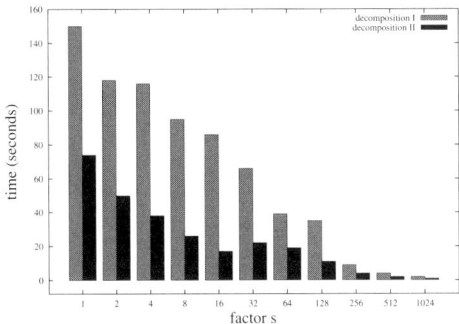

Fig. 11.6. Run times for different schedules.

11.6.3 Extensions

Figures 11.7 and 11.8 show results computed with Algorithm 3 for the joint reconstruction–parameter estimation problems (11.27) and (11.28), respectively. These results prove the stability of our approach and enables us to cope with such inverse problems.

11.7 Conclusion

We presented an overview over recent results obtained with a novel approach to binary tomography. Ingredients of this approach are (1) a least-squares error criterion for reconstruction, (2) a variational prior enforcing spatially homogeneous solution, (3) relaxation of 0/1-constraints and adding a concave penalty term, and (4) iterative optimization by DC-programming. The approach is essentially free of tuning parameters and applicable to large-scale

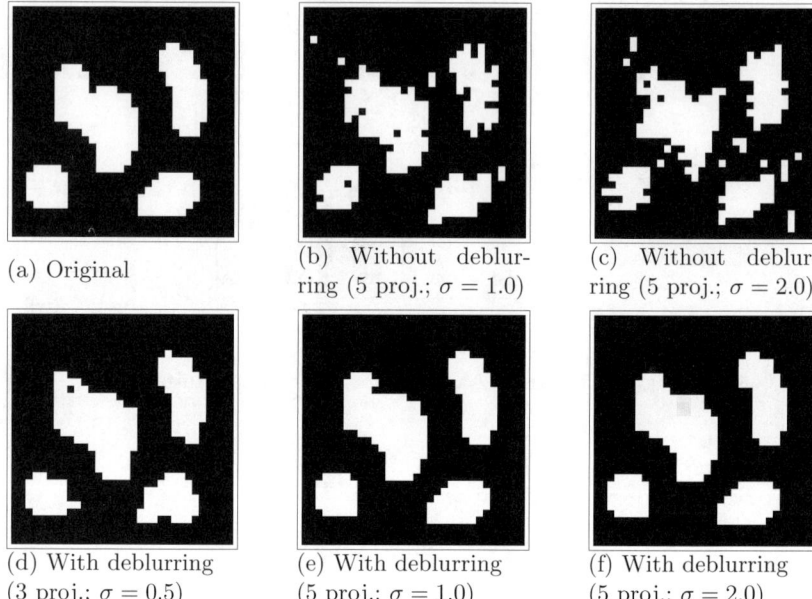

(a) Original

(b) Without deblur-ring (5 proj.; $\sigma = 1.0$)

(c) Without deblur-ring (5 proj.; $\sigma = 2.0$)

(d) With deblurring (3 proj.; $\sigma = 0.5$)

(e) With deblurring (5 proj.; $\sigma = 1.0$)

(f) With deblurring (5 proj.; $\sigma = 2.0$)

Fig. 11.7. Reconstruction from blurred objects. (a) Original image (32×32) convolved with a Gaussian kernel ($\sigma \in \{1.0, 2.0\}$) and projected along five directions ($0°$, $22.5°$, $45°$, $67.5°$, $90°$). (b) and (c): Reconstructions without deblurring. (e) and (f): Reconstructions with deblurring. (d) Reconstruction from three projections only ($0°$, $45°$, and $90°$). Parameter $\alpha = 0.01$ in all experiments.

3D reconstruction problems. Experimental results demonstrate promising optimization performance. The reconstruction process can be extended to include the estimation of parametric models of the imaging process.

Our further work will focus on various applications of binary tomography, and on the inclusion of prior knowledge about object structure beyond the elementary property "spatial smoothness."

Acknowledgments

We gratefully acknowledge support from Siemens Medical Solutions (Forchheim, Germany).

Appendix: Derivation of (11.17)

Applying Woodbury's formula [10], we compute

$$Q_{\mu'}^{-1} = (Q_0 - \delta_\mu I)^{-1} = Q_0^{-1} + \delta_\mu Q_0^{-1} (I - \delta_\mu Q_0^{-1})^{-1} Q_0^{-1}. \qquad (11.29)$$

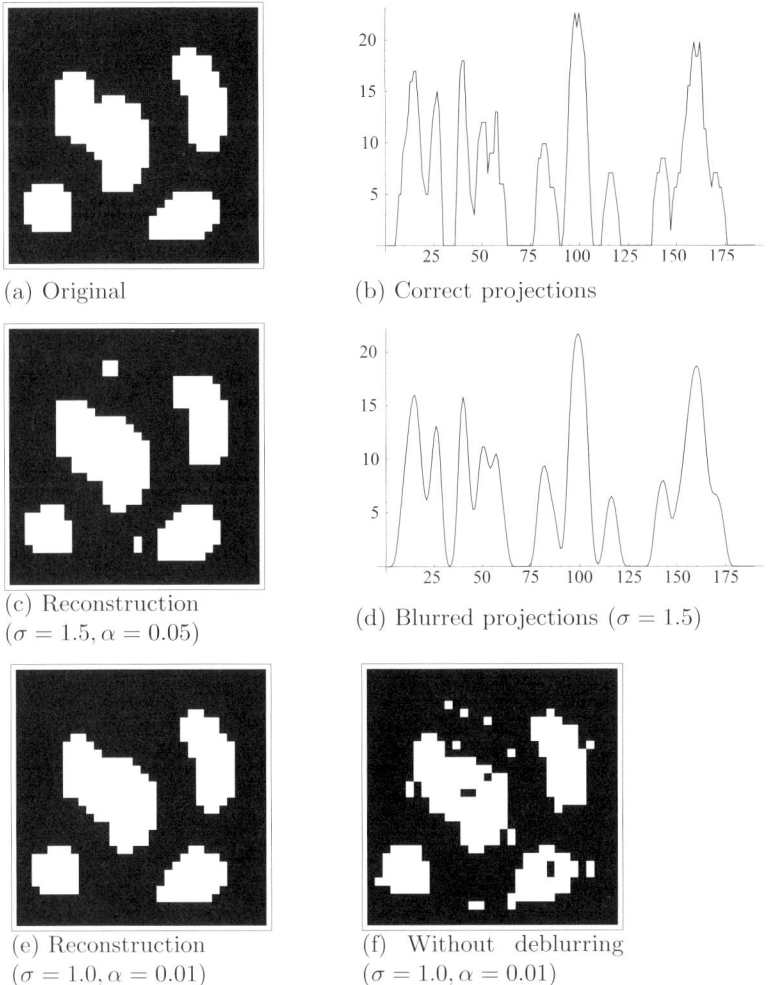

(a) Original

(b) Correct projections

(c) Reconstruction
$(\sigma = 1.5, \alpha = 0.05)$

(d) Blurred projections $(\sigma = 1.5)$

(e) Reconstruction
$(\sigma = 1.0, \alpha = 0.01)$

(f) Without deblurring
$(\sigma = 1.0, \alpha = 0.01)$

Fig. 11.8. Reconstruction from blurred projections. The image shown in (a) was projected along $0°$, $45°$, $90°$, $135°$ and convolved with a Gaussian kernel ($\sigma = 1.5$). (b) and (d): Correct and blurred projection data, respectively. (c) Reconstruction from the data shown in (d), $\alpha = 0.05$. (e) Reconstruction from projection data that were blurred with $\sigma = 1.0$. The accuracy of estimating the unknown parameter σ during the reconstruction is about 6%. (f) Erroneous reconstruction without taking deblurring into account.

Because $\delta_\mu < \lambda_{\min}(\mathbf{Q}_0)$ — see (11.18) and the corresponding discussion — we have $\|\delta_\mu \mathbf{Q}_0^{-1}\| = \delta_\mu \|\mathbf{Q}_0^{-1}\| < 1$ and, as a consequence, the valid representation (Neumann series)

$$Q_{\mu'}^{-1} = Q_0^{-1} + \delta_\mu Q_0^{-1} \left(\sum_{k=0}^{\infty} (\delta_\mu Q_0^{-1})^k \right) Q_0^{-1} \approx Q_0^{-1}(I + \delta_\mu Q_0^{-1}) . \qquad (11.30)$$

Insertion into (11.16) and ignoring the quadratic term in δ_μ give, using (11.15),

$$\mathbf{x} + \delta\mathbf{x} \approx Q_0^{-1}(I + \delta_\mu Q_0^{-1})(\mathbf{q}_0 - \frac{\delta_\mu}{2}\mathbf{e}) \approx \mathbf{x} + \delta_\mu Q_0^{-1}(\mathbf{x} - \frac{1}{2}\mathbf{e}). \qquad (11.31)$$

Taking the norm and the Cauchy–Schwarz inequality result in (11.17).

References

1. Baumeister, J.: *Stable Solution of Inverse Problems*. F. Vieweg & Sohn, Braunschweig/Wiesbaden, Germany (1987).
2. Bauschke, H.H., Borwein, J.M.: On projection algorithms for solving convex feasibility problems. *SIAM Review*, **38**, 367–426 (1996).
3. Beck, A., Teboulle, M.: Global optimality conditions for quadratic optimization problems with binary constraints. *SIAM J. Optimiz.*, **11**, 179–188 (2000).
4. Birgin, E.G., Martínez, J.M., Raydan, M.: Algorithm 813: SPG-software for convex-constrained optimization. *ACM Trans. Math. Softw.*, **27**, 340–349 (2001).
5. Censor, Y., Zenios, S.A.: *Parallel Optimization: Theory, Algorithms, and Applications*. Oxford Univ. Press, New York, NY (1998).
6. Demoment, G.: Image reconstruction and restoration: Overview of common estimation structures and problems. *IEEE Trans. Acoustics, Speech, Signal Proc.*, **37**, 2024–2036 (1989).
7. Engl, H.W., Hanke, M., Neubauer, A.: *Regularization of Inverse Problems*. Kluwer, Dordrecht, The Netherlands (1996).
8. Floudas, C.A., Visweswaran, V.: Quadratic optimization. In: Horst, R., Pardalos, R.M. (eds.): *Handbook of Global Optimization*, Kluwer Acad. Publ., Dordrecht, The Netherlands, pp. 217–269 (1995).
9. Giannessi, F., Niccolucci, F.: Connections between nonlinear and integer programming problems. In *Symposia Mathematica*, Vol. 19, Academic Press, Orlando, FL, pp. 161–176 (1976).
10. Golub, G.H., van Loan, C.F.: *Matrix Computations*, 3rd ed., Johns Hopkins Univ. Press, Baltimore, MD (1997).
11. Gordon, R., Bender, R., Herman, G.T.: Algebraic reconstruction techniques (ART) for three-dimensional electron microscopy and x-ray photography. *J. Theor. Biol.*, **29**, 471–481 (1970).
12. Hackbusch, W.: *Iterative Solution of Large Sparse Systems of Equations*. Springer, Berlin, Germany (1993).
13. Herman, G.T.: *Mathematical Methods in Tomography*. Springer, Berlin, Germany (1992).
14. Herman, G.T., Kuba, A. (eds.): *Discrete Tomography: Foundations, Algorithms, and Applications*. Birkhäuser, Boston, MA (1999).
15. Herman, G.T., Kuba, A.: Discrete tomography in medical imaging. *Proc. IEEE*, **91**, 1612–1626 (2003).

16. Horst, R., Tuy, H.: *Global Optimization: Deterministic Approaches*, 3rd ed., Springer, Berlin, Germany (1996).
17. Kaczmarz, S.: Angenäherte Auflösung von Systemen linearer Gleichungen. *Bull. Acad. Polon. Sci. et Let. A*, pp. 355–357 (1937).
18. McLachlan, G.J., Krishnan, T.: *The EM Algorithm and Extensions*. Wiley, New York, NY (1996).
19. Pham Dinh, T., Elbernoussi, S.: Duality in d.c. (difference of convex functions) optimization subgradient methods. In: Hoffmann, K.-H., Hiriart-Urruty, J.-B., Lemarechal, C., Zowe, J. (eds.), *Trends in Mathematical Optimization*, Birkäuser, Basel, Switzerland, pp. 277–293 (1988).
20. Pham Dinh, T., Hoai An, L.T.: A D.C. optimization algorithm for solving the trust-region subproblem. *SIAM J. Optim.*, **8**, 476–505 (1998).
21. Popa, C., Zdunek, R.: Kaczmarz extended algorithm for tomographic image reconstruction from limited data. *Math. Comput. Simul.*, **65**, 579–598 (2004).
22. Rockafellar, R.T., Wets, R.J.-B.: *Variational Analysis*. Springer, Berlin, Germany (1998).
23. Schüle, T., Schnörr, C., Weber, S., Hornegger, J.: Discrete tomography by convex-concave regularization and D.C. programming. *Discr. Appl. Math.*, **151**, 229–243 (2005).
24. Schüle, T., Weber, S., Schnörr, C.: Adaptive reconstruction of discrete-valued objects from few projections. *Electr. Notes Discr. Math.*, **20**, 365–384 (2005).
25. Vogel, C.R.: *Computational Methods for Inverse Problems*. SIAM, Philadelphia, PA (2002).
26. S. Weber, Schüle, T., Schnörr, C., Kuba, A.: Binary tomography with deblurring. In: Reulke, R., Eckardt, U., Flach, B., Knauer, U., Polthier, K. (eds.), *Combinatorial Image Analysis*. Springer, Berlin, Germany, pp. 375–388 (2006).

Part III

Applications of Discrete Tomography

12

Direct Image Reconstruction-Segmentation, as Motivated by Electron Microscopy

H.Y. Liao and G.T. Herman

Summary. Our aim is to produce a tessellation of space into small voxels and, based on only a few tomographic projections of an object, assign to each voxel a label that indicates one of the components of interest constituting the object. Examples of application are in the areas of electron microscopy, industrial nondestructive testing, cardiac imaging, etc.

Current approaches first reconstruct the density distribution from the projections and then segment (label) this distribution. We instead postulate a low-level prior knowledge regarding the underlying distribution of label images and then directly estimate the label image based on the prior and the projections. In particular, we show, in the binary (i.e., two labels) case, that the marginal posterior mode estimator outperforms the widely known maximum a posteriori probability estimator.

As measured by label misclassification in the reconstructions, our direct labeling method was experimentally proved (in the binary case) to be superior to current approaches. However, when a detectability measure was used, its relative performance was less satisfactory. We discuss possible improvements.

12.1 Introduction

The essence of discrete tomography is to make use of the knowledge that the reconstruction should contain only a few values to make up for the lack of availability of a large number of projections [25]. For example, in industrial nondestructive testing, each voxel in the reconstruction can be labeled as containing either (the presence of) the scanned object or air; the number of projections should be small for containment of cost. Another example is in electron microscopy of biological macromolecules, in which the labels (components) could be, e.g., ice, protein, and RNA; and because of the damage by radiation, only a very limited dose can be applied to the specimen.

Traditionally, in all applications that use a discrete tomography method, a label is determined by the density within the corresponding component. Under this assumption, partial volume effects along the boundaries between components are ignored. Examples of application areas are cardiac imaging

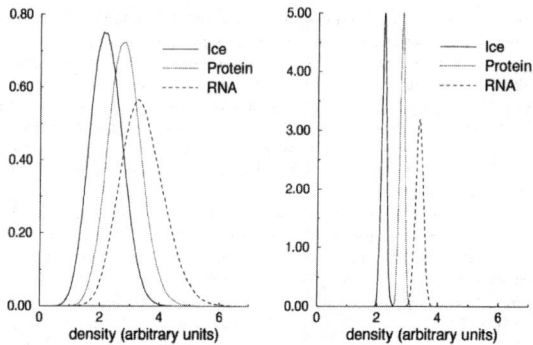

Fig. 12.1. Histograms of the densities corresponding to volumes sampled using voxels of edge length equal to 2.5 (left) and 7.5 (right), obtained from volumes composed only of ice, only protein, or only RNA; from [7].

[8, 11, 41], angiography [14], attenuation map correction [1, 2, 11, 13], etc. In contrast to these applications and in addition to the partial volume effect, in electron microscopy the range of densities that may occur in a voxel may overlap for the different labels that may be assigned to that voxel. As the resolution increases, this overlap of densities becomes higher, as indicated by the histograms of densities in Fig. 12.1.

The understanding of the macromolecular mechanisms of the key cell functions has great impacts; for example, it may be essential for the discovery of a new drug. Since these mechanisms are highly correlated with the three-dimensional (3D) structure, an accurate reconstruction of the 3D volume is vital for the inference of the biological functions [16, 30]. To improve on existing reconstruction methods that ignore the phenomenon indicated on the left of Fig. 12.1, we propose new techniques directly applicable to the case of overlapping density ranges.

We postulate that *Gibbs priors* [48] enable us to model the underlying distribution of label images. Such priors, which allow us to "encode" the general shapes and sizes of characteristic structures [33, 37], need to be learned from a training set of typical correctly labeled images [33]. Our approaches are statistical: The reconstruction is considered to be a minimizer of a *Bayes risk*. A popular choice for the optimizer is the well-known *maximum a posteriori probability* (MAP) estimator [48]. However, we also study the *marginal posterior mode* (MPM) estimator, as it has been suggested [15] that, for image denoising purposes, it would not cause "oversmoothing," as would the MAP estimator. Here we show experimentally that this is also the case in image reconstruction.

In Section 12.2, we introduce our statistical model, and in Section 12.3, we define the two estimators (MAP and MPM). Because of the complicated form of the true estimators, in Section 12.4, we propose approximations to both of them, and in Section 12.5, we introduce our algorithms that search for the approximated estimators. All the experimental results, shown in Section 12.6, are demonstrated for the binary (i.e., two labels) case for 2D and 3D images. A methodology for objective comparison of algorithms is also treated. We make some discussions and give the conclusions in the last section.

12.2 The Model

Based on a Bayesian viewpoint, we combine the information coming from the measurement data with the Gibbs prior and then minimize a *Bayes risk* that is defined to be the expectation of some *loss function* with respect to the *posterior probability*. The posterior probability is proportional to the product of the (Gibbs) prior probability and the *likelihood* that is defined to be the conditional probability of the measurement data given the label image. The optimizer of the Bayes risk (or *Bayes estimator*) is adopted as the solution of the reconstruction problem. Our model is hierarchical: At the bottom are the *label images*, which are assumed to obey a Gibbs probability distribution; on top of the label images, we have the *gray-value* (or density) *images*, which model the uncertainty of the density at each voxel. Finally, on top of the gray-value images are the *measurements*, which are defined to be a noisy version of the projections of a gray-value image. Our task is to estimate the label image from the measurements.

12.2.1 The Label Image

For simplicity in the discussions, we concentrate for now on two-dimensional (2D) label images. Later, in Section 12.6, we consider 3D images. Let D be the domain, which is defined to be a fixed nonempty square subset of the square lattice (i.e.,

$$D = \left\{ (v_1, v_2) \in \mathbb{Z}^2 \mid 0 \le v_1, v_2 < V \right\}, \tag{12.1}$$

where $\mathbb{Z}$ denotes the set of all integers). An element $d \in D$ is called a *point* in D. Any nonempty subset of D is called a *clique*. Given a clique q, a *configuration* (over q) is defined as a mapping from q into the set of labels $\Lambda = \{\lambda_1, \lambda_2, \ldots, \lambda_K\}$. In the special case where $q = D$, a configuration $g : D \to \Lambda$ is called a *label image* and will be denoted by x. Sometimes, for computational purposes, it is convenient to express images as vectors. Thus, we allow x to denote either an image with domain D or a column vector of dimension $|D| = V^2$; i.e., the elements of the corresponding vector $x = (x_0, \ldots, x_{|D|-1})^t$ are defined by $x_{v_2 V + v_1} = x(v_1, v_2)$, $0 \le v_1, v_2 < V$. Since the Voronoi neighborhood [23] on the plane of a point in $\mathbb{Z}^2$ is a unit square (commonly referred to as a *pixel*), we also call a label image a labeling of the set of pixels corresponding to D.

We assume that there is a prior distribution that assigns to every label image $x \in \Lambda^D$ a probability $\pi(x)$. Typically, this prior distribution is a *Gibbs distribution* (GD), which means that

$$\pi(x) = Z^{-1} \exp[-H(x)], \qquad (12.2)$$

where $\pi(x)$ is the probability of occurrence of the image x, Z is the normalizing factor, and $H(x)$ is referred to as the *energy* of x (see, e.g., [48]). The energy is the negative of sum of *local potentials*, each of which is a real number assigned to the configuration on a clique. As a result, $\pi(x)$ is a product of terms, each of which depends on only one clique. Typically, the local potential depends on the labels in the cliques in a way that is invariant under various transformations (such as translations, rotations, and reflections); this results in having only a few possible values for the local potentials, which are the *parameters* of the GD. In the examples with 2D images, we consider two labels [i.e., $|\Lambda| = 2$, and the labels are black (or 0) and white (or 1)] and use a GD that has five parameters. Each parameter corresponds to 3×3 clique configurations that are considered to contain one of the following five "local features": a black region, a white region, an edge, a convex corner, or a concave corner. (See Fig. 12.2. More details can be found in [33].) To see how the general shapes and sizes of characteristic structures in images can be "encoded" by these parameters, Fig. 12.3 shows typical random samples from four GDs, whose parameters were conveniently adjusted for illustration purposes.

For electron microscopy applications, we can think of ice as corresponding to black and protein to white. The nature of the boundaries between ice an protein is modeled by the local features. To obtain the parameters of the GD, there are standard techniques for estimating them from typically correctly segmented images (see, e.g., [31] for a survey). In [33], we applied the best-known techniques to our models with the five parameters. Here we use the estimation method we found to be the best (the *pseudo-likelihood method* [3, 4]) in these experiments.

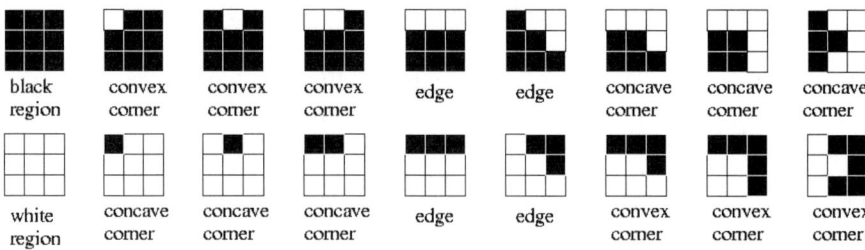

Fig. 12.2. Configurations of a 3×3 clique that specify local features referred to as: a black region, a convex corner, a concave corner, an edge, and a white region.

Fig. 12.3. Sample images (63×63) from four different Gibbs distributions modeled by five parameters, each one of which is assigned to a local feature of Fig. 12.2.

12.2.2 The Gray-Value Image

Let $\mathbf{Y}$ be a set of *gray-value images*, each of which is an I-dimensional vector $y = (y_0, \ldots, y_{I-1})^t$, where $y_i \in Y$ (the set of *gray values*, $Y \subseteq \mathbb{R}$), for $0 \leq i \leq I - 1$. We assume that there is a conditional distribution that, given a label image x, assigns a probability $\phi(y|x)$ to every gray-value image y. [Since $\mathbf{Y}$ is not necessarily finite, it would be more precise to say that $\phi(y|x)$ is the probability density function defining the conditional distribution of the gray value image y given the label image x. For the sake of brevity, we will continue to refer to a notation such as $\phi(y|x)$ as a "probability" rather than as a "probability density function."] Unless otherwise stated, we work with the special case in which $I = |D|$ and, for every label x_i, there is a distribution that assigns (independently) a probability $\varphi(y_i|x_i)$ to every gray-value y_i, for $0 \leq i \leq I - 1$. Consequently,

$$\phi(y|x) = \prod_{i=0}^{I-1} \varphi(y_i|x_i). \tag{12.3}$$

For example, in electron microscopy applications, a gray value y_i is the density of the Voronoi neighborhood of the lattice point i, for $0 \leq i \leq I - 1$; and the probabilities $\varphi(y_i|x_i)$ intend to model the histograms in Fig. 12.1; i.e., the uncertainty of the density around the average density, denoted by μ_{x_i}, corresponding to the label x_i.

12.2.3 The Measurements

Let $\mathbf{W}$ be a set of *measurement vectors*, each of which is a J-dimensional column vector $w = (w_0, \ldots, w_{J-1})^t$, where $w_j \in W \subseteq \mathbb{R}$, for $0 \leq j \leq J - 1$. We assume that there is a conditional distribution that, given a gray-value image y, assigns a probability $\chi(w|y)$ to every measurement vector w. Usually, w is related to a linear transformation z of the gray-value image

$$z = Ry, \tag{12.4}$$

where R is of size $J \times I$ with fixed coefficients and none of the rows of R is a null vector. Here two cases are studied: one in which R is the identity matrix (thus, $J = I$) and the other one in which R is the *projection matrix* [21].

The first case is based on current approaches of first reconstructing the gray-value image followed by a segmentation. If the gray-value reconstruction were perfect; i.e., the measurement is the gray-value image itself ($w = y$), then the resulted segmented image would be the best one can expect from current techniques. This idealistic situation provides us with an "upper bound" on the quality of the label reconstruction by a current approach.

The second case reflects real tomography applications, in which the measurement data are a set of *projections*, each of which is usually modeled as the measured (hence, noisy) integrals of the density of the object being reconstructed along lines that either are parallel to each other or share a point. In our framework, this can be modeled by setting the entry r_{ji} of R to be the length of intersection between the line j and the Voronoi neighborhood of the point i.

For the experiments reported here, we work with the special case in which $\chi(w|y)$ has a product form; i.e., given a gray-value image y, there is (for $0 \le j \le J - 1$) a conditional probability $\psi_j(w_j|y)$ of the jth measurement being w_j, and

$$\chi(w|y) = \prod_{j=0}^{J-1} \psi_j(w_j|y). \tag{12.5}$$

12.2.4 The Posterior Probability

The *likelihood* $\eta(w|x)$ of measuring w given a label image x, assuming (as reasonable) that w does not depend on x given y, is the integral (or sum if Y is discrete)

$$\eta(w|x) = \int_{\mathbf{Y}} \chi(w|y)\phi(y|x)dy. \tag{12.6}$$

By invoking Bayes' rule, the posterior probability $\theta(x|w)$ of x given the measurement w is proportional to the product of the prior probability $\pi(x)$ and the likelihood $\eta(w|x)$:

$$\theta(x|w) = \frac{\pi(x)\eta(w|x)}{Prob(w)} \propto \pi(x)\eta(w|x). \tag{12.7}$$

12.3 Optimization Criteria: The MAP and the MPM Estimators

Because the exact or perfect solution rarely exists, inexact but optimal (in some sense) solutions are usually sought instead. Since the model for the prior as well as the model for likelihood of the data are available to us by assumption, it seems natural to seek a solution from the Bayesian point of view. In Bayesian estimation theory, estimators are studied in terms of *loss functions* [48].

For a given measurement w, let $\widehat{x}(w)$ denote an estimator that hopefully is "close" to the unknown x. The loss of estimating a true x by $\widehat{x}$ is measured by a symmetric "distance" or loss function $\widetilde{C}(x, \widehat{x}) \geq 0$ with the convention that $\widetilde{C}(x, x) = 0$. Given a loss function $\widetilde{C}(x, \widehat{x})$, a posterior probability $\theta(x|w)$, and a measurement vector w, the Bayes risk is defined as

$$\widetilde{R}(\widetilde{C}, \widehat{x}, w) = \sum_{x \in \Lambda^D} \widetilde{C}(x, \widehat{x}(w))\,\theta(x|w). \qquad (12.8)$$

An estimator $\widehat{x}(w)$ that minimizes this risk is known as a *Bayes estimator*.

Two much-used loss functions are the *all-or-none loss function* $[\widetilde{C}_0(x, \widehat{x})$, which equals 0 if $\widehat{x} = x$ and is 1 otherwise], and the *Hamming loss function* $[\widetilde{C}_0(x, \widehat{x})$, which is the number of points at which $\widehat{x}$ and x differ]. The former gives rise to the popular *maximum a posteriori probability* (MAP) estimator

$$x^{MAP}(w) = \arg \max_{x \in \Lambda^D} [\theta(x|w)], \qquad (12.9)$$

whereas the latter corresponds to the *marginal posterior mode* (MPM) estimator, whose ith element is the label that maximizes the marginal posterior

$$x_i^{MPM} = \arg \max_{x_i^* \in \Lambda} \theta(x_i^*|w), \qquad (12.10)$$

for $i = 0, \dots, |D| - 1$.

12.4 Approximation to the Posterior Probability

Two challenges concern the estimation. First, computing the exact MAP or the MPM estimators implies, respectively, the finding of the maximum of the posterior probability or its marginal. Unfortunately, closed and explicit forms for these optima do not exist and neither do efficient deterministic algorithms for finding them. In such a situation, *Markov Chain Monte Carlo* (MCMC) [6] methods might be the only feasible recourse. In particular, for the MAP estimator, because of the nonlinearity and the nonconvexity of the posterior probability, the optimum cannot be obtained via local search techniques, unless a suboptimal estimator is sought. We found that a local method, such as the one known as *iterated conditional mode* [5], yields results that are not nearly as good as those provided by our approaches. As for other local methods, such as *relaxation labeling* [42], it has been suggested in [31] that it often produces solutions with risk that is well above the attainable minimal risk. As a consequence, we restrict our attention to global methods. In addition to nonconvexity, the posterior (probability) is defined on discrete labels; therefore, a combinatorial optimization technique needs to be used.

The second challenge has to do with the fact that the complicated nature of the posterior (specifically, the likelihood term involves a multidimensional integration) does not make possible an efficient sampling in the MCMC method; or at least we are not aware of such. Therefore, we investigated the existence of alternative approaches that not only can be efficiently implemented but also deliver good reconstructions. We propose the *pseudo-likelihood* (PL) approximation. We also investigated the *mean-by-the-mode likelihood* approximation, but we do not show its results because they are not better than those produced by PL when noise is high (which is likely to be the case in our applications). It is, however, a good approximation only when the noise is low [32].

Prior to introducing the PL approximation, we study the case when the probabilities involved are normally distributed, because then there is a closed form for the likelihood, and the approximation error can be easily calculated.

12.4.1 Normality Assumption

In practice, it is not unreasonable to assume normally distributed gray values and measurements. Thus, in all the discussions (although some of them do not require this assumption) and the experiments, the probabilities $\phi(y|x)$ in (12.3) and $\chi(w|y)$ in (12.5) are restricted to be normally distributed.

Let $\phi(y|x)$ be a normal distribution with mean vector μ_x and covariance matrix Σ_x; i.e.,

$$\phi(y|x) = Normal\,(\mu_x, \Sigma_x) \tag{12.11}$$

and $Y = \mathbb{R}$. We work with the special case in which $\Sigma_x = \mathrm{diag}_{0 \le i \le I-1}(\sigma_{x_i}^2)$ is positive definite. We assume that the measurement is a (Gaussian) noisy linear transformation, as in (12.4), of the gray-value image; i.e.,

$$\chi(w|y) = Normal\,(Ry, \Sigma_w), \tag{12.12}$$

where Σ_w is the covariance matrix of the noise; we consider the case in which $\Sigma_w = \mathrm{diag}_{0 \le j \le J-1}(\sigma_{w_j}^2)$ is also positive definite.

It is convenient to view the gray-value image y and the measurement vector w as instances, respectively, of the associated random vectors $\mathbf{y}$ and $\mathbf{w}$. Accordingly, (12.11) implies that

$$\mathbf{y} \sim Normal\,(\mu_x, \Sigma_x), \tag{12.13}$$

and (12.12) implies that

$$\mathbf{w} = R\mathbf{y} + \mathbf{n}, \tag{12.14}$$

where $\mathbf{n}$ is the random vector associated with the measurement noise; i.e., $\mathbf{n} \sim Normal\,(0, \Sigma_w)$.

A result in probability theory [27] establishes that $R\mathbf{y}$ is a normally distributed random vector with mean $R\mu_x$ and covariance $R\Sigma_x R^t$. Knowing this and assuming (as reasonable) that $R\mathbf{y}$ and $\mathbf{n}$ are uncorrelated, we have the probability law for the likelihood

$$\eta(w|x) = Normal\left(R\mu_x, R\Sigma_x R^t + \Sigma_w\right). \tag{12.15}$$

More explicitly, if we set $\mu_w = R\mu_x$ and $\Sigma_{wx} = R\Sigma_x R^t + \Sigma_w$, then

$$\eta(w|x) = \frac{1}{(2\pi)^{J/2} |\Sigma_{wx}|^{1/2}} \exp[-\frac{1}{2}(w - \mu_w)^t \Sigma_{wx}^{-1}(w - \mu_w)], \tag{12.16}$$

where Σ_{wx} is also positive definite, because so are Σ_x and Σ_w by assumption.

12.4.2 The Pseudo-Likelihood (PL) Approximation

We approximate the likelihood in (12.6) by the *pseudo-likelihood* (PL) that is defined as

$$\eta_{PL}(w|x) \doteq \prod_{j=0}^{J-1} \varsigma_j(w_j|x), \tag{12.17}$$

where $\varsigma_j(w_j|x)$, for $j = 0, \ldots, J-1$, is the likelihood (probability) of observing w_j given x; i.e., it is the marginal

$$\varsigma_j(w_j|x) = \int_{W_j} \eta(w'|x)dw', \tag{12.18}$$

where

$$W_j = \left\{w' \mid w'_j = w_j\right\} \tag{12.19}$$

[the integral in (12.18) is replaced by a sum if $\mathbf{W}$ is discrete]. The *pseudo-posterior* $\theta_{PL}(x|w)$ is obtained by replacing $\eta(w|x)$ by $\eta_{PL}(w|x)$ in (12.7). The introduction of the PL in (12.9) and (12.10) by replacing $\eta(w|x)$ by $\eta_{PL}(w|x)$ in (12.7) gives rise to, respectively, the *pseudo-MAP* (P-MAP) *estimator*

$$x^{PMAP} = \arg\max_x \theta_{PL}(x|w), \tag{12.20}$$

and the *pseudo-MPM* (P-MPM) *estimator*

$$x_i^{PMPM} = \arg\max_{x_i \in \Lambda} \theta_{PL}(x_i|w), \tag{12.21}$$

for $i = 0, \ldots, I - 1$.

The PL approximation is justified when, e.g., the measurements are very noisy. It assumes they are statistically independent. This is valid in many tomography problem settings [24, 45, 46], but unfortunately it is not so in our framework, because of the dependencies coupled by the gray values. Intuitively, however, it is reasonable to argue that these dependencies are rather "weak" when noise is high. We now establish a relationship between the true likelihood and the PL under the normality assumption.

In this case, the marginal distributions $\varsigma_j(w_j|x)$ in (12.18) becomes, noting (12.15),

$$\varsigma_j(w_j|x) = Normal\left(\mu_{w_j}, \sigma^2_{PLj}\right), \tag{12.22}$$

where, for $0 \leq j \leq J-1$, μ_{w_j} is the jth element of $\mu_w = R\mu_x$ and $\sigma^2_{PLj} = r_j^t \Sigma_x r_j + \sigma^2_{w_j} > 0$, with r_j being the transpose of the jth row of R. Hence, the PL becomes

$$\eta_{PL}(w|x) = Normal\left(\mu_w, \Sigma_{PL}\right), \tag{12.23}$$

where we have set $\Sigma_{PL} = \mathrm{diag}_{0 \leq j \leq J-1}(\sigma^2_{PLj})$. A closer look tells us that Σ_{PL} is, in fact, the diagonal part of Σ_{wx} in (12.16); thus, we can set $\Sigma_{wx} = \Sigma_{PL} - \Re$, where the entries of $\Re$ are the off-diagonal elements of Σ_{wx} but with negative sign. If $\eta_{PL}(w|x)$ were a good approximation to $\eta(w|x)$, then Σ_{PL} should be also a good approximation to Σ_{wx}. Assuming that $\left|\Sigma_{PL}^{-1}\Re\right| < 1$, one can think of Σ_{PL}^{-1} as the 0th-order approximation to $\Sigma_{wx}^{-1} = (\Sigma_{PL} - \Re)^{-1}$ in the series expansion

$$\Sigma_{wx}^{-1} = \Sigma_{PL}^{-1}\left(I_J - \Sigma_{PL}^{-1}\Re\right)^{-1} = \Sigma_{PL}^{-1}\left(I_J + \Sigma_{PL}^{-1}\Re + \cdots\right). \tag{12.24}$$

The condition $\left|\Sigma_{PL}^{-1}\Re\right| < 1$ is generally true when, e.g., the noise level is high, which is the case in electron tomography; hence, the PL is a good approximation to the true likelihood.

12.5 Reconstruction Algorithms

As already mentioned in Section 12.4, we resort to MCMC types of algorithms if we are interested in finding global optima. In particular, for MAP estimators, *simulated annealing* [9, 29] are suitable for searching in a high-dimensional discrete space. For the MPM estimator, the modes can be estimated simply by sampling the posterior probability. In fact, both simulated annealing and sampling can be carried out by MCMC algorithms.

12.5.1 Metropolis Algorithm for Finding the MAP and the MPM Estimators

Since simulated annealing can be considered a sequence of sampling algorithms, each of which is at a fixed temperature that slowly decreases according to an *annealing schedule* [18], our optimization task becomes a sampling task that can be carried out, e.g., via the *Metropolis algorithm* [6, 38]. In each step of this algorithm, the ratio $\gamma(x^{(n')})/\gamma(x^{(u)})$ is calculated, where γ is the target distribution and $x^{(u)}$ and $x^{(n')}$ are, respectively, the current state (image) and a "tentative" image for the next state. Here $x^{(n')}$ and $x^{(u)}$ differ at only one randomly selected point. The next state $x^{(n)}$ is equal to $x^{(n')}$ with probability $\min\{1, \gamma(x^{(n')})/\gamma(x^{(u)})\}$. A *cycle* of the Metropolis algorithm consists of $|D|$ (the size of the image) such steps. Since typically a large number of cycles is required, it is highly desirable that the ratio can be computed efficiently. The distribution γ in our case is proportional to $[\pi(x)\eta_{PL}(w|x)]^{1/T}$: T either changes according to an annealing schedule (for MAP estimators) or is fixed at 1 (for MPM estimators). For efficiency, we adopt a strategy very similar to that in [47], in which the value of T is absorbed into the computation of (pre-generated pseudo-) random numbers needed during the sampling. Thus, we only need to be concerned with the distribution γ itself for both estimators. In translating [47] to our problem, we have to precalculate and store all the possible values of the log-ratio of the likelihood term

$$\log\left[\frac{\eta_{PL}(w|x^{(n')})}{\eta_{PL}(w|x^{(u)})}\right]. \tag{12.25}$$

12.5.2 Implementation of the Reconstruction Algorithms

Following the discussions in Subsection 12.5.1, here we concentrate on the target distribution $\theta_{PL}(x|w) \propto \pi(x)\eta_{PL}(w|x)$ for both the MAP and the MPM estimators. Using (12.23), the log ratio in (12.25) under the normality assumption is

$$\log\left[\frac{\eta_{PL}\left(w|x^{(n')}\right)}{\eta_{PL}\left(w|x^{(u)}\right)}\right] = \sum_{j:r_{ij}\neq 0} \log\frac{\sigma_{PLj}\left(x^{(u)}\right)}{\sigma_{PLj}\left(x^{(n')}\right)} \tag{12.26}$$

$$+ \sum_{j:r_{ij}\neq 0}\left[\frac{\left(r_j^t\mu_{x^{(u)}} - w_j\right)^2}{2\sigma_{PLj}^2\left(x^{(u)}\right)} - \frac{\left(r_j^t\mu_{x^{(n')}} - w_j\right)^2}{2\sigma_{PLj}^2\left(x^{(n')}\right)}\right],$$

where $x^{(n')}$ and $x^{(u)}$ differ only at the ith point and, from Subsection 12.4.2,

$$\sigma_{PLj}^2 = r_j^t\Sigma_x r_j + \sigma_{w_j}^2. \tag{12.27}$$

   In order for the the log ratio in (12.27) to be precalculated exactly and efficiently stored, we let the elements of r_j (for $0 \leq j \leq J - 1$) have only a few (one, in our experiments) possible nonzero values (see later in Subsection 12.6.2). Specifically, suppose that there are exactly T_j nonzero elements of r_j, all having a same value. Then, since we are dealing with binary images, there can be only $T_j + 1$ possible values for the expressions $r_j^t\mu_{x^{(u)}}$, $r_j^t\mu_{x^{(n')}}$, and $r_j^t\Sigma_x r_j$ in (12.27) and (12.27). Each value depends solely on the number of grid points (ranging from 0 to T_j) that are labeled black or white along the line corresponding to the jth measurement. Therefore, given w_j and $\sigma_{w_j}^2$, we need only to precalculate and store $T_j + 1$ values for the jth measurement.

12.6 Experiments

Given some (2D or 3D) phantoms that are label images, we generated their corresponding gray-value images (one gray-value image for each phantom) and simulated the projections taken from the gray-value images. Our task is to estimate the label images from the projections and to evaluate the reconstruction quality, which in this case is indicated by the average percentage of misclassified labels as well as (in the 3D case) by the area under a *receiver operating characteristic* (ROC) curve [40, 49].

We tested our estimators and compared them with the iterated conditional mode (ICM) approach [5] and a current method [using an *algebraic reconstruction technique* (ART) [19, 21]] of first reconstructing the gray-value image and then segmenting it to obtain the label image. ART has proven to outperform several algorithms for various tasks [22, 28, 35, 44]. We also investigated the approach discussed in Subsection 12.2.3 in which we assume a perfect reconstruction of the gray-value image and then segment it using an optimal threshold. Both 2D and 3D reconstructions were studied, and a methodology for objective comparison of algorithms [17, 26] was applied.

12.6.1 The General Setting

In all the experiments we took binary (two-label) images: We used black (or 0) to represent ice and white (or 1) to represent protein. The product structure of $\phi(y|x)$ implies that for a label image, a gray-value image can be obtained by sampling at each pixel according to the probability $\varphi(y_i|x_i)$, for $0 \leq i \leq I-1$. Normality is assumed in all the experiments. The $\varphi(y_i|x_i)$, for $0 \leq i \leq I-1$, is taken to be normally distributed with mean μ_{x_i} and variance $\sigma_{x_i}^2$, where $\mu_{x_i} = \sigma_{x_i}^2$, $\mu_0 = 4$, and $\mu_1 = 9$. However, for the projection data simulation, to avoid negative densities (gray values), the value of y at a pixel was set to zero whenever it was negative according to $\varphi(y_i|x_i)$; this happens only with probability less than 0.028 if $x_i = 0$ and less than 0.01 if $x_i = 1$. There is no particular reason for choosing these values of mean and variance, except for the fact that they reflect the idea of overlapping histograms in Fig. 12.1.

The significance of the differences in reconstruction quality (as measured by the average percentage of misclassified labels) between two estimators is measured using the t-test, which produces the P-value [39]. A low P-value (usually less than 0.05) indicates that the null hypothesis that the two estimators have the same performance can be rejected in favor of the alternative hypothesis, which states that the respective qualities do differ.

12.6.2 2D Experimental Details

To assess the usefulness of Gibbs priors, we first took phantoms of size $I = 63 \times 63$, which are true random samples from a GD, namely, the one that

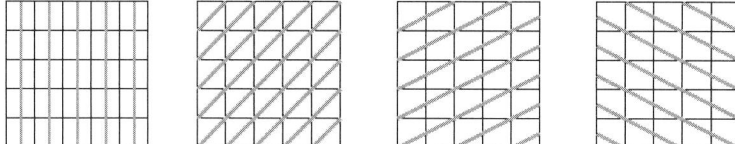

Fig. 12.4. Illustration on a 5×5 image of the chosen projection lines, so that the length of intersection of a line with a pixel is the same in the direction with tangent equal to (respectively from left to right) infinity, 1, 0.5, and -0.5. Ninety-degree rotations of these directions give the directions with tangents equal to, respectively, $0, -1, -2$, and 2.

generated the leftmost image of Fig. 12.3. We then also considered label images that represent the cross section of a macromolecule.

The projections forming the measurement vector w were simulated as follows. There were either four or eight projections using parallel lines in each projection, such that the tangent of the angle, denoted by α, between these lines and the "positive horizontal direction" is 0, infinity, -1, and 1 in the case of four projections and it is 0, infinity, -1, 1, -0.5, 0.5, -2, and 2 in the case of eight projections. We chose parallel lines so that the nonzero lengths of intersections of a line with the pixels are all the same in one direction; see Fig. 12.4.

This choice is not a necessary condition for validity of the our approaches, but it simplifies their implementation. For each experiment we formed a J-dimensional column vector $z = (z_1, \ldots, z_J)^t$ from the sums of the pixel values in the gray-value image along the J lines in all the projections.

We chose $\psi_j(w_j|y)$, for $0 \le j \le J - 1$, to be normally distributed with mean z_j, and we initially intended to set the variance to be $\sigma_{wj}^2 = N \cdot z_j$. We call N the *noise level*, whose values were chosen to be $0.25, 1.0$, or 4.0. Since it is possible that $z_j = 0$, which would not produce a positive definite (diagonal) covariance matrix Σ_w in (12.12), we replace σ_{wj}^2 by $N \cdot \tilde{w}_j = N \cdot \max(\mu_0, w_j)$, where w_j is sampled from $\psi_j(w_j|y)$. The preceding is how we modeled $\psi_j(w_j|\mathbf{y})$ in the algorithms. For the simulated noisy projections, to avoid negative w_j we set $w_j = \tilde{w}_j$, for $j = 0, \ldots J - 1$. For a justification, see [32].

For the P-MAP estimators, we ran $5 \cdot 10^4$ cycles of the Metropolis algorithm for each temperature T, where $1/T$ ranged from 0.5 to 1.4 in increments of 0.05. We did not observe significant improvements by increasing the range (from 0.5 to up to 2) of $1/T$. For the P-MPM estimator, we took a total of 1000 samples for computing the mode, and each sample was obtained by running $2 \cdot 10^4$ cycles (which is sufficient for the burn-in). A mode based on 1000 samples was practically the same as that based on 5000 samples.

Table 12.1. Percentage of Misclassification in the PL Approximation (N is the Noise Level)

Method	$N = 0.25$	$N = 1.0$	$N = 4.0$
P-MAP with 4 projections	7.0 ± 4.0	9.4 ± 5.1	14.9 ± 6.5
P-MPM with 4 projections	5.4 ± 2.2	7.2 ± 3.3	11.9 ± 4.3
P-MAP with 8 projections	3.4 ± 1.4	4.8 ± 1.8	9.8 ± 3.5
P-MPM with 8 projections	2.8 ± 1.0	4.0 ± 1.4	7.7 ± 2.7

12.6.3 2D Experimental Results

Table 12.1 reports on the quality of the two estimators for the three noise levels. It demonstrates the superiority of the P-MPM estimator to the P-MAP estimator with P-values (see Subsection 12.6.1) that are less than 10^{-4} for all the noise levels. Figure 12.5 shows some actual reconstructions.

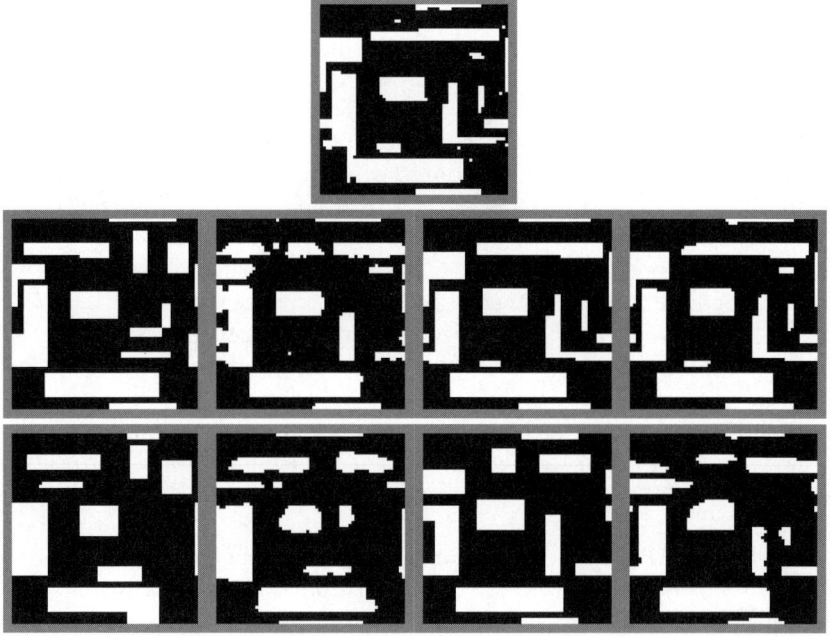

Fig. 12.5. Reconstructions of label images from a true Gibbs distribution. The top image is a phantom. From left to right in the second row are its P-MAP and P-MPM estimates from four projections, and the P-MAP and P-MPM estimators from eight projections; all the reconstructions correspond to the noise level $N = 0.25$, and the number of misclassifications are 600, 391, 182, and 186, respectively. The bottom row, in the same arrangement, corresponds to $N = 4.0$, with the number of misclassification being 893, 719, 482, and 480.

Table 12.2. Percentage of Misclassification (N is the Noise Level)

Method	8 projections, $N = 1.0$
Optimal thresholded gray-value image	6.8 ± 0.2
Optimal thresholded gray-value reconstruction	7.7 ± 0.2
ICM	9.5 ± 0.1
P-MAP	4.1 ± 0.3
P-MPM	3.5 ± 0.2

We also reconstructed binary images that represent a cross section of a macromolecule in four conformations, based on eight projections and with noise level $N = 1.0$. Our approaches require the knowledge of the GD from which the unknown image is a typical sample. To that end, for each of the four images, we estimated the Gibbs prior parameters using the other three images.

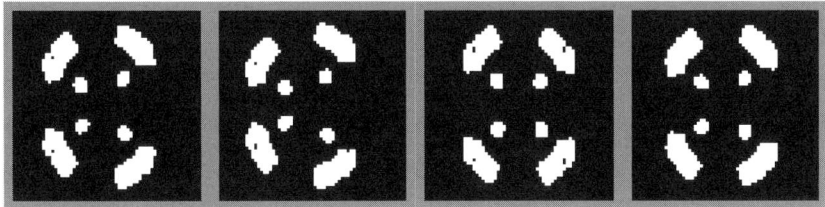

Fig. 12.6. A cross section of a macromolecule in four conformations.

The four conformations are depicted in Fig. 12.6, Table 12.2 reports on the quality of the estimators, and Fig. 12.7 shows actual reconstructions of one phantom. We note that in terms of misclassification, current techniques perform worse than our methods. However, our P-MPM estimator, which has the fewest misclassification, does not fully recover all the features in the original image. Therefore, a different quality indicator ought to be used, such as the area under a ROC curve (see our experiments with 3D images). We also note that, in general, P-MAP estimates are better at recovering small features, but the reconstructed structures are more blocky, a property described as "oversmoothing" in [15].

12.6.4 3D Experimental Details

In the single-axis data-collection scheme [16, 30] in electron microscopy, a main advantage of a fully 3D reconstruction using 3D cliques (as opposed to using 2D cliques and doing a slice-by-slice reconstruction) is the smoothness imposed across neighboring slices. In our discussion ahead, we will, in fact, deal with a set of viewing directions adjusted to the grid points.

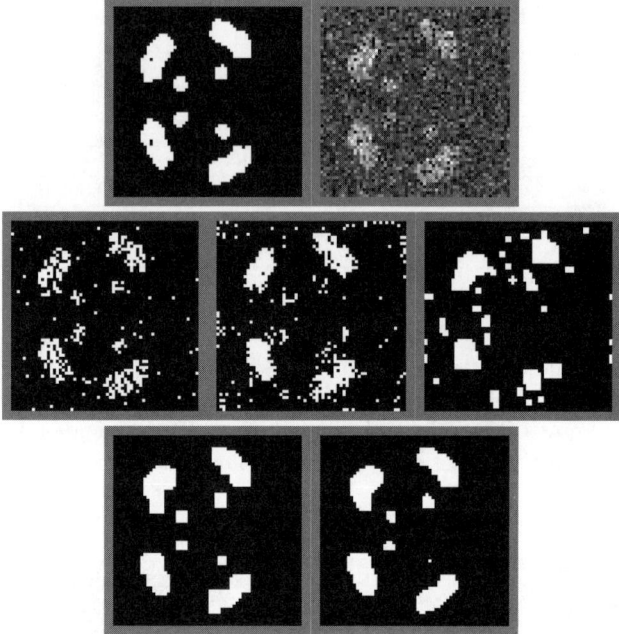

Fig. 12.7. Reconstructions of an image representing the cross section of a macro-molecule. From left to right, in the top row are one phantom and its gray-value image. In the central row are an optimal thresholding of the gray-value image (corresponding to an "ideal" reconstruction by current approaches), the reconstruction by the an ART-with-pixel current approach, and that by the ICM method. The number of misclassification are respectively 272, 319, and 387. In the bottom row are the reconstructions using the estimators P-MAP and P-MPM, whose number of misclassification are, respectively, 147 and 130.

For 3D label images, we define the domain D as a subset of the *face-centered cubic* (FCC) grid F

$$D = \{v = (v_1, v_2, v_3) \mid v \in F \text{ and } 0 \leq v_p < V_p \text{ for } p = 1, 2, 3\}, \qquad (12.28)$$

where

$$F = \left\{ v = (v_1, v_2, v_3) \mid v \in \mathbb{Z}^3, \sum_{p=1}^{3} v_p \equiv 0 (\text{mod} 2) \right\}, \qquad (12.29)$$

and the V_p are positive integers. Apart from a smoother graphic display of a surface [23] when using a FCC grid, its grid points are more "evenly" distributed, and each has fewer (only 12) face-or-edge neighboring grid points than a cubic grid point (that has 18 face-or-edge neighbors). This implies less computational burden in the sampling of Gibbs distributions. Here a grid point and its 12 neighbors constitute a clique. The local features (i.e., configurations on a clique) that we are interested in are black regions, white regions,

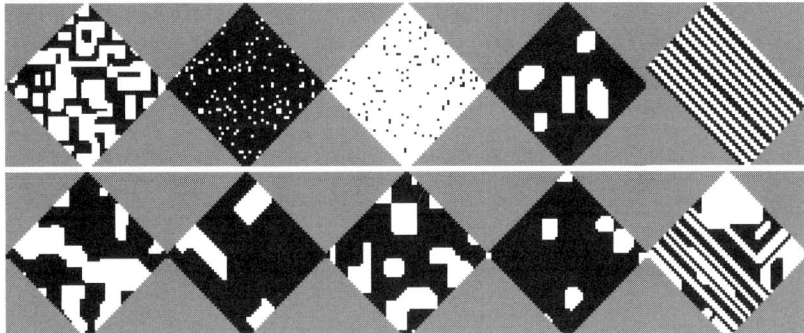

Fig. 12.8. Cross sections (the 30th slice) of typical images corresponding to 10 of our 3D GD models. The first nine cross sections are normal to the direction 3, and the last one is normal to the direction 1.

Cartesian and regular walls, small and large convex corners, and small and large concave corners; see [34] for details. Figure 12.8 shows the cross sections of typical 3D sample images from 10 different GDs, and surface renderings of 4 of the 10 samples are depicted in Fig. 12.9.

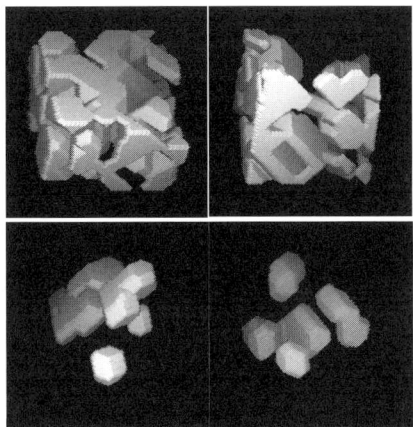

Fig. 12.9. Surface rendering of the samples 1, 3, 4, and 9 of Fig. 12.8 (from left to right and top to bottom).

Phantoms

We considered 3D binary images with domain size such that $V_1 = V_2 = 64$ and $V_3 = 42$ (so that $|D| = 86,016$). Ten phantoms represented biological macromolecules, each of which is a discretization of nine spheres. Near the surface of the top and bottom spheres are four possible locations for a little

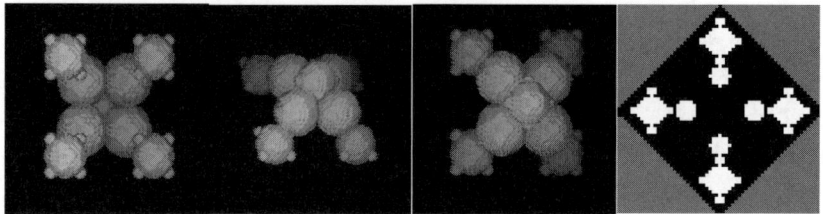

Fig. 12.10. Surface renderings of a phantom and one of its cross sections.

sphere that can be either present or absent with probability 0.5 (so the total number of distinct phantoms is $2^{5 \times 4}$, but we randomly selected 10 of them for the experiments). Figure 12.10 shows the case when all the little spheres are present. The discretization was done by labeling white a grid point (in D) if it is inside or on a sphere, and it is labeled black otherwise. The purpose of introducing the little spheres is to evaluate the detectability of small structures.

For the estimation of the parameters of the GD, we used the 3D model described above and randomly took 100 (different from the previous 10) training phantoms. The number of training images turned out to be more than sufficient, since the estimates do not differ significantly from those based on 1000 or even on 10 training images.

Projection Data

In each projection we took parallel lines that pass through all the grid points in the domain D, and the lengths of intersection with a rhombic-dodecahedron voxel have all the same value. Nine projections with such a property are in the direction $(0, 1, 1)$, $(0, -1, 1)$, $(1, 0, 1)$, $(-1, 0, 1)$, $(1, 1, 0)$, $(-1, 1, 0)$, $(1, 0, 0)$, $(0, 1, 0)$, and $(0, 0, 1)$. Neither the condition of passing through all the grid points, nor the condition that the intersection length must be equal in one projection, is necessary for the validity of the our approaches, but together they simplify the implementation. For the jth line ($j = 0, \ldots, J - 1$), we computed the line integral z_j of the gray values inside the mathematically described images as follows. Let l_0 and l_1 be, respectively, the lengths of intersection of the line with the spheres and with the background. Then z_j was assumed to come from a normal distribution with mean and variance equal to $\mu_0 l_0 + \mu_1 l_1$, where $\mu_0 = 4$ and $\mu_1 = 9$. To avoid negativity, we set z_j to 0 whenever it was sampled negative (with probability less than 0.028 in only a few measurements). Our $\psi_j(w_j|y)$ in the algorithms was considered to be normally distributed with mean z_j, and we initially intended to set the variance to be $\sigma_{wj}^2 = N \cdot z_j$. To avoid nonpositive variance, we replaced σ_{wj}^2 by $N \cdot \widetilde{w}_j = N \cdot \max(\mu_0, w_j)$, where w_j is sampled from $\psi_j(w_j|y)$. Finally, the simulated measurement was taken to be $\widetilde{w}_j$, similarly to what we did with 2D images.

Reconstruction Methods

Our proposed approaches were compared with conventional approaches of first reconstructing the gray-value image followed by a segmentation. We used ART with blobs [22, 35] for the gray-value reconstruction, followed by an optimal thresholding. The sequence of projections in ART is the same as the one given in the previous subsubsection, and the sequence of lines in one projection was such that no blob intersects two consecutive lines. The parameters for the blobs were obtained based on the *equivalent-grids* criterion of [36] (which determined the grid sampling distance) and the (first and fifth) zero-crossing criterion of [20] (which gave the radius and the rate of decay of the blobs); see [34] for details. The thresholding level was chosen to yield the "correct" relative concentration of the black and white region. Such a concentration was estimated from the training phantoms.

In our methods, we found that we can run fewer cycles for the samplings than in the 2D case. In particular, we ran 3000 cycles to obtain one sample (in total, 500 samples were taken for one P-MPM estimate). We observed that typical energy does not significantly change even if we increased the number of cycles to $5 \cdot 10^5$. We ran 10^4 cycles for each temperature of the simulated annealing for one P-MAP estimate. The annealing schedule was such that $1/T$ ranged from 0.1 to 1.25 with intervals of 0.05. The number of cycles and the annealing schedule were not optimized.

Evaluation

The average percentage of misclassification, which will be denoted by δ, can be regarded to as a *figure of merit* (FOM) in the context of statistical-hypothesis-testing-based methodology [17, 26] for the evaluation of the relative efficacy of two reconstruction methods. A FOM measures how helpful a reconstructed image is for solving a specific problem (or achieving a task) in the application area. (Strictly speaking, the FOM in this case should be $100 - \delta$ instead.)

Here we are interested not only in the "appearance" of the reconstructions but in the detectability of small structures as well. To that end, for each reconstruction we use two measures: One is δ and the other is 100 times the area under a ROC curve. For details on the latter applied to our 3D phantoms, see [32].

12.6.5 3D Experimental Results

In Table 12.3, we report on the quality of the reconstructions using nine projections by the current ART-based approach, the P-MPM estimator, and the P-MAP estimator. Figure 12.11 shows the actual reconstructions of one phantom in one cross section. As far as the measure δ is concerned, in the case $N = 0.01$, the P-MPM estimator is significantly (P-value less than 0.001; see Subsection 12.6.1) the best, followed by the P-MAP estimator, and then the

Table 12.3. Quality of Reconstruction Using Nine Projections, According to δ (percentage of misclassification averaged over the ten testing phantoms; left side) and the Detectability Measure (100× area under a ROC curve; right side) (N is the noise level)

Method	$N = 0.01$	$N = 1.0$	$N = 4.0$	$N = 0.01$	$N = 1.0$	$N = 4.0$
ART	1.36 ± 0.04	1.61 ± 0.05	2.15 ± 0.08	98 ± 4	95 ± 5	95 ± 4
P-MPM	0.97 ± 0.04	1.35 ± 0.07	2.33 ± 0.06	98 ± 3	85 ± 7	73 ± 9
P-MAP	1.19 ± 0.05	1.64 ± 0.08	2.62 ± 0.09	97 ± 4	84 ± 8	68 ± 6

ART estimator. For $N = 1.0$, the P-MPM estimator is still significantly the best, while the comparison between the other two estimators is not significant. For $N = 4.0$, the ART estimator is significantly the best, followed by the P-MPM estimator, and then the P-MAP estimator.

According to the detectability measure (by the area under a ROC curve), for $N = 0.01$, the differences among the three estimators are not significant, and neither are the differences between the P-MPM and the P-MAP estimators at the three noise levels. For $N = 1.0$ and $N = 4.0$, the ART estimator is significantly the best.

12.7 Conclusions and Discussions

We have created 2D and 3D Gibbs prior models that allow us to directly recover the label image from the projection data. We have shown that an MPM type of estimator performs better than an MAP type of estimator.

Our experiments on 2D images indicate that our proposed techniques outperform an ART-with-pixel-based current approach and even an "ideal" current approach (in which the gray-value image is perfectly reconstructed), in terms of misclassification. The P-MPM estimator proved to be the best in general, under that measure.

The results of our experiments on 3D images indicate that although the P-MPM estimator is superior to an ART-with-blob-based current approach in terms of misclassifications (except at the higher noise level), it is not so under a detectability measure.

The main differences between the two sets of experiments are (i) ART with pixel basis was used in 2D and ART with blob basis in 3D, and (ii) the nature of the Gibbs prior. Our 3D reconstructions may be improved by "enhancing" our Gibbs prior model. For example, the cliques of our 3D models are relatively smaller (when looking at a cross section) than those of our 2D models, and (as mentioned in [10, 33]) the reconstruction quality using small cliques can be poor compared to that when using larger ones.

In this work, for estimating the Gibbs distribution from which typical images of an application area are assumed to be samples, we first created a

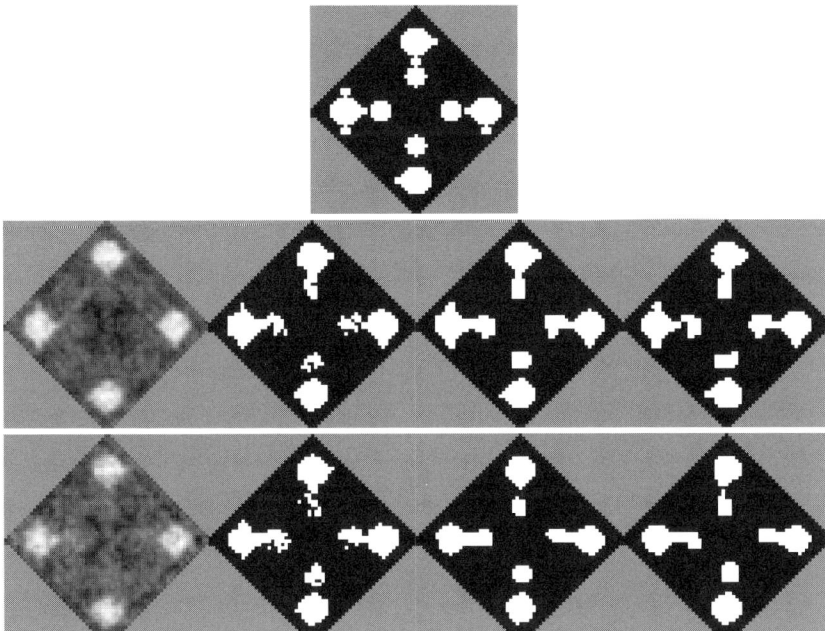

Fig. 12.11. Reconstructions of a 3D phantom (one cross-section). The top image is the phantom. From left to right in the second row are its reconstruction using ART, an optimal segmentation of the ART reconstruction, the P-MPM and P-MAP estimators; all the reconstructions correspond to the noise level $N = 0.01$ and the number misclassification (in the 3D object) are 1231, 888, and 1083. The bottom row, with the same arrangement, corresponds to $N = 4.0$ with 1922, 2069, and 2339 misclassifications. The size of a phantom is 86,016.

model and then estimated the parameters of the Gibbs prior for that model from the images. An interesting open problem is to determine also the model from the images; this means choosing an appropriate set of cliques and local features.

A disadvantage of the MAP estimator is oversmoothing. A weakness of the MPM criterion is the lack of distinction between "scattered" and "aggregated" misclassifications: A modest number of misclassifications are rather harmless if they are scattered, as they would be interpreted as isolated misclassifications, which is not the case if they aggregate into some artifact. Therefore, it is important to develop and study new estimators that would not present such undesirable properties [43].

Acknowledgment

This work was supported by the NIH grant HL70472, by the NSF grant DMS0306125, and by a Mina Rees Fellowship.

References

1. Battle, X.L., Le Rest, A., Turzo, C., Bizais, Y.: Three-dimensional attenuation map reconstruction using geometrical models and free-form deformations. *IEEE Trans. Med. Imag.*, **19**, 404–411 (2000).
2. Battle, X.L., Le Rest, A., Turzo, C. Bizais Y.: Free-form deformation in tomographic reconstruction. Application to attenuation map reconstruction. *IEEE Trans. Nucl. Sci.*, **47**, 1065–1071 (2000).
3. Besag, J.: Statistical analysis of non-lattice data. *The Statistician*, **24**, 179–195 (1975).
4. Besag, J.: Efficiency of pseudo-likelihood estimation for simple Gaussian fields. *Biometrika*, **64**, 616–618 (1977).
5. Besag, J.: On the statistical analysis of dirty pictures. *J. Roy. Statist. Soc. Ser. B*, **48**, 259–302 (1986).
6. Brémaud, P.: *Markov Chains: Gibbs Fields, Monte Carlo Simulation, and Queues*. Springer, New York, NY (1999).
7. Carazo, J.M., Sorzano, C.O., Rietzel, E., Schröder R., Marabini, R.: Discrete tomography in electron microscopy. In: Herman, G.T., Kuba, A. (eds.), *Discrete Tomography: Foundations, Algorithms, and Applications*, Birkhäuser, Boston, MA, pp. 405–416 (1999).
8. Carvalho, B.M., Herman, G.T., Matej, S., Salzberg, C., Vardi, E.: Binary tomography for triplane cardiography. In: Kuba, A., Sámal, M., Todd-Pokropek, A. (eds.) *Information Processing in Medical Imaging*, Springer, Berlin, Germany, pp. 29–41 (1999).
9. Cerney, V.: Thermodynamical approach to the traveling salesmen problem: An efficient simulation algorithm. *J. Optimiz. Theory Appl.*, **45**, 41–51 (1985).
10. Chan, M.T., Herman, G.T., Levitan, E.: Probabilistic modeling of discrete images. In Herman, G.T., Kuba, A. (eds.), *Discrete Tomography: Foundations, Algorithms, and Applications*, Birkhäuser, Boston, MA, pp. 213–235 (1999).
11. Cunningham, G.S., Hanson, K.M, Battle, X.L.: Three-dimensional reconstructions from low-count SPECT data using deformable models. *Opt. Express*, **2**, 227–236 (1998).
12. Dempster, A.P., Laird, N.M., Bubin,D.B.: Maximum likelihood from incomplete data via the EM algorithm. *J. Royal Stat. Soc., Series B*, **39**, 1–38 (1977).
13. Fessler, J.A.: Segmented attenuation correction for PET. In *Proc. IEEE Nuc. Sci. Symp. and Med. Imag. Conf.*, Orlando, FL, pp. 1182–1184 (1992).
14. Fessler, J.A., Macovski, A.: Object-based 3D reconstruction of arterial trees from magnetic resonance angiograms. *IEEE Trans. Med. Imag.*, **10**, 25–39 (1991).
15. Fox, C., Nicholls, G.K.: Exact MAP states and expectations from perfect sampling: Greig, Porteous and Seheult revisited. In Mohammad-Djafari, A. (ed.), *Bayesian Inference and Maximum Entropy Methods in Science and Engineering*, AIP Conference Proceedings, Melville, NY, pp. 252–263 (2001).

16. Frank, J. *Three-Dimensional Electron Microscopy of Macromolecular Assemblies: Visualization of Biological Molecules in Their Native State.* Oxford University Press, New York, NY (1996).

17. Furuie, S.S., Herman, G.T., Narayan, T.K., Kinahan, P., Karp, J.S., Lewitt, R.M., Matej, S.: A methodology for testing for statistically significant differences between fully 3D PET reconstruction algorithms. *Phys. Med. Biol.*, **39**, 341–354 (1994).

18. Geman, S., Geman, D.: Stochastic relaxation, Gibbs distributions, and the Bayesian restoration of images. *IEEE Trans. Pattern Anal. Mach. Intell.*, **6**, 721–741 (1984).

19. Gordon, R., Bender, R., Herman, G.T.: Algebraic reconstruction techniques (ART) for three-dimensional electron microscopy and X-ray photography. *J. Theoret. Biol.*, **29**, 471–482 (1970).

20. Green, J.J.: Approximation with the radial basis functions of Lewitt. In: Leversley, J., Anderson, I., Mason, J.C. (eds.), *Algorithms for Approximation IV*, University of Huddersfield, Huddersfield, UK, pp. 212–219 (2002).

21. Herman, G.T.: *Image Reconstruction from Projections: The Fundamentals of Computerized Tomography.* Academic Press, New York, NY (1980).

22. Herman, G.T.: Algebraic reconstruction techniques in medical imaging. In: Leondes, C.T. (ed.), *Medical Imaging, Systems Techniques and Applications — Computational Techniques*, Gordon and Breach Science Publishers, Amsterdam, The Netherlands, pp. 1–42 (1997).

23. Herman, G.T.: *Geometry of Digital Spaces.* Birkhäuser, Boston, MA (1998).

24. Herman, G.T., De Pierro, A.R, Gai, N.: On methods for maximum a posteriori image reconstruction with a normal prior. *J. Visual Comm. Image Represent.*, **3**, 316–324 (1992).

25. Herman, G.T., Kuba, A. (eds.): *Discrete Tomography: Foundations, Algorithms, and Applications.* Birkhäuser, Boston, MA (1999).

26. Herman, G.T., Meyer, L.B.: Algebraic reconstruction techniques can be made computationally efficient. *IEEE Trans. Med. Imag.*, **12**, 600–609 (1993).

27. Jacobs, I.M., Wozencraft, J.M.: *Principles of Communication Engineering.* Waveland Press, Prospect Hights, IL (1990).

28. Kinahan, P.E., Matej, S., Karp, J.S., Herman, G.T., Lewitt, R.M.: A comparison of transform and iterative reconstruction techniques for a volume-imaging PET scanner with a large acceptance angle. *IEEE Trans. Nucl. Sci.*, **42**, 2281–2287 (1995).

29. Kirkpatrick, S., Gelatt, C.D., Vecchi, M.P.: Optimization by simulated annealing. *Science*, **220**, 671–680 (1983).

30. Kyte, K. (ed.): *Structure in Protein Chemistry.* Garland Publishers, New York, NY (1995).

31. Li, S.Z.: *Markov Random Field Modeling in Image Analysis.* Springer, Tokyo, Japan (2001).

32. Liao, H.Y.: *Reconstruction of Label Images Using Gibbs Priors.* Ph.D. Thesis, City University of New York, New York (2005).

33. Liao, H.Y., Herman, G.T.: Automated estimation of the parameters of Gibbs priors to be used in binary tomography. *Discrete Appl. Math.*, **139**, 149–170 (2004).

34. Liao, H.Y., Herman, G.T.: Discrete tomography with a very few views, using Gibbs priors and a marginal posterior mode. *Electr. Notes Discr. Math.*, **20**, 399-418 (2005).

35. Matej, S., Herman, G.T., Narayan, T.K., Furuie, S.S., Lewitt, R.M., Kinahan, P.: Evaluation of task-oriented performance of several fully 3D PET reconstruction algorithms. *Phys. Med. Biol.*, **39**, 355–367 (1994).

36. Matej, S., Lewitt, R.M.: Efficient 3D grids for image reconstruction using spherically-symmetric volume elements. *IEEE Trans. Nucl. Sci.*, **42**, 1361–1370 (1995).

37. Matej, S., Vardi, A., Herman, G.T., Vardi, E.: Binary tomography using Gibbs priors. In: Herman, G.T., Kuba, A. (eds.), *Discrete Tomography: Foundations, Algorithms, and Applications*, Birkhäuser, Boston, MA, pp. 191–212 (1999).

38. Metropolis, N., Rosenbluth, A.W., Rosenbluth, M.N., Teller, A.H., Teller, E.: Equation of state calculations by fast computing machines. *J. Chem. Phys.*, **21**, 1087–1092 (1953).

39. Montgomery, D.C., Runger, G.C.: *Applied Statistics and Probability for Engineers*, 3rd ed. John Wiley & Sons, New York, NY (2002).

40. Narayan, T.K.: *Evaluation of Image Reconstruction Algorithms by Optimized Numerical Observers*. Ph.D. Thesis, University of Pennsylvania, Philadelphia, PA (1998).

41. Prause, G.P.M., Onnasch, D.G.W.: Binary reconstruction of the heart chamber from biplane angiographic image sequence. *IEEE Trans. Med. Imag.*, **15**, 532–559 (1996).

42. Rosenfeld, A., Hummel, R., Zucker, S.: Scene labeling by relaxation operations. *IEEE Trans. Syst. Man Cyber.*, **6**, 420–433 (1976).

43. Rue, H.: New loss function in Bayesian imaging. *J. Am. Stat. Assoc.*, **90**, 900–908 (1995).

44. Scheres, S.H.W., Marabini, R., Lanzavecchia, S., Cantele, F., Rutten, T., Fuller, S.D., Carazo, J.M., Burnett, R.M., San Martin, C.: Classification of single projection reconstructions for cryo-electron microscopy data of icosahedral viruses. *J. Struct. Biol.*, **151**, 79–91 (2005).

45. Shepp, L.A., Vardi, Y.: Maximum likelihood reconstruction in positron emission tomography. *IEEE Trans. Med. Imag.*, **1**, 113–122 (1982).

46. Sotthivirat, S., Fessler, J.A.: Image recovery using partitioned-separable paraboloidal surrogate coordinate ascent algorithms. *IEEE Trans. Image Process.*, **11**, 306–317 (2002).

47. Vardi, E., Herman, G.T., Kong, T.Y.: Speeding up stochastic reconstructions of binary images from limited projection directions. *Linear Algebra Appl.*, **339**, 75–89 (2001).

48. Winkler, G.: *Image Analysis, Random Fields and Dynamic Monte Carlo Methods*, 2nd ed., Springer, Berlin, Germany (2003).

49. Zhou, X., Obuchowski, N.A., McClish, D.K.: *Statistical Methods in Diagnostic Medicine*. John Wiley & Sons, New York, NY (2002).

13

Discrete Tomography for Generating Grain Maps of Polycrystals

A. Alpers, L. Rodek, H.F. Poulsen, E. Knudsen, and G.T. Herman

Summary. The determination of crystalline structures is a demanding and fundamental task of crystallography. Most crystalline materials, natural or artificial, are in fact polycrystals, composed of tiny crystals called grains. Every grain has an associated average orientation that determines the spatial configuration of the crystalline lattice. Typically, the structure of a polycrystal is rendered via an orientation map or a grain map, in which individual pixels/voxels are assigned a grain orientation or a grain label. We present two related approaches to reconstructing a 2D grain map of a polycrystal from X-ray diffraction patterns. The first technique makes the assumption that each grain is actually a perfect crystal, i.e., that the specimen is not deformed. The other method can be applied also when the sample has been exposed to moderate levels of deformation. In both cases, the grain map is produced by a Bayesian discrete tomographic algorithm that uses Gibbs priors. The optimization of the objective function is accomplished via the Metropolis algorithm. The efficacy of the techniques is demonstrated by simulation experiments.

13.1 Introduction

In nature most materials such as rocks, ice, sand, and soil appear as aggregates comprised of a set of small crystals. Similarly, modern society is built on applications of metals, ceramics and other "hard materials," which are also polycrystalline.

An example of an undeformed *polycrystal* is shown in Fig 13.1. The individual crystals are known as *grains*. Each grain is characterized by its position and shape as well as by the orientation of the 3D *crystalline lattice* (the discrete lattice of atom positions). The latter property is known as the *grain orientation*. The physical, chemical, and mechanical properties of the material are to a large extent governed by the geometrical features of this 3D complex, including neighboring effects (such as the correlation between the orientation of two neighboring grains and the morphology of the boundary separating them). Remarkably, until recently, no nondestructive methods existed for visualizing the grains in 3D. Studies of grains could be performed

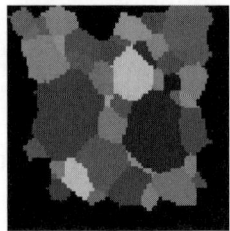

Fig. 13.1. Grain map of an undeformed aluminum polycrystal. The orientation of the crystalline lattice (represented by a gray scale) within each grain is constant.

only by sectioning the sample and characterizing the surface by, e.g., optical or electron microscopy. This way does not allow us to follow the evolution of the 3D complex as function of time, e.g., to visualize the growth or shrinkage of a grain when the sample is heated. As a consequence of this lack of experimental studies, existing models of basic industrial processes, such as deformation and annealing, are grossly simplified and typically only deal with average properties of the grains.

Three-dimensional X-ray diffraction (3DXRD) is a novel experimental method for characterization of polycrystalline materials [24]. Its primary goal is to provide 3D grain maps (3D equivalents of Fig. 13.1) and even 3D movies by repeated in situ acquisitions of 3D grain maps during the relevant treatment of the sample. The method is based on reconstruction using X-rays with a set-up similar to that of conventional transmission tomography. The vital difference is that in computerized tomography the absorption of the incident beam through the sample is probed, while in 3DXRD the diffracted beam is probed as it diverges from the sample on the exit side. The *diffraction pattern* on the detector typically is composed of a set of distinct *diffraction spots*. Acquiring images at a set of rotation angles, each grain gives rise to ≈5–30 spots, with positions and intensity distributions determined by the local orientation of the crystalline lattice. A sketch of the data collection methodology is shown in Fig. 13.2.

Note that the data acquisition is similar to what is usual in discrete tomography (DT), with the important difference that the diffraction spots do not correspond to measured sums along straight lines, but rather correspond to measured sums taken over more general sets. Our approach differs in this sense from approaches formerly known in the DT literature.

The first 3DXRD grain maps were reconstructed in 2003 by applying a constrained variant of the algebraic reconstruction technique (ART) [25]. From these and other studies [20, 23], it has become clear that this approach has severe limitations:

(a) The grain map is generated by patching together reconstructions for individual grains. Each of these reconstructions is originally represented as a real-valued function, and subsequently binarized by using a threshold.

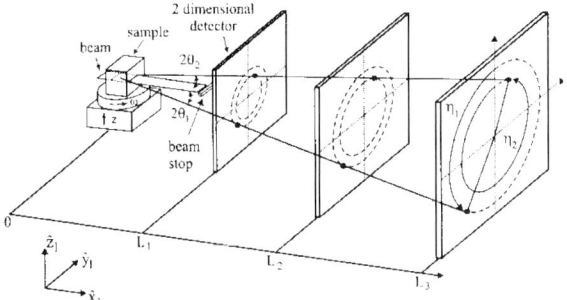

Fig. 13.2. Sketch of the 3DXRD geometry. Detectors are positioned perpendicular to the beam at distances L_1, L_2, and L_3.

The resulting grain maps often show unphysical ambiguous areas near the grain boundaries, where some parts may be associated with more than one grain and some with none.

(b) For each grain, the nature of the diffraction process implies that there is only a finite set of possible projections. The exact number depends on the experiment, but it may be as low as 5. This sparsity of data interferes with the aim of obtaining high-quality grain maps.

(c) It is of major interest to extend the concept of 3D mapping to deformed materials. While the ART formalism can be generalized to this case [23], the demands for computer power have so far prohibited such solutions.

Fortunately, the grain structure exhibits additional properties, which may be exploited in the reconstruction:

(a) The grains can be approximated by discrete objects in the sense that a given voxel in the sample belongs either fully to a given grain or not at all.

(b) The grains are simply-connected 3D space-filling objects within the borders given by the sample geometry.

(c) The grain boundaries are smooth.

(d) The physics underlying the generation of the structure implies that grain maps tend to resemble each other, once they have been scaled to the average grain size. Hence, it is possible to describe local properties statistically.

These arguments suggest that tools from discrete tomography [15] should be well suited for the reconstruction of grain maps. In this work, we investigate the prospect of using Bayesian discrete tomographic algorithms that employ Gibbs priors. Our exposition is based on the papers [1, 2, 26].

The outline of this chapter is as follows. We define the concepts of orientation maps and grain maps in Section 13.2. Unit quaternions are shown to be appropriate for representing orientations. In Section 13.3, we present our approach for undeformed specimens. The quality of the reconstructed maps is demonstrated and quantified by simulation studies. Similarly, in Section 13.4, the formalism and simulation results for the moderately deformed case are given. Section 13.5 concludes with a discussion and outlook.

13.2 Orientations and Grains

In a crystalline material, the atoms are arranged in a three-dimensional discrete lattice. The grain can be fully characterized by two properties:

(a) The *lattice*, $\mathcal{L} = \{x\mathbf{a} + y\mathbf{b} + z\mathbf{c} \mid x, y, z \in \mathbb{Z}\}$, where $\mathbf{a}, \mathbf{b}, \mathbf{c} \in \mathbb{R}^3$ are given vectors not all lying in the same plane and $\mathbb{Z}$ is the set of all integers. Notably, for a given lattice, a number of symmetry operations may exist (such as inversions, rotations, and mirror operations) that map the lattice onto itself. Lattices that are invariant under such operations are said to exhibit *crystal symmetries*.

(b) The *orientation* of the lattice. Notably, due to crystal symmetries, distinct rotations of the lattice may result in the same orientation.

Most crystalline materials are polycrystals. In case of an *undeformed specimen*, the lattice within each grain is near-perfect. As such, each grain can be associated with exactly one orientation. Let a 2D section of the specimen of interest, D, be discretized into a set of pixels. We define a *grain map* f as a function mapping the finite domain $D \subseteq \mathbb{Z}^2$ into $\{1, \ldots, l\}$, where the integer l is the number of grains in the map. Clearly, if i and j are pixels in the same grain, then $f(i) = f(j)$. We further define an *orientation map* o as a function mapping D into the set of unit quaternions (see Subsection 13.2.1). For undeformed specimens, o has to fulfill $f(i) = f(j) \Rightarrow o(i) = o(j)$ for all pixels i and j within the same grain, whereas this need not be true in the deformed case.

If an initially undeformed specimen is deformed, the boundaries between grains get distorted. At the same time, the lattice is no longer homogeneous within each grain, but there is a spatial variation of orientation. With increasing amount of deformation, these distortions become larger and larger. In the following we confine ourselves to *moderate* degrees of *deformation*, which refers to the case in which it is possible to derive the corresponding grain map from a given orientation map.

Algorithms producing grain maps from given orientation maps are standard in the analysis of electron microscopy data [4]. They are based on the class of image analysis tools known as *connected component* or *labeling* routines. These techniques classify the pixels of an image into so-called regions by assigning a unique region label to every pixel.

The aim of this chapter is to establish algorithms that—given 3DXRD data—reconstruct both grain maps and orientation maps. The simultaneous reconstruction has several advantages, such as speed of computation and the fact that DT tools can be applied. Additionally, many applications demand an accurate determination of both orientation maps and grain maps.

In the following, we will assume throughout that the sample is a monophase polycrystal of a known material, implying that all grains have the same a priori known crystal structure.

13.2.1 Representation of Orientations by Unit Quaternions

Different kinds of formalisms exist to describe orientations. A common approach is to describe an orientation by a rotation in 3D space—the rotation that has to be performed to obtain the actual arrangement of grain atoms, starting from a fixed reference system. In this way, orientations and rotations seem to be synonyms of the same idea. The issue of crystalline orientations is, however, more complicated: The same orientation can sometimes be achieved by two or more quite different rotations, due to the crystal symmetries.

It is critical to choose an appropriate representation for orientations. For example, it is important that every orientation of interest can indeed be represented. Furthermore, the scheme should provide a simple and useful way of visualization; it should include a notion of "distance" or "dissimilarity" $d(o_1, o_2)$ between a pair (o_1, o_2) of orientations, and it should allow easy/fast computations, for example, for the "composition" of two orientations.

Representation by unit quaternions has several well-known advantages, such as that there is a metric based on the norm of the 4D vectors of quaternion components (see Subsection 13.2.2) and there is a continuous correspondence between unit quaternions and points on a 4D sphere of unit radius. In the following, we summarize the most important properties of unit quaternions, mainly focusing on how they represent 3D rotations. Before proceeding with the exposition, however, a few notes are in order concerning different aspects of orientations.

It is a well-known fact that any rigid transformation of 3D space into itself can be described by a translation of the origin followed by a rotation around an axis through the translated origin. Since from the point of view of orientations, the translation part of this process is irrelevant, every orientation is describable by a unit vector $\mathbf{n}$ (specifying the axis of rotation) and an angle θ (specifying the amount of counterclockwise rotation around the directed axis). However, such a description $(\mathbf{n}, \theta)$ of orientations is not unique: $(-\mathbf{n}, -\theta)$ or $(\mathbf{n}, \theta + 2\pi)$ will result in the same orientation.

What is the "distance" between the orientations defined by $(\mathbf{n}_1, \theta_1)$ and $(\mathbf{n}_2, \theta_2)$? Heuristically, we may argue that it should be (a monotonic function of) the smallest positive angle θ_3 such that the rotation $(\mathbf{n}_1, \theta_1)$ followed by the rotation $(\mathbf{n}_3, \theta_3)$, for some unit vector $\mathbf{n}_3$, will result in the orientation defined by $(\mathbf{n}_2, \theta_2)$. At this stage, it is far from obvious how such a distance should be computed. Quaternions provide us with a natural way of achieving that, as discussed in Subsection 13.2.2.

There is an inherent difficulty with the definition of crystalline orientation: Even with the knowledge of the location of the crystal lattice points in space (relative to some fixed coordinate system), the *average orientation* of the grain (in the sense of how it had to be rotated relative to some reference position in order to get into its current position) is not defined in an obvious and unambiguous manner. Consider, for example, the *simple cubic lattice* whose lattice points are at locations (x, y, z) with x, y, and z integers. Suppose further that we rotate the lattice by $\frac{3\pi}{4}$ radians counterclockwise about the positive z-axis. The resulting arrangement of lattice points is indistinguishable from what would be obtained by rotating the lattice by $\frac{\pi}{4}$ radians counterclockwise (or, for that matter, clockwise) about the positive z-axis. Thus, due to the lattice structure (more specifically, the rotational crystal symmetries), the same observable arrangement of lattice points can be obtained by very different rotations; which of these should then be selected for the definition of "orientation"? We return to this important point in Subsection 13.2.2, but we will ignore its consequences in the discussion until then.

Quaternions and their applications to rotations and orientations have a well-developed theory [3, 8, 9, 18, 22]. In this subsection, we give only a skeleton development, restricting our attentions to those definitions and facts that we absolutely need for our purpose.

A *quaternion* $\mathbf{q}$ is a 4-tuple (a, b, c, d) of real numbers. The product of two quaternions is defined by

$$(a_1, b_1, c_1, d_1)(a_2, b_2, c_2, d_2) = (a_3, b_3, c_3, d_3), \tag{13.1}$$

where

$$\begin{aligned}
a_3 &= a_1 a_2 - b_1 b_2 - c_1 c_2 - d_1 d_2, \\
b_3 &= a_1 b_2 + b_1 a_2 + c_1 d_2 - d_1 c_2, \\
c_3 &= a_1 c_2 - b_1 d_2 + c_1 a_2 + d_1 b_2, \\
d_3 &= a_1 d_2 + b_1 c_2 - c_1 b_2 + d_1 a_2.
\end{aligned} \tag{13.2}$$

It is easy to check that multiplication is associative, and so one can use unambiguously the notation $\mathbf{pqr}$ for the product of the three quaternions $\mathbf{p}$, $\mathbf{q}$, and $\mathbf{r}$. Note also that $(1, 0, 0, 0)$ is an *identity element*; i.e., for any quaternion $\mathbf{q}$, we have

$$(1, 0, 0, 0)\mathbf{q} = \mathbf{q} = \mathbf{q}(1, 0, 0, 0). \tag{13.3}$$

The *norm* of the quaternion (a, b, c, d) is defined by

$$|(a, b, c, d)| = \sqrt{a^2 + b^2 + c^2 + d^2}. \tag{13.4}$$

We now specify two useful subsets of the set of quaternions. For both of these, it is helpful to introduce the notation $(a, \mathbf{b})$, where $\mathbf{b}$ is the 3D vector (b, c, d), to abbreviate the quaternion (a, b, c, d). The *conjugate* of the quaternion $\mathbf{q} = (a, \mathbf{b})$ is defined to be $\bar{\mathbf{q}} = (a, -\mathbf{b})$. Note that the conjugate of the product of two quaternions is the reversed product of their conjugates; i.e., $\overline{\mathbf{q_1 q_2}} = \bar{\mathbf{q}}_2 \bar{\mathbf{q}}_1$.

The set of *pure quaternions* consists of quaternions of the form $(0, \mathbf{b})$. Note that there is an obvious 1-to-1 mapping of the 3D Euclidean space onto the set of pure quaternions.

The set of *unit quaternions* consists of quaternions whose norm is 1. It is easy to check that the product of two unit quaternions is a unit quaternion, and that the conjugate of a unit quaternion is also a unit quaternion, and it is, in fact, the case that, for every unit quaternion $\mathbf{q}$, $\mathbf{q}\bar{\mathbf{q}} = (1, 0, 0, 0) = \bar{\mathbf{q}}\mathbf{q}$. Another useful property is that if $\mathbf{q}_3 = \bar{\mathbf{q}}_1 \mathbf{q}_2 \mathbf{q}_1$, where $\mathbf{q}_1$ is a unit quaternion and $\mathbf{q}_2$ is any quaternion, then the first component of $\mathbf{q}_3$ is the same as that of $\mathbf{q}_2$.

Every unit quaternion $\mathbf{q}$ can be written as

$$\mathbf{q} = (a, \mathbf{b}) = \left(\cos \left(\tfrac{1}{2}\theta \right), \mathbf{n} \sin \left(\tfrac{1}{2}\theta \right) \right), \tag{13.5}$$

for some real number θ and 3D unit vector $\mathbf{n}$. We are now going to discuss that this unit quaternion can be used to achieve a *rotation* in 3D about the directed axis $\mathbf{n}$ by the counterclockwise angle θ. Let $\mathbf{b}$ be a 3D vector. Then $\mathbf{q}(0, \mathbf{b})\bar{\mathbf{q}}$ will be a pure quaternion $(0, \mathbf{b}')$, where $\mathbf{b}'$ is the vector obtained from $\mathbf{b}$ by the rotation about the directed axis $\mathbf{n}$ by the counterclockwise angle θ.

As an example, consider the rotation by $\frac{3\pi}{4}$ radians counterclockwise about the positive z-axis. According to the discussion above, this is represented by the quaternion

$$\mathbf{q} = \left(\sqrt{\tfrac{1}{2} - \tfrac{\sqrt{2}}{4}}, 0, 0, \sqrt{\tfrac{1}{2} + \tfrac{\sqrt{2}}{4}} \right); \tag{13.6}$$

see (13.5). It is easy to check, using (13.1) and (13.2), that for this $\mathbf{q}$

$$\mathbf{q}(0, 0, 1, 0)\bar{\mathbf{q}} = \left(0, -\tfrac{1}{\sqrt{2}}, -\tfrac{1}{\sqrt{2}}, 0 \right), \tag{13.7}$$

corresponding to the fact that the specified rotation maps the 3D vector $(0, 1, 0)$ into $\left(-\tfrac{1}{\sqrt{2}}, -\tfrac{1}{\sqrt{2}}, 0 \right)$.

Note that the unit quaternion $\mathbf{q}$ does not determine $(\mathbf{n}, \theta)$ uniquely, but all the $(\mathbf{n}, \theta)$ that satisfy (13.5) describe the same transformation of the 3D space onto itself, since any of them can be obtained from any other by steps consisting of changing θ by 4π or simultaneously taking the negative of both $\mathbf{n}$ and θ. The transformation of the 3D space also does not change by adding 2π to θ, but this changes the quaternion $\mathbf{q}$ of (13.5) into $-\mathbf{q}$. Thus, the unit quaternions $\mathbf{q}$ and $-\mathbf{q}$ define the same rotational transformation of the 3D space into itself; there is a 2-to-1 mapping of the set of unit quaternions onto the set of such rotational transformations.

A particularly useful and elegant consequence of this approach is that the rotation represented by the unit quaternion $\mathbf{q}_1$ followed by the rotation represented by the unit quaternion $\mathbf{q}_2$ is the *composite rotation* represented by $\mathbf{q}_2\mathbf{q}_1$, since for any quaternion $\mathbf{p}$ we have

$$\mathbf{q}_2(\mathbf{q}_1\mathbf{p}\bar{\mathbf{q}}_1)\bar{\mathbf{q}}_2 = (\mathbf{q}_2\mathbf{q}_1)\mathbf{p}(\bar{\mathbf{q}}_1\bar{\mathbf{q}}_2) = (\mathbf{q}_2\mathbf{q}_1)\mathbf{p}(\overline{\mathbf{q}_2\mathbf{q}_1}). \tag{13.8}$$

13.2.2 Distance in Orientation Space

We now continue with the central issue of how to define the distance $d(o_1, o_2)$ between the orientations o_1 and o_2. Initially, we ignore the underlying crystalline lattice and consider only the distance, denoted by r, between rotations.

According to the heuristic stated in Subsection 13.2.1, such a distance between two rotations should be a monotonic function of the smallest nonnegative angle θ_3 such that the first rotation followed by a third rotation $(\mathbf{n}_3, \theta_3)$, for some unit vector $\mathbf{n}_3$, will result in the second rotation. If the first rotation is represented by the unit quaternion $\mathbf{q}_1$, and the second by the unit quaternion $\mathbf{q}_2$, then a unit quaternion $\mathbf{q}_3$ that corresponds to the desired third rotation is $\mathbf{q}_2\bar{\mathbf{q}}_1$, since

$$\mathbf{q}_3\mathbf{q}_1 = (\mathbf{q}_2\bar{\mathbf{q}}_1)\mathbf{q}_1 = \mathbf{q}_2(\bar{\mathbf{q}}_1\mathbf{q}_1) = \mathbf{q}_2(1,0,0,0) = \mathbf{q}_2. \tag{13.9}$$

Since $\mathbf{q}_3$ and $-\mathbf{q}_3$ define the same rotation, the first component a_3 is nonnegative for at least one of them, and the corresponding smallest nonnegative θ_3 must lie between 0 and π. This is the value that indicates the dissimilarity, and so $r(\mathbf{q}_1, \mathbf{q}_2) := 1 - |a_3|$ can be used as the definition of distance. Looking at the first row of (13.2) for the product $\mathbf{q}_2\bar{\mathbf{q}}_1$, with $\mathbf{q}_1 = (a_1, b_1, c_1, d_1)$ and $\mathbf{q}_2 = (a_2, b_2, c_2, d_2)$, we see that

$$a_3 = a_1a_2 + b_1b_2 + c_1c_2 + d_1d_2. \tag{13.10}$$

It is clear that a_3 is nothing but the dot product of $\mathbf{q}_1$ and $\mathbf{q}_2$ when they are considered as 4D unit vectors. In particular, $|a_3|$, and hence $r(\mathbf{q}_1, \mathbf{q}_2)$, does not depend on the choice of the unit quaternions used to represent the first two rotations: If one used the alternative representations $-\mathbf{q}_1$ and $-\mathbf{q}_2$ for one or both of these rotations, then the value of $|a_3|$ would remain the same. It can be verified that $r(\mathbf{q}_1, \mathbf{q}_2) = 0$ if, and only if, $\mathbf{q}_1 = \pm\mathbf{q}_2$, and that $r(\mathbf{q}_1, \mathbf{q}_2) = r(\mathbf{q}_2, \mathbf{q}_1)$ (in other words, we have the desirable property that the distance from $\mathbf{q}_1$ to $\mathbf{q}_2$ is the same as the distance from $\mathbf{q}_2$ to $\mathbf{q}_1$). Also, it is the case that $r(\mathbf{q}_1, \mathbf{q}_2) = r(\bar{\mathbf{q}}_1, \bar{\mathbf{q}}_2) = r((1,0,0,0), \bar{\mathbf{q}}_2\mathbf{q}_1)$.

Now we return to the issue raised in Subsection 13.2.1, namely that orientations are associated with a crystal structure, and hence the rotational crystal symmetries have to be taken into account. To illustrate this problem, let $\mathbf{q}$ denote a fixed unit quaternion describing an arbitrary rotation, and $\mathbf{s}$ be a unit quaternion describing a symmetry rotation of the crystalline lattice (i.e., a rotation that maps every lattice point onto a lattice point). It is easy to see that the rotation $\mathbf{q}\mathbf{s}$ results in the same orientation of the lattice as the rotation $\mathbf{q}$. Thus, $\mathbf{q}$ and $\mathbf{q}\mathbf{s}$ are said to be *crystallographically equivalent*.

As an example, let us consider the three *cubic crystal lattices*: the simple cubic, the face-centered cubic, and the body-centered cubic lattice. These lattices have the same crystal symmetries: There are 48 symmetry operations, 24 of which are pure rotations. So, for every rotation $\mathbf{q}$, there are 23 other rotations that are crystallographically equivalent with it. Many important metals have a cubic lattice. For instance, iron has a body-centered cubic lattice, while gold, silver, aluminum, copper, and lead all have a face-centered one. Indeed, the study of relative orientations in the presence of crystal symmetries has been an active field of research in the analysis of the *texture of materials* for over 30 years [12, 13, 14, 17, 22].

We are now ready to define the *distance* $d(\mathbf{q}_1, \mathbf{q}_2)$ between two orientations of the lattice brought about by rotations represented by unit quaternions $\mathbf{q}_1$ and $\mathbf{q}_2$. If the quaternions $\mathbf{q}_1$ and $\mathbf{q}_2$ correspond to the orientations of two neighboring grains, or of two neighboring pixels in the orientation map, then $d(\mathbf{q}_1, \mathbf{q}_2)$ should measure the size of the disorientation between the grains/pixels, taking into consideration the underlying crystal symmetries. Following the methodology presented in [12, 14], this can be done as follows: Let S denote the set of all symmetry rotations of the lattice. (Since inversions, translations, and reflections are irrelevant from the point of view of equivalent orientations, it is enough to restrict S to rotational operations.) Then, by definition,

$$d(\mathbf{q}_1, \mathbf{q}_2) = \min_{\mathbf{s}_1, \mathbf{s}_2 \in S} r(\mathbf{q}_1 \mathbf{s}_1, \mathbf{q}_2 \mathbf{s}_2), \tag{13.11}$$

i.e., the smallest distance between a quaternion that is crystallographically equivalent to $\mathbf{q}_1$ and another quaternion that is crystallographically equivalent to $\mathbf{q}_2$.

Sometimes it is intuitively informative to refer to the distance as if it were measured in degrees. This can be done by associating a *disorientation angle* with every distance value. The following is the precise definition: We say that distance d (recall that $0 \leq d \leq 1$) is equivalent to the disorientation θ if, and only if, $0 \leq \theta \leq 180$ and $\cos\left(\frac{1}{2}\theta\right) = 1 - d$. Note that there is one, and only one, such θ for any d such that $0 \leq d \leq 1$. That this is a reasonable convention follows from the definition of $r(\mathbf{q}_1, \mathbf{q}_2)$. In the material presented below, whenever we specify that a disorientation is θ, then we mean by this the corresponding distance $d = 1 - \cos\left(\frac{1}{2}\theta\right)$.

We are now going to show that, in fact,

$$d(\mathbf{q}_1, \mathbf{q}_2) = \min_{\mathbf{s} \in S} r\left((1,0,0,0), \mathbf{s}\mathbf{q}_2\bar{\mathbf{q}}_1\right). \tag{13.12}$$

We first recall that $r(\mathbf{q}_1\mathbf{s}_1, \mathbf{q}_2\mathbf{s}_2) = r((1,0,0,0), \bar{\mathbf{s}}_2\bar{\mathbf{q}}_2\mathbf{q}_1\mathbf{s}_1)$. To evaluate the right-hand side, we need the first component of $\bar{\mathbf{s}}_2\bar{\mathbf{q}}_2\mathbf{q}_1\mathbf{s}_1 = \bar{\mathbf{s}}_1\mathbf{s}_1\bar{\mathbf{s}}_2\bar{\mathbf{q}}_2\mathbf{q}_1\mathbf{s}_1$. Recalling a previously stated property of this product, we see that its first component is the same as that of $\mathbf{s}_1\bar{\mathbf{s}}_2\bar{\mathbf{q}}_2\mathbf{q}_1$. Since the conjugate of a crystal symmetry is a crystal symmetry and the product of two crystal symmetries is also a crystal symmetry, the claim (13.12) follows.

Though it would be possible to determine the value of r in (13.12) for each $\mathbf{s}$ one by one, and then to choose the smallest one, this would really slow down the reconstruction procedure. (For example, S has 24 elements for cubic lattices.) A more efficient method is to use a look-up table of the values of $\min_{\mathbf{s} \in S} r((1,0,0,0), \mathbf{sq})$, based on quantization of the unit quaternion $\mathbf{q}$. We now show that there is a fairly easy way to implement such a look-up table.

First, it should be recalled that the components of a unit quaternion have magnitudes less than or equal to 1. For any rotation, the first component a of $\mathbf{q}$ can be chosen to be nonnegative. Since a is uniquely determined by the other components, it can be ignored for the construction of the look-up table. For the sake of simplicity, let us suppose that the whole range $[-1, 1]$ of the other three components is sampled using M values. This way we get a table T of M^3 values such that, at those locations for which $b^2 + c^2 + d^2 \leq 1$, the element t_{bcd} is the needed value for the unit quaternion $\mathbf{q} = (a, b, c, d)$ for the corresponding nonnegative a. If $b^2 + c^2 + d^2 > 1$, the value of t_{bcd} is undefined. This convention makes the table easily addressable, at the cost of some wasted memory. The sampling resolution M may simply be chosen based on memory considerations. For example, having $M = 101$ and using 8 bytes to represent real numbers, T consumes $8.24 \cdot 10^6$ bytes (about 7.86 megabytes).

To find the desired $d(\mathbf{q}_1, \mathbf{q}_2)$, we calculate $\mathbf{q}_3 = (a_3, b_3, c_3, d_3)$ according to (13.9). If a_3 is negative, we replace $\mathbf{q}_3$ with $-\mathbf{q}_3$. Then $d(\mathbf{q}_1, \mathbf{q}_2)$ is approximated by $t_{b'_3 c'_3 d'_3}$, where b'_3, c'_3, and d'_3 are the sampling points nearest to b_3, c_3, and d_3, respectively.

13.3 The Undeformed Case

In this section we present an algorithm for grain map reconstruction. Note that in the undeformed case the orientation map follows from the grain map once the orientation of one pixel of every grain has been determined.

Until recently, the following method has been used for grain map reconstruction [25]. A program called GRAINDEX, based on ray tracing, analyzes the diffraction spots on the detector and identifies subsets of those spots in such a way that all spots in a single subset originate from a single grain. GRAINDEX also provides the orientation of these grains, so in this undeformed case there remains only the task of reconstructing the grain map. Data from the spots of a single subset form a real-valued vector $\mathbf{b}$, and then an algebraic reconstruction technique (ART) [11] is applied to solve a system of linear equations $\mathbf{Ax} = \mathbf{b}$, where $\mathbf{A}$ is a real-valued matrix describing the experimental geometry and $\mathbf{x}$ is a 0/1–vector identifying the pixels in this particular grain. These separately reconstructed grains are patched together to form a grain map, but due to several reasons (e.g., noise in the data and the "real-valued" nature of the ART algorithm) one finds that there are many "ambiguous pixels" in such maps, i.e., some are assigned to multiple grains or to no grains at all.

The algorithm that we present in this section was originally designed to work on such reconstructed grain maps, which had a small number of "ambiguous pixels." In this sense it is a *restoration algorithm*. Surprisingly, as demonstrated in the next section, we can successfully apply the algorithm to grain maps where initially only one pixel of each grain is known in advance, i.e., where all other pixels were considered as "ambiguous." Since GRAIN-DEX provides such information, one can work directly on such low-quality grain maps without invoking the ART routine. Our exposition in this section, however, discusses an approach for assigning to grains those pixels that are not unambiguously assigned by ART.

13.3.1 Algorithmic Overview

The central idea of the approach is to take as input a 2D grain map f (generated by ART as described above) and the diffraction data. Our proposed algorithm only changes pixels of the grain map that are classified "ambiguous." The task is to assign these pixels to the "correct" grains. To this end, we utilize a Markov-chain-based Monte Carlo method, namely the *Metropolis algorithm* [21], which has proved to be useful in other applications of DT, such as the reconstruction of binary (or gray-leveled) images from projections [15].

We assume that the grain maps are random samples from a *Gibbs distribution* [5, 10] defined by

$$\pi(f) = \frac{1}{Z}e^{-\beta H(f)}, \tag{13.13}$$

where $\pi(f)$ is the probability of occurrence of the grain map f, $\beta > 0$ is a parameter analogous to the inverse of the *temperature*, Z corresponds to the *partition function* in statistical mechanics, and $H(f)$ is the energy of f. This energy $H(f)$ is based only on local 3×3 features (called *configurations*) of the image. The local features of interest are partitioned into equivalence classes (for example, one of these is associated with edges) $G_0, \ldots, G_C$ and

$$H(f) = -\sum_{c=0}^{C} N(G_c, f)U_c, \tag{13.14}$$

where $N(G_c, f)$ counts the number of times a configuration from G_c occurs in f, and the number U_c is the *potential* associated with the class G_c (for $0 \leq c \leq C$) [19]. These potentials are chosen so that random samples from the Gibbs distribution resemble the arrangement of grains in polycrystals.

We also need to take the diffraction data $\mathbf{P}$ into account. (Such data can be modeled as a real-valued vector.) Let $\mathbf{P}_f$ denote the simulated diffraction data given the image f, and let $\alpha, \beta \in \mathbb{R}$ be given positive parameters. We apply the Metropolis algorithm to the nonzero-valued distribution γ defined by

$$\gamma(f) = \frac{1}{Z}e^{-\beta\left(H(f)+\alpha\|\mathbf{P}_f - \mathbf{P}\|_1\right)}, \tag{13.15}$$

where $\|\cdot\|_1$ denotes the ℓ_1-norm. The reason for choosing γ as in (13.15) is that we want to find the grain map f that minimizes $H(f) + \alpha \|\mathbf{P}_f - \mathbf{P}\|_1$. This can be provided within an adequate running time by the Metropolis algorithm.

A single step of the Metropolis algorithm may be described as follows. One of the originally ambiguous pixels is randomly selected together with an alternative assignment of the pixel to a grain. Then we calculate $p = \frac{\gamma(f')}{\gamma(f)}$, the ratio of the probabilities of the new grain map f' (which we obtain by the alternative assignment of the selected pixel) and the old grain map f. We accept the alternative assignment with probability $\min\{1, p\}$. One *cycle* of the Metropolis algorithm consists of n Metropolis steps, where n is the total number of originally ambiguous pixels in the grain map.

Note that our Gibbs distributions are defined on multicolored images. However, in order to keep the number of parameters low, we compute $H(f)$ by suitably resorting to binary configurations, as explained in the next subsection.

13.3.2 Algorithmic Details

For each pixel in the multicolored grain map, we define its *local configuration* as a 3×3 array of black and white pixels as follows: The central pixel is always white and any other pixel is white if, and only if, it belongs to the same grain as the central pixel. These configurations are partitioned into seven classes $G_0, G_1, \ldots, G_6$, each containing configurations of similar morphology, such as "grain interior," "grain edge," etc. For $1 \le i \le 6$, the class G_i consists of the configurations illustrated in Fig. 13.3 and all the configurations that can be obtained from it by a sequence of $90°$ rotations around the center and mirror images about the central vertical line. Configurations not in any of $G_1, \ldots, G_6$, are put into G_0.

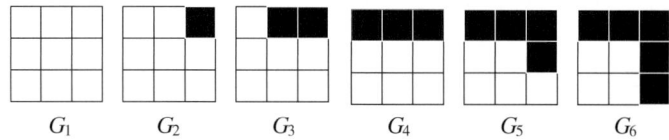

G_1 G_2 G_3 G_4 G_5 G_6

Fig. 13.3. The configurations $G_1, \ldots, G_6$ of a 3×3 clique that we use in our model.

Next we approximate the distribution of grain maps by a Gibbs distribution (13.13). For this we need to define the potentials U_i of (13.14). We use an approach based on counting 3×3 configurations in typical microstructures (the training set) for determining the potentials.

The restoration algorithm seeks to maximize (13.15). Both α and β are system parameters to be optimized by simulations. The maximization is performed by the Metropolis algorithm [21], which is directly applicable to (13.15).

Evidently, different samples will give rise to different estimated Gibbs distributions. It would be cumbersome, in some cases even impossible, to establish the required potentials prior to every 3DXRD experiment. However, grain microstructures are, broadly speaking, similar (e.g., grain growth is often associated with self-similar patterns). Hence, we predict that the algorithm is sufficiently robust with respect to the choice of the potentials, and so one set of parameters can be used for a large set of samples.

To test the robustness of our algorithm, we used six different sets of potentials $U^i = (U_1, U_2, U_3, U_4, U_5, U_6)$, where U_0 was always set to 0:

$U^1 = (1.4, 0.71, 0.61, 0.79, 0.5, 0.61)$, a medium-scale grain structure;

$U^2 = (1.4, 0.8, 0.8, 0.94, 0.19, 0.82)$, a coarse-grained structure;

$U^3 = (1.4, 0.94, 0.94, 1.09, 0.12, 1.01)$, a fine-grained structure;

$U^4 = (1.4, 0.91, 0.91, 1.08, 0.02, 1.0)$, a partially recrystallized sample;

$U^5 = (1.5, 1.2, 0.84, 1, 1.25, 0.6)$ displays grain-like features;

$U^6 = (0.5, 0.4, 1.0, 0.8, 0.1, 0.6)$ does not produce grain-like features.

The potentials $U^1, \ldots, U^5$ were determined by methods from [6] using a training set of aluminum grain samples; U^6 was chosen arbitrarily. Unless stated otherwise, we use the Gibbs prior defined by U^1.

13.3.3 Results

Figure 13.4 shows one aluminum grain map of 128×128 pixel size containing 44 grains (left image), and its reconstruction using ART (right image). The right image contains 1490 white pixels, which correspond to ambiguous points that ART was unable to reconstruct. Our approach tries to resolve the ambiguous white pixels; an ideal output of our algorithm would be the retrieval of the left image. We remark that the ART reconstruction is not perfect; even among the nonwhite pixels, 682 pixels are incorrectly assigned in Fig. 13.4 (right). Since our algorithm processes only white pixels, there is no possibility of correcting those wrong assignments.

Taking the original image, we simulated noiseless detector data and ran our algorithm on the image with ambiguities using a 3 GHz Pentium 4 processor. Initially, the white points were randomly assigned to the grains that surround the white region in which they occurred. The size of the detector (in pixels) was 1024×1536, and we used 91 projections provided by equally spaced rotation angles ω between -45 and 45 degrees. In our simulations, it turned out that only roughly 0.02% of the pixels on the detectors were actually hit by diffraction beams (resulting in a nonzero value), and most grains produced approximately a total of eight spots on the detector. Every diffracted beam recorded on the detector hits only one detector pixel and adds a uniform amount to its intensity.

Based on the set of Gibbs potentials U^1, the diffraction images, and the ambiguity areas defined above, a series of restorations was made with varying system parameters α, β, the number of Monte Carlo cycles (MCC), as well as the additive noise term. The noise was implemented by adding a value of

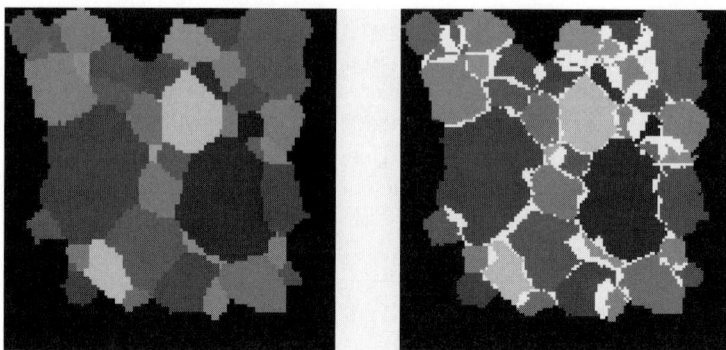

Fig. 13.4. The left image shows a typical grain map, which was experimentally determined by electron microscopy. The right image shows the grain map (produced by ART) where ambiguities have to be resolved (white points).

1 to randomly chosen detector pixels. In the following, noise levels will be indicated in percent as the ratio of the total number of added 1's to all the detector pixels. The quality of the restorations is determined by the "number of errors," which is the number of pixels in the white areas that have been assigned to a grain in the restored map that is different from the grain in the original map. To improve the statistics, each simulation was repeated 10 times with different initial seeds to the Metropolis algorithm. The restorations were found to converge rapidly. The running time for each restoration (based on 1000 MCC) was 10 seconds.

The variation in the number of errors as a function of α and β using the Gibbs prior associated with U^1 is shown in Fig. 13.5. For noise levels clearly below 100% — as expected for the level of noise in real 3DXRD experiments — a broad optimal range is around $(\alpha, \beta) = (1, 1)$. In the experiments that follow, we use these values.

The variation with noise of such optimized restorations is compared to results for projections only in Fig. 13.6. "Projections only" implies no use of Gibbs priors, i.e., based on $\gamma(f) = \frac{1}{Z}e^{-\|\mathbf{P}_f - \mathbf{P}\|}$, instead of (13.15). Also shown is the result of a pure 2D-ART reconstruction based on the simulated diffraction images. Ambiguous pixels were in this case allocated to the grain yielding the highest rational value among the single-grain reconstructions. There are significant differences in performance among the three methods.

Based on the six sets of potentials $U^1, \ldots, U^6$, but otherwise with the same settings of system parameters ($\alpha = \beta = 1$), restorations were made to the grain map shown on the right in Fig. 13.4. The results are shown in Fig. 13.7. Evidently, the quality of reconstruction based on the five sets of potentials related to grain-like features is nearly identical. This is seen as a strong indication that reconstructions of reasonably similar samples with unknown microstructures can be based on a set of Gibbs potentials derived from electron microscopic investigations of one representative.

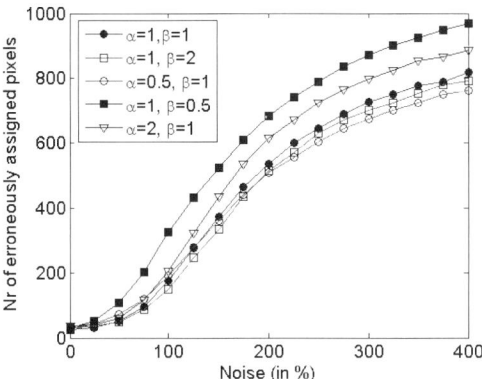

Fig. 13.5. Optimization of system variables α and β. For various (α, β), the variation in restoration quality—determined as the total number of ambiguous pixels in the reconstructed map assigned to the wrong grain—is shown as a function of the noise in the simulated detector images.

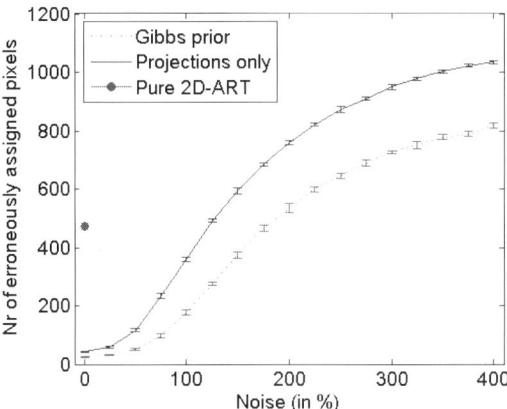

Fig. 13.6. Reconstruction quality as a function of the amount of additive noise in the simulated detector images. Two map restoration methods are compared: restoration from projections only and restoration from projections plus the Gibbs prior based on U^1. The result for reconstruction from noiseless data based purely on 2D-ART is also indicated.

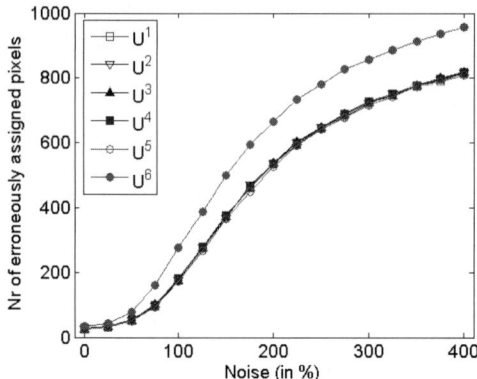

Fig. 13.7. Test of robustness. The quality of restoration is shown as a function of noise for six sets of Gibbs potentials U^1, U^2, U^3, U^4, U^5, and U^6.

Additionally, we investigated the effect of varying the average number of useful diffraction spots per grain (at a noise level of 0% and 100%; see Fig. 13.8 left and right, respectively). The number of spots was varied by removing spots from the simulated detector images. The removal was carried out arbitrarily, by terminating the spot simulation (favoring no particular kind of spots) after a prescribed amount of spots occurred on the detector. Again the superior quality of the mapping based on the restoration algorithm with Gibbs priors over the pure 2D-ART approach is evident.

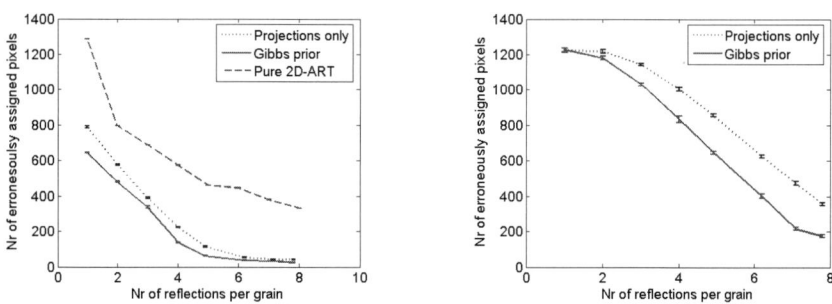

Fig. 13.8. Reconstruction quality as a function of the average number of useful spots per grain. Left: At a noise level of 0%, two map restoration methods are compared with pure 2D-ART: restoration by projection only and restoration by projections plus the optimized Gibbs priors. Right: Results for a noise level of 100%.

Finally, we tested the extreme approach in which simulations were repeated with an initial grain map with all the 10,299 (except for 44) nonblack pixels of the grain map in Fig. 13.4 assigned to be white points. The 44 assigned pixels corresponded to 1 pixel per grain—namely the pixels closest to the individual centers of mass. These pixels may be thought of as seeds for the algorithm. The running time was six times longer than for the results presented before. The total number of incorrectly assigned pixels in the three cases of reconstruction from noiseless data with Gibbs priors, "Projections only" and 2D-ART, respectively, are 120, 586 and 5482. Notably, the total number of errors is smaller than the corresponding result with an initial map provided by 2D-ART, while the number of errors in the ambiguous parts is larger. The results for the 100% noise case are much worse than those obtained using an initial map, due to the fact that the Metropolis algorithm gets stuck at a local maximum, which might be resolved by vastly increasing the number of MCC. These results indicate that an optimal trade-off between the accuracy of initial map and the presented method with respect to running time, noise, and reconstruction quality has to be found. This optimum may depend on specifics of the grain map and is a topic of current research.

13.4 The Moderately Deformed Case

Now we proceed toward the more general problem of reconstructing orientation maps of deformed samples. This procedure is of high relevance for many industrial applications that seek to assess the effects of structural deformation and of stress on the physical and mechanical properties of polycrystalline materials. The ultimate goal is to obtain orientation maps of highly strained specimens by means of reconstruction, but this turns out to be a complicated task. Instead, we restrict the discussion to *moderate deformations*. We have coined this term to indicate levels of deformation at which it is possible to deduce the (deformed) grain map from the orientation map. This restriction is expected to allow reconstructions of acceptable quality even under unfavorable circumstances (e.g., high background radiation level or low photon count).

The approach presented below is again a kind of restoration algorithm that is an extension of the technique introduced in Section 13.3. The method was originally designed as a "post-processing" tool that can recover the complete orientation map from a partially reconstructed map obtained via some other procedure, but it turned out that it can be successfully utilized as a *reconstruction algorithm*.

13.4.1 Algorithm Overview

The aim is to reconstruct simultaneously a 2D orientation map/grain map pair of a cross section of the specimen from a set of diffraction patterns acquired by 3DXRD.

The algorithm described here is strongly motivated by the technique discussed in Subsection 13.3.1. In particular, one is looking for an orientation map whose simulated projections approximate the measured ones as closely as possible, and for a grain map that exhibits typical features of moderately deformed polycrystals. As mentioned in Section 13.2, the classic way to construct grain maps from deformed orientation maps (as derived from electron microscopy) employs connected component techniques. These are based on the fact that orientations of neighboring pixels within any grain are related to each other, as can be observed in real-life polycrystals. In other words, the orientation map reveals a sort of *homogeneity* or *smoothness* inside every grain, and we make use of this principle.

Our approach is superior to the techniques just mentioned in the sense that it is assisted by 3DXRD diffraction measurements, hence making non-destructive dynamic studies feasible. Also, in comparison to, e.g., ART-based 3DXRD reconstructions, the solutions are determined by using the original (unaltered) projections, that is, diffraction spots need not be discarded in case of spot overlap. The latter may prove useful for larger grain maps and for higher levels of deformation, since these usually give rise to many overlapping diffraction spots.

As before, our aim is to associate with each pixel $i \in D \subset \mathbb{Z}^2$ in the area of interest both a grain label $f(i) \in \{1, \ldots, l\}$ and an orientation $o(i)$ represented by a unit quaternion (see Subsection 13.2.1). The notation f_ℓ will be used to designate the set $\{i \in D \mid f(i) = \ell\}$ of indices of all the pixels associated with the grain labeled $\ell \in \{1, \ldots, l\}$. In addition, the special grain label 0 will also be employed during the course of reconstruction in order to indicate *ambiguous pixels* whose grain membership is not yet decided.

Two more concepts need to be established before proceeding. Recalling the definition of distance between orientations, cf. (13.11) and (13.12), the *average orientation* of a set of orientations represented by the unit quaternions $\mathbf{q}_1, \ldots, \mathbf{q}_R$ is represented by a unit quaternion $\mathbf{q}$ that minimizes $\sum_{r=1}^{R} d(\mathbf{q}_r, \mathbf{q})$. The *orientation spread* of grain f_ℓ is defined as the maximal distance between the average orientation of f_ℓ and the orientation of any pixel constituting f_ℓ.

The following requirements have to be satisfied for a successful application of the algorithm:

(a) The number l of grains should be fixed and known beforehand.
(b) An initial guess of average orientations, orientation spread, centers of mass, and approximate morphologies of grains should be available. A program called GRAINSWEEPER [24] is under development; its specific purpose is to provide such information on grain maps and orientation maps via the analysis of 3DXRD diffraction patterns.
(c) The statistical distribution of typical grain morphologies in moderately deformed orientation maps is available.

As explained at the end of Subsection 13.2.2, orientations are discretized using an appropriate quantization step. (This is not only an issue of memory requirements or reconstruction speed. Specifically, it is a fundamental property of 3DXRD that the obtainable spatial resolution—with respect to grain position inside the specimen — and the angular resolution — related to the precision with which orientations can be measured — of detectors are not independent. See [24] for a deeper discussion.) This effectively means that the set of possible orientations is known and finite. Since there are finitely many grains in the cross section, the problem becomes a DT reconstruction task.

Our reconstruction procedure is an extension of the Bayesian technique described in Section 13.3 for the undeformed case, but was also inspired by a similar approach for gray-valued images described in [7]. Since the orientation of a pixel within a particular grain is likely to be similar to that of its neighbors, and all moderately deformed grain maps show similar morphological features (depending on the material and the magnitude of deformation, of course), we decided to model both maps simultaneously by a Gibbs distribution. This has the advantage that only *local* features need to be specified, making the description compact and the algorithm efficient.

The probability of occurrence of a grain map/orientation map pair (f, o) is given by, similar to (13.13),

$$\pi(f, o) = \frac{1}{Z} e^{-\beta H(f, o)}. \tag{13.16}$$

It is the construction of the *energy functional* $H(f, o)$ that carries the desired properties of a grain map f and of an orientation map o. As presented more precisely below, this functional is calculated as a weighted sum of *clique potentials*. It is defined as

$$H(f, o) = H_1(f, o) + H_2(f). \tag{13.17}$$

The first term establishes a *homogeneity* condition:

$$H_1(f, o) = -\sum_{\ell=1}^{l} \left(\sum_{C \in \mathcal{C}_{+,\ell}} \lambda_1 \Phi_C(o) + \sum_{C \in \mathcal{C}_{\times,\ell}} \lambda_2 \Phi_C(o) \right), \tag{13.18}$$

with

$$\Phi_{\{i,j\}}(o) = e^{-\frac{(d(o(i), o(j)))^2}{2\delta^2}}. \tag{13.19}$$

By $\mathcal{C}_{+,\ell}$ we denote the set of all horizontal and vertical pair cliques (i.e., pairs of pixel indices) within grain f_ℓ, while $\mathcal{C}_{\times,\ell}$ is that of all diagonal pair cliques inside grain f_ℓ. The real-valued coefficients λ_1 and λ_2 determine the contribution of each type of interaction, and the free real parameter $\delta > 0$, together with the λ_i, controls the degree of homogeneity. (In fact, δ is related to the maximal orientation spread over all the grains, or, more explicitly, to the maximal distance between the orientations of adjacent pixels within any grain.) As discussed in Subsection 13.2.2, the nonnegative function $d(o(i), o(j))$ measures the distance of two orientations; a smaller value indicates more similar orientations [see (13.12)].

The second term in $H(f, o)$, namely $H_2(f)$, models the *borders* between neighboring grains. That is, the purpose of this term is to capture typical grain-like features of moderately deformed maps. We used an $H_2(f)$ that is defined exactly as in (13.14). As demonstrated in Subsection 13.3.3, the effects of such a term are very robust with respect to the choice of clique potentials. Moreover, moderately deformed grains, by definition, used to be undeformed before deformation. As the morphology changes during deformation are relatively small, we claim that the set of configurations shown in Fig. 13.3 is appropriate for moderately deformed grain maps, too. The clique potentials U^1 introduced in Subsection 13.3.2 were used for implementation.

Having defined the desired distribution of grain maps and orientation maps, we can now formulate the posterior distribution in terms of the physical measurements. Analogously to (13.15), we end up with the goal of maximizing the *objective functional*

$$\gamma(f, o) := \frac{1}{Z} e^{-\beta \left(H_1(f,o) + H_2(f) + \alpha \| \mathbf{P}_o - \mathbf{P} \|_1 \right)}. \tag{13.20}$$

[Note the replacement of $\mathbf{P}_f$ in (13.15) by $\mathbf{P}_o$. This is necessary, since orientation is not unambiguously determined by the label in the deformed case.] In the present implementation, the *Metropolis algorithm* [21] is being employed for this purpose. A major advantage of this iterative Monte Carlo approach is that it does not need the value of $\gamma(f, o)$ itself during optimization.

At every iteration of the Metropolis algorithm, a new pair (f', o') of maps is devised from the current (f, o) as described ahead. The new pair is accepted, as explained in Subsection 13.3.1, based on the ratio:

$$\frac{\gamma(f', o')}{\gamma(f, o)} = e^{-\beta \left(H(f',o') - H(f,o) + \alpha \left(\| \mathbf{P}_{o'} - \mathbf{P} \|_1 - \| \mathbf{P}_o - \mathbf{P} \|_1 \right) \right)}. \tag{13.21}$$

The new approximations (f', o') are constructed according to three principles:

(a) An ambiguous pixel may only be given the label and orientation of an adjacent nonambiguous pixel.
(b) A nonambiguous pixel may retain its association with a grain while its orientation may be replaced with one of its nearest neighbors in orientation space.
(c) A nonambiguous pixel at a grain boundary may be given the same label and orientation as a neighboring pixel associated with an adjacent grain.

More specifically, (f', o') is generated from (f, o) as follows:

Let $f'(i) := f(i)$ and $o'(i) := o(i)$ for all $i \in D$;
Randomly choose a pixel $i \in D$;
if at least one neighbor of i is nonambiguous
   Randomly choose a nonambiguous neighbor, pixel j;
   if pixel i is ambiguous
      Set $f'(i) := f(j)$ and $o'(i) := o(j)$;
      Accept (f', o') unconditionally;
   else
      if $f(i) = f(j)$
         $o'(i) := \mathbf{q}$, where $\mathbf{q}$ is one of the orientations that are adjacent
                   to either $o(i)$ or $o(j)$ in orientation space;
         Decide on whether to accept (f', o');
      else
         $f'(i) := f(j)$, $o'(i) := o(j)$;
         Decide on whether to accept (f', o');
      endif
   endif
endif

The optimization procedure can, in theory, be started from an arbitrary pair (f, o) of maps, but f is usually initialized so that most of the pixels are assigned the ambiguous label. The exact way of their construction is discussed in the next subsection.

The relaxation parameter β (inverse of the temperature) is used to control the acceptance ratio: A lower β increases the probability of accepting (f', o') even when the value of the objective functional declines, while a higher β "freezes" the system into accepting only those (f', o') that result in an improvement of $\gamma(f, o)$. The results we are going to report in the next subsection were produced by keeping β constant all the time, and stopping optimization after a certain number of iterations. This is a trade-off between adequate running speed and the possibility of unwanted local optima. Considering the good quality of the present reconstructions, we postulate that only a slight improvement would be gained by employing more elaborate techniques such as the Gibbs Sampler [10] in conjunction with simulated annealing (SA) [10, 16].

13.4.2 Results

The algorithm described above has been implemented as a program written in C. All the timings mentioned later were measured under Linux on a state-of-the-art PC having 1.25 GB RAM and a 2.8 GHz processor.

Stochastic methods are renowned not only for their ability to easily solve complicated problems, but also because they tend to be slow as compared to deterministic approaches. Therefore, considerable effort has been invested in optimizing the program code. For reference purposes, we summarize some of these.

(a) As explained in Subsection 13.2.2, the continuous orientation space is discretized into finitely many quantized orientations.
(b) Several look-up tables are utilized throughout the program to store pre-computed values of certain functions whose evaluation should be as fast as possible. One example is the table containing approximate values of

$d(\mathbf{q}_1, \mathbf{q}_2)$, described in Subsection 13.2.2. In addition, the potentials associated with any 3×3 binarized grain map configurations are stored in a
9D look-up table.

(c) The objective functional $\gamma(f, o)$ needs to be completely evaluated only
once, right before optimization is started. Whenever a pair (f', o') of maps
is to be tested for acceptance as the new approximation of the optimal
maps [with (f, o) being the current pair of maps], $\gamma(f', o')$ is computed by
updating $\gamma(f, o)$ according to the changes caused by switching from (f, o)
to (f', o'). In particular, terms $H_1(f, o)$, $H_1(f', o')$, $H_2(f)$, and $H_2(f')$ are
affected by only those 3×3 cliques that contain the pixel i being modified.
(There are only 9 such cliques.) Furthermore, the simulated projections
$\mathbf{P}_{o'}$, and thus the error $\|\mathbf{P}_{o'} - \mathbf{P}\|_1$, can be directly derived from $\mathbf{P}_o$ by
subtracting the projections on the detector generated by the old orien-
tation $o(i)$ and then by adding those obtained with the new orientation
$o'(i)$.

Numerous simulations have been performed to optimize the free parameters of the algorithm and to quantitatively characterize the quality of the
reconstructions as functions of magnitude of orientation spread within grains,
those of degree of morphological complexity of grain maps, and of the artificial
noise.

Four 64×64-pixel test maps of aluminum samples of varying complexity
were used. In all cases, the *reference orientation map* was generated by electron microscopy; these maps are depicted in the upper left corners of Figs. 13.9
to 13.12, respectively. They represent different complexities in terms of the
number of grains and of the orientation spread inside grains:

Case I: This map comprises 11 grains; on average, the orientation spread
within grains is 0.0003427 (i.e., equivalent to the disorientation angle of
$\approx 3°$), while one grain has a spread of 0.0018652 ($7°$).

Case II: This map comprises 26 grains; the average orientation spread is
around 0.0018652 ($7°$), but the spread within grains varies from 0.0003427
up to 0.0183728 ($3°$–$22°$). The subdivision of some grains into subgrains
is also noticeable.

Case III: This map comprises 3 grains; the average orientation spread is
0.0074538 ($14°$).

Case IV: The material is, in this case, too deformed to comply with being
"moderately deformed" as defined in the introduction of this section.
Grains cannot be identified in an unambiguous way, and the orientation
spread sometimes surpasses 0.0109841 ($17°$). This case is included to test
the limitations of the algorithm.

We remark that the gray scale used in Figs. 13.9 to 13.14 makes it difficult to
see the orientation differences inside the grains for Cases I–III.

For each case, first a *reference grain map* was determined from the reference orientation map via a connected component technique. The next step

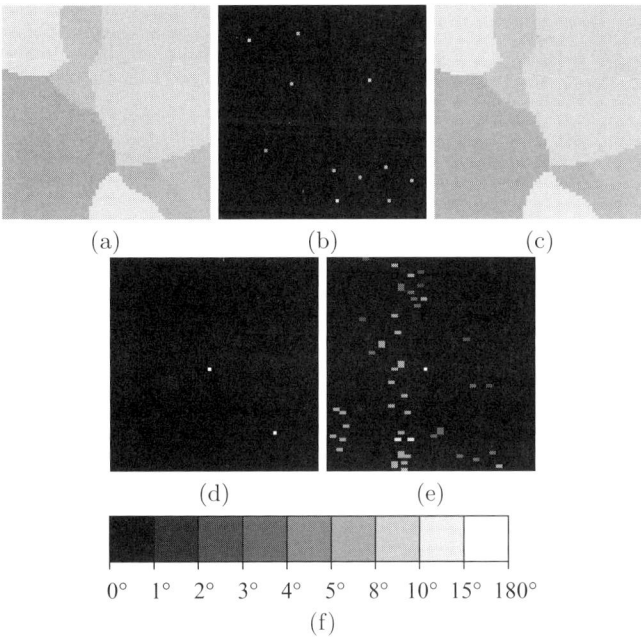

Fig. 13.9. The reconstruction of Test Case I using noiseless projections. **(a)** Reference orientation map. **(b)** Initial orientation map. **(c)** Reconstructed orientation map. **(d)** Difference of the reference and the reconstructed grain maps. Black pixels denote identical grain labels; white pixels represent mismatching ones. **(e)** Difference of the reference and the reconstructed orientation maps. The intensity of the pixels is determined by the distance (rotation angle) of corresponding orientation pairs, as shown in **(f)**.

consisted of the determination of the center-of-mass pixel and the average orientation of each of the grains. These were later used to initialize (f, o) by assigning a grain label and the corresponding average orientation to every center-of-mass pixel (called *seed points*), and by setting the labels of the remaining pixels to ambiguous. (The orientations of the latter were simply left undefined.) This procedure was meant to mimic the minimal outcome of an external method (e.g., GRAINSWEEPER [24]) to be used to retrieve such information by the preprocessing of 3DXRD diffraction patterns. For Case IV, somewhat arbitrarily a set of 31 seeds was determined.

Next for every test case, 3DXRD diffraction patterns associated with the reference orientation maps were simulated, optionally applying some synthetic noise as well. We generated 91 projections corresponding to equally spaced rotation angles from the interval $[-45°, 45°]$. The acquisition set-up imitated that of the 3DXRD microscope at the European Synchrotron Radiation Facility (ESRF) at the time.

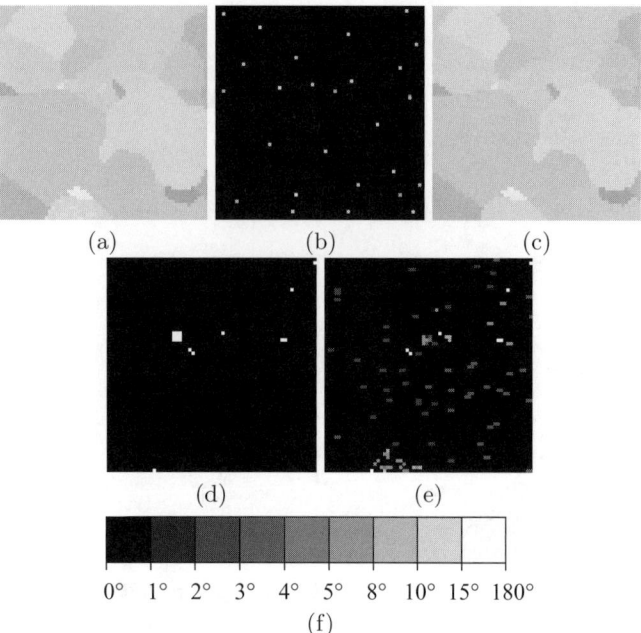

Fig. 13.10. The reconstruction of Test Case II using noiseless projections. Map arrangement and gray scales as for Fig. 13.9.

In order to come close to the quality of real diffraction patterns, varying levels of artificial noise were applied to the simulated projections. The distortions of measurements are caused by different kinds of phenomena: scattering, fluctuation of the intensity of the X-ray beam, statistical error (the so-called Poisson or quantum noise), cross-talk between neighboring detector pixels, etc. Out of these, perhaps the Poisson noise is the most prominent; therefore, only this sort of deviation was taken into account. Let us suppose that the intensity (photon count) I_0 of every detector pixel is to be distorted by $L\%$ of noise. The noisy intensity I_{noisy} was then, as an approximation to the Poisson distribution, defined as a uniformly distributed random number taken from $\left[I_0\left(1 - \frac{L}{100}\right), I_0\left(1 + \frac{L}{100}\right)\right]$, subject to the constraint of nonnegativity. A trivial property of such noise is that $I_{\text{noisy}} = 0$ whenever $I_0 = 0$. It should be stressed that this definition of noise is considerably different than that used for the simulation experiments in Section 13.3 (and in [1, 2]), so the results and conclusions cannot be directly compared.

The Gibbs potentials were fixed to the values U^1 introduced in Subsection 13.3.2. The ratio $\frac{\lambda_1}{\lambda_2}$ was also held constant at $\sqrt{2}$, as suggested in [7]. The only remaining free parameters of the objective functional were the relaxation scalar β, the two weights λ_1 and α that determine the relative importance of the three terms in (13.20), and the measure δ of the orientation spread appearing in (13.19).

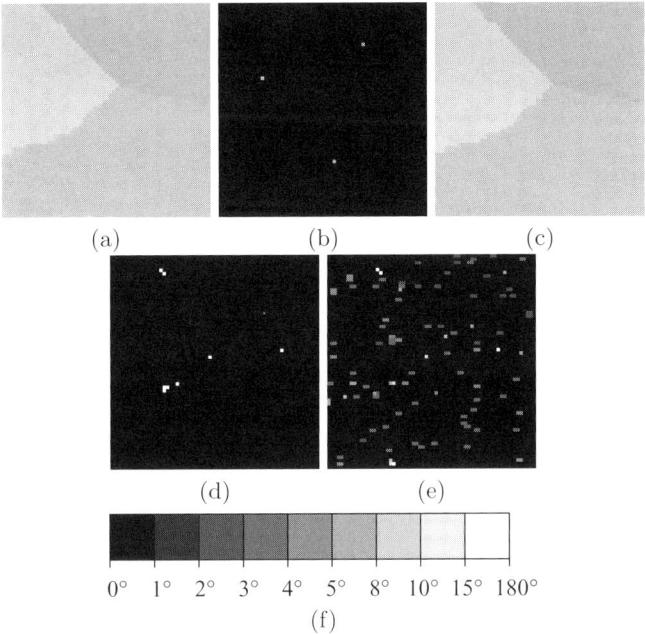

Fig. 13.11. The reconstruction of Test Case III using noiseless projections. Map arrangement and gray scales as for Fig. 13.9.

Based on the four test cases, associated input projections, and initial maps as defined above, a series of reconstructions was performed with varying system parameters α, β, λ_1, and number of Metropolis steps, as well as different noise levels. (The value of δ was always guessed from the reference orientation map and kept constant all the time. In particular, δ was set to 0.005 [11.5°], 0.01 [16.2°], 0.008 [14.5°], and 0.021 [23.5°] for Test Cases I–IV, respectively.)

The quality of the results were measured by two figure-of-merit functions, FOM_G and FOM_O.

$$\text{FOM}_\text{G} := 1 - \frac{M}{|D|}, \qquad (13.22)$$

where M denotes the number of mismatching grain labels between corresponding pixels of the reference and reconstructed grain maps, and $|D|$ is the number of pixels. The second figure-of-merit is related to the distance between the original orientation $o^{\text{orig}}(i)$ and the resulting orientation $o^{\text{rec}}(i)$ for each pixel i:

$$\text{FOM}_\text{O} := 1 - \frac{1}{d_{\max}|D|} \sum_{i \in D} d\left(o^{\text{orig}}(i), o^{\text{rec}}(i)\right), \qquad (13.23)$$

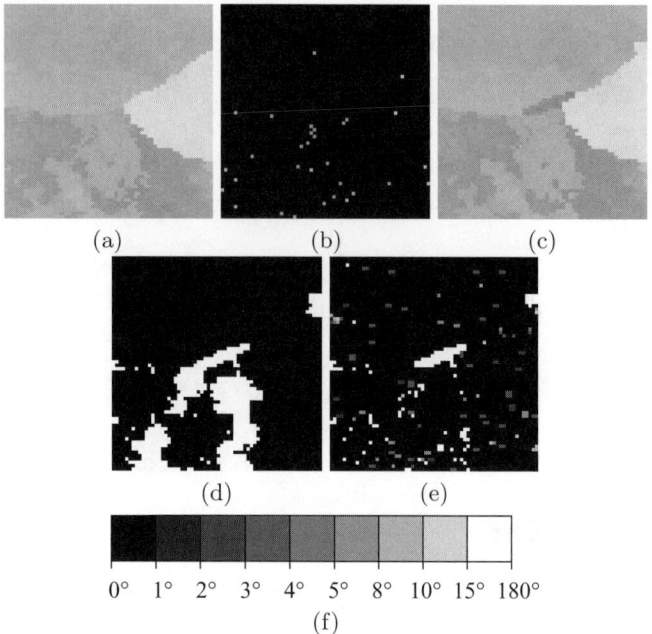

Fig. 13.12. The reconstruction of Test Case IV using noiseless projections. Map arrangement and gray scales as for Fig. 13.9.

where, for $i \in D$, $o^{\mathrm{orig}}(i)$ and $o^{\mathrm{rec}}(i)$ denote the orientations at pixel i in the original and in the reconstructed maps, and $d_{\max}$ represents the maximal possible value of $d(\cdot, \cdot)$, which equals about 0.1464466 (62.8°) for the face-centered cubic lattice. Evidently, $\mathrm{FOM_G} = \mathrm{FOM_O} = 1$ for perfectly reconstructed maps, while $\mathrm{FOM_G} \approx 0$ and $\mathrm{FOM_O} \approx 0.5$ for a random reconstruction.

Reconstructions tended to converge quite rapidly, needing not more than 2.5 million iterations (corresponding to about 8 minutes of computer time, and to approximately 600 MCC as defined in Subsection 13.3.3). The variations of the FOMs with respect to the aforementioned free parameters turned out to be small, implying that the algorithm is robust. For the following, the values $\alpha = \beta = \lambda_1 = 1$ have been employed.

Figures 13.9 through 13.12 present the results for the four test cases using ideal diffraction patterns. The qualities of the reconstructions in the first three cases are all very good, with both FOM values being at or above 0.99. Remarkably, a high-quality orientation map—with $\mathrm{FOM_O} = 0.986$—is derived also for Case IV. (In this case, the grain map is deteriorated and thus $\mathrm{FOM_G}$ is irrelevant.)

Similar reconstructions for 100% of noise are shown in Figs. 13.13 and 13.14, and figures-of-merit are summarized in Fig. 13.15. (The latter plot was acquired by repeating every reconstruction 10 times using different seeds for the pseudo-random number generator, where the error bars indicate the standard error due to this variability.) The noise in experimental data is estimated to be of order 10%, so the effect is clearly exaggerated in these simulations. Nevertheless, the FOM values of the reconstructions remain high.

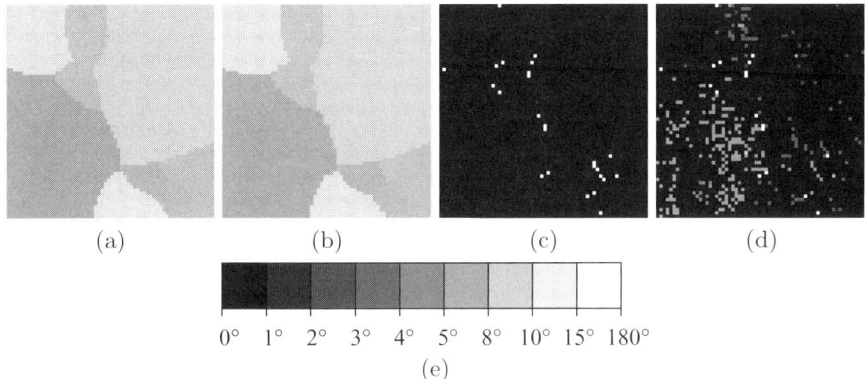

(a)   (b)   (c)   (d)

0° 1° 2° 3° 4° 5° 8° 10° 15° 180°

(e)

Fig. 13.13. The reconstruction of Test Case I at 100% noise level. **(a)** Reference orientation map. **(b)** Reconstructed orientation map. **(c)** Difference of the reference and the reconstructed grain maps. Black pixels denote identical grain labels; white pixels represent mismatching ones. **(d)** Difference of the reference and the reconstructed orientation maps. The intensity of the pixels is determined by the distance (rotation angle) of corresponding orientation pairs, as shown in **(e)**.

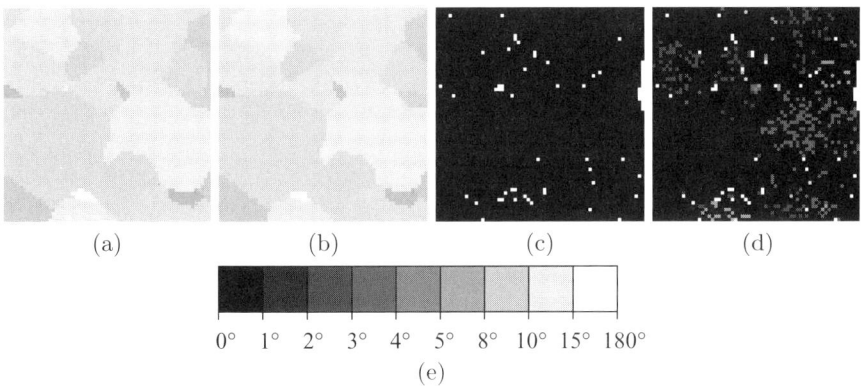

(a)   (b)   (c)   (d)

0° 1° 2° 3° 4° 5° 8° 10° 15° 180°

(e)

Fig. 13.14. The reconstruction of Test Case II at 100% noise level. Map arrangement and gray scales as for Fig. 13.13.

The impact of terms $H_1(f, o)$ and $H_2(f)$ was investigated by performing some experiments for Case II when one or both of these terms had been disabled. To get reliable statistics, all simulations were repeated 10 times

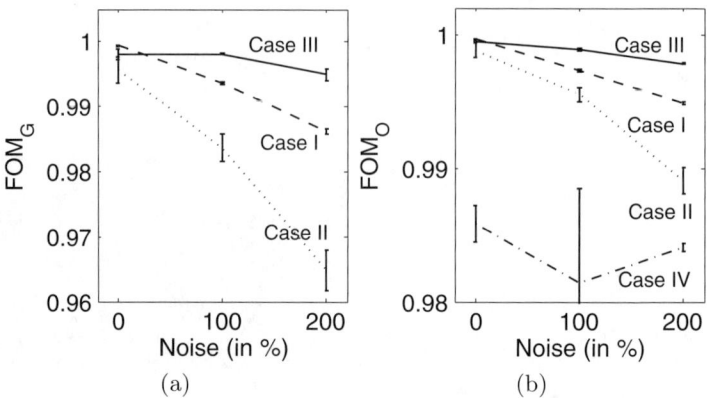

Fig. 13.15. Quality of the reconstructions as the function of noise level. (**a**) FOM_G versus the level of noise. (**b**) FOM_O versus the level of noise.

using different seeds for the pseudo-random number generator. The results are presented in Fig. 13.16. It is evident that including at least one of the additional terms is beneficial at higher noise levels.

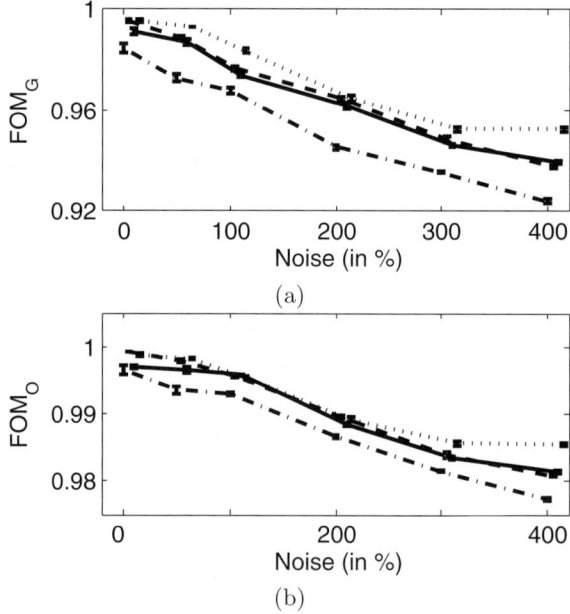

Fig. 13.16. Importance of various terms of the objective functional as the function of noise level. (**a**) FOM_G versus the level of noise. (**b**) FOM_O versus the level of noise. (**Legend**) Dotted: all terms; solid: $H_1(f, o)$ + projections; dashed: $H_2(f)$ + projections; dashdot: projections only.

13.5 Discussion and Outlook

We have demonstrated that the discrete tomography approach yields substantial improvements over the continuous approach (such as ART) when grain map and orientation map reconstructions are desired. The discrete nature of the reconstruction task was exploited in two ways:

(a) By introducing labels and discrete grain maps. This has reduced the size of solution space by orders of magnitude, thereby enabling the use of stochastic routines. We showed that we provide reconstructions of a quality that is clearly superior to previous approaches. The stochastic routines do need a priori information in terms of initial maps. However, this requirement is not that demanding; for the case of undeformed grains, even the output from an indexing program may do.

(b) By use of priors. To enable this, the methodology has been generalized from a two-phase (binary) to multiphase systems. The priors were shown to provide better maps in the cases where the reconstructions based only on the projections deteriorated (few projections, high noise, initial maps with little information).

Work on reconstructions of real experimental data is currently pending for both the undeformed and the moderately deformed cases.

The presented work serves as a basis for further improvements. We conclude with briefly stating some important further directions.

(a) The presented reconstructions were 2D. Three-dimension reconstructions are also of great interest; in producing them we will make use of (3D) Gibbs priors.

(b) It is unclear how to make a trade-off among the accuracy of the initial grain map (with ambiguous areas), the running time of the restoration algorithm, and the actual noise level.

(c) Real samples are usually not rectangular, so some pixels in the maps may correspond to air where there is no material to cause diffracted photons. The current implementation has some limited support for such *void pixels*, but their full-fledged handling will be a subject of future development

Acknowledgments

The authors would like to thank S. Schmidt, H.Y. Liao, Z. Kiss, and S.W. Rowland for helpful discussions. The European Synchrotron Radiation Facility is acknowledged for provision of beamtime. This work was partially supported by NIH grant HL070472 and NSF grant DMS0306215, by the Danish National Research Foundation, and by the Danish Natural Science Research Council (via Dansync). The first author was partially supported by a Feodor Lynen fellowship of the Alexander von Humboldt Foundation (Germany).

References

1. Alpers, A., Knudsen, E., Poulsen, H.F., Herman, G.T.: Resolving ambiguities in reconstructed grain maps using discrete tomography. *Electr. Notes Discr. Math.*, **20**, 419–437 (2005).
2. Alpers, A., Poulsen, H.F., Knudsen, E., Herman, G.T.: A discrete tomography algorithm for improving the quality of 3DXRD grain maps. *J. Appl. Cryst.*, **39**, 281–299 (2006).
3. Altmann, S.L.: *Rotations, Quaternions, and Double Groups.* Clarendon Press, Oxford, UK (1986).
4. Bässmann, H., Besslich, P.W.: *Bildverarbeitung Ad Oculos.* Springer, Berlin, Germany (1991).
5. Brémaud, P.: *Markov Chains: Gibbs Fields, Monte Carlo Simulations, and Queues.* Springer, New York, NY (1999).
6. Carvalho, B.M., Herman, G.T., Matej, S., Salzberg, C., Vardi, E.: Binary tomography for triplane cardiography. In: Kuba, A., Samal, M., Todd-Pokropek, A. (eds.), *Information Processing in Medical Imaging.* Springer, Berlin, Germany, pp. 29–41 (1999).
7. Chan, M.T., Herman, G.T., Levitan, E.: Probabilistic modeling of discrete images. In: Herman, G.T., Kuba, A. (eds.), *Discrete Tomography: Foundations, Algorithms, and Applications.* Birkhäuser, Boston, MA, pp. 213–235 (1999).
8. Conway, J.H., Smith, D.A.: *On Quaternions and Octonions: Their Geometry, Arithmetic, and Symmetry.* A. K. Peters, Natick, MA (2003).
9. Frank, F.C.: Orientation mapping. *Met. Trans.*, **A19**, 403–408 (1988).
10. Geman, S., Geman, D.: Stochastic relaxation, Gibbs distributions, and the Bayesian restoration of images. *IEEE Trans. PAMI*, **6**, 721–741 (1984).
11. Gordon, R., Bender, R., Herman, G.T.: Algebraic reconstruction techniques (ART) for three-dimensional electron microscopy and X-ray photography. *J. Theor. Biol.*, **29**, 471–482 (1970).
12. Grimmer, H.: Disorientations and coincidence rotations for cubic lattices. *Acta Cryst.*, **A30**, 685–688 (1974).
13. Hansen, L., Pospiech, J., Lücke, K.: *Tables of Texture Analysis of Cubic Crystals.* Springer, Berlin, Germany (1978).
14. Heinz, A., Neumann, P.: Representation of orientation and disorientation data for cubic, hexagonal, tetragonal and orthorombic crystals. *Acta Cryst.*, **A47**, 780–789 (1991).
15. Herman, G.T., Kuba, A. (eds.): *Discrete Tomography: Foundations, Algorithms, and Applications.* Birkhäuser, Boston, MA (1999).
16. Kirkpatrick, S., Gelatt, C.D., Vecchi, M.P.: Optimization by simulated annealing. *Science*, **220**, 671–680 (1983).
17. Kocks, U.F., Tomé, C.N., Wenk, H.R.: *Texture and Anisotropy.* Cambridge University Press, Cambridge, UK (1998).
18. Kuipers, J.B.: *Quaternions and Rotation Sequences: A Primer with Applications to Orbits, Aerospace and Virtual Reality.* Princeton University Press, Princeton, NJ (1999).
19. Liao, H.Y., Herman, G.T.: Automated estimation of the parameters of Gibbs priors to be used in binary tomography. *Discrete Appl. Math.*, **139**, 149–170 (2004).

20. Markussen, T., Fu, X., Margulies, L., Lauridsen, E.M., Nielsen, S.F., Schmidt, S., Poulsen, H.F.: An algebraic algorithm for generation of three-dimensional grain maps based on diffraction with a wide beam of hard X-rays. *J. Appl. Cryst.*, **37**, 96–102 (2004).
21. Metropolis, N., Rosenbluth, A.W., Rosenbluth, M.N., Teller, A.H., Teller, E.: Equation of state calculations by fast computing machines. *J. Chem. Phys.*, **21**, 1087–1092 (1953).
22. Morawiec, A.: *Orientations and Rotations. Computations in Crystallographic Textures*. Springer, Berlin, Germany (2004).
23. Poulsen, H.F.: A six-dimensional approach to microstructure analysis. *Phil. Mag.*, **83**, 2761–2778 (2003).
24. Poulsen, H.F.: *Three-Dimensional X-Ray Diffraction Microscopy: Mapping Polycrystals and Their Dynamics*. Springer, Berlin, Germany (2004).
25. Poulsen, H.F., Fu, X.: Generation of grain maps by an algebraic reconstruction technique. *J. Appl. Cryst.*, **36**, 1062–1068 (2003).
26. Rodek, L., Knudsen, E., Poulsen, H.F., Herman, G.T.: Discrete tomographic reconstruction of 2D polycrystal orientation maps from X-ray diffraction projections using Gibbs priors. *Electr. Notes Discr. Math.*, **20**, 439–453 (2005).

14

Discrete Tomography Methods for Nondestructive Testing

J. Baumann, Z. Kiss, S. Krimmel, A. Kuba, A. Nagy, L. Rodek, B. Schillinger, J. Stephan

Summary. The industrial nondestructive testing (NDT) of objects seems to be an ideal application of discrete tomography. In many cases, the objects consist of known materials, and a lot of a priori information is available (e.g., the description of an ideal object, which is similar to the actual one under investigation). One of the frequently used methods in NDT is to take projection images of the objects by some transmitting ray (e.g., X- or neutron-ray) and reconstruct the cross sections. But it can happen that only a few number of projections can be collected, because of long and/or expensive data acquisition, or the projections can be collected only from a limited range of directions. The chapter describes two DT reconstruction methods used in NDT experiments, shows the results of a DT procedure applied in the reconstruction of oblong objects having projections only from a limited range of angles, and, finally, suggests a few further possible NDT applications of DT.

14.1 Introduction

Many industrial applications need a procedure to get information about the structure of the object to be investigated in a nondestructive manner. X-ray tomography is such a technique, performing reconstructions of cross sections of the object from X-ray transmission projections. Nevertheless, the acquisition of such projection images can be an expensive and time-consuming procedure, and it is also possible that projections from certain directions cannot be taken. It is therefore important to be able to reconstruct from as few views as possible. An approach to achieving this is the application of discrete tomographic (DT) methods, in which only a special class of objects can be reconstructed, namely those comprising only a few homogeneous materials that can be characterized by known, discrete absorption values. Accordingly, the result of a DT reconstruction is an image having values only corresponding to the few known absorption coefficients. An overview of theory, algorithms, and applications of DT can be found in [4].

A substantial difference between classical computed tomography (CT) and discrete tomography (DT) is that in the latter it is assumed that the range of the image function consists of finitely many *known values*. Moreover, in many cases, some *a priori information* is also available about the object under investigation; for example, the structure of the object is similar to that of a given template. An important application of discrete tomography is the industrial *nondestructive testing* (NDT), in which the internal structure of a specimen is to be determined without causing any damage.

This chapter describes DT reconstruction algorithms used in NDT in Section 14.2. Also, the test results of the simulation and physical experiments are presented. In Section 14.3, we show that the application of these DT methods is suitable, for example, to increase the possible inspection size of single-material oblong objects. The increase of the object's size with DT reconstruction compared to filtered back-projection (FBP) used in X-ray computed tomography (CT) was estimated to be above 50%. Finally, in Section 14.4, we suggest some further possible NDT applications of DT.

14.2 Reconstruction of Pixel-based and Geometric Objects

This section introduces two kinds of DT techniques, which can be applied to reconstruct two-level and even multilevel images (i.e., their range contains only two or even more than two values, respectively) from their projections. Both algorithms consider the reconstruction problem as an optimization problem to be solved by a method called *simulated annealing* (SA). The difference between the reconstruction algorithms is the representation of the object under investigation.

One of the reconstruction techniques is a pixel-based method that considers the object as a set of pixels, i.e., as a usual digital image. The main advantage of the pixel-based method is that it is general in the sense that it can be used for reconstructing any shape. This method is described in Subsection 14.2.3.

The other algorithm reconstructs objects consisting of circles, cylinders, and spheres made of homogeneous materials only. Such 2D and 3D geometric objects can be represented by a few parameters like radii, positions, heights, etc. In this case, the reconstruction means the determination of the parameters of the geometric objects; in other words, the optimization carries out a search in the space of parameters. This parameter-based method is presented in Subsection 14.2.4.

In order to assess the efficiency of these techniques, we performed several simulation experiments. We were also interested in how certain reconstruction parameters (e.g., the number of projections) or the amount of noise affect the reconstructed image. These results and conclusions are shown in Subsection 14.2.5. We had the opportunity to test both algorithms also for reconstructing real, not necessarily binary, objects. The results of these X-ray experiments are given in Subsection 14.2.6.

The physically measured projections are not suitable for immediate reconstruction due to several properties and defects of the image acquisition system (e.g., nonuniform sensitivity during acquisition and on the detector plate, bright specks, presence of statistical noise, etc.). Hence, some preprocessing steps are necessary to reduce these effects. These correction steps are summarized in Subsection 14.2.6.

The algorithms presented here have been incorporated into the system called DIRECT (discrete reconstruction techniques) [17], which is a framework for testing and visualizing various DT methods. For more details about implementation, see [7, 10].

14.2.1 Reconstruction as an Optimization Problem

The usual tomographic imaging procedure is to collect projections of the object using some transmission rays, like X- or neutron rays. The rays transmitted through the object are partially absorbed by the materials comprising the object. The relation between the initial and transmitted (unabsorbed) ray intensities, I_S and I_D, respectively, can be expressed as a function that depends on the absorption coefficient (μ) of the object, that is,

$$I_D\left(s, \vartheta\right) = I_S \cdot e^{-\int\limits_{S}^{D} \mu(u)du} , \qquad (14.1)$$

where the integral is taken on the line between the source (S) and detector (D). This equation is a basic relation in *transmission tomography*, in which the cross sections of the object are to be determined from such measurements.

Mathematically, transmission tomography is modeled by the *Radon transform*, $\mathcal{R}f$, which gives the line integrals of a two-dimensional integrable function f. Formally,

$$[\mathcal{R}f]\left(s, \vartheta\right) = \int\limits_{-\infty}^{\infty} f(x, y)\, du , \qquad (14.2)$$

where s and u denote the variables of the coordinate system rotated by ϑ. The function $\mathcal{R}f$ for a fixed value of ϑ is also called the ϑ-angle *projection* of f.

Returning to the physical model of transmission tomography, hereafter let f denote the absorption coefficient of the 2D object being studied. Then the ϑ-angle projection of f, $[\mathcal{R}f](s, \vartheta)$ can be computed from the transmission measurements, $I_D(s, \vartheta)$ after a suitable *logarithmic transform*. That is, we are looking for an f such that

$$[\mathcal{R}f]\left(s, \vartheta\right) = \log \frac{I_S}{I_D\left(s, \vartheta\right)} . \qquad (14.3)$$

Now the *reconstruction problem* can be posed as one where the goal is to find a function f such that its projections are equal to the right side of

(14.3). In other words, we are looking for the inverse of $\mathcal{R}$. The function f is sometimes called the *image function* or, briefly, the *image*.

Let $P_\vartheta(s)$ denote the acquired projection of angle ϑ [i.e., the right side of (14.3)] as a function of s for a given direction ϑ. Similarly, let $[\mathcal{R}f](\vartheta)$ denote the projection of the image f taken at angle ϑ, which is also a function of s. Both methods to be presented consider the reconstruction problem as an optimization task that minimizes the *objective functional*

$$C(f) = \sum_\vartheta \| [\mathcal{R}f](\vartheta) - P_\vartheta \|^2 , \qquad (14.4)$$

where $\|.\|$ denotes the usual Euclidean norm. So, using the formalism of (14.4), the aim of this optimization is to find the image function f, whose corresponding projections are the most suitable for the input data.

To solve the optimization tasks associated with the different kind of representations, we used the method of simulated annealing (SA).

14.2.2 Simulated Annealing (SA)

Simulated annealing (SA) is a random-search technique that is based on the physical phenomenon of metal cooling. The system of metal particles gradually reaches the minimum energy level where the metal freezes into a crystalline structure.

The algorithm (see Fig. 14.1) starts from an arbitrary initial binary image $x = x^{(0)}$ and an initial (high) temperature $T^{(0)}$, and calculates the objective functional value $C(x)$. Then a position j is randomly chosen in the reconstructed image x. Let x' be the image that differs from x only by changing the value of x in position j to the other binary value, i.e., $x'_j = 1 - x_j$. This change is accepted by the algorithm, i.e., x is replaced by x', if $C(x') < C(x)$. Even if the objective functional does not get smaller, the change is accepted with a probability depending on the difference $\Delta C = C(x') - C(x)$.

Formally, the change is accepted even in that case when

$$\exp(-\Delta C/\kappa T) > z, \qquad (14.5)$$

where κ, T, and z are, respectively, the Boltzmann constant ($11.3805 \times 10^{-23} \times$ m^{2}kg s$^{-2}K^{-1}$), current temperature, and a randomly generated number from a uniform distribution in the interval $[0, 1]$. Otherwise, the change is rejected, i.e., x does not change in this iteration step. If a change is rejected, then we test the level of *efficiency* of changes in the image in the last iterations. It means that we count the number of rejections in the last N_{iter} iterations. If this number is greater than a given threshold value R_{thr}, then the efficiency of changes is too low and the SA optimization algorithm will be terminated.

We calculate the variance of the cost function in the last N_{var} iterations. A so-called equilibrium state is said to be attained if the present estimate of the current ΔC variance is greater than the previous variance estimate. If the

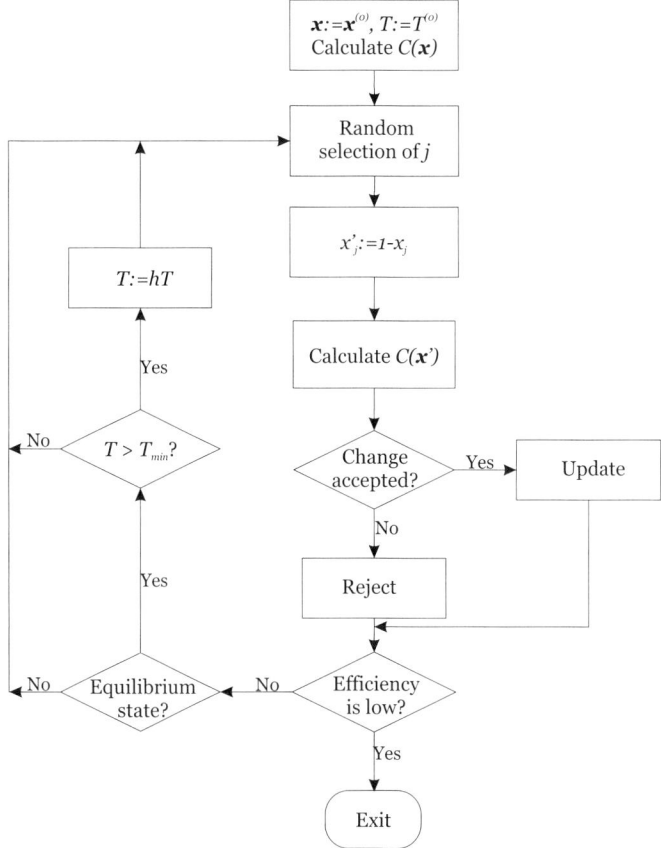

Fig. 14.1. Flowchart of the implemented SA algorithm.

equilibrium state is achieved, we reduce the current temperature (allowing changes with smaller probabilities when the value of the objective functional is greater) and let the algorithm run with a lower temperature value (T is replaced by $h \cdot T$, where h is the *cooling factor*). In our experiments, we chose the same value for this parameter as in [12], namely $h = 0.9$.

Finally, we implemented the SA as follows. We change all the x-vector elements from 0 to 1 or vice versa in one iteration step. The changes are accepted or rejected as it is described. When one iteration has been done, we reduce the current temperature and start a new iteration step. The algorithm stops when the ratio of the value of the current objective function and that of the starting objective function fall below a given threshold value ($C(x')/C(x^{(0)}) < C_{\text{thr}}$) or the current temperature is less then a given temperature ($T < T_{\text{thr}}$).

14.2.3 The Pixel-based Reconstruction Method

Since industrial objects are often made of more than two materials, it was desirable to enable the technique to reconstruct not only binary but multi-level images as well. In this case, the pixels can take their intensity values from $D = \{d_1, \ldots, d_l\}$, i.e., $l \geq 2$ denotes the number of possible intensity values (levels). The obvious extension of the binary modification rule to multilevel image is a uniformly distributed random choice of an intensity level from D.

In order to improve the efficiency, we add to (14.4) a regularization term $\phi(f)$ that includes the a priori information about the image function to be reconstructed. So the objective that we used in our pixel-based method is

$$C(f) = \sum_{\vartheta} \| [\mathcal{R}f](\vartheta) - P_\vartheta \|^2 + \gamma \cdot \phi(f), \tag{14.6}$$

where $\gamma \geq 0$ is the so-called regularization parameter, which determines the weight between the two terms. A small γ prefers a result that matches better the input projections, a big γ yields an outcome that is more appropriate for the a priori information. If the image to be reconstructed contains a few large regions made of homogeneous materials, this information may be modeled by *smoothness*, provided by the functional

$$\phi(f) = -\sum_{x,y} \sum_{u,v} f(x - u, y - v) \frac{\exp\left(-\frac{(u-\mu_1)^2 + (v-\mu_2)^2}{2\sigma_1\sigma_2}\right)}{\sqrt{2\pi}\sigma_1\sigma_2}, \tag{14.7}$$

where $\sigma_1, \sigma_2, \mu_1$, and μ_2 are suitable constants.

14.2.4 The Parameter-based Method

Our second reconstruction method takes the assumption that the object is composed of a tube encompassing a solid cylinder called the interior (i.e., the inner space of the tube), which contains a known number of disjoint solid spheres or cylinders made of homogeneous materials. Furthermore, it is also assumed that at most four different homogeneous materials constitute the object, namely,

(a) the material of the tube,
(b) the material of the interior,
(c) the material of the spheres and cylinders, and
(d) the background surrounding the object, which is usually air or vacuum.

Since spheres as well as cylinders can be described by a few parameters like center, height, and radius, each object can be represented as a vector of parameters called a *configuration*. In order to perform a truly 3D recon-struction, the optimization of the objective functional $C(f)$ is performed in the parameter space iteratively. Starting off from an initial configuration, the current configuration is altered at every iteration step to produce a better approximation of the object to be reconstructed. The modified configuration may be accepted only if it satisfies certain geometric restrictions. A more detailed description of the algorithm can be found in [7, 10].

14.2.5 Simulation Studies

Reconstruction of Pixel-based Objects

We reconstructed several multilevel phantom objects. One of the phantoms and one of its projections can be seen in Fig. 14.2(a) and (b). The reconstructions using the objective functionals (14.4) and (14.6) with the regularization term (14.7) are shown in Fig. 14.2(c) and (d), respectively. Clearly, the smoothness term improved the quality by preferring images having connected regions with constant values.

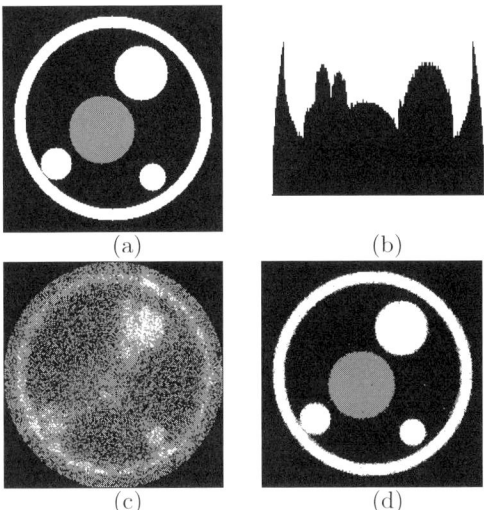

Fig. 14.2. The three-level phantom image and its reconstructions. (**a**) The phantom image used for simulation studies. (**b**) One of the projections of the object in (a). Reconstruction results from 12 noiseless projections, 400 measurements/projection (**c**) using the objective functional (14.4), and (**d**) using the objective functional of (14.6) and (14.7).

Reconstruction of Parameter-based Objects

The aim of this simulation experiment was to examine the effects of geometric complexity of the 3D object when using only two noisy projections. The object was a tube containing spheres with different diameters. The complexity of the object was determined by the number of spheres in the tube. As Fig. 14.3 shows, it is, generally, hard to produce an acceptable result from two projections if there are five or more spheres. The objects are presented using the virtual reality modeling language (VRML97 [19]) and reconstructed by DIRECT [17].

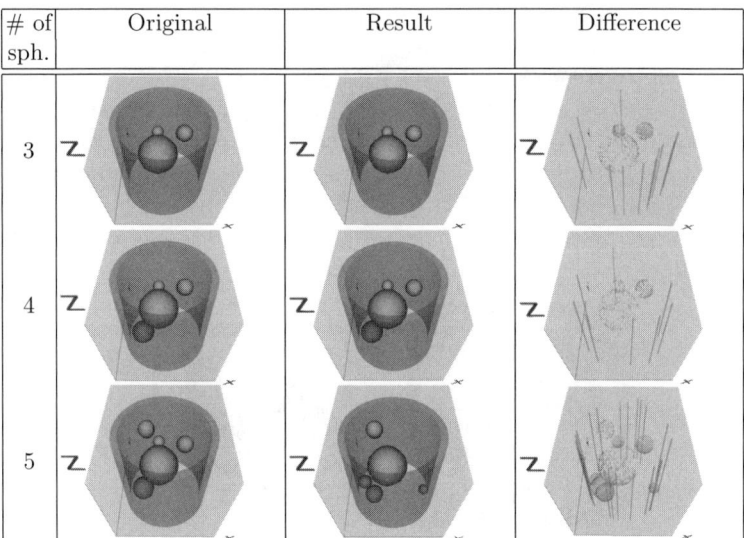

Fig. 14.3. Reconstruction by parameter-based method using different numbers of spheres (parameters: 10% noise, two 2D projections, 100 × 100 measurements/projection). First column: number of spheres. Second column: original objects. Third column: reconstructed objects. Fourth column: differences between the reconstructed and original objects (only mismatching voxels are painted).

The influence of the noise can be observed in the reconstructed images in Fig. 14.4.

14.2.6 Experimental Results

We had the opportunity to test our techniques using X-ray projection data of real physical phantoms. One of these physical experiments is presented in this subsection.

Test Object

The object was a *reference cylinder*; a solid cylinder made of plexiglas, containing three cylindrical bores of different diameters and depths in an asymmetric arrangement [see Fig. 14.5(a)]. The lower part of the deepest hole was filled with aluminium screws, as shown in Fig. 14.5(b).

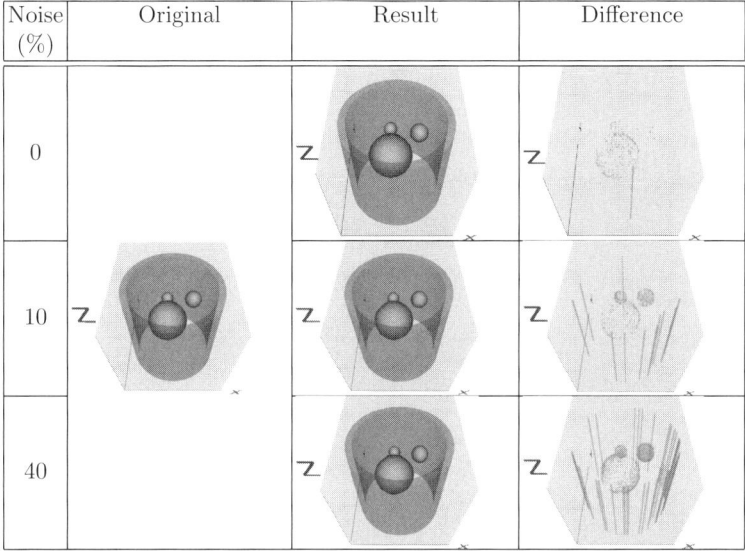

Noise (%)	Original	Result	Difference
0			
10			
40			

Fig. 14.4. Reconstructions by the parameter-based method from noise-free and noisy projections (parameters: three spheres, two 2D projections, 100×100 measurements/projection). First column: noise level. Second column: original object. Third column: reconstructed objects. Fourth column: differences between the reconstructed and the original object.

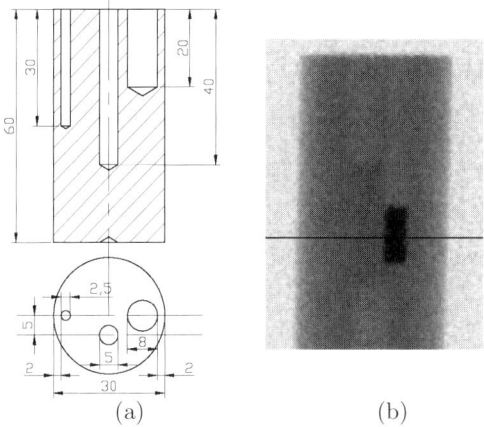

Fig. 14.5. Reference cylinder. (**a**) Structure of the reference cylinder used in the X-ray experiments. (**b**) One of its projections.

Data Acquisition

The apparatus was suitable to collect not only X-rays but also other kinds of rays (neutron or gamma) as well (see Fig. 14.6). The object to be investigated is placed on a table rotated by a stepper motor, thus letting the beams transmit through the object in different directions. The beams attenuated by the object impact into a scintillator, which transforms the detected radiation into visible light detected by a CCD camera. Since the camera can be damaged by direct exposure to radiation, an optical mirror system conveys the light from the scintillator to the CCD camera. The images taken by the camera are stored temporarily by the camera controller, and finally a dedicated PC reads out the raw image data from this storage. A more detailed description of the imaging apparatus can be found in [1].

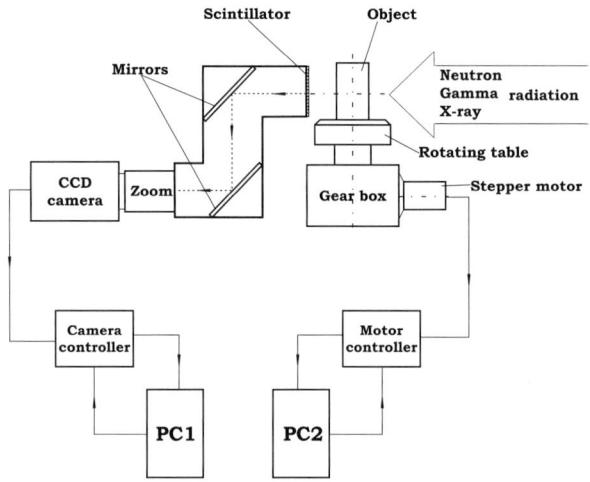

Fig. 14.6. Imaging apparatus for collecting projections.

Preprocessing

Due to several distorting effects of the data acquisition system, the measured projections of the physical objects were not suitable for immediate reconstruction. In order to diminish the effects of these distortions, some corrections (preprocessing steps) were performed on the projection data. In the case of the reference cylinder, these steps were the following:

(a) *Logarithmic transformation* of the measured data according to (14.3). This step is necessary to get the line integrals of the absorption function to be reconstructed.

(b) Due to the fluctuating flux of the rays and/or the changing sensitivity of the imaging system in time, the average intensity of the projections varied from projection to projection. In order to eliminate this effect, we performed *intensity correction* by multiplying the projections by suitable constants.

(c) A further distorting effect was caused by white points randomly distributed in the projections. To reduce their effects, we applied a *thresholded median filtering*.

Further details about the correction steps and their effects on the reconstruction can be found in [10].

Determination of Intensity Levels

The next problem to be solved before reconstruction was that the exact intensity levels of the cross-section images (i.e., the exact absorption values) were unknown. Anyway, in real physical experiments, only approximative absorption values can be given, since only average absorption coefficients could be used for polychromatic X-rays. This fact violated one of our basic assumptions, namely, the absorption coefficients of the few materials making up the object should have been known exactly. So we had to find a technique to approximate the right absorption values.

In the case of the parameter-based method, the absorption values could be calculated in virtue of the object geometry. In the pixel-based case, our idea was that we approached the image f of the right (but unknown) values with another image f' having more given values approximating the right ones from both directions. As a first approximation of the right intensity values, we could take the local maxima in the histogram of f'. The set of the increased number of intensity levels of f' was produced by the equidistant division of the interval of the possible levels of f. For example, if the intensity levels are from the interval $[0, 1]$, and 41 intensity levels are picked from that, the increased set of levels is $\{0, 1/40, 2/40, \ldots, 1\}$.

In the case of the reference cylinder, even the background was subtracted, because it was very noisy, and it degraded the result. Despite this step, the image still remained a three-level one (having a background value near 0). A reconstruction result, which was done by using 41 intensity levels from 18 projections, can be seen in Fig. 14.7. The obtained intensity levels can be considered only as an approximation of the right ones. As a following step, we took the local maxima of the histogram of this reconstruction result as the intensity levels that could be used for the multilevel DT reconstruction. In Fig. 14.8, the histogram of Fig. 14.7 is presented. It can be seen that there are three peeks in the histograms (see pointers in Fig. 14.8). The corresponding intensity levels were used in the multilevel DT reconstruction.

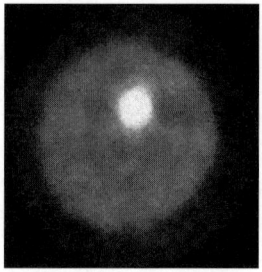

Fig. 14.7. A reconstruction result (155 × 155) of the pixel-based method using 41 intensity levels.

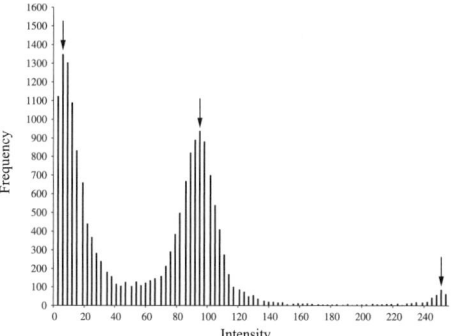

Fig. 14.8. Histogram of the reconstructed cross section in Fig. 14.7.

Pixel-based Reconstruction Results

With the preprocessed projections and intensity values described so far, we performed the pixel-based reconstruction. Its result may be seen in Fig. 14.9(a). For the sake of comparison, we performed ART reconstruction (1000 iterations, relaxation parameter 0.001), which yielded the outcome visible in Fig. 14.9(b).

Parameter-based Reconstruction Results

In addition to the software experiments mentioned in Subsection 14.2.5, we had the opportunity to try the parameter-based reconstruction method on physically measured data too. In the experiments, we used the reference cylinder introduced in Subsection 14.2.6. [One of its X-ray projections is shown in Fig. 14.10(a).] Because of the assumption that every cylindrical hole is filled with the same material, the lower half of the projections had to be discarded [see Fig. 14.10(b)]. The model reconstructed from four projections and the difference of the original and the reconstructed model are seen in Fig. 14.10(c)-(f), respectively. For a more detailed description of these physical experiments, see [7, 10, 11].

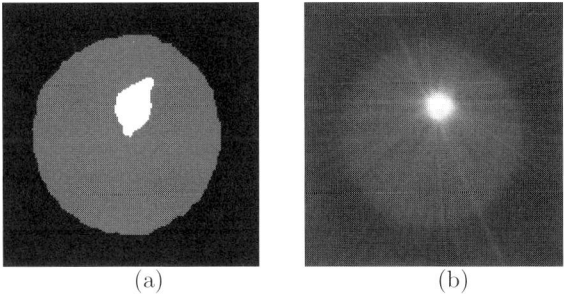

Fig. 14.9. Reconstruction results. (**a**) A pixel-based reconstruction result of the cross section denoted in Fig. 14.5(b) using three intensity levels. (**b**) An ART reconstruction yielded by SNARK93 [18].

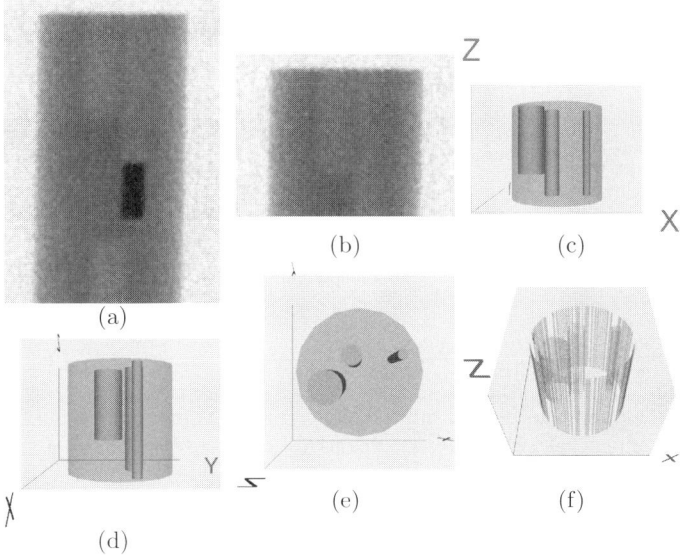

Fig. 14.10. Projection and reconstruction results of the Plexiglas object given in Fig. 14.5. (**a**) One of the projection images of the whole object. (**b**) One of the projection images of the upper half of the object. (**c**) 0° view of the reconstructed model. (**d**) 90° view of the reconstructed model. (**e**) Top-down view of the reconstructed model. (**f**) Difference between the reconstructed and original models.

14.3 Reconstruction from Limited View Angles

The scope of this section is to point out a further potential of DT for NDT
with X-ray CT. A key problem for X-ray CT in NDT is the strong absorption
in metal objects. We aim to increase the inspection size of oblong objects that
are made of a single material and for which X-ray penetration is limited for a
few directions [see Fig. 14.11(a)]. This is a special case of *limited view angle
tomography*. It is clear that filtered back-projection (FBP) is not suitable as
a reconstruction method because it requires projection data from many view
angles on a circular source trajectory, i.e., usually a 180° scan for parallel beam
geometry and a 360° scan for fan beam geometry. If we use FBP despite the
lack of data, limited view angle artifacts will arise. A compensation is possible
with DT using the preknowledge about the material composition of the object.

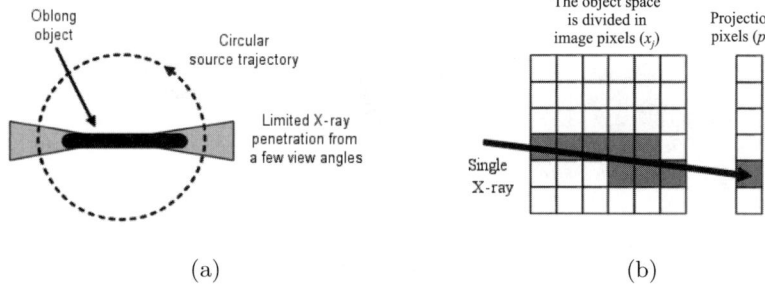

(a)   (b)

Fig. 14.11. (a) Special case of limited view angle tomography for oblong objects.
(b) Illustration of one projection equation: It is a projection along a single X-ray
onto one detector pixel. The image pixels that contribute to the projection are drawn
shaded.

Nevertheless, FBP is the most popular technique in NDT because of its
high image quality, fast implementation, and robustness against distortions in
the data, e.g., noise, polychromatic X-rays, and scattering. The ultimate goal
of this work is the reconstruction of experimental data with DT for which
high data quality is crucial. Before starting with the experiments, we simulated projection data and analyzed the sensitivity of DT to distortions. For the
experiment itself, we compared a micro-focus CT system with a *flat-panel image* (FPI) detector at Siemens to a special line detector set up at the EMPA.[1]
All investigations were performed with 2D tomography and a special phantom
that features relevant NDT tasks like crack and void detection as well as dimensional measuring. A beam-hardening correction was also performed. The

---

[1] Eidgenössische Materialprüfungs- und Forschungsanstalt, Dübendorf, Switzerland.

simulations and experiments were performed by Siemens. The reconstructions using discrete tomography were done at the University of Szeged.

Let us consider again the optimization task given in (14.6) using the smoothing regularization term (14.7) and the optimization method simulated annealing described in Subsection 14.2.2.

14.3.1 Experimental Issues

Investigated Object: Bat Phantom

We designed a phantom that is a model for a number of nondestructive testing problems. It is made of copper (strong absorber) with gaps (*crack detection*), drills (void detection), curved and linear shapes (dimensional measuring). Figure 14.12 shows a photo of the manufactured phantom. This "bat phantom" has a cross-sectional size of 70 mm × 16 mm, and the smallest drill diameter and gap height are 0.5 mm. The phantom length of 70 mm is a critical size for X-ray penetration in copper at 200 kV. This size was defined with the help of simulated data for different conditions (namely, object size, voltage, and dynamic range).

Fig. 14.12. Photo of the investigated bat phantom (cross section 70 mm × 16 mm).

Selecting an Appropriate Experimental Set-up to Avoid Scattering and to Achieve a High Dynamic Range

Experimental measurements were done at two different setups for CT. The first one is a 225 kV micro-focus system with a 2D FPI detector at Siemens CT PS9. The other is a 450 kV mini-focus X-ray tube with a 1D line detector at the EMPA. The principal configuration of the two systems is sketched in Fig. 14.13.

The 225 kV micro-focus system is designed for high-resolution 3D cone beam computed tomography of small parts. The object is usually magnified by a large factor, and the spatial resolution is defined by the focal spot size of the X-ray tube (typ. ∅ 1–100 μm). At the same time, the tube power is limited (typ. < 100 W), and the acquisition time for one projection is rather large. A 2D area detector is necessary to achieve reasonable scanning times in 3D micro-focus CT. The advantages of our FPI detector are a high spatial resolution (in our case, 2048 × 2048 pixels of 0.2-mm pixel size) and good noise properties. A disadvantage is that strong internal scattering affects the image quality if large and strong absorbing objects are investigated at higher energies, e.g. the bat phantom at 200 kV. This is a commonly known problem for FPI detectors in NDT [15], and the usable dynamic range (maximum detectable intensity/minimum detectable intensity) is significantly reduced for such experiments. Scattering from the object plays a minor role for this set-up because the object–detector distance is quite large (0.5–1 m).

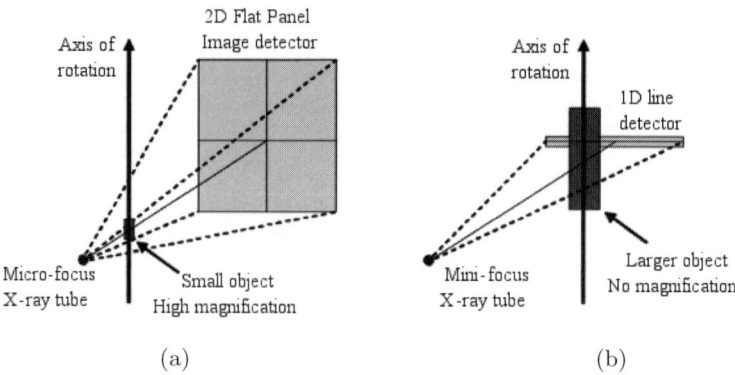

Fig. 14.13. Geometric configuration of the investigated CT systems. **(a)** Micro-focus CT with FPI detector and **(b)** mini-focus CT with line detector.

The 450 kV mini-focus system uses 2D fan beam geometry and a line detector whose pixels are spaced in equal angular increments (Fig. 14.14). It is designed for the inspection of larger parts with a lower resolution. To enhance penetration possibilities, voltages up to 450 kV can be used. A high tube power (1 kW) allows reasonably fast scanning, but the focal spot size is large (⌀ 2.5 mm). If the investigated object is not magnified (or a small magnification is used), the spatial resolution will be determined by the detector pixel size. As the detector pixel spacing (2.1 mm) is large and the number of detector channels (125) is small, subpositions are scanned to achieve a resolution of 0.1–1 mm. For our experiments, an acquisition mode has been used that yielded parallel beam projection data[2] with 0.23-mm resolution. The most important advantage of the EMPA system is its special line detector that avoids X-ray scattering. It has a tungsten collimator to suppress scattering coming from the object (important because of a small object–detector distance). Moreover, it uses large and strong absorbing scintillator cells (6-mm $CdWO_4$) such that almost no radiation can pass into the detector housing and cause internal scattering. Therefore, the data are not distorted, which is a prerequisite for

---

[2] This is possible by a translational movement of the object parallel to the detector, rotation by the fan angle and resorting of the projection rays.

DT reconstruction. Furthermore, the usable dynamic range and the possible material thickness for inspection are much larger as compared to the FPI detector.

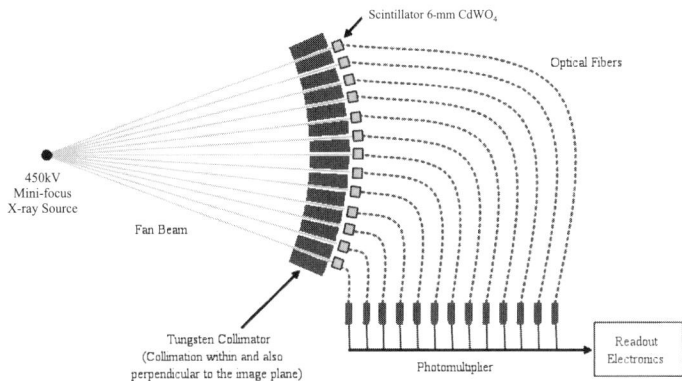

Fig. 14.14. Schematic of EMPA set-up. Scattering is avoided by a special line detector.

In order to study the effects of polychromatic X-ray and its correction, a special phantom object was designed and used in the experiments. The details of these experiments are given in [8].

14.3.2 Results

Simulation Results

To analyze the performance of discrete tomography, simulated projections have been used. We started with ideal monochromatic data and then investigated how noise and polychromatic X-rays affected the reconstruction. Scattering has not been considered in the simulations. The simulation was done for ideal fan beam geometry, i.e., a point source and a linear detector (400 detector pixels, 360 projections in 360°, image pixel size for reconstruction 0.32 mm). The detected intensities were computed by line integrals and the exponential absorption law. Using floating-point arithmetic, the dynamic range was infinite at first, i.e., no views with limited number of digits occurred. In order to produce views with a limited number of digits, we reduced the dynamic range by setting all values below a certain threshold to this minimum value. For all monochromatic examples, the energy was 160 keV. For the polychromatic case, a linearly approximated tube spectrum at 160 kV was used with an additional beam-hardening filter of 1.5-mm copper. This approximation is sufficient here because the spectrum is not too different from a real one and we look at the problem from a qualitative point of view.

The reconstructions were performed with filtered back-projection (FBP) and discrete tomography (i.e., reconstruction of pixel-based objects). The execution of FBP needed 5 sec on a 2 GHz CPU. This compares to 10 min for one DT reconstruction (10^5 iterations). Furthermore, the DT reconstructions were repeated 50 times and averaged to give a better and more stable result (repeated reconstructions do not give identical results with DT thanks to the stochastic behavior of SA). The total reconstruction time for 50 repetitions was 8 hr. As an additional feature, a smoothness penalty term has been used. Different settings will be mentioned explicitly.

Simulation for the Ideal Case

The first result we show is for the ideal case, i.e., monochromatic data, no noise, and infinite dynamic range. In Fig. 14.15, the FBP reconstruction for a high sampling with 800 detector pixels and 2880 projections is shown. No artifacts are visible in this image, and we can take it as a reference for comparison with the other results. To point out deviations between different reconstructions, we will frequently use vertical line profiles across the most critical region of the bat phantom as indicated by the arrow.

For the investigation with DT, we used a low sampling of 400 detector pixels and 360 projections. This optimized the reconstruction time, and for DT it is expected to produce no errors (DT is also suitable to reconstruct objects from a very small number of projections). The reconstructions from low sampling with FBP and DT are comparable on Figs. 14.16(a) and (b). A closer look at the vertical line profiles [Fig. 14.16(c) and (d)] reveals ripples (aliasing artifacts) for FBP due to the low sampling, but the geometric shape does not change. The profiles are compared to FBP with high sampling, for which only some minor spikes remain (the sampling is still not high enough). The DT result is exact within the pixel resolution. This result was computed without a smoothness penalty term as it did not change anything here. Note that the line profiles for the low sampling were resampled to match the high sampling case.

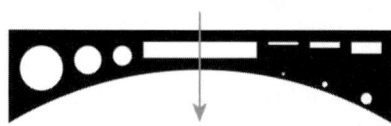

Fig. 14.15. FBP reconstruction for the ideal case with high sampling. The arrow indicates the position where line profiles will be taken.

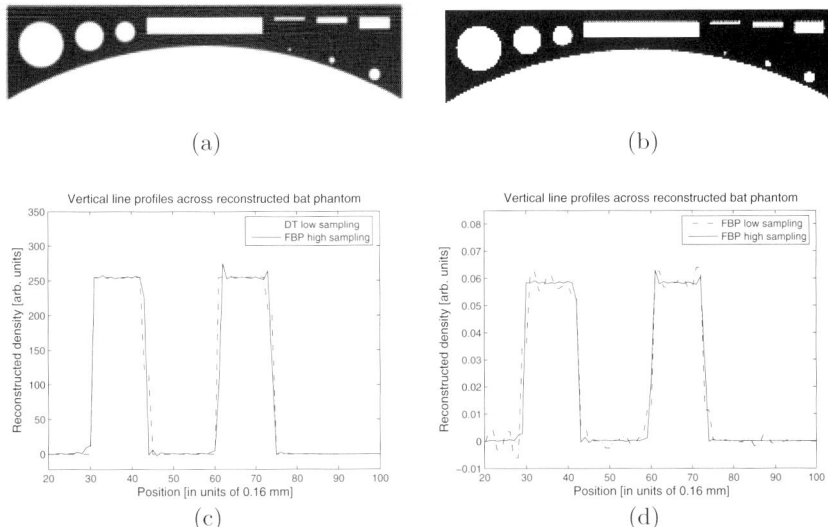

Fig. 14.16. (a) FBP and (b) DT (no smoothness penalty term) reconstruction for the ideal case (with low sampling). The corresponding vertical line profiles are shown in (c) and (d). They are compared to FBP with high sampling.

Simulation with Reduced Dynamic Range

To simulate a real detector, we reduced the dynamic range to 8.5 bits, which was found in first experiments. Figure 14.17(a) shows the formation of limited view angle artifacts for the FBP reconstruction. The number of artifacts is quite large here, and the problem can be seen as difficult to solve. For discrete tomography, we tested reconstructions with different options (see the details in [8]). In this case, a solution could be found only with the help of a smoothness penalty term [Fig. 14.17(b)]. The implementation of the smoothness penalty term was a major success of our work. It is suitable not only to suppress branches but also reduces the sensitivity to other distortions, for example, to noise. The overall stability of the algorithm was significantly enhanced.

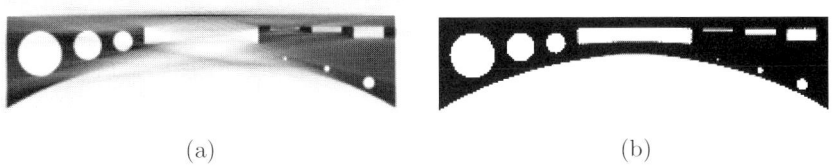

Fig. 14.17. Reconstructions for 8.5-bit reduced dynamic range. (a) FBP, (b) DT (50 repetitions, with smoothness penalty term).

Comparing the vertical line profile of this result (with smoothness penalty term) to the ideal case with infinite dynamic range [Fig. 14.18(a)], we observe some remaining deviations of the object shape. Here the limits for reduced data can be seen. The maximum penetration length for X-rays in copper at 160 keV and 8.5-bit dynamic range is 32 mm. This is also the maximum object length for which FBP reconstruction is exact. Considering that the investigated object length was 70 mm, the DT result is quite impressive. This proves that DT is suitable to increase the possible object length for inspection.

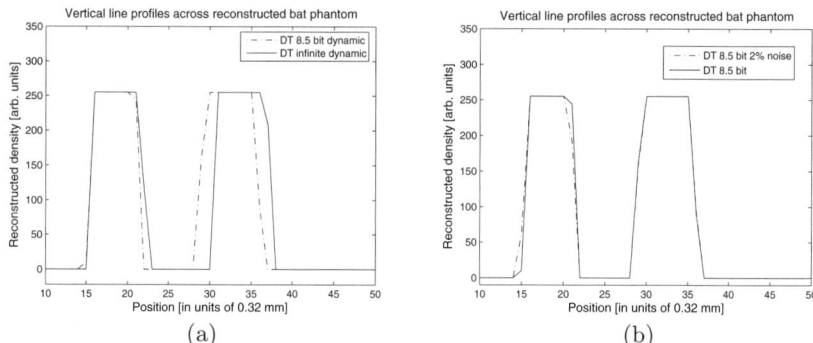

Fig. 14.18. Vertical line profiles for DT reconstructions. (**a**) 8.5-bit reduced dynamic range compared to infinite dynamic range. (**b**) 2% noise compared to no noise for 8.5-bit reduced dynamic range.

Simulation with Noise and Reduced Dynamic Range

In Fig. 14.19, we show the impact of 2% (relative to the free ray intensity) quantum noise that was added to the projection data in the case of 8.5-bit reduced dynamic range. An impression for the amount of noise can be obtained from the FBP reconstruction [Fig. 14.19(a)]. The DT reconstruction [Fig. 14.19(b)] is almost unchanged compared to the case without noise. This is clearly visible in the vertical line profile [Fig. 14.18(b)]. Only for larger noise levels, e.g., 5%, we observed deformations and distortions of the object

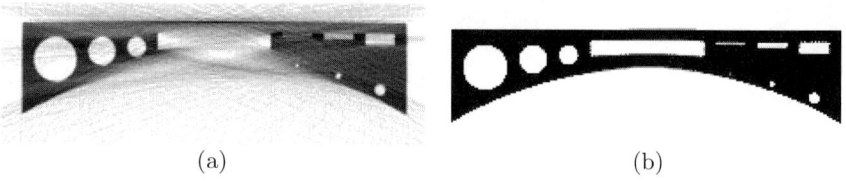

Fig. 14.19. (**a**) FBP and (**b**) DT reconstruction from noisy data (2% noise added to the case of 8.5-bit reduced dynamic range).

(not shown). The stability against moderate noise is an important capability considering experimental data. An explanation may be that the distortions are statistically distributed and the correct object is still the best fit to the projection data.

Experimental Results

From the simulation studies we found that a beam-hardening correction was necessary for good reconstructions with DT. Furthermore, we can expect that scattering is also very critical because it is a systematic distortion as polychromatic X-rays are. The measurements were taken with two different set-ups (Subsection 14.3.1). One was at Siemens (micro-focus X-ray tube and FPI detector) and the other at the EMPA (mini-focus X-ray tube and special line detector). If not explicitly mentioned, we used 200 kV and a 1.5-mm Cu filter for our experiments. The acquired data were down-sampled for reconstruction: EMPA (parallel beam geometry, 330 detector pixels, 312 projections in 180°, image pixel size for reconstruction 0.23 mm) and Siemens (fan beam geometry, 400 detector pixels, 360 projections in 360°, image pixel size for reconstruction 0.23 mm). The DT reconstructions were performed as described for the simulation part.

Reconstruction Results from Experimental Data

First we will show the reconstruction results for the FPI detector. From the discussion above, we expect a strong impact because of the massive scattering effects. For FBP [Fig. 14.20(a)] we observe huge limited view angle artifacts and a strong smearing in the reconstructed image. With continuously increasing distortions, the quality of the FBP result decreases continuously. This kind of stability is a major strength of FBP. The behavior of DT is different, however. Due to the large amount of distortions, the reconstruction with DT is not possible any longer [Fig. 14.20(b)]. The object "breaks up" at some level of distortions. A beam-hardening correction was not feasible here.

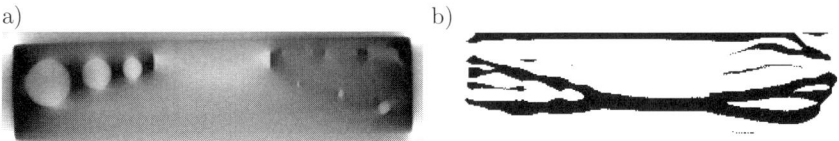

a)   b)

Fig. 14.20. Attempt to reconstruct data from FPI detector (200 kV) with (**a**) FBP and (**b**) DT.

For the EMPA line detector, the data quality is much better. With FBP reconstruction of the raw data, we observed only very small limited view angle

artifacts (not shown). To make the problem a bit more challenging, we reduced
the dynamic range in a preprocessing step to 10 bits. In a second preprocessing
step, the beam-hardening correction, which was described in [8], was carried
out. The FBP result is shown in Fig. 14.21(a). Now the reconstruction with
DT is also possible [Fig. 14.21(b)]. Up to this point, all experiments were
performed at 200 kV. Another way to solve the problem is to increase the
voltage. At 450 kV the limited view angle artifacts in FBP disappeared almost
completely (Fig. 14.22).

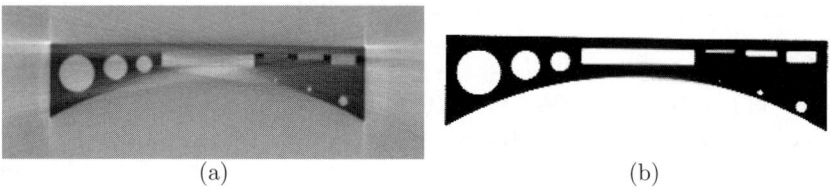

(a)   (b)

Fig. 14.21. (a) FBP and (b) DT reconstruction with beam-hardening correction
for line detector (200 kV).

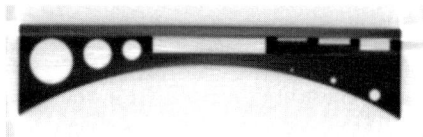

Fig. 14.22. FBP reconstruction with beam-hardening correction for line detector
(450 kV, high sampling).

For a precise analysis, we compared the vertical line profiles of the DT
result at 200 kV to the FBP result at 450 kV (Fig. 14.23). The positions of the
profiles relative to the object were the same as in the simulation part and were
indicated in Fig. 14.16. Considering the shape of the reconstructed object, we
found that DT (200 kV) and FBP (450 kV) are in good agreement. A closer
look reveals that the FBP case is not perfect, because the X-ray penetration is
still not fully possible and some artifacts remain in the reconstructed image.
The upper center bar is brighter in the image, and the corresponding first
peak in the vertical line profile is widened a little bit. The geometric shape
for the DT reconstruction appears to be quite good. The full width at half
maximum of the peaks in the vertical profile is 2 mm for the first peak and
2.1 mm for the second peak as compared to 2.1 mm in the original object. As
the spatial resolution was only 0.23 mm, the accuracy was not very high at
this stage. This might also be the reason why the smallest drill hole appears
slightly too small here. The final result clearly shows that DT can be applied in

experiments with high data quality to increase the possible inspection size of oblong objects. To quantize the improvement, the object size (70 mm) can be compared to the penetration limit (37 mm). But FBP may also be suitable to reconstruct objects that are a bit larger than 37 mm, because small artifacts can be tolerated. We estimate that the improvement in object size of DT compared to FBP was above 50%.

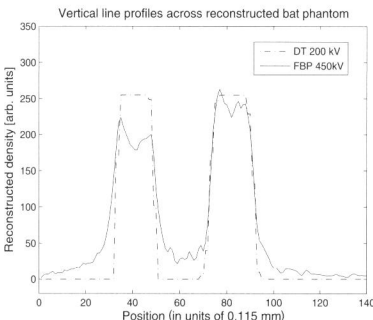

Fig. 14.23. Plot for line detector: comparison of vertical line profiles for DT (200 kV) and FBP (450 kV, high sampling) reconstructions.

14.3.3 Discussion and Further Research

We implemented two methods. The pixel-based one seems to be promising for the reconstruction of industrial objects (made of a few materials) from a small number of projections. It gave good results even in nonideal, for example, in noisy circumstances using a priori information. Since the absorption coefficients were not known exactly we implemented a technique to retrieve their approximative values.

If the object to be reconstructed is known to be mathematically representable by some parametric functions (e.g., simple geometric primitives like spheres or cylinders), the usage of such a priori information may greatly improve the quality of the reconstructed image, even when fewer projections are available. This is demonstrated by the fact that the parameter-based reconstruction method shows high robustness even if the projections are degraded by 40% of the additive noise.

It is also clear that the parameter-based algorithm is inapplicable if the object cannot be described in a simple geometric way, or when the materials of which the specimen is made are not homogeneous. On the other hand, the pixel-based method is unaffected by these circumstances, so it can again be employed successfully. Furthermore, the pixel-based algorithm may benefit from using more intensity levels, whereas the parameter-based one is limited to four absorption values only.

Though the techniques presented here gave promising and acceptable results, we are planning to improve their effectiveness in the future. It would be desirable, for both methods, to speed up the optimization procedure and to test them on more physically measured projections. The pixel-based technique should be made less sensitive to noise by incorporating a noise model. Finally, some practical extensions of the parameter-based algorithm would be to allow for more than four materials and to use more complex prior knowledge (model) of the object.

We proved that DT is suitable to increase the possible object size of oblong, single-material objects. The dimensions for the bat phantom were chosen according to similar NDT problems that are difficult to solve. The limits for DT reconstruction were analyzed via simulations. For the best results, the implementation of a smoothness penalty term was an important step. Adding moderate noise of 2% did not change the result, but polychromatic X-rays caused deviations in the object's shape. We concluded that a beam-hardening correction is necessary for experimental data. In the experimental part, we investigated a micro-focus CT system with a FPI detector at Siemens and a mini-focus CT system with a special line detector at the EMPA. The EMPA line detector very efficiently avoids scattering and acquires high-quality data, while the data of the FPI detector are strongly distorted by scattering for this type of experiment (large and strong absorber at high energy). As expected, DT reconstruction was not possible for the FPI detector data. In contrast to this, the EMPA system delivered good results. The improvement in object size, compared to FBP, was estimated to be above 50%.

14.4 Proposed Combination of CAD Data and DT

There are many problems in technological applications of tomography, such as the examination of turbine blades for geometrical perfection and for obstruction either by remaining wax after the casting process or by coking after extended use. The detection of such a third material only makes sense using neutron radiography, where metals can be well penetrated while keeping a high sensitivity for hydrogenous materials such as wax and coking, which is not possible with X-rays. For measurement of deviations of the ideal shape, either radiation can be employed.

High-quality neutron computed tomography is available at Paul-Scherrer-Institute, Switzerland, at Technische Universität München, Germany [2], and also at NIST, USA.

14.4.1 Turbine Blades and Machine Parts

Modern turbine blades are hollow and contain channels for gas cooling by the centrifugal force. Gas (air) enters the blade at the bottom, flows through a zigzag channel, and is drained through small-diameter bores at the trailing edge of the fin. This internal cooling allows the blade to run at an external gas temperature well above the melting point of its alloy, which enables the turbine to run with higher efficiency. Figure 14.24 shows the neutron radiography of a large turbine blade with cooling channels and particles used for internal cleaning after production, which had not been completely removed.

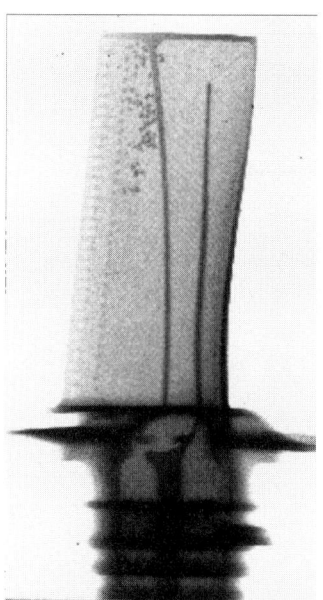
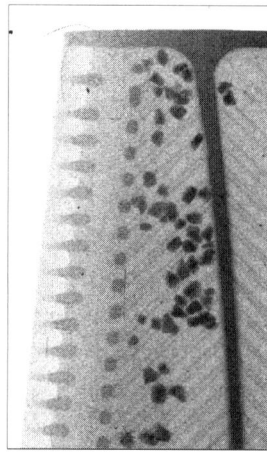

Fig. 14.24. Neutron radiography of a large turbine blade with cooling channels and particles used for internal cleaning after production. Images courtesy of PSI.

For small turbine blades, the complete bulk can be well penetrated, and a complete reconstruction is possible. Figure 14.25 shows a section of a neutron computed tomography of a small turbine blade of about 4-cm diameter. The blade contains several large-diameter cooling channels and several rows of small-diameter draining bores for the cooling gas.

Due to the half-moon cross section of the turbine blades, the inner chord is never accessible for tangential rays. All rays penetrating this area travel a long distance through solid material, and for large turbine blades, they are attenuated close to zero. This leads to a fuzzy reconstruction in that area, whether neutrons or high-energy X-rays are used for imaging.

Figure 14.26 presents filtered back-projection reconstructions from simulated ideal X-ray projection data of a phantom at 200kV. In Fig. 14.26(a), the dynamic range was infinite, while it was reduced to 7 bits in Fig. 14.26(b). The latter case is an approximation for a real X-ray tomography experiment. Fuzzy reconstruction appears both on the inner chord of the shape and also

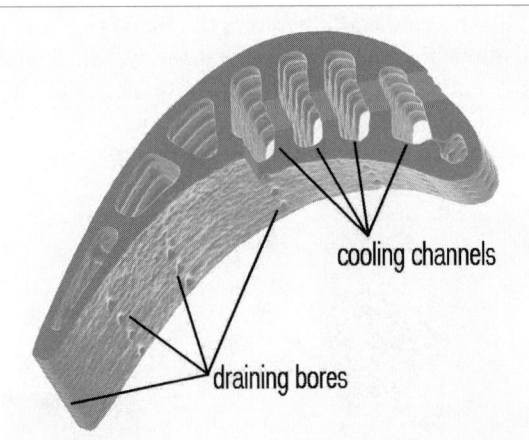

Fig. 14.25. Neutron computed tomography of a small turbine blade of about 4-cm diameter with large-diameter cooling channels and small-diameter draining bores.

on the long, straight outer section, where rays have to penetrate a long path of bulk material.

Figure 14.27 shows a stroboscopic neutron radiography of a combustion engine running at 1000 rpm, measured by a joint research team PSI, TU München, Uni Heidelberg, and ILL at the Institut Laue-Langevin, France [13]. A sensor on the cam shaft is used to trigger the camera at a defined position of the pistons. For the first time, the oil cooling of the pistons was made visible: An oil jet is ejected from below to the bottom of the piston, lowering its temperature by more than 200° during operation. The oil jet and the oil dome at the piston bottom are clearly visible. Standard back-projection tomography is not possible, as the engine cannot be penetrated along the large dimension parallel to the crank shaft.

14.4.2 Proposed DT Research Project

The examples shown above demonstrate some very real technical problems with high possible merit, since large turbine blades are manufactured as single crystals and may cost more than 100,000 Euros each, so the development of this new method may prove to be very profitable.

Both in the case of the turbine blades and in the case of the combustion engine, the ideal shape of the parts is available in the form of original design CAD data in the computer, and manufacturing is usually accurate within small fractions of a millimeter.

Every modern CAD software can output the original CAD data in the format of an STL triangular surface mesh. At the software company Volume Graphics [16], a software tool is available to generate a voxel data set out

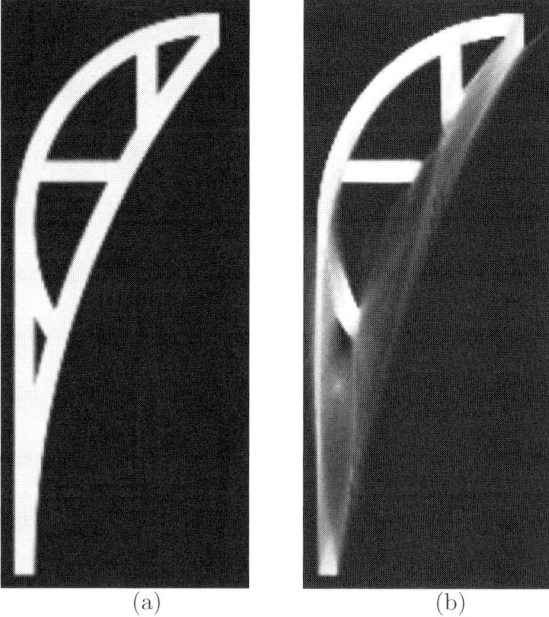

(a)   (b)

Fig. 14.26. Reconstruction of a phantom from simulated ideal data: (**a**) infinite dynamic range and (**b**) 7 bits. Fuzzy reconstruction appears where rays have to penetrate a long path of bulk material.

of STL data to any scale and resolution, so the ideal reconstruction of the turbine blade (and in the long run, of the engine) can be calculated from the original design data.

We propose to use this perfect reconstruction data set as a priori information in order to detect any deviation from this ideal shape, caused either by production defects (only two materials existent), or by obstructions by wax or coking, or lubricant in the case of the engine, which would mean a third material in the data set. Apart from detecting the third material, the main task of DT would be to enable tomographic reconstruction either from projections with limited angular range when some angles are not accessible or when the shape of the sample causes insufficient data for some angles.

In the latter case, both neutrons and X-rays can be employed, but the detection of the third material is especially feasible for neutron tomography. TU München proposes to take over the physics part in a joint research project together with Volume Graphics and an institute of mathematics to be defined.

We are aware that there is still a long way to go until the very recent method of discrete tomography can be applied to these actual physical problems, but we also believe that the possible merit, both scientific and economic, will be very high and is well worth the effort of a joint research project.

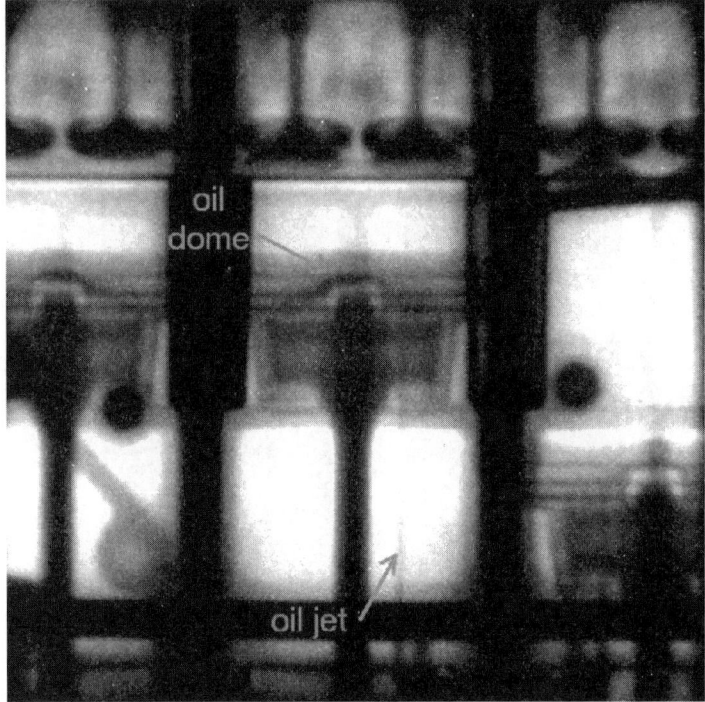

Fig. 14.27. Stroboscopic neutron radiography of a combustion engine running at 1000 rpm. An oil jet is ejected from below to the bottom of the piston. The oil jet and the oil dome at the piston bottom are clearly visible.

Acknowledgments

Research supported in part by the grants DMS 0306215 (National Science Foundation, USA) and T 048476 (Hungarian Research Foundation, OTKA). S. Krimmel gives thanks to P. Böni, who is one of his advisers at the Technische Universität München, to A. Flisch for supporting the measurements at the EMPA, and to M. Goldammer for perusal of the manuscript. A. Kuba thanks the support of the Alexander von Humboldt Foundation (Bonn, Germany) during the preparation of this chapter during his stay in München and Mannheim.

References

1. Balaskó, M., Kuba, A., Nagy, A., Kiss, Z., Rodek, L., Ruskó, L.: Neutron-, gamma- and X-ray three-dimensional computer tomography at the Budapest research reactor, *Nucl. Inst. & Meth.*, A, **542**, 22–27 (2005).

2. Calzada, E., Schillinger, B., Grünauer, F.: Construction and assembly of the neutron radiography and tomography facility ANTARES at FRM-II. *Nucl. Inst. & Meth., A*, **542**, 38–44 (2005).

3. Geman, S., Geman, D.: Stochastic relaxation, Gibbs distributions, and the Bayesian restoration of images. *IEEE Trans. PAMI*, **6**, 721–741 (1984).

4. Herman, G. T., Kuba, A. (eds.): *Discrete Tomography: Foundations, Algorithms, and Applications.* Birkhäuser, Boston, MA (1999).

5. Kak, A.C., Slaney, M.: *Principles of Computerized Tomographic Imaging.* IEEE Press, New York, NY (1987).

6. Kirkpatrick, S., Gelatt, C. D., Vecchi, M. P.: Optimization by simulated annealing. *Science*, **220**, 671–680 (1983).

7. Kiss, Z., Rodek, L. Kuba, A.: Image reconstruction and correction methods in neutron and X-ray tomography. *Acta Cybernetica*, **17**, 557–587 (2006).

8. Krimmel, S., Baumann, J., Kiss, Z., Kuba, A., Nagy, A., Stephan, J.: Discrete tomography for reconstruction from limited view angles in non-destructive testing. *Electr. Notes Discr. Math.*, **20**, 455–474 (2005).

9. Krimmel, S., Stephan, J., Baumann, J.: 3D computed tomography using a microfocus X-ray source: Analysis of artifact formation in the reconstructed images using simulated as well as experimental projection data. *Nucl. Inst. & Meth, A*, **542**, 399–407 (2005).

10. Kuba, A., Rodek, L., Kiss, Z., Ruskó, L., Nagy, A., Balaskó, M.: Discrete tomography in neutron radiography. *Nucl. Inst. & Meth., A*, **542**, 376–382 (2005).

11. Kuba, A., Ruskó, L., Rodek, L., Kiss, Z.: Preliminary studies of discrete tomography in neutron imaging, *IEEE Trans. Nucl. Sci.*, **52**, 380–385 (2005).

12. Robert, N., Peyrin, F., Yaffe, M. J.: Binary vascular reconstruction from a limited number of cone beam projections. *Med. Phys.*, **21**, 1839–1851 (1994).

13. Schillinger, B., Abele, H., Brunner, J., Frei, G., Gähler, R., Gildemeister, A., Hillenbach, A., Lehmann, E., Vontobel, P.: Detection systems for short-time stroboscopic neutron imaging and measurements on a rotating engine. *Nucl. Inst. & Meth., A*, **542**, 142–147 (2005).

14. Schillinger, B.: Proposed combination of CAD data and discrete tomography for the detection of coking and lubricants in turbine blades or engines. *Electr. Notes Discr. Math.*, **20**, 493–499 (2005).

15. Zscherpel U., Osterloh, K., Ewert, U.: Unschärfeprobleme beim Einsatz digitaler Detektoren in der Durchstrahlungsprüfung. *DGZfP Annual Meeting* (2003). With associated web site
http://www.ndt.net/article/dgzfp03/papers/v22/v22.htm.

16. http://www.volumegraphics.com.

17. http://www.inf.u-szeged.hu/direct/, homepage of DIRECT framework.

18. http://mipgsun.mipg.upenn.edu/snark/index.html, homepage of SNARK93 software system.

19. http://www.web3d.org/x3d/vrml/, homepage of VRML97, Virtual Reality Modeling Language.

15

Emission Discrete Tomography

E. Barcucci, A. Frosini, A. Kuba, A. Nagy, S. Rinaldi, M. Samal, S. Zopf

Summary. Three problems of emission discrete tomography (EDT) are presented. The first problem is the reconstruction of measurable plane sets from two absorbed projections. It is shown that Lorentz theorems can be generalized to this case. The second is the reconstruction of binary matrices from their absorbed row and columns sums if the absorption coefficient is $\mu_0 = \log((1+\sqrt{5})/2)$. It is proved that the reconstruction in this case can be done in polynomial time. Finally, a possible application of EDT in single photon emission computed tomography (SPECT) is presented: Dynamic structures are reconstructed after factor analysis.

15.1 Introduction

In the classical physical model of *transmission tomography*, some rays are emitted from a source and *transmitted* through the object to be imaged. The intensity of the transmitted rays is measured, and these data are the input for reconstructing the object. In this chapter, we deal with an alternative physical model used in *emission tomography*, where we measure rays *emitted* from the object itself. In our special case, we suppose that all points of the object emit rays into all directions of the space with unit intensity. It is also supposed that the whole space is filled with some homogeneous material having known absorption. The projections of the ray-emitting object are acquired by detectors placed outside the object. We are interested in the reconstruction of objects from such *absorbed projections*.

Emission discrete tomography (EDT) is when the object to be reconstructed is represented by a function having a known, discrete range. Many results of EDT concern reconstruction of finite 2D subsets of points having nonnegative integer coordinates, called discrete sets. These sets can also be represented by binary matrices. In the special case when the absorption coefficient is $\log((\sqrt{5}+1)/2)$ and the horizontal and vertical absorbed projections are given, there is a necessary and sufficient condition of uniqueness [14, 15, 16], and reconstruction methods [2, 13] have been published. It has been proved [3] that two opposite absorbed projections determine a discrete set uniquely. A general algebraic characterization of discrete sets being nonuniquely determined from a finite number of given absorbed projections is shown in [7]. There are results also in the more general class of measurable plane sets. It is proved that Lorentz theorems can be extended also in the case of absorbed projections [12].

In this chapter, we discuss three EDT problems: a pure theoretic, an algorithmic, and an application one. The very first problem in Section 15.2 is the generalization of Lorentz theorems when the two projections depend not on a constant absorption coefficient, but on some given separable functions, and these functions can be different in different directions. The next problem to be discussed in Section 15.3 is to reconstruct binary matrices from absorbed row and column sums if the absorption coefficient is $\log((\sqrt{5}+1)/2)$. The algorithm shows that this reconstruction problem can be solved in polynomial time (cf. [2]). Finally, we show a possible application of EDT in medical imaging in Section 15.4. In nuclear medicine, there are imaging devices [e.g., single photon emission tomography (SPECT) cameras with two or more heads] to collect sequences of images simultaneously from a small number of projections. That is, a 4D image (three spatial and one temporal dimensions) can be reconstructed from such data. The base of discrete tomography in this case is that before reconstruction the image sequences can be expressed as linear combinations of the projections of so-called factor images (the factors can be computed by factor analysis). Here the factors are 3D homogeneous objects to be reconstructed from their projections by some EDT method. The results of the first simulation experiences are given in the last part of Section 15.4.

15.2 Generalization of Lorentz Theorems

The reconstruction of measurable plane sets from their projections is a classical problem with several applications. The projections are usually defined as the integral values of the characteristic function of the set along straight lines in different directions. One of the most frequently studied cases is that of the horizontal and vertical projections, i.e., the line integrals along horizontal and vertical directions are given. The measurable plane sets can be classified with respect to the projections as uniquely and nonuniquely determined ones. A set is *uniquely determined* or, shortly, *unique* if there is no essentially different set with the same horizontal and vertical projections. Otherwise, the set is said to be *nonuniquely determined* or, shortly, *nonunique*. Even function-pairs can be classified from the viewpoint of reconstruction as unique, nonunique, and inconsistent ones. A pair of functions is *unique/nonunique* if they are essentially the horizontal and vertical projections of a unique/nonunique plane set. It is also possible that there is no measurable plane set having projections essentially the same as the function-pair; in this case, the function-pair is called *inconsistent*.

The very basic result related to such classification of measurable plane sets is due to Lorentz, who published necessary and sufficient conditions on uniqueness/nonuniqueness/inconsistency of function-pairs in 1949 [19]. He also gave a characterization of the uniquely determined sets. Other results about the reconstruction of plane sets appear in [9, 17, 18].

A new kind of projection can be defined in the case of emission computed tomography, where the projections of the set also contain the effect of the constant absorbing space. This absorption problem is studied in the case of discrete plane sets [4, 7, 14]. There is also a result [12] that similar theorems can be proved for absorbed projections as for nonabsorbed projections in the case of measurable plane sets.

Let us suppose that the object to be reconstructed is given by a measurable subset in the first quadrant of the plane. The absorption in the plane is represented by a known constant μ. The detectors are placed in the points of the positive parts of the x-, respectively, y-axis so that they measure the activities along the vertical, respectively, horizontal half-lines of the first quadrant of the plane.

We are going to show that the EDT defined above can be transformed into the classical *transmission discrete tomography* (TDT), where the sets are to be reconstructed from nonabsorbed projections. In this way, the problems of EDT can be reformulated as TDT problems. For example, uniqueness and existence in EDT can be reduced to the case solved by Lorentz theorems, and the uniquely determined plane sets in EDT can be reconstructed and characterized in a similar way to TDT.

15.2.1 Preliminaries

Projections without Absorption

Let F be a measurable plane set of finite measure, i.e., $\lambda_2(F) < \infty$ (λ_2 is the Lebesgue measure on the plane). Let χ_F denote the characteristic function of $F \subseteq \mathbb{R}^2$.

The functions

$$[\mathcal{P}_X F](y) = \int_{-\infty}^{\infty} \chi_F(x, y) \, \mathrm{d}x = f_X(y) \qquad (15.1)$$

and

$$[\mathcal{P}_Y F](x) = \int_{-\infty}^{\infty} \chi_F(x, y) \, \mathrm{d}y = f_Y(x) \qquad (15.2)$$

are said to be the (*nonabsorbed and nongeneralized*) *horizontal* and *vertical projections* of F, respectively (see Fig. 15.1). Two measurable plane sets F and F' of finite measure are said *tomographically equivalent* (*with respect to their projections*), mathematically denoted by $F \sim F'$, if

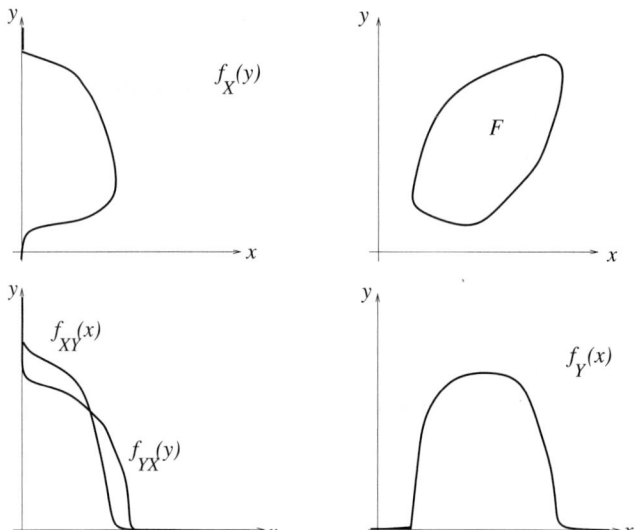

Fig. 15.1. The plane set F, its horizontal (f_X), vertical (f_Y), and second projections.

$$\mathcal{P}_X F \;=\; \mathcal{P}_X F' \quad \text{and} \quad \mathcal{P}_Y F \;=\; \mathcal{P}_Y F' \text{ a.e.,} \qquad (15.3)$$

where "a.e." abbreviates "almost everywhere."

The following problems are studied in connection with the reconstruction of measurable plane sets.

UNIQUENESS U_2.

    Given: *A measurable plane set F.*

    Question: *Does there exist a measurable plane set F' essentially different from F such that F and F' are tomographically equivalent with respect to their (nonabsorbed and nongeneralized) horizontal and vertical projections?*

CONSISTENCY (or EXISTENCE) C_2.

    Given: *Two functions, p and $q : \mathbb{R} \longrightarrow \mathbb{R}_+$.*

    Question: *Does there exist a measurable plane set F such that*

$$[\mathcal{P}_X F](y) \;=\; q(y) \quad \text{and} \quad [\mathcal{P}_Y F](x) \;=\; p(x) \quad \text{a.e.} \quad (15.4)$$

RECONSTRUCTION R_2.

    Given: *Two functions, p and $q : \mathbb{R} \longrightarrow \mathbb{R}_+$.*

    Task: *Construct a measurable plane set F such that*

$$[\mathcal{P}_X F](y) \;=\; q(y) \quad \text{and} \quad [\mathcal{P}_Y F](x) \;=\; p(x) \quad \text{a.e.} \quad (15.5)$$

Considering the plane sets

$$\{(x, y) \mid 0 \le x \le [\mathcal{P}_X F](y)\} \tag{15.6}$$

and

$$\{(x, y) \mid 0 \le y \le [\mathcal{P}_Y F](x)\} \tag{15.7}$$

and taking their projections, we get the *second projections* of F, formally,

$$f_{XY}(x) \;=\; \int_{-\infty}^{\infty} \chi\{y \mid f_X(y) \ge x\} \, dy \tag{15.8}$$

and

$$f_{YX}(y) \;=\; \int_{-\infty}^{\infty} \chi\{x \mid f_Y(x) \ge y\} \, dx \tag{15.9}$$

(see Fig. 15.1).

For the *third projections* of F, we have

$$f_{XYX}(y) \;=\; \int_{-\infty}^{\infty} \chi\{x \mid f_{XY}(x) \ge y\} \, dx \tag{15.10}$$

and

$$f_{YXY}(x) \;=\; \int_{-\infty}^{\infty} \chi\{x \mid f_{YX}(y) \ge x\} \, dy \,. \tag{15.11}$$

Then, using this notation, the Lorentz theorem has the following form.

Theorem 1. *Let $f_X(y)$ and $f_Y(x)$ be nonnegative integrable functions such that*

$$\int_{-\infty}^{\infty} f_X(y) \, dy \;=\; \int_{-\infty}^{\infty} f_Y(x) \, dx. \tag{15.12}$$

(i) There exists an $F \subseteq \mathbb{R}^2$ measurable plane set having these functions as its horizontal and vertical projections if, and only if,

$$\int_0^c f_{XY}(x) \, dx \;\ge\; \int_0^c f_{YXY}(x) \, dx \quad \text{for all } c > 0. \tag{15.13}$$

(ii) There exists a uniquely determined $F \subseteq \mathbb{R}^2$ measurable plane set having these functions as its horizontal and vertical projections if, and only if,

$$\int_0^c f_{XY}(x) \, \mathrm{d}x = \int_0^c f_{YXY}(x) \, \mathrm{d}x \qquad \text{for all } c > 0. \qquad (15.14)$$

(iii) The functions f_X and f_Y are inconsistent, i.e., no plane set F exists with these functions as its (nonabsorbed and nongeneralized) projection functions, if, and only if,

$$\int_0^c f_{XY}(x) \, \mathrm{d}x < \int_0^c f_{YXY}(x) \, \mathrm{d}x \qquad \text{for some } c > 0. \qquad (15.15)$$

15.2.2 Reconstruction of Measurable Sets from Two Generalized Projections

Our goal in this subsection is to show that the definition of projections can be even more general and that Lorentz theorems are still valid. Emission computed tomography will be considered again, i.e., all the points of the set that is to be reconstructed are emitting unit intensity rays in all directions. The whole plane is supposed to modify these rays—following different laws in different directions. We will show that the sets, and also the function-pairs in case of generalized modification, can be characterized in a similar way as it was done in the classical case or with a homogeneous μ-absorption [27].

Generalized Projections

Consider a measurable plane set $G \subseteq \mathbb{R}_+^2$ with finite measure. Suppose that the intensity of a ray being transmitted through set G changes by

$$I = I_0 \cdot \int \omega_r(x, y), \qquad (15.16)$$

where I_0 is the ray's initial intensity and ω_r is a strictly positive function defined on $\mathbb{R}_+^2$ that additionally depends on the ray's direction r. In the following, we are interested in the horizontal and vertical directions only, i.e., $r = (1, 0)$ and $r = (0, 1)$, respectively. Thus, for the horizontal and vertical projections, we have

$$\mathcal{P}_X^{(\omega)}(y) = \int_0^\infty \chi_G(x, y) \cdot \omega_{(1,0)}(x, y) \, \mathrm{d}x \qquad (15.17)$$

and

$$P_Y^{(\omega)}(x) = \int_0^\infty \chi_G(x, y) \cdot \omega_{(0,1)}(x, y) \, \mathrm{d}y. \qquad (15.18)$$

We suppose that $\omega_{(1,0)}$ and $\omega_{(0,1)}$ are the products of two strictly positive integrable functions each, i.e.,

$$\omega_{(1,0)}(x, y) = \alpha(x) \cdot \beta(y) \quad \text{and} \quad \omega_{(0,1)}(x, y) = \gamma(x) \cdot \delta(y), \qquad (15.19)$$

where α, β, γ, and δ are strictly positive functions defined on $\mathbb{R}_+$. We define the *generalized first projections* of a measurable plane set $G \subseteq \mathbb{R}_+^2$ by

$$[\mathcal{P}_X^{(\alpha,\beta)} G](y) = \int_0^\infty \chi_G(x, y) \cdot \alpha(x) \cdot \beta(y) \, \mathrm{d}x \qquad (15.20)$$

and

$$[\mathcal{P}_Y^{(\gamma,\delta)} G](x) = \int_0^\infty \chi_G(x, y) \cdot \gamma(x) \cdot \delta(y) \, \mathrm{d}y. \qquad (15.21)$$

We also suppose that these projections (integrals) exist almost everywhere.

Two measurable plane sets G and G' are said to be *tomographically equivalent with respect to their generalized projections* if

$$\mathcal{P}_X^{(\alpha,\beta)} G = \mathcal{P}_X^{(\alpha,\beta)} G' \quad \text{and} \quad \mathcal{P}_Y^{(\gamma,\delta)} G = \mathcal{P}_Y^{(\gamma,\delta)} G' \quad \text{a.e.,} \qquad (15.22)$$

shortly, $G \sim_{(\alpha,\beta,\gamma,\delta)} G'$.

The following problems are to be investigated again.

UNIQUENESS UG$_2$.

Given: A measurable plane set $G \subseteq \mathbb{R}_+^2$.

Question: Does there exist a measurable plane set $G' \subseteq \mathbb{R}_+^2$ essentially different from G such that G and G' are tomographically equivalent with respect to their generalized horizontal and vertical projections?

CONSISTENCY (or EXISTENCE) CG$_2$.

Given: Two functions, p and $q : \mathbb{R}_+ \longrightarrow \mathbb{R}_+$.

Question: Does there exist a measurable plane set $G \subseteq \mathbb{R}_+^2$ such that

$$[\mathcal{P}_X^{(\alpha,\beta)} G](y) = q(y) \quad \text{and} \quad [\mathcal{P}_Y^{(\gamma,\delta)} G](x) = p(x) \quad \text{a.e.?} \qquad (15.23)$$

RECONSTRUCTION RG$_2$.

Given: Two functions, p and $q : \mathbb{R}_+ \longrightarrow \mathbb{R}_+$.

Task: Construct a measurable plane set $G \subseteq \mathbb{R}^2_+$ such that

$$[\mathcal{P}_X^{(\alpha,\beta)}G](y) \; = \; q(y) \quad \text{and} \quad [\mathcal{P}_Y^{(\gamma,\delta)}G](x) \; = \; p(x) \quad \text{a.e.}$$
$$(15.24)$$

15.2.3 Transformation

Similarly to the μ-absorption, let us define two transformations of the plane into itself and the composition of these transformations.

Let T_X and T_Y be defined by

$$T_X(x,y) \; = \; (t_\alpha(x), y), \quad \text{where} \quad t_\alpha(x) \; = \; \int_0^x \alpha(\xi) \, \mathrm{d}\xi, \quad x \geq 0, \quad (15.25)$$

and

$$T_Y(x,y) \; = \; (x, t_\delta(y)), \quad \text{where} \quad t_\delta(y) \; = \; \int_0^y \delta(\eta) \, \mathrm{d}\eta, \quad y \geq 0, \quad (15.26)$$

and for the composition $T = T_X \circ T_Y = T_Y \circ T_X$, we have

$$T(x,y) \; = \; (t_\alpha(x), t_\delta(y)). \quad (15.27)$$

Since α and δ are supposed to be strictly positive functions, T_X and T_Y, and, thus, T are injective transformations of the plane $\mathbb{R}^2_+$ into itself. This can be shown with the help of the following lemma (the proof is omitted here).

Lemma 1. *Let ε be an everywhere strictly positive integrable function $\mathbb{R} \to \mathbb{R}_+$. For each E measurable subset of $\mathbb{R}$, which has a positive measure, the integral of ε over E is positive, formally,*

$$\int_E \varepsilon(x) \, \mathrm{d}x > 0. \quad (15.28)$$

Lemma 2. *Let ε be an everywhere strictly positive integrable function $\mathbb{R} \to \mathbb{R}_+$. The integral function of ε,*

$$E(x) = \int_0^x \varepsilon(\xi) \, \mathrm{d}\xi, \quad (15.29)$$

is an injective function $\mathbb{R} \longrightarrow \mathbb{R}$.

The transformation T plays a very important role in the following. It gives the possibility to reduce the reconstruction problem of generalized projections to the classical reconstruction problem in such a way that we consider the measurable plane set

$$F \; = \; TG. \quad (15.30)$$

Generalized First Projections

We define the following two functions from which the original generalized projections can be calculated by

$$g_X^{(\alpha)}(y) = [\mathcal{P}_X^{(\alpha)}G](y) = \int_0^\infty \chi_G(x,y) \cdot \alpha(x) \, dx \qquad (15.31)$$

and

$$g_Y^{(\delta)}(x) = [\mathcal{P}_Y^{(\delta)}G](x) = \int_0^\infty \chi_G(x,y) \cdot \delta(y) \, dy \,. \qquad (15.32)$$

Then for the generalized projections, we have

$$[\mathcal{P}_X^{(\alpha,\beta)}G](y) = \beta(y) \cdot [\mathcal{P}_X^{(\alpha)}G](y) \quad \text{and} \quad [\mathcal{P}_Y^{(\gamma,\delta)}G](x) = \gamma(x) \cdot [\mathcal{P}_Y^{(\delta)}G](x). \qquad (15.33)$$

For any measurable sets $I \subseteq \mathbb{R}$ and $J \subseteq \mathbb{R}$, we know that

$$\int_I 1 \cdot \alpha(x) \, dx = \int_{t_\alpha I} 1 \, dx \quad \text{and} \quad \int_J 1 \cdot \delta(y) \, dy = \int_{t_\delta J} 1 \, dy, \qquad (15.34)$$

in other forms,

$$\int_0^\infty \chi_I(x) \cdot \alpha(x) \, dx = \int_0^\infty \chi_{t_\alpha I}(x) \, dx \quad \text{and} \quad \int_0^\infty \chi_J(y) \cdot \delta(y) \, dy = \int_0^\infty \chi_{t_\delta J}(y) \, dy. \qquad (15.35)$$

Using all these facts, we can calculate the generalized first projections of G:

$$\begin{aligned} g_X^{(\alpha)}(y) &= [\mathcal{P}_X^{(\alpha)}G](y) = \int_{-\infty}^\infty \chi_G(x,y) \cdot \alpha(x) \, dx = \int_{-\infty}^\infty \chi_{T_X G}(x,y) \, dx \\ &= [\mathcal{P}_X T_X G](y) = [\mathcal{P}_X T G](t_\delta(y)) \\ &= f_X(t_\delta(y)) \end{aligned} \qquad (15.36)$$

and

$$\begin{aligned} g_Y^{(\delta)}(x) &= [\mathcal{P}_Y^{(\delta)}G](x) = \int_{-\infty}^\infty \chi_G(x,y) \cdot \delta(y) \, dy = \int_{-\infty}^\infty \chi_{T_Y G}(x,y) \, dy \\ &= [\mathcal{P}_Y T_Y G](x) = [\mathcal{P}_Y T G](t_\alpha(x)) \\ &= f_Y(t_\alpha(x)). \end{aligned} \qquad (15.37)$$

This shows that the generalized first projections of G can be calculated from the (nonabsorbed and nongeneralized) projections of the transformed sets $T_X G$ and $T_Y G$ and from those of the transformed set $F = TG$. Note that the functions β and γ do not play a role when we calculate these equalities and transformations.

Generalized Second Projections

For the *generalized second projections* of the plane set $G \subseteq \mathbb{R}_+^2$, we do not take into account the β- and γ-functions. These projections are defined by

$$g_{XY}^{(\alpha\delta)} = \mathcal{P}_Y^{(\delta)}\{(x,y)\,|\,g_X^{(\alpha)}(y) \geq x\} \tag{15.38}$$

and

$$g_{YX}^{(\delta\alpha)} = \mathcal{P}_X^{(\alpha)}\{(x,y)\,|\,g_Y^{(\delta)}(x) \geq y\}. \tag{15.39}$$

Let us calculate the generalized second projections,

$$
\begin{aligned}
g_{XY}^{(\alpha\delta)} &= \mathcal{P}_Y^{(\delta)}\{(x,y)\,|\,g_X^{(\alpha)}(y) \geq x\} = \mathcal{P}_Y T_Y\{(x,y)\,|\,g_X^{(\alpha)}(y) \geq x\} \\
&= \mathcal{P}_Y T_Y\{(x,y)\,|\,f_X(t_\delta(y)) \geq x\} = \mathcal{P}_Y\{(x,y)\,|\,f_X(y) \geq x\} \\
&= f_{XY}
\end{aligned}
\tag{15.40}
$$

and, similarly,

$$
\begin{aligned}
g_{YX}^{(\delta\alpha)} &= \mathcal{P}_X^{(\alpha)}\{(x,y)\,|\,g_Y^{(\delta)}(x) \geq y\} = \mathcal{P}_X T_X\{(x,y)\,|\,g_Y^{(\delta)}(x) \geq y\} \\
&= \mathcal{P}_X T_X\{(x,y)\,|\,f_Y(t_\alpha(x)) \geq y\} = \mathcal{P}_X\{(x,y)\,|\,f_Y(x) \geq y\} \\
&= f_{YX}.
\end{aligned}
\tag{15.41}
$$

From these equations we see that the generalized second projections of a set G are identical to the second (nonabsorbed and nongeneralized) projections of the transformed set $F = TG$.

Generalized Third Projections

The *generalized third projections* are defined by

$$g_{XYX}^{(\alpha\delta)} = \mathcal{P}_X\{(x,y)\,|\,g_{XY}^{(\alpha\delta)}(x) \geq y\} \tag{15.42}$$

and

$$g_{YXY}^{(\delta\alpha)} = \mathcal{P}_Y\{(x,y)\,|\,g_{YX}^{(\delta\alpha)}(y) \geq x\}, \tag{15.43}$$

and, thus, we get

$$
\begin{aligned}
g_{XYX}^{(\alpha\delta)} &= \mathcal{P}_X\{(x,y)\,|\,g_{XY}^{(\alpha\delta)}(x) \geq y\} = \mathcal{P}_X\{(x,y)\,|\,f_{XY}(x) \geq y\} \\
&= f_{XYX}
\end{aligned}
\tag{15.44}
$$

and

$$
\begin{aligned}
g_{YXY}^{(\delta\alpha)} &= \mathcal{P}_Y\{(x,y)\,|\,g_{YX}^{(\delta\alpha)}(y) \geq x\} = \mathcal{P}_Y\{(x,y)\,|\,f_{YX}(y) \geq x\} \\
&= f_{YXY}.
\end{aligned}
\tag{15.45}
$$

Theorem about Generalized Projections

We are going to prove a theorem about the existence and uniqueness of a measurable set G for given generalized projection functions similar to the cases without absorption and with μ-absorption.

Theorem 2. *Let $\alpha(x) > 0$, $\beta(y) > 0$, $\gamma(x) > 0$, and $\delta(y) > 0$ a.e. be four strictly positive functions $\mathbb{R}_+ \to \mathbb{R}_+$. Given $g_X^{(\alpha,\beta)}(y)$ and $g_Y^{(\gamma,\delta)}(x)$, two non-negative integrable functions, such that*

$$\int_0^\infty \frac{g_X^{(\alpha,\beta)}(y)}{\beta(y)} \cdot \delta(y) \, \mathrm{d}y \;=\; \int_0^\infty \frac{g_Y^{(\gamma,\delta)}(x)}{\gamma(x)} \cdot \alpha(x) \, \mathrm{d}x. \tag{15.46}$$

(i) *There exists a $G \subseteq \mathbb{R}_+^2$ measurable plane set of finite measure having these functions as its horizontal and vertical generalized projections if, and only if,*

$$\int_0^c g_{XY}^{(\alpha\delta)}(x) \, \mathrm{d}x \;\geq\; \int_0^c g_{YXY}^{(\delta\alpha)}(x) \, \mathrm{d}x, \quad \text{for all } c > 0. \tag{15.47}$$

(ii) *There exists a uniquely determined $G \subseteq \mathbb{R}_+^2$ measurable plane set of finite measure having these functions as its horizontal and vertical generalized projections if, and only if,*

$$\int_0^c g_{XY}^{(\alpha\delta)}(x) \, \mathrm{d}x \;=\; \int_0^c g_{YXY}^{(\delta\alpha)}(x) \, \mathrm{d}x, \quad \text{for all } c > 0. \tag{15.48}$$

(iii) *The functions $g_X^{(\alpha,\beta)}$ and $g_Y^{(\gamma,\delta)}$ are inconsistent, i.e., no plane set G exists with these functions as its generalized projection functions, if, and only if,*

$$\int_0^c g_{XY}^{(\alpha\delta)}(x) \, \mathrm{d}x \;<\; \int_0^c g_{YXY}^{(\delta\alpha)}(x) \, \mathrm{d}x, \quad \text{for some } c > 0. \tag{15.49}$$

Proof. Consider the plane transformation

$$T(x,y) \;=\; (t_\alpha(x), t_\delta(y)) \;=\; \left(\int_0^x \alpha(\xi) \, \mathrm{d}\xi, \int_0^y \delta(\eta) \, \mathrm{d}\eta \right). \tag{15.50}$$

Let us define the functions f_X and f_Y by

$$f_X(t_\delta(y)) = \frac{g_X^{(\alpha,\beta)}(y)}{\beta(y)} \quad \text{and} \quad f_Y(t_\alpha(x)) = \frac{g_Y^{(\gamma,\delta)}(x)}{\gamma(x)}. \tag{15.51}$$

These functions are defined in $t_\delta\mathbb{R}_+$ and $t_\alpha\mathbb{R}_+$, respectively. Let us define them to be 0 out of these sets. Since t_α and t_δ are injective (see Lemma 2), these definitions make sense. From the definitions of f_X and f_Y and from the assumption, we know that

$$\int_0^\infty f_X(y)\, dy = \int_0^\infty \frac{g_X^{(\alpha,\beta)}(y)}{\beta(y)} \cdot \delta(y)\, dy = \int_0^\infty \frac{g_Y^{(\gamma,\delta)}(x)}{\gamma(x)} \cdot \alpha(x)\, dx = \int_0^\infty f_Y(x)\, dx.$$

(15.52)

We are going to use Theorem 1 in the proof of the three cases.

(i) There exists a measurable plane set F with (nonabsorbed and non-generalized) given projections f_X and f_Y if, and only if, the condition $\int_0^c f_{XY}(x)dx \geq \int_0^c f_{YXY}(x)\, dx$ is satisfied, for all $c > 0$. Consider (15.40) and (15.45). If there exists a set G with the generalized projections $g_X^{(\alpha,\beta)}$ and $g_Y^{(\gamma,\delta)}$, then f_X and f_Y are the (nonabsorbed and nongeneralized) projections of $F = TG$ and thus, the inequality holds. If the inequality holds, there exists a set $F \subseteq \mathbb{R}^2$ with the (nonabsorbed and nongeneralized) projections f_X and f_Y. The set $F \cap T\mathbb{R}_+^2$ has the same (nonabsorbed and nongeneralized) projections (almost everywhere) since the projections are 0 outside $t_\delta\mathbb{R}_+$ and $t_\alpha\mathbb{R}_+$, respectively. Thus, $G = T^{-1}(F \cap T\mathbb{R}_+^2)$ is a measurable set with the generalized projections $g_X^{(\alpha,\beta)}$ and $g_Y^{(\gamma,\delta)}$.

(ii) The set F is unique if, and only if, $\int_0^c f_{XY}(x)\, dx = \int_0^c f_{YXY}(x)\, dx$, for all $c > 0$. Since T is an injective transformation of the plane into itself and $F \cap (T\mathbb{R}^2)^c$ has measure 0, the set G is also unique with respect to its generalized projections if, and only if, $\int_0^c g_{XY}(x)\, dx = \int_0^c g_{YXY}(x)\, dx$, for all $c > 0$. (M^c denotes the complement of the set M.)

(iii) No set F exists if, and only if, there exists a $c > 0$ with $\int_0^c f_{XY}(x)\, dx < \int_0^c f_{YXY}(x)\, dx$. As a similar consequence, there is no set G with the generalized projections $g_X^{(\alpha,\beta)}$ and $g_Y^{(\gamma,\delta)}$ if, and only if, there exists a $c > 0$ with $\int_0^c g_{XY}(x)\, dx < \int_0^c g_{YXY}(x)\, dx$.

$\square$

An Example for Generalized Absorption

Let us assume a material with anisotropic absorption. This means that different absorption coefficients have to be taken into account in the x- and y-directions. A ray's intensity will change by the equation

$$I = I_0 \cdot \int_G e^{-\langle \mu, r\rangle}\, dr,$$

(15.53)

where $\mu = (\mu_x, \mu_y)$ is the vector of the absorption coefficients. Calculating the intensities along the x- and y-directions, we get

$$P_X^{(\alpha,\beta)}(y) = \int_G e^{-\mu_x \cdot x}\, dx \quad \text{and} \quad P_Y^{(\gamma,\delta)}(x) = \int_G e^{-\mu_y \cdot y}\, dy$$

(15.54)

or, equivalently,

$$P_X^{(\alpha,\beta)}(y) = \int_0^\infty \chi_G(x,y) \cdot e^{-\mu_x \cdot x} \, dx \quad \text{and} \quad P_Y^{(\gamma,\delta)}(x) = \int_0^\infty \chi_G(x,y) \cdot e^{-\mu_y \cdot y} \, dy.$$

(15.55)

Setting $\alpha(x) = e^{-\mu_x \cdot x}$, $\beta(y) = 1$, $\gamma(x) = 1$, and $\delta(y) = e^{-\mu_y \cdot y}$, we get an example of the generalized case. The ray intensities in each direction change by the same law as they do in case of the μ-absorption, but for given functions we will get different sets having these functions as generalized projections. Applying the transformation

$$T(x,y) = (\frac{1 - e^{-\mu_x \cdot x}}{\mu_x}, \frac{1 - e^{-\mu_y \cdot y}}{\mu_y})$$

(15.56)

on the plane, we can reduce the problem of generalized projections to the classical (nongeneralized) case and vice versa.

Uniqueness in the Case of Generalized Projections

As a consequence of Theorem 2, we get directly

Theorem 3. *Let α, β, γ, and δ be four strictly positive, integrable functions $\mathbb{R} \to \mathbb{R}_+$. Let $G \subset \mathbb{R}^2$ be a measurable plane set having a finite measure. G is uniquely determined by its generalized projections $g_X^{(\alpha,\beta)}$ and $g_Y^{(\gamma,\delta)}$, if and only if,*

$$g_{XY}^{(\alpha\delta)}(x) = g_{YXY}^{(\delta\alpha)}(x), \quad \text{for all } x \in \mathbb{R}.$$

(15.57)

Remark 1. It is easy to see that Theorem 3 is true also if (15.57) is replaced by

$$g_{YX}^{(\delta\alpha)}(y) = g_{XYX}^{(\alpha\delta)}(y), \quad \text{for all } y \in \mathbb{R}.$$

(15.58)

Theorem 2 also indicates that whenever a measurable plane set G is unique in the generalized case, its transformed set TG is also unique in the nongeneralized case and vice versa: Whenever a measurable set $F \subseteq T\mathbb{R}^2$ is unique with respect to its (nonabsorbed and nongeneralized) projections, the set $G = T^{-1}F$ is unique with respect to its generalized projections $P_X^{(\alpha,\beta)}G$ and $P_Y^{(\gamma,\delta)}G$. The transformation T is defined by

$$T(x,y) = (\int_0^x \alpha(\xi) \, d\xi, \int_0^y \delta(\eta) \, d\eta).$$

(15.59)

Finally, let us mention that a characterization of the measurable plane sets, which are unique with respect to their generalized projections, is given in [27].

15.3 An Algorithm for Reconstructing Binary Matrices from Absorbed Row and Column Sums

In this section, we move from the general class of characteristic functions to the special class of binary matrices. We consider a reconstruction problem when the absorption coefficient is just $\mu = \mu_0 = \log((1 + \sqrt{5})/2)$ and the projections are the absorbed row and column sums. We are going to prove that this reconstruction problem can be solved in polynomial time and even such an algorithm is presented here. Let us remark that a polynomial reconstruction algorithm is published also in the case when the two absorbed projections are the opposite row/column projections of the binary matrix to be reconstructed [4].

15.3.1 Definitions and Notation

Using the notations of [15], let $A = (a_{ij})_{m \times n}$ be the binary matrix to be reconstructed (i.e., $a_{ij} \in \{0, 1\}$ for $i = 1, 2, \ldots, m$, $j = 1, 2, \ldots, n$). In order to make the notation simple, let $\beta_0 = e^{\mu_0} = (1 + \sqrt{5})/2$. Then the ($\mu_0$-absorbed) *horizontal and vertical projections* of A are defined as

$$R_{\beta_0}(A) = R = (r_1, \ldots, r_m), \quad \text{where} \quad r_i = \sum_{j=1}^{n} a_{ij} \beta_0^{-j} \tag{15.60}$$

and

$$C_{\beta_0}(A) = C = (c_1, \ldots, c_n), \quad \text{where} \quad c_j = \sum_{i=1}^{m} a_{ij} \beta_0^{-i}, \tag{15.61}$$

respectively, for each $1 \le i \le m$ and $1 \le j \le n$.

The selected β_0 has the following important property:

$$\beta_0^{-i} = \beta_0^{-i-1} + \beta_0^{-i-2}. \tag{15.62}$$

Equation (15.62) means that if three consecutive elements in a row of a binary matrix are 100, then they can be changed (switched) to 011 (or vice versa) without changing the absorbed row sum. Of course, an analogue statement is true also for columns. This switching property is the base of the whole uniqueness problem. A switching theory for this scenario has already been provided in [15, 16]; we only recall some useful basic definitions and results.

A binary word $w = a_1 \ldots a_n$, with $n \in \mathbb{N}$, is called a *finite n-length representation in base β_0* (briefly, a *β_0-representation*) of $r \in \mathbb{R}$ if

$$r = a_1 \cdot \beta_0^{-1} + a_2 \cdot \beta_0^{-2} + \cdots + a_n \cdot \beta_0^{-n}, \tag{15.63}$$

while r is said to be the *value* of w. A β_0-representation is a *β_0-expansion* if it does not contain any 011 subword. Naturally, a number r can have several

n-length β_0-representations, but there is only one β_0-expansion of length n. As an example, the following words are β_0-representations of length 11 of the same number:

$$
\begin{aligned}
w_1 &= 0\ 1\ 0\ 1\ 1\ 0\ 1\ 0\ 0\ 0\ 0, \\
w_2 &= 0\ 1\ 0\ 1\ 1\ 0\ 0\ 1\ 1\ 0\ 0, \\
w_3 &= 0\ 1\ 1\ 0\ 0\ 0\ 0\ 1\ 1\ 0\ 0, \\
w_4 &= 1\ 0\ 0\ 0\ 0\ 0\ 1\ 0\ 0\ 0\ 0,
\end{aligned}
\tag{15.64}
$$

but only the last one is a β_0-expansion.

Using the concept of β_0-representation, we can say that if r_i and c_j are the ith row sum and jth column sum, respectively, of an $m \times n$ binary matrix A ($1 \le i \le m$ and $1 \le j \le n$), then the words created from the binary digits of the binary matrix A in row i, i.e., $a_{i1}a_{i2} \ldots a_{in}$ and in column j, i.e., $a_{1j}a_{2j} \ldots a_{mj}$, are n-length and m-length β_0-representations of r_i and c_j, respectively.

It is easy to see on the base of (15.62) that not only 100 can be replaced by 011, but also any subsequence $1(0x)^k 00$ by $0(1x)^k 11$ ($k \ge 0$), and vice versa, in a β_0-representation without changing the value of the represented number (x stands in the positions of binary digits, which do not change their values during the replacement). We call such a replacement a *1D switching* and denote it by $1(0x)^k 00 \leftrightarrow 0(1x)^k 11$. Specially, the simplest 1D switching, $100 \leftrightarrow 011$, is called (*1D*) *elementary switching*.

It is easy to see that each 1D switching can be obtained by the consecutive application of 1D elementary switchings. As an example, the 1D switching

$$
1010100 \leftrightarrow 0111111 \tag{15.65}
$$

can be obtained by the application of three 1D elementary switchings:

$$
1010100 = 1010011 = 1001111 = 0111111. \tag{15.66}
$$

More generally, it is also true [16] that any n-length β_0-representation of a number can be obtained from any other n-length β_0-representation of the same number by consecutive applications of 1D switchings.

15.3.2 Reconstruction from μ_0-Absorbed Row and Column Sums

Now, we consider the reconstruction problem in the case when the μ_0-absorbed row and column sums of the binary matrix are given.

RECONSTRUCTION RA.

Given:	*Two nonnegative real vectors, R and C.*
Task:	*Construct a binary matrix A such that its μ_0-absorbed row and column sums, i.e., $R(A)$ and $C(A)$, are R and C, respectively.*

Before giving a reconstruction algorithm, we extend the concept of 1D switching to that of 2D switching, i.e., a transformation that changes some elements of the binary matrix A, without modifying its horizontal and vertical μ_0-absorbed projections. A complete study of 2D switchings from a tomographical point of view can be found in [15, 16].

2D Switching

Using the notation of [15], let

$$S_{ij} = \{i-1, i, i+1\} \times \{j-1, j, j+1\} \tag{15.67}$$

be the 3×3 discrete square set of positions of A such that $1 < i < m$ and $1 < j < n$. Two squares S_{ij} and $S_{i'j'}$ are said to be *side-connected* if either $i = i'$ and $|j - j'| = 2$, or $|i - i'| = 2$ and $j = j'$. A collection Σ of discrete squares is side-connected if each couple of its elements S_{ij} and $S_{i'j'}$ is connected by a *side chain*, i.e., by a sequence of elements of Σ starting with S_{ij}, ending with $S_{i'j'}$, and such that any two consecutive elements of the sequence are side-connected. The side-connected set Σ is *strongly side-connected* if, whenever two of its elements intersect, then either they are side-connected or they have a common side-connected neighbor. By definition, a single square is a side-connected set. Examples of not side-connected, side-connected, and strongly side-connected sets are given in Fig. 15.2(a)–(c).

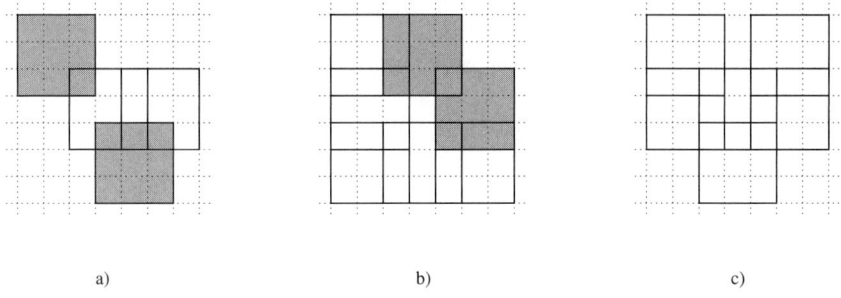

a)   b)   c)

Fig. 15.2. Examples of not side-connected, side-connected, and strongly side-connected sets of discrete 3×3 squares. The squares indicated by their borders are the elements of the sets. (**a**) A not side-connected set. (The highlighted squares are not side-connected with any other squares of the set.) (**b**) A side-connected set, which is not strongly side connected. (The highlighted squares have a common position, but they are not side-connected.) (**c**) A strongly side-connected set.

Lemma 3. *The elements of a (strongly) side-connected set Σ can be rearranged in Σ' so that each prefix of Σ' is a (strongly) side-connected set itself.*

Proof. Let $\Sigma = \{S_1, S_2, \ldots, S_k\}$ be a (strongly) side-connected set. We rearrange Σ in the sequence $\Sigma' = \{S_1', S_2', \ldots, S_k'\}$ so that $S_1' = S_1$, and, for each $1 < i \le k$, the element S_i' is the first element of Σ not yet belonging to Σ' and is (strongly) side-connected with at least one of the elements of Σ'. The existence of such a Σ' can be proved indirectly. Let us assume that there exists an index l $(1 < l \le k)$ such that none of the elements of $\Sigma \setminus \{S_1', S_2', \ldots, S_l'\}$ is (strongly) side-connected with any element of $\{S_1', S_2', \ldots, S_l'\}$. Then there is no side chain between any two elements of these sets, which is a contradiction. □

From now on, each time when we deal with (strongly) side-connected sets, we consider the sets rearranged according to Lemma 3.

We define the *pattern* as a binary-valued function defined on an arbitrary subset of the positions of A. The domain of the pattern P is denoted by $\mathrm{dom}(P)$. Furthermore, we say that a pattern P contains a pattern P', denoted as $P' \subseteq P$, if P is the extension of P' according to the usual analytical meaning.

Let the two patterns

$$E_{ij}^{(0)} = \begin{matrix} 0 & 1 & 1 \\ 1 & 0 & 0 \\ 1 & 0 & 0 \end{matrix} \qquad \text{and} \qquad E_{ij}^{(1)} = \begin{matrix} 1 & 0 & 0 \\ 0 & 1 & 1 \\ 0 & 1 & 1 \end{matrix} \qquad (15.68)$$

be defined on the discrete square S_{ij}. It is easy to check that the substitution of $E_{ij}^{(0)}$ with $E_{ij}^{(1)}$ in a binary matrix or vice versa is a 2D switching, i.e., it does not change the μ_0-absorbed horizontal and vertical projections. Furthermore, such a switching is minimal with respect to the number of elements involved. We refer to the patterns $E_{ij}^{(0)}$ and $E_{ij}^{(1)}$ as 0-*type* and 1-*type 2D elementary switching patterns*, respectively.

The *composition* of patterns P and P' is denoted by $\odot$ and is defined on the set

$$\mathrm{dom}(P \odot P') = \mathrm{dom}(P) \triangle \mathrm{dom}(P') \qquad (15.69)$$

($\triangle$ denotes the symmetric difference) by

$$[P \odot P'](i,j) = \begin{cases} p(i,j) & \text{if } (i,j) \in \mathrm{dom}(P), \\ p'(i,j) & \text{if } (i,j) \in \mathrm{dom}(P'). \end{cases} \qquad (15.70)$$

Figure 15.3 shows the composition of two patterns P and P' having nondisjoint domains.

Two patterns, P and P', are *strongly linked* in a pattern P'' if

$$\mathrm{dom}(P) \cup \mathrm{dom}(P') \subseteq \mathrm{dom}(P''), \quad P \odot P' \subsetneqq P'', \quad P \not\subseteq P'', \quad \text{and} \quad P' \not\subseteq P''. \qquad (15.71)$$

It is important to remark that if P and P' are strongly linked in P'', then $\mathrm{dom}(P) \cap \mathrm{dom}(P') \ne \emptyset$. Figure 15.4 shows two different cases. In the first case, the patterns P and P' of Fig. 15.3 are strongly linked in the pattern

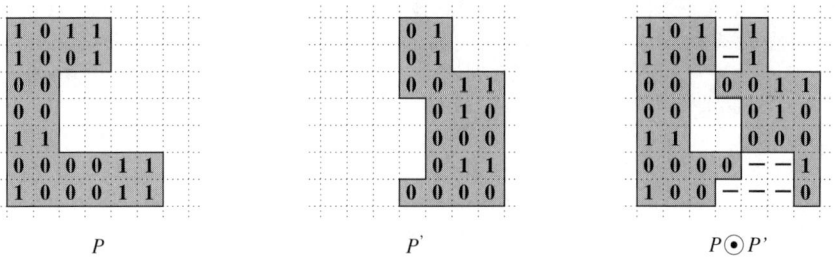

Fig. 15.3. The composition of the patterns P and P'. The symbol "$-$" indicates the positions of undefined elements in $\operatorname{dom}(P) \cup \operatorname{dom}(P')$.

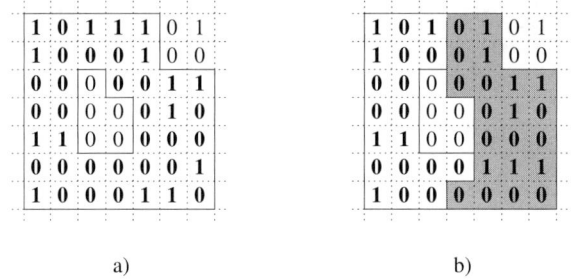

a)   b)

Fig. 15.4. The patterns P and P' in Fig. 15.3 are strongly linked in pattern (**a**), while they are not in pattern (**b**).

of Fig. 15.4(a). The same patterns are not strongly linked in the pattern of Fig. 15.4(b), because it contains the highlighted pattern P'.

In the sequel, we indicate with $p : E_1, \ldots, E_k$ the sequence of the 2D elementary switching patterns $E_1, \ldots, E_k$ of the same type, whose domains form a strongly side-connected set. Furthermore, let $\bigodot_{i=1}^{k} E_i$ denote the successive compositions of the elements of p, formally,

$$\bigodot_{i=1}^{k} E_i = [\ldots [[E_1 \odot E_2] \odot E_3] \odot \cdots \odot E_k] . \qquad (15.72)$$

($\bigodot_{i=1}^{1} E_i = E_1$ by definition.) As an example of the successive compositions of $E_{ij}^{(1)}, E_{i-2,j}^{(1)}, E_{i-2,j+2}^{(1)}$, and $E_{i,j-2}^{(1)}$; see Fig. 15.5.

It is easy to check the following property.

Property 1. Let E_1 and E_2 be two elementary switching patterns, strongly linked in a pattern P. The sequence of the three consecutive elements of the pattern P in positions $\operatorname{dom}(E_1) \cap \operatorname{dom}(E_2)$ is different from both 100 and 011.

We now define the general notion of the *2D composite switching pattern*, which plays a central role in the algorithm for solving RECONSTRUCTION

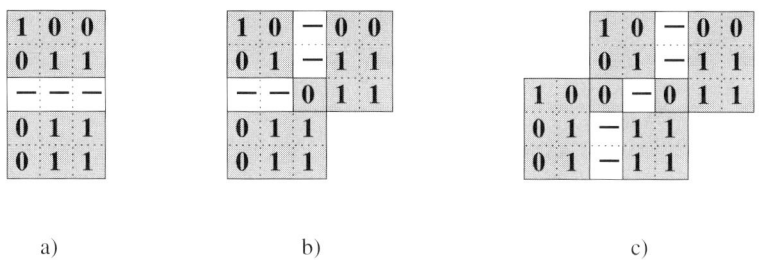

a)   b)   c)

Fig. 15.5. The steps (**a**), (**b**), and (**c**) giving the successive composition of $E_{ij}^{(1)}$, $E_{i-2,j}^{(1)}$, $E_{i-2,j+2}^{(1)}$, and $E_{i,j-2}^{(1)}$.

RA. Given a sequence $p : E_1, \ldots, E_k$, the *2D composite switching pattern* E is defined so that

(i) $\mathrm{dom}(E) = \bigcup_{i=1}^{k} \mathrm{dom}(E_i)$,

(ii) $\bigodot_{i=1}^{k} E_i \subset E$,

(iii) there exists a sequence $p' : E'_1, \ldots, E'_k$ whose elements are a permutation of those of p such that $\bigodot_{l=1}^{i-1} E'_l$ and E'_i are strongly linked in E for each $1 < i \le k$ (see Fig. 15.6).

Any 2D elementary switching component is also a 2D composite switching component by definition ($k = 1$). The elements of sequence p are said to be the *components* of the composite switching pattern E, which also inherits its type from its components. Figure 15.6 shows two patterns E' and E'' containing the composition of the elements of the sequence

$$p : E_{ij}^{(1)}, E_{i,j+2}^{(1)}, E_{i-2,j}^{(1)}, E_{i-2,j+2}^{(1)} . \tag{15.73}$$

At first sight, it may seem that both E' and E'' do not satisfy condition (iii) of the definition of the elementary switching pattern. But if we consider the sequence

$$p' : E_{ij}^{(1)}, E_{i-2,j}^{(1)}, E_{i-2,j+2}^{(1)}, E_{i,j+2}^{(1)}, \tag{15.74}$$

we notice that it is a rearrangement of the elements of p preserving the side connectedness and satisfying condition (iii), as desired. Hence E' is a composite switching pattern, while no such rearrangement can be found for E''.

Lemma 4. *A 2D composite switching pattern does not contain any other 2D composite switching patterns.*

Proof. Let us assume that E and E' are two 2D composite switching patterns whose components are the elements of the sequences p and p', respectively, such that $E' \subsetneq E$. It is easy to see that E and E' have the same type and p' is a subsequence of p. By definition, there are $E_i \in p \setminus p'$ and $E_j \in p'$, which are strongly linked in E. Since E' does not contain E_i, the sequence of

E' :

1	0	0	0	0
0	1	0	1	1
1	0	1	1	0
0	1	0	1	1
0	1	0	1	1

E'' :

1	0	0	0	0
0	1	0	1	1
1	0	1	0	0
0	1	0	1	1
0	1	0	1	1

Fig. 15.6. Pattern E' is a 2D composite switching pattern, while E'' does not satisfy condition (iii) of the definition. The highlighted elements indicate the positions for which the 2D elementary switching components containing these positions are not strongly linked in E' and E''.

the three consecutive positions of $\mathrm{dom}(E_i) \cap \mathrm{dom}(E_j)$ have values 100 or 011 in E'. At the same time, by Property 1, the same consecutive positions have values being different from 100 and 011 in E, which is a contradiction.   □

In [15], it is proved that a 2D composite switching pattern is defined up to the order of its components. Furthermore, it has the following remarkable result.

Theorem 4. *Let E and E' be two 2D composite switching patterns obtained from the two sequences*

$$p : E^{(0)}_{i_1,j_1}, \ldots, E^{(0)}_{i_k,j_k} \quad and \quad p' : E^{(1)}_{i_1,j_1}, \ldots, E^{(1)}_{i_k,j_k}, \qquad (15.75)$$

respectively. If E coincides with E' in $\mathrm{dom}(E \setminus \bigodot^k_{t=1} E^{(0)}_{i_t,j_t})$, then the substitution of E with E' or vice versa in any binary matrix does not change the μ_0-absorbed horizontal and vertical projections of the matrix, i.e., it is a switching operator.

The switching operator defined in Theorem 4 is also called *composite switching*, while the pair (E, E') is called *composite switching pair*. The composite switching is the most general switching as it is shown in [15] by the following result.

Theorem 5. *Each 2D switching can be obtained by the successive application of composite switchings.*

Given a composite switching pattern E, two complementary sets of positions can be defined on its domain: the *core*, which contains the positions being all elements of its 8-neighborhood in $\mathrm{dom}(E)$, and the *boundary* containing the rest of the positions of $\mathrm{dom}(E)$.

Lemma 5. *Two 2D composite switching patterns contained in a binary matrix can intersect each other only along their boundaries.*

Proof. This immediately follows from Lemma 4, since if two 2D composite switching patterns share some positions in their cores, then they also share some 3×3 elementary switching pattern and, consequently, they contain the same 2D elementary switching pattern.

An Algorithm for Solving RECONSTRUCTION RA

If there is no absorption, then the reconstruction algorithms usually do not deal with the search of possible 2D switchings. The reason is that the (unabsorbed) 2D switchings in a binary matrix can constitute a very complicated structure and it cannot be handled simultaneously by a polynomial-time process. On the contrary, in the case of absorbed projections, as it is shown, the domain of a switching becomes a connected area, and this property provides the possibility of detecting all switchings in a binary matrix easily and reconstructing it efficiently by handling all its possible ways of growing, without slipping into nonpolynomial computations [2].

It is clear that the μ_0-absorbed row and column sums of an $m \times n$ binary matrix are nonnegative real numbers having n-length and m-length, respectively, β_0-representations. Let us call such vectors *compatible*. So, the $m \times n$ binary matrix is reconstructed from compatible vectors R and C, entry by entry, in a process that exhaustively searches for all possible elementary switching pairs. Once one of them is supposed to be found, the algorithm tries to follow its evolution by means of two different lines of computation (only two lines are sufficient by Lemma 4). Finally, if no inconsistencies are found, the two patterns are fixed in A, and their core positions will not be changed by the computation any more.

The algorithm relies on two binary $m \times n$ matrices ROW and COL, which are initialized with the β_0-expansions of the elements of R and C, respectively. During the process, they are updated according to the part of the matrix that has been already reconstructed, and they eventually can be duplicated if a switching pair is detected.

REC2DSWITCH.

Input:	Vectors $R = (r_1, \ldots, r_m)$ and $C = (c_1, \ldots, c_n)$ with nonnegative real numbers.
Output:	A binary matrix A, whose horizontal and vertical μ_0-absorbed projections are R and C, respectively, if such a matrix exists, else failure.
Step 1:	Create the $m \times n$ binary matrices ROW, COL, and A such that
	- the ith row of ROW is the β_0-expansion of r_i ($i = 1, 2, \ldots, m$),
	- the jth column of COL is the β_0-expansion of c_j ($j = 1, 2, \ldots, n$),
	- all the elements of A are undefined.
Step 2:	**for** $1 \leq j \leq n$ and $1 \leq i \leq m$,
	if (i, j) is not a position in the core of an already detected 2D composite switching pattern, **then**
	2.1 **if** $ROW[i, j] = 0$ and $COL[i, j] = 0$, **then** set $A[i, j] = 0$;

2.2 **if** $ROW[i,j] = 1$ and $COL[i,j] = 0$, **then** set $A[i,j] = 0$
and perform the shortest 1D switching in the ith row of
ROW starting from position (i,j). If there is no such 1D
switching, then halt and failure;

2.3 **if** $ROW[i,j] = 0$ and $COL[i,j] = 1$, **then** set $A[i,j] = 0$
and perform the shortest 1D switching in the jth column
of COL starting from position (i,j). If there is no such
1D switching, then halt and failure;

2.4 **if** $ROW[i,j] = 1$ and $COL[i,j] = 1$, **then** HUNT-
SWITCH(i,j);

Step 3:   *Give the matrix A as output.*

Now, we briefly sketch the subprocedure mentioned in Step 2.4, hunting
for elementary switching pairs:

HUNT-SWITCH (i,j).

Step A: *Create the local matrices ROW', ROW''', COL', and COL''
initialized as*

$$ROW' = ROW'' = ROW \quad and \quad COL' = COL'' = COL.$$
$$(15.76)$$

Step B: *We are going to check the possibility of two composite switching patterns $E^{(0)}$ and $E^{(1)}$ in A forming a switching pair.
Their components will be denoted by $p^{(0)}$ and $p^{(1)}$, respectively. Let $i' = i + 1$, and $j' = j + 1$.*

*Step B.A: Assume that $E^{(0)}_{(i',j')}$ belongs to $p^{(0)}$. Try to create
$E^{(0)}_{(i',j')}$ in ROW' and COL' by performing the shortest
1D switchings in the rows from $i' - 1$ to $i' + 1$ of ROW'
and in the columns from $j' - 1$ to $j' + 1$ of COL'. If
such switchings are not possible (no $E^{(0)}$ in A), then set
$A[i,j] = 1$ and exit the subprocedure;*

*Step B.B: Assume that $E^{(1)}_{(i',j')}$ belongs to $p^{(1)}$. Try to create
$E^{(1)}_{(i',j')}$ in ROW'' and COL'' by performing the shortest
1D switchings in the rows from $i' - 1$ to $i' + 1$ of ROW''
and in the columns from $j' - 1$ to $j' + 1$ of COL''. If
such switchings are not possible (no $E^{(1)}$ in A), then set
$A[i,j] = 0$ and exit the subprocedure;*

*Step B.C: Check the boundary of $E^{(0)}_{(i',j')}$ [respectively, of
$E^{(1)}_{(i',j')}$] for other 0-type [respectively, 1-type] 3×3 elementary switching patterns, which are strongly linked
with it, and which have to be inserted in $p^{(0)}$ [respectively,
$p^{(1)}$]. For each elementary switching pattern, apply Steps*

> B.A and B.B recursively, after uploading i' and j' to the central position of the elementary switching pattern;

Step C: Copy those entries of ROW' whose positions belong to $dom(E^{(0)})$ in the corresponding positions of A and update the entries of ROW and COL with those of ROW' and COL', then exit the subprocedure.

Remark 2. In Step C of HUNT-SWITCH(i, j), the choice of updating the matrices ROW and COL with the entries of ROW' and COL' instead of with those of ROW'' and COL'' is arbitrary. However, once the choice has been made, it has to be maintained all over the reconstruction process in order to prevent inconsistencies that may arise when two composite switching patterns intersect.

The proof of the correctness of REC2DSWITCH is immediate, since it performs an exhaustive search of all the composite switching pairs contained inside each solution.

Theorem 6. *Let R and C be compatible vectors. Algorithm REC2DSWITCH reconstructs a binary matrix having the μ_0-absorbed row and column sums R and C, respectively, if such a matrix exists; otherwise, it returns with failure.*

With the following theorem, it is proved that the reconstruction problem RECONSTRUCTION RA can be solved in polynomial time with algorithm REC2DSWITCH.

Theorem 7. *The problem RECONSTRUCTION RA can be solved in polynomial time with respect to the dimensions m and n.*

Proof. The complexity of REC2DSWITCH is computed from the complexities of each of its steps.

Step 1: The matrices ROW, COL, and A are created in $O(mn)$ time.
Step 2: It requires at most mn calls of its substeps. The complexities of Step 2.1 and Step 2.2 are constant, while Step 2.3 involves the call of the procedure HUNT-SWITCH. This procedure simply scans and compares part of the positions of the matrices ROW', ROW'', COL' and COL'', in $O(mn)$ time.
Step 3: It requires again $O(mn)$ time.

So, the total time complexity of the procedure is $O(m^2n^2)$. $\square$

Let us conclude this section with a remark and an example.

Remark 3. Algorithm REC2DSWITCH detects all the switching pairs present inside each of its solutions, so it allows us to solve the related uniqueness problem also.

Example 1. As an example, we show how algorithm REC2DSWITCH reconstructs a solution when the input vectors are

$$R = (\beta_0^{-1}, \beta_0^{-1} + \beta_0^{-2} + \beta_0^{-3}, \beta_0^{-1} + \beta_0^{-6}, \beta_0^{-1} + \beta_0^{-5}, \beta_0^{-1} + \beta_0^{-3}) \quad (15.77)$$

and

$$C = (\beta_0^{-2} + \beta_0^{-3}, \beta_0^{-1} + \beta_0^{-2} + \beta_0^{-3}, \beta_0^{-1} + \beta_0^{-5}, \beta_0^{-1}, \beta_0^{-4}, \beta_0^{-1} + \beta_0^{-3}, \beta_0^{-1}). \quad (15.78)$$

In Step 1 the matrices

$$ROW = \begin{array}{l} 1\,0\,0\,0\,0\,0\,0 \\ 1\,1\,1\,0\,0\,0\,0 \\ 1\,0\,0\,0\,0\,1\,0 \\ 1\,0\,0\,0\,1\,0\,0 \\ 1\,0\,1\,0\,0\,0\,0 \end{array}, \qquad COL = \begin{array}{l} 1\,1\,1\,1\,0\,1\,1 \\ 0\,1\,0\,0\,0\,0\,0 \\ 0\,1\,0\,0\,0\,1\,0 \\ 0\,0\,0\,0\,1\,0\,0 \\ 0\,0\,1\,0\,0\,0\,0 \end{array}, \quad (15.79)$$

and A are created.

Since $ROW[1,1] = COL[1,1] = 1$, Step 2.4 calls Hunt-Switch$(1,1)$, which returns failure, because it is not able to find a switching pattern in this position. Then Step 2.4 proceeds in two parallel computations, setting the entry in position $(1,1)$ both to the value 0 and to the value 1. Since the process for the value 1 fails in position $(1,2)$, then $A[1,1] = 0$ and ROW and COL are updated with the performed 1D switchings, i.e., $ROW[1,2] = ROW[1,3] = 1$, and $COL[2,1] = COL[3,1] = 1$.

In position $(2,1)$, similar steps are performed and $A[2,1]$ is set to 1 with no further changes in ROW and COL.

The analysis of position $(3,1)$ starts and HUNT-SWITCH $(3,1)$ is called. The entries in dom$(E_{(4,2)}^{(0)})$ in ROW' and COL' have to be modified with a series of 1D switchings involving rows 3, 4, and 5 of ROW' and columns 1, 2, and 3 of COL'. The process is successfully completed and then it is applied to ROW'' and COL'' as well. At this stage, the four matrices are the following:

$0\,1\,1\,0\,0\,0\,0$	$0\,1\,0\,1\,0\,1\,1$	$0\,1\,1\,0\,0\,0\,0$	$0\,1\,1\,1\,0\,1\,1$
$1\,1\,1\,0\,0\,0\,0$	$1\,1\,1\,0\,0\,0\,0$	$1\,1\,1\,0\,0\,0\,0$	$1\,1\,0\,0\,0\,0\,0$
$0\,1\,1\,0\,0\,1\,0$	$0\,1\,1\,0\,0\,1\,0$	$1\,0\,0\,0\,0\,1\,0$	$1\,0\,0\,0\,0\,1\,0$
$1\,0\,0\,0\,1\,0\,0$	$1\,0\,0\,0\,1\,0\,0$	$0\,1\,0\,1\,1\,1\,1$	$0\,1\,0\,0\,1\,0\,0$
$1\,0\,1\,0\,0\,0\,0$	$1\,0\,1\,0\,0\,0\,0$	$0\,1\,1\,1\,1\,0\,0$	$0\,1\,1\,0\,0\,0\,0$
ROW'	COL'	ROW''	COL''

where the boldface entries are those involved in the 1D switchings.

Now Step $B.C$ checks the boundaries of $E_{(4,2)}^{(0)}$ and $E_{(4,2)}^{(1)}$ for the presence of strongly linked elements present in $p^{(0)}$ and $p^{(1)}$. In this case, only the positions $(3,3)$, $(4,3)$, and $(5,3)$ allow one, so Steps $B.A$ and $B.B$ are performed again after updating $i' = 4$ and $j' = 4$.

The process goes on without finding inconsistences until all the components of the elementary switching pair are detected. The four matrices computed at the end of Step 2 are shown in Fig. 15.7, where the elements of $E^{(0)}$ and $E^{(1)}$ are indicated by 3×3 boxes.

0	1	0	1	0	1	1
1	1	1	0	0	0	0
0	1	1	0	0	1	0
1	0	0	0	1	0	0
1	0	1	0	0	0	0

$ROW' = COL'$

0	1	1	0	0	0	0
1	1	0	1	0	1	1
1	0	0	0	0	1	0
0	1	0	1	1	1	1
0	1	1	1	0	1	1

$ROW'' = COL''$

Fig. 15.7. The matrices $ROW' = COL'$ and $ROW'' = COL''$, and the composite switching patterns $E^{(0)}$ and $E^{(1)}$.

Matrices ROW, COL, and A are updated, and HUNT-SWITCH $(3, 1)$ terminates. Step 2 of REC2DSWITCH finishes by scanning ROW and COL without making any further change, and matrix A, which is equal to ROW, is given as output.

15.4 Reconstruction of Factor Structures Using the DT Method

In the last section of this chapter, we consider the following problem. Let us suppose that there is a 3D dynamic object, which can be represented by a nonnegative function $f(r,t)$, where r and t denote the position in space and the time, respectively. Suppose that f can be expressed as a weighted composition of a number of (so far unknown) binary-valued functions $f_k(r)$, $k = 1, 2, \ldots, K$ $(K \geq 1)$, being constant in time, such that

$$f(r,t) = c_1(t) \cdot f_1(r) + c_2(t) \cdot f_2(r) + \cdots + c_K(t) \cdot f_K(r) + \eta(r,t), \quad (15.80)$$

where $c_k(t)$ denotes the kth weighting coefficient, which depends on time, and $\eta(r,t)$ represents the noise or residual in (r,t). Given the assumption that η and f are uncorrelated, $c_k(t)$ and $f(r)$ are to be determined so that the f_k are independent of the f_j, for all $k \neq j$. If the values of $f(r,t)$ are available, then the problem can be solved by factor analysis.

However, in reality, we cannot always measure the function f in the points of the space, but we can measure certain projections only. This is frequently the case, for example, in nuclear medicine, where the object is the radioactivity distribution in an organ and the projections are the gamma camera images from different directions. In such a case, SPECT imaging is applied to collect projection data for reconstructing tomographic slices of the object.

Furthermore, we deal with a special *emission tomography* model, where the object is considered as a set of points emitting rays into all directions of the space, and the space is filled with some material attenuating the rays. It is important that the absorption is included into the definition of a projection.

Let $f(r, t)$ denote the intensity function of the object to be reconstructed. Suppose that the absorption in the space is constant; $\mu \geq 0$ everywhere. All half-lines in the space can be described as $\ell(S, v) = \{S + u \cdot v \mid u \geq 0\}$, where S and v are the point and the direction of the half-line, respectively. Then the *absorbed projections* of f in time t can be measured along half-lines by so-called point detectors:

$$[\mathcal{P}^{(\mu)} f](S, v, t) = \int_0^\infty f(S + u \cdot v, t) \cdot e^{-\mu u} \, du. \tag{15.81}$$

For the sake of simplicity, let us suppose that the support of f is the 3D unit cube, and the detectors sit on the left, right, up, and down sides of the cube, and measure the absorbed projections along half-lines, which are perpendicular to the corresponding side of the cube.

The problem is to reconstruct f from a small number of *absorbed projections*, especially if we have only four projections, $\mathcal{L}^{(\mu)} f$, $\mathcal{R}^{(\mu)} f$, $\mathcal{U}^{(\mu)} f$, and $\mathcal{D}^{(\mu)} f$, defined as

$$[\mathcal{L}^{(\mu)} f](y, t) = \int_0^1 f(u, y, t) \cdot e^{-\mu u} \, du,$$

$$[\mathcal{R}^{(\mu)} f](y, t) = \int_0^1 f(1 - u, y, t) \cdot e^{-\mu u} \, du,$$

$$[\mathcal{U}^{(\mu)} f](x, t) = \int_0^1 f(x, 1 - u, t) \cdot e^{-\mu u} \, du,$$

$$[\mathcal{D}^{(\mu)} f](x, t) = \int_0^1 f(x, u, t) \cdot e^{-\mu u} \, du. \tag{15.82}$$

That is, we are given two opposite horizontal and two opposite vertical *absorbed projections* (see Fig. 15.8). Let us call the first two projections *left* and *right* ones, and the other two projections *up* and *down* ones. (In the emission tomography model, opposite projections are not identical because of attenuation.)

The task can be divided into two parts: First we have to separate the projections of the individual structures f_k from the linear combination of the projections of the 3D dynamic object f [see (15.80)]. Next we reconstruct the cross sections of each 3D factor structure independently.

In order to test the possible application of EDT in such cases, a phantom model was selected and the reconstruction performed.

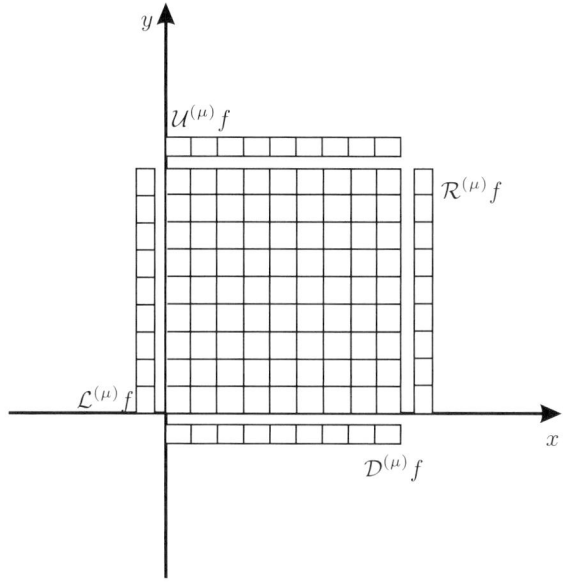

Fig. 15.8. The arrangement of the opposite absorbed projections.

15.4.1 Phantom

We implemented and tested a two-step procedure for reconstructing physiologically separable factors of a simulated renal system (the simplified 3D mathematical model of the kidney was provided by Dr. W. Backfrieder, AKH Vienna, Austria [1]). The phantom satisfies the assumption of factor analysis that the structures are homogeneous, i.e., each structure is a composition of identical voxels. The system consists of five factors representing two vascular and two renal structures and the urinary bladder (i.e., $K = 5$). They are in a discrete space of 64^3 voxels (voxel size is $6 \times 6 \times 6$ mm). Each structure is defined by a geometric object (e.g., by discrete spheres, tubes). Table 15.1 shows some information about these structures.

Table 15.1. Structures of the Given Phantom

Structure name	Organ	Volume
Vascular structure 1	heart, aorta	2652 voxels
Vascular structure 2	liver, spleen	10603 voxels
Renal parenchymas	two identical items	1350 voxels
Renal pelvis	two identical items	606 voxels
Urinary bladder	bladder	2094 voxels
Background		rest of the 64^3 cube

The background represents the rest of the cube. Absorption, scatter, depth-dependent resolution, partial volume effects, and also Poisson noise have been taken into account in this simulation in order to approximate a real nuclear medicine SPECT study. The factors change their weights (intensities) with time according to some given functions $c_k(t)$, $k = 1, 2, \ldots, 5$. Four absorbed projections with size 64×64 are taken at 120 discrete-time moments. The simulated structures have specific dynamics (radioactivity changes with time) so that they can be separated from each other by factor analysis.

15.4.2 Factor Analysis

Factor analysis (FA) was performed for each sequence of projections (left, right, up, and down) by the method using spatial constraints, e.g., nonnegativity of the factors [24, 25]. For each direction, the results of the FA are five 64×64 factor images and the corresponding five vectors with 120 factor coefficients. However, the output factor images are not necessarily the projections of the factors. What we obtained as factor images are the projections of the factors up to some multiplicative constants only. That is, we have five images $\mathcal{U}^{(\mu)} f_k^{(u)}$ (see Fig. 15.9) and five vectors $c_k^{(u)}$, $k = 1, 2, \ldots, 5$, at the end of the FA step applied to the projection up. The relation between f_k, c_k and $f_k^{(u)}$, $c_k^{(u)}$ is $c_k(t) \cdot f_k(r) = c_k^{(u)}(t) \cdot f_k^{(u)}(r)$, for all $k = 1, 2, \ldots, 5$. Similar relations can be set up for the results of the FA applied to the images taken in other directions. The curves containing the resulting coefficients are given in Fig. 15.10.

15.4.3 Reconstruction

Although $f_k^{(u)}$ and the factors computed by FA are not necessarily binary functions, they are still two-valued [the range of function $f(u)_k$ contains the 0 and another real number, say $I_k^{(u)}$]. In order to reduce the problem to binary reconstruction problems, we have to find the values $I_k^{(u)}$. This pre-reconstruction step was done by a heuristic algorithm described in [21].

Knowing the four absorbed projections of each factor, we can try to reconstruct them by some EDT reconstruction method. Let us suppose that the 2D cross sections of the factor functions can be represented by $n \times n$ binary matrices, or—equivalently—by binary vectors $x \in \{0, 1\}^J$, $J = n^2$.

Our EDT reconstruction problem can be described as a linear equation system

$$Ax = b, \quad \text{such that } x \text{ is binary.} \tag{15.83}$$

Instead of solving the equation system (15.83) directly, it is reformulated as an optimization problem. Formally, find the minimum of the objective function

$$C(x) = \|Ax - b\|^2 + \gamma \cdot \Phi(x), \quad \text{such that } x \text{ is binary.} \tag{15.84}$$

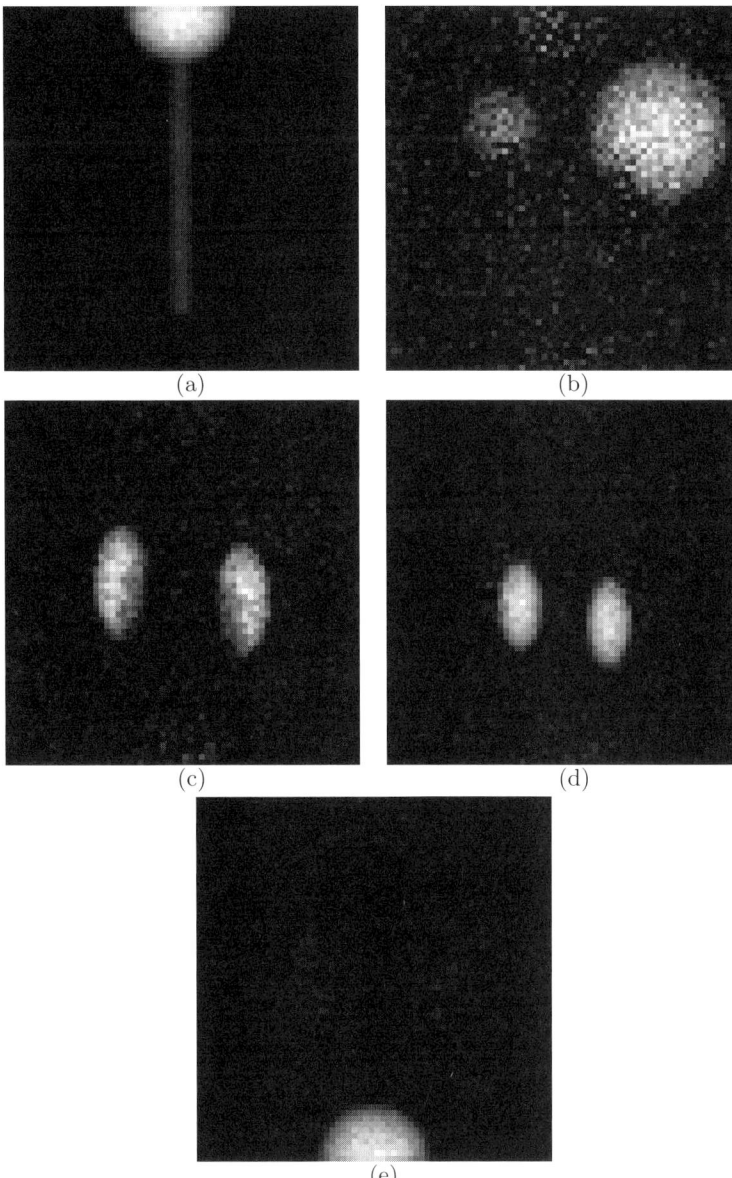

Fig. 15.9. The up-projections of the factor structures. (**a**) Heart and aorta. (**b**) Liver and spleen. (**c**) Renal parenchymas. (**d**) Renal pelvis. (**e**) Bladder.

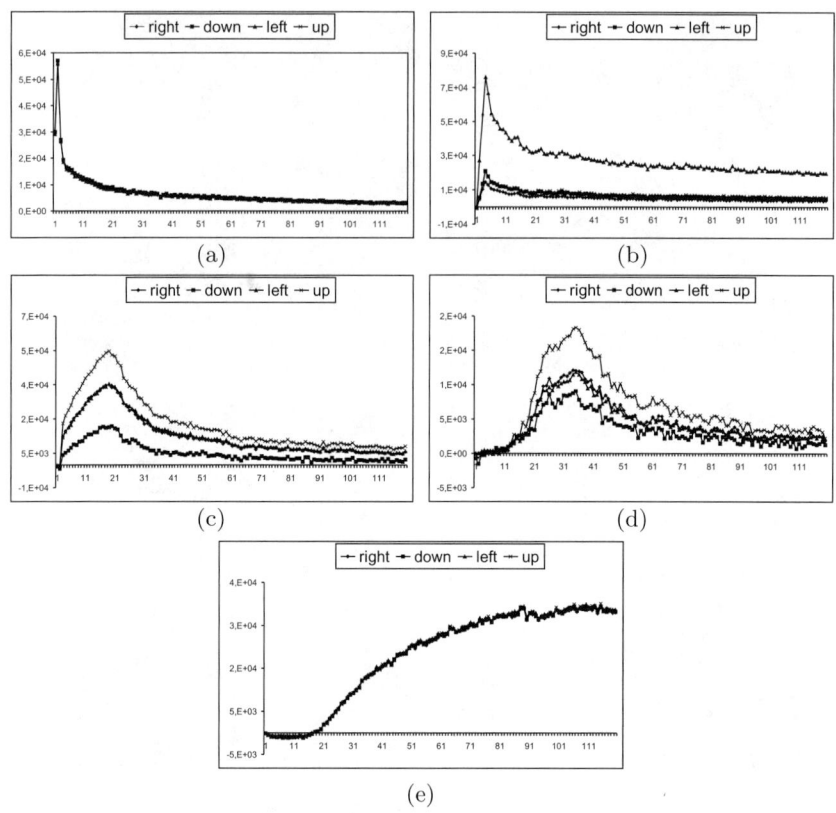

Fig. 15.10. Curves computed by FA and showing the changes of factor coefficients in time in all four projections. (**a**) Heart and aorta. (**b**) Liver and spleen. (**c**) Renal parenchymas. (**d**) Renal pelvis. (**e**) Bladder.

The first term in (15.84) controls that we have an x satisfying (15.83) at least approximately. The second term gives us the possibility to include a priori knowledge about x into the optimization. In our case, we have used the function

$$\Phi(x) = \sum_{j=0}^{J}\sum_{\ell=0}^{J} G_\sigma(d(j,\ell)) \cdot |x_j - x_\ell| , \qquad (15.85)$$

where G_σ is the Gaussian function with parameter σ and $d(j,\ell)$ denotes the distance between the jth and ℓth pixels. This regularization term forces the optimization procedure to find images having possibly large connected regions that have the same binary values.

For solving (15.84), the *simulated annealing* (SA) optimization method [20] was implemented.

15.4.4 Results

The factor analysis successfully separates the projections of individual dynamic objects; see Fig. 15.9 demonstrating the separated up-projections and Fig. 15.10 showing the factor weights (coefficients) changing in time in all four projections. It is interesting that the structures in the center of the 3D cube space [heart and aorta, Fig. 15.10(a) and bladder Fig. 15.10(e)] have almost the same curves in all projections (absorption has the same effect in all four directions). The effects of absorption in the case of other structures located off-center of the 3D cube are different in different directions.

For the reconstruction, we had to choose a proper regularization scalar γ in (15.84), then we could perform the reconstructions slice by slice for each structure (see Fig. 15.11). After reconstruction, we could calculate the volumes of each structure (see Table 15.2). The percentages in Table 15.2 give the values relative to the real volumes (see Table 15.1).

Table 15.2. The Volumes of the Reconstructed Structures

Structure name	Original volume	Reconstructed volume
Vascular structure 1	2652 voxels	2546 voxels (96%)
Vascular structure 2	10603 voxels	9629 voxels (90%)
Renal parenchymas	1350 voxels	1450 voxels (107%)
Renal pelvis	606 voxels	513 voxels (85%)
Urinary bladder	2094 voxels	1932 voxels (92%)

Having reconstructed all sections of all structures, we could make a 3D visualization by the program package Slicer [26]. The result can be seen in Fig. 15.12.

During reconstruction we observed that the liver and spleen (vascular structure 2) were considerably less smooth than other structures. This error can have two likely reasons:

(a) Factor analysis error — due to
   (i) complete overlaps of the liver and spleen in the left and right projections, and
   (ii) high attenuation of both structures in all four projections. One of the two structures is lost in each of the two lateral ($\mathcal{L}$ and $\mathcal{R}$) projections. Such data represent a difficult task for factor analysis.
(b) Reconstruction error — factor images of the liver and spleen are of low contrast and noisy in all projections. This is a likely reason for "blurriness" or poor smoothness of those structures in our reconstructions. In fact, it is not a reconstruction error as such — the result is a realistic reconstruction of noisy factor objects.

Looking at Table 15.2, we can conclude that the volume of the factor structures was near the expected values (with an error less then 10%), the worst

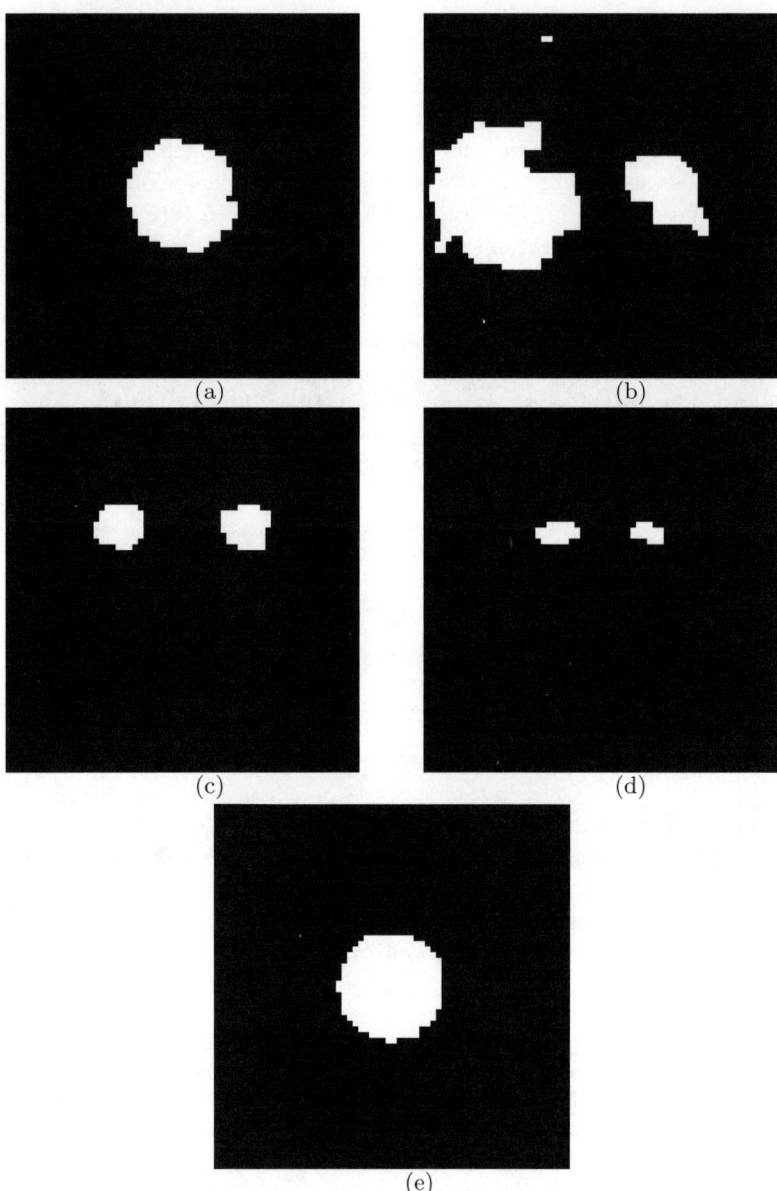

Fig. 15.11. Representative reconstructed slices of the structures. (**a**) Heart and aorta. (**b**) Liver and spleen. (**c**) Renal parenchymas. (**d**) Renal pelvis. (**e**) Bladder.

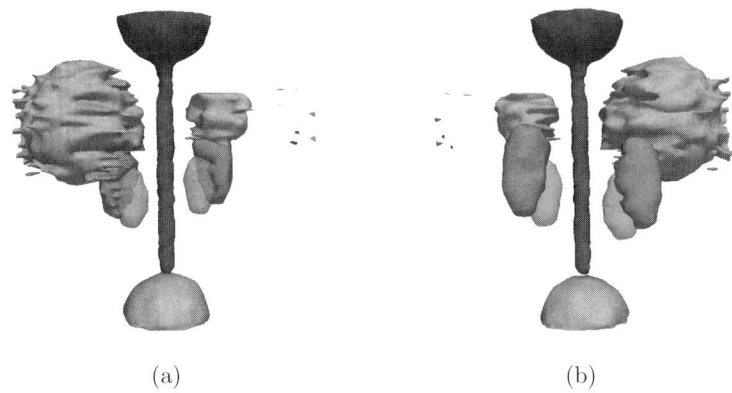

(a)   (b)

Fig. 15.12. 3D visualization of the reconstructed structures from two views.

value is in the relatively small renal pelvis, which could be recostructed with an error of 15 %. It is important to remark here that during the reconstruction we considered the absorption without any correction of scatter and noise.

In essence, our method provides a solution to a general problem of reconstructing 3D dynamic binary structures from a small number of projections.

References

1. Backfrieder, W., Samal, M., Bergmann, H.: Toward estimation of compartment volumes and radionuclide concentrations in dynamic SPECT using factor analysis and limited number of projections. *Physica Medica*, **15**, 160 (1999).
2. Balogh, E., Kuba, A., Del Lungo, A., Nivat, M.: Reconstruction of binary matrices from absorbed projections. In: Braquelaire, A., Lachaud, J.-O., Vialard, A. (eds.), *Discrete Geometry in Computer Imagery*, Springer, Berlin, Germany, pp. 392–403 (2002).
3. Barcucci, E., Frosini, A., Rinaldi, S.: Reconstruction of discrete sets from two absorbed projections: An algorithm. *Electr. Notes Discr. Math.*, **12** (2003).
4. Frosini, A., Barcucci, E., Rinaldi, S.: An algorithm for the reconstruction of discrete sets from two projections in present of absorption. *Discr. Appl. Math.*, **151**, 21–35 (2005).
5. Frosini, A., Rinaldi, S., Barcucci, E., Kuba, A.: An efficient algorithm for reconstructing binary matrices from horizontal and vertical absorbed projections. *Electr. Notes Discr. Math.*, **20**, 347–363 (2005).
6. Gardner, R.J.: *Geometric Tomography*. Cambridge University Press, Cambridge, UK (1995).
7. Hajdu, L., Tijdeman, R.: Algebraic aspects of emission tomography with absorption. *J. Reine Angew. Math.*, **534**, 119–128 (2001).
8. Herman, G.T., Kuba, A. (eds.): *Discrete Tomography: Foundations, Algorithms, and Applications*. Birkhäuser, Boston, MA (1999).

9. Kaneko, A., Huang, L.: Reconstruction of plane figures from two projections. In: Herman, G.T., Kuba, A. (eds.), *Discrete Tomography. Foundations, Algorithms, and Applications*. Birkäuser, Boston, MA, pp. 115–135 (1999).

10. Kellerer, H.: Masstheoretische Marginalprobleme. *Math. Ann.*, **153**, 168–198 (1964).

11. Kuba, A.: Reconstruction of two-directionally connected binary patterns from their two orthogonal projections. *Comp. Vision Graph. Image Proc.*, **27**, 249–265 (1984).

12. Kuba, A.: Reconstruction of measurable sets from two absorbed projections. Techn. Rep., University of Szeged, Szeged, Hungary (2004).

13. Kuba, A., Nagy, A., Balogh, E.: Reconstruction of *hv*-convex binary matrices from their absorbed projections. *Discr. Appl. Math.*, **139**, 137–148 (2004).

14. Kuba, A., Nivat, M.: Discrete tomography with absorption. In: Borgefors, G., di Baja, S. (eds.), *Discrete Geometry in Computer Imagery*, Springer, Berlin, Germany, pp. 3–34 (2000).

15. Kuba, A., Nivat, M.: Reconstruction of discrete sets with absorption. *Lin. Algebra Appl.*, **339**, 171–194 (2001).

16. Kuba, A., Nivat, M.: A sufficient condition for non-uniqueness in binary tomography with absorption. *Discr. Appl. Math.*, **346**, 335–357 (2005).

17. Kuba, A., Volčič, A.: Characterization of measurable plane sets which are reconstructable from their two projections. *Inverse Problems*, **4**, 513–527 (1988).

18. Kuba, A., Volčič, A.: The structure of the class of non-uniquely reconstructible sets. *Acta Sci. Szeged*, **58**, 363–388 (1993).

19. Lorentz, G.G.: A problem of plane measure. *Amer. J. Math.*, **71**, 417–426 (1949).

20. Metropolis, N., Rosenbluth, A., Rosenbluth, A.T.M., Teller, E.: Equation of state calculation by fast computing machines. *J. Chem. Phys.*, **21**, 1087–1092 (1953).

21. Nagy, A., Kuba, A., Samal, M.: Reconstruction of factor structures using discrete tomography method. *Electr. Notes Comput. Sci.*, **20**, 519–534 (2005).

22. Reeds, J.A., Shepp, L.A., Fishburn, P.C., Lagarias, J.C.: Sets uniquely determined by projections. I. Continuous case. *SIAM J. Applied Math.*, **50**, 288–306 (1990).

23. Ryser, H.R.: Combinatorial properties of matrices of zeros and ones. *Canad. J. Math.*, **9**, 371–377 (1957).

24. Samal, M., Karny, M., Surova, H., Marikova, E., Dienstbier, Z.: Rotation to simple structure in factor analysis of dynamic radionuclide studies. *Phys. Med. Biol.*, **32**, 371–382 (1987).

25. Samal, M., Nimmon, C.C., Britton, K.E., Bergmann, H.: Relative renal uptake and transit time measurements using functional factor images and fuzzy regions of interest. *Eur. J. Nucl. Med.*, **25**, 48–54 (1998).

26. Slicer program: http://www.slicer.org.

27. Zopf, S., Kuba, A.: Reconstruction of measurable sets from two generalized projections. *Electr. Notes Discr. Math.*, **20**, 47–66 (2005).

Application of a Discrete Tomography Approach to Computerized Tomography

Y. Gerard and F. Feschet

Summary. Linear programming is used in discrete tomography to solve the relaxed problem of reconstructing a function f with values in the interval $[0, 1]$. The linear program minimizes the uniform norm $||Ax - b||_\infty$ or the 1-norm $||Ax - b||_1$ of the error on the projections. We can add to this objective function a linear penalty function $p(x)$ for trying to obtain smooth solutions.

The same approach can be used in computerized tomography. The question is if it can provide better images than the classical methods of computerized tomography. The aim of this chapter is to provide a tentative answer. We present a preliminary study on real acquisitions from a phantom and provide reconstructions from a few projections, with qualities similar to the traditional methods.

16.1 Introduction

Computerized tomography (CT) is a technology of major importance in medical imaging and in several other fields related to nondestructive material testing. Although there has been considerable progress since the 1970s, improving the methods remains an important aim. The two important features of a reconstruction algorithm are its time of computation and the quality of the reconstructed images. The time of computation has been a decisive consideration in CT, but the improvement of CPUs now allows us to investigate methods that used to be considered too time-consuming. The hope is to enhance significantly the quality of the reconstructed images.

The notion of quality of an image is essential. What is a satisfying image and what is a nonsatisfying one? The answer to this question determines the operational details of many CT algorithms. If the question is put to a physician, he will answer in terms of diagnosis: The best image is the one that allows the best diagnosis. Unfortunately, medical knowledge can be hardly translated into numerical data. The usual way to express the quality of an image in regard to the data is to evaluate the physical adequacy between the image and the measurements. This value is called the *likelihood* of the image. Its mathematical expression involves a model of the physical process of the measurement. According to this point of view, the problem of tomographic reconstruction becomes the problem of computation of the most likely image given the data (if we add some constraints of speed, the problem is to compute in a bounded time the most likely image as possible). This is a problem of optimization. A description of a reconstruction algorithm requires in this framework three specifications:

(a) What is the chosen mathematical model of the physical process of the measurement?
(b) What is the mathematical expression of the likelihood of an image given the data?
(c) What is the method of optimization used for obtaining an image of maximal likelihood?

There are as many tomographic methods as replies, and we are going to present a method by answering, briefly in this introduction and with more details in the following, these three questions as follows:

(a) Regarding the mathematical model of the physical process of the measurements, it is possible to take into account the probabilistic laws that govern emission or absorption of particles [20], but we use a more basic model: a Dirac model, where the measurements are assumed to be the sums of the values of points belonging to digital lines.
(b) Regarding the second question, we express the likelihood of an image using the norm of the error vector, where the error vector is the difference between the real measurements (the data) and the measurements simulated from the image (with sums according to discrete lines).
(c) The chosen method of optimization is linear programming (LP). This approach, although novel in the framework of CT, comes from DT, where LP has been used since the 1990s [1, 4]. LP requires a linear form for the likelihood. In spite of this constraint, Weber et al. [22] have shown that a linear regularization term can be added to the objective function in order to obtain smooth reconstructed images.

The fact that LP has been first used in DT can perhaps be explained by the time of computation and the size of the reconstruction instances, which are smaller in DT than in CT, since binary constraints make the problem harder. The converse is, however, more usual: Many ideas of DT have been first investigated in CT [16, 21]. This is, for instance, the case with Bayesian methods. A methodology for obtaining a DT algorithm from a CT method is discussed in [2]. The idea is here to do the converse: Obtain a CT algorithm from an approach that has been first developed for DT.

The use of LP for DT goes back to the early days of the field. The relaxation of the binary constraint $x \in \{0, 1\}^d$ to $x \in [0, 1]^d$ has been introduced in DT by R. Aharoni, G.T. Herman, and A. Kuba in [1], who showed that with this relaxed constraint the problem of reconstruction could be solved by LP. Their idea was to use this routine for obtaining binary images, and the technique has been followed up by several authors [4, 8, 22, 23]. By using the same kind of method in CT, we are only returning the approach to its domain of origin with the hope that it can be helpful for providing nice reconstructed images.

We focus in Section 16.2 on a short presentation of CT classical algorithms. Sections 16.3 and 16.4 are devoted to the presentation of the new method by answering in detail the three previous questions. Section 16.5 considers the various methods of optimization to solve our LP problem. Section 16.6 presents the experimental results on a phantom.

16.2 CT Reconstruction Methods

The first kind of CT methods are based on Fourier analysis. They are said to be *analytical*. The physical process of the measurements is modeled by a continuous Radon transform [17]. No notion of likelihood is used in this framework, and no optimization step is required since Fourier slice theorem provides an exact formula for inverting the Radon transform. Thus, the main theoretical difficulty of this kind of method is the conversion of the discrete data (there are only a finite number of detectors in a camera) into a continuous function. After this first step, the application of the inversion formula of the Radon transform provides a continuous function that can be digitized in order to obtain the reconstructed image. The fact that no optimization is needed reduces the time of computation. This kind of method is fast, but the conversion from the discrete data into a continuous function requires relatively dense sampling. It compels the number of directions to be greater than 30 and a low ratio between the noise and the signal amplitude. We can say that X-ray scanners satisfy these experimental conditions, but not emission tomography. This explains why the main analytical reconstruction method called filtered back-projection (FBP) is used in X-ray scanners, but also that its application in nuclear medicine [single photon emission computed tomography (SPECT) or positron emission tomography (PET)] is more problematic.

The analytical approach is fortunately not the only option. Other methods have been developed. They are said to be *iterative*, since their principle is to increase iteratively the likelihood of a current image given the data. Several models can be considered, but due to time of optimization, the rivalry between analytical and iterative methods has first turned to the advantage of analytical approach. The development of emission tomography in medical imaging, the enhancement of mathematical knowledge of optimization, and the improvement of CPUs have reverted this tendency and provided a large reemergence of interest in the iterative approach [13].

The oldest iterative method is the algebraic reconstruction technique (ART) [6, 7, 10, 11]. The physical model considered in this approach is discrete. There is the choice between partitioning the environment in a lattice of cells (pixels, voxels) or representing it by a lattice of points (a Dirac model). The problem of reconstruction becomes that of attributing to each cell or each point a value that can be considered to be its gray level. The mathematical model of the measurements assumes that each measurement corresponds to a linear combination of these values (the attribution of the coefficients of the linear combination is discussed in the next section). Thus, the problem of reconstruction is reduced to solving a large system of linear equations $Ax = b$ (one variable per pixel of the resulting image). The large size of the linear system is not the only reason to avoid the classical Gauss method: The feasibility of the linear system is not guaranteed, but it is unthinkable that due to our reconstruction algorithm we have to say to a physician, "sorry, the data do not provide any solution." Thus, it is more natural to use iterative algorithms to solve the linear system $Ax = b$, since they always provide an approximate solution. There exist several well-known methods in numerical analysis: Jacobi, Gauss-Seidel, or their relaxed versions. The principle of ART is quite similar to the one of the Jacobi approach, with the difference that it takes advantage of the properties of the tomographic linear systems to accelerate convergence. In this framework, we consider that the likelihood is monotonic in the difference between Ax and b. This leads to a class of iterative algorithms for $\|Ax - b\|$ minimization, a classical approach used in numerical analysis for solving linear systems. Several gradient methods can be used in this framework. All these algebraic methods are based on approximating a solution of the linear system of equations by using iterations on a current image (or a current vector).

Another approach is expectation maximization (EM) and its faster variant-ordered subset expectation maximization (OSEM). The mathematical model of the measurements uses Poisson statistics, namely "exact" probabilistic laws of emission and absorption of a particle [20]. This results in a nonlinear mathematical expression for the likelihood of an image and a process to improve iteratively its value for a current image.

All the iterative methods, from ART to OSEM, have been improved by adding the possibility of taking into account information in addition to the measurements. This can be an arbitrary choice (for instance, that an image should be quite regular) or knowledge coming from other equipment. This interaction with external data is modeled mathematically by Bayes' theorem. The likelihood becomes the product between the consistency of the image with prior information and its consistency with the measurements. It is also possible to compute their sum instead of their product (with or without adding a *log*), so that the total likelihood is the sum of the consistency with the measurements and a second term penalizing inconsistency with the prior information. This modification of the likelihood has, of course, important consequences on the iteration process; the resulting iterative methods are called "Bayesian." The algebraic method that we present in this chapter is from this class.

16.3 Dirac Model with Digital Lines

Any mathematical model of the measurement is based on a sequence of more or less arbitrary choices. The first important choice is between models with a lattice of pixels and those with a lattice of points. Although the material investigated by CT is usually continuous, the Dirac model (with points) can provide good results.

16.3.1 Pixel Model

In the case of a pixel model, it is often considered that a measurement by a detector of the camera is a linear combination of the gray levels of the pixels crossed by the corresponding straight line. The contribution of a pixel to the measurement is weighted by the length of its intersection with the line. This is the principle of the *length ray model* (Fig. 16.1).

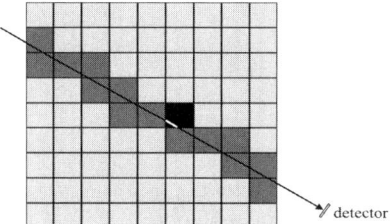

Fig. 16.1. In the length ray model, the measurement of a detector is the linear combination of the gray levels of the pixels crossed by the corresponding line. The contribution of each pixel is weighted by the length of its intersection with the line.

16.3.2 Notation

In the following, we consider a lattice of points that is embedded in a real Euclidean space. The lattice consists of all points that are integer linear combinations of two vectors i and j. The Euclidean scalar product of vectors specified by (u, v) and (x, y) (i.e., $ui + vj$ and $xi + yj$) is denoted by $(u, v).(x, y)$. The Euclidean norm associated with this dot product is denoted by $||(x, y)||$. We notice that, generally speaking, $(u, v).(x, y)$ is different from $ux + vy$ and $||(x, y)||$ is different from $\sqrt{x^2 + y^2}$, since we do not assume that i and j are vectors of norm 1 perpendicular to each another. If they are perpendicular and their lengths are both equal to l, then the dot product can be expressed directly by $(u, v).(x, y) = l^2(ux+vy)$, and it follows that $||(x, y)|| = l\sqrt{x^2 + y^2}$.

16.3.3 Basic Dirac Model with Digital Lines

We consider in our Dirac model that the measurement of a detector is the sum of the gray levels corresponding to lattice points belonging to a strip (Fig. 16.2). Such a structure is called *digital line*: A digital line consists of those lattice points (x, y) that are solutions of an equation of form $h \leq (u, v).(x, y) < h + \delta$ [18], where the vector of coordinates (u, v) [assumed different from $(0, 0)$] is normal to the direction of the line. The value $\sqrt{|h|}$ is the shift of the digital line with respect to the origin, and the value $\delta/\|(u, v)\|$ is the thickness of the digital line [$\sqrt{|h|}$ and $\delta/\|(u, v)\|$ are lengths].

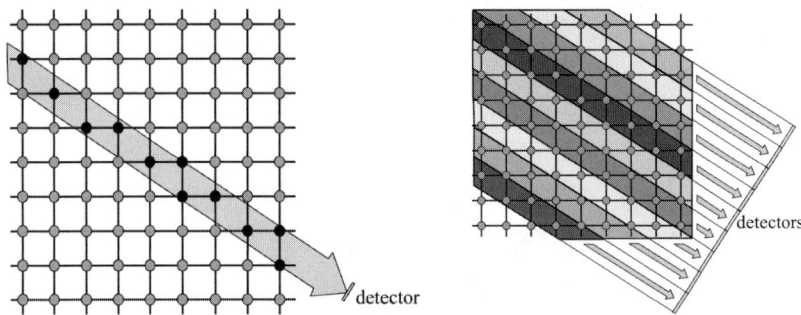

Fig. 16.2. On the left, the measurement of a detector is the sum of the gray levels of the pixels belonging to a digital line, namely the sum of the values of the points belonging to a strip (the weight of each point is 1 if it belongs to the corresponding digital line and 0 otherwise). On the right, the tiling of the lattice points by parallel digital lines. This model guarantees a uniform contribution of all points to the measurements in any direction.

It seems natural in this framework to choose digital lines, where the thickness $\delta/\|(u, v)\|$ is equal to the width of any detector (Fig. 16.2). By assuming that the detectors are placed contiguously (without spaces between them), this provides in each direction a set of digital lines tiling the lattice. This model is our basic Dirac model with digital lines.

16.3.4 Advantages and Drawbacks

The first advantage of the previous model is that it provides linear combinations with only 0s and 1s as coefficients. As each point in the image belongs to exactly one digital line of the tiling, the contributions of all the points are equal in all directions (Fig. 16.3). To this advantage, there is a drawback. Let us assume, for instance, that all the points belonging to a region of interest (ROI) have a gray level equal to 1, while all the others have a null gray level. Thus, the value measured on a detector is equal to the number of points in the intersection between one digital line and the ROI. Due to the definition of digital lines, the simulated measurements have unrealistic structural variations (Fig. 16.3). This drawback comes from the variation in the number of lattice points in consecutive digital lines. The first part of this variation is due to the length of the segment cutting the lattice (an equivalent variation is also observed in the length ray model), but there is also a second term: A given digital line has more or less thin sections. By considering the intersection between parallel digital lines of constant thickness and the rectangular support of the image, some digital lines have a thin section in the rectangle while others can have a thicker one. It provides an unrealistic variance in the simulated measurements. This detrimental effect can be important in the two diagonal directions (the ratio between the cardinalities of parallel digital segments of same length can be equal to 2) and even in the horizontal and vertical directions of the lattice.

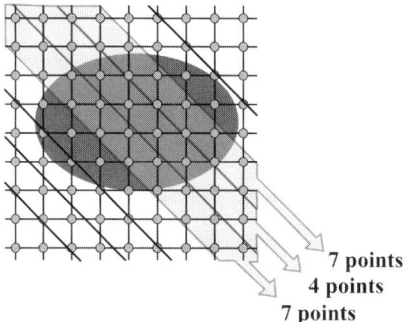

7 points
4 points
7 points

Fig. 16.3. A region of interest is represented in gray. If we assume that the points in this region have a gray level equal to 1 while all other gray levels are null, this provides us with a sequence 7, 4, 7 in the simulated measurements, which is not realistic.

16.3.5 Improving the Model

We could hope that previous detrimental effect of cardinalities variance remains quite small in practice, but we prefer investigating different ways of improving the model by introducing some corrections:

(a) Choose a starting angle for the reconstruction that restricts cardinalities variance. This becomes difficult if the number of directions of the measurements becomes large.
(b) Use digital lines that do not have a fixed thickness $\delta/\|(u,v)\|$. This means that the thickness of the digital lines will not always be equal to the width of the detectors. One consequence is that the set of digital lines considered in one direction does not tile the lattice anymore. *Naive digital*

lines ($\delta = max\{|(u, v).(1, 0)|, |(u, v).(0, 1)|\}$) or *standard digital lines* ($\delta = |(u, v).(1, 0)| + |(u, v).(0, 1)|$) [18] can be used. We call this model a Dirac model with naive or standard digital lines.

(c) Weigh the contribution of the points by the total number of points in the digital line. We call this reasonable option the *cardinal correction* in the experiments.

The two last corrections destroy the property that all points have the same contribution to all measurements. They favor another property that is verified by the length ray model: The sum of the coefficients for computing each simulated measurement according to all detectors is proportional to the length of the intersection between the corresponding line and the lattice. We can ask for a perfect model to conciliate perfectly both requests (such a model would be perfect, but it seems hard to obtain).

The three models tested in the experimental section are the (basic) Dirac model with digital lines, the Dirac model with naive digital lines (which do not tile the lattice), and the Dirac model with digital lines corrected by weights associated with cardinalities (*cardinal correction*).

16.4 Likelihood

Regardless of the choice of the algebraic model (length ray model or Dirac model with digital lines), it provides a linear operator A that allows us to express the simulated measurements from a gray-level image x as the linear product Ax.

Denoting the vector of the experimental measurements by b, the problem of reconstruction is to compute a gray-level image x satisfying $Ax = b$. There may not be an exact solution, and it is necessary to compute an approximative one. This is the idea that we have introduced with the term "likelihood". Any image x may be more or less likely with respect to the measurements b. The ideal image satisfies $Ax = b$, while an unlikely image is characterized by an Ax far from b. Thus, it is natural to consider that the likelihood of x can be evaluated from $||Ax - b||$ with a norm chosen between $||.||_\infty$, $||.||_1$ and $||.||_2$.

This approach is efficient, but better results can be obtained by adding a Bayesian correction: We add to the norm of the error $Ax - b$ a second term based on a smoothness prior.

The idea to consider a smoothness prior in conjunction with the norm of the residual error was already present in Chapter 13 of [9], while the introduction of a regularization term goes back to 1976 [12]. This approach with the Euclidean norm has been, for instance, investigated in CT in 1992 by L. Kaufman [14, 15] ($||Ax - b||$ minimization is the classical least-squares method), while an approach with $||.||_1$ or $||.||_\infty$ norms has been investigated by S. Weber et al. in the framework of DT in [23]. Our contribution to this technique starts in [3, 5].

The principle is to express the likelihood as the sum of $||Ax - b||$ and a penalty term $p(x)$ penalizing an irregular x. One choice is to express $p(x)$ as the sum of quadratic terms $\sum_{i \in I} (x_{i'} - x_{i''})^2$, where I is the set of the edges between neighboring points or pixels in the lattice, and where i' and i'' denote the vertices of edge i. Thus, $p(x)$ is null if, and only if, the gray level of x is constant. This term provides a measure of the local homogeneity (the smoothness) of the image x, but, its expression being quadratic, it cannot be used in our linear approach. A method to obtain a linear equivalent of this value of homogeneity is presented in [22]. It consists of introducing one auxiliary variable (denoted y_i) for each edge i between neighboring pixels or points i' and i''. By imposing the two constraints (1) $y_i \geq x_{i'} - x_{i''}$ and (2) $y_i \geq x_{i''} - x_{i'}$, we can be sure that $y_i \geq |x_{i'} - x_{i''}|$. We consider that the value $|x_{i'} - x_{i''}|$ expresses the local homogeneity of x around the edge i. Thus, the sum $\sum_{i \in I} |x_{i'} - x_{i''}|$ expresses the overall smoothness of x. The sum of auxiliary variables $\sum_{i \in I} y_i$ is necessarily greater than the smoothness value $\sum_{i \in I} |x_{i'} - x_{i''}|$, but, as there is no other constraint on y than (1) and (2), $\sum_{i \in I} y_i$ minimization guarantees equality $\sum_{i \in I} y_i = \sum_i |x_{i'} - x_{i''}|$. This provides a way to incorporate the smoothness of x in an objective function without using any absolute value or quadratic expression but with auxiliary variables. Some other penalty terms can also be expressed linearly with the trick of using an auxiliary variable, but in order to reduce the number of parameters of the method, we have focused our experiments on the edge penalty.

Now that we have expressed the penalty $p(x)$ by a linear term that can be incorporated in an objective function, it remains to do the same with the norm $||Ax - b||$. This is, of course, not possible in the case of Euclidean norm, but for $||.||_1$ and $||.||_\infty$, we use the same kind of technique.

We start with the $||.||_1$ norm by introducing a vector of auxiliary variables h related to x by the linear constraints (3) $-h \leq Ax - b \leq h$. This guarantees the inequality $||Ax - b||_1 \leq \mathbb{1}.h$, where $\mathbb{1}.h$ is the dot product between h and the vector $\mathbb{1}$ of constant coordinate equal to 1. If no other constraint on h is introduced, $\mathbb{1}.h$ minimization guarantees equality $||Ax - b||_1 = \mathbb{1}.h$. Thus, we consider the likelihood of x as the sum $likelihood_1(x) = ||Ax - b||_1 + K \sum_{i \in I} |x_{i'} - x_{i''}|$, where K is a positive constant controlling the weight of regularization (also referred to as the "entropy" ahead) with respect to the error on the measurements. This nonlinear value can be minimized on x by minimizing the linear objective function $\mathbb{1}.h + K \sum_{i \in I} y_i$ under linear constraints (1), (2), and (3).

With the $||.||_\infty$ norm, we use the same principle, but instead of bounding $Ax - b$ with a vector h, we use a real number h. The linear constraints (4) $-h\mathbb{1} \leq Ax - b \leq h\mathbb{1}$ imply the inequality $||Ax - b||_\infty \leq h$. If we introduce no other constraint on h, the minimization of h leads to the equality $||Ax - b||_\infty = h$. Thus, we express the uniform likelihood of x as $likelihood_\infty(x) = ||Ax - b||_\infty + K \sum_{i \in I} |x_{i'} - x_{i''}|$, where K is again a positive constant controlling the relative weight of smoothness penalty. This nonlinear expression can be minimized on x by minimizing the linear objective function $h + K \sum_{i \in I} y_i$ under linear constraints (1), (2), and (4).

16.5 Optimization

As we have reduced the problem of minimization of the two Bayesian expressions of likelihood $likelihood_1(x)$ and $likelihood_\infty(x)$ (a low value corresponds to a likely image) to a problem of minimization of a linear objective function under linear constraints (a linear program), it remains only to solve it by using an LP algorithm. Several methods can be used: primal or dual or even primal-dual simplex algorithms [19] or interior points methods [25]. Special techniques could also be used, but we believe that standard methods in LP are efficient enough to solve our problem. We tested the solution of our LP problem using both soplex [24], which is freely available, and the solver Cplex 9.1, which is probably the best commercial solver available today. All tests were done on a Pentium IV Xeon machine with hyperthreading and 1 GByte of main memory. soplex furnishes an implementation of the primal simplex method, whereas Cplex offers the primal and dual simplex methods and an implementation of an interior points method. All optimization methods are iterative. It should be noted that simplex-based methods are exact, whereas interior points methods are approximate in the sense that they find only approximations to the optimal solutions. However, interior points methods could be pursued until a guaranty of optimality is reached. As this feature is implemented in Cplex, we choose to always optimize until optimality is reached. This means that our running time will be higher for interior points methods than what is really needed to provide a good solution. We have estimated that times could be divided by two if we were interested in an approximate solution that does not differ much from the optimal one.

Since we provide the possibility to solve the tomographic reconstruction problem with either the $||.||_\infty$ or the $||.||_1$ norm, we tested both reconstructions with the different optimization method. It should be noted that with the $||.||_\infty$ norm, we sometimes obtain problems that are not solved with the interior points algorithm (it terminates with an infeasibility error), while the dual simplex algorithm always works. Such problems with interior points methods never happen with the $||.||_1$ norm, and we believe that they are related to the use of the $||.||_\infty$ norm.

To appreciate the times of the different optimization methods, we mention that a typical LP problem has 15,000 constraints and 11,000 variables for a reconstruction with 16 projections on a 64×64 matrix. The LP system is always sparse for the $||.||_1$ norm but contains at least one dense column for the $||.||_\infty$ norm, which means that the latter optimization problem is harder to attack and is less efficient. In a previous paper [5], experiments done with soplex took 6 hours, which was prohibitive for clinical use. When switching to Cplex and the dual simplex method, our running times reduced to less than

10 minutes. This is already progress. When using the $||.||_1$ norm, with which we always reach an optimality condition with interior points methods, our running times reduced to 25 seconds. In the last experiments presented in the next section, no computation took more than 25 seconds to be completed with a certificate of optimality of the solution. It is, of course, much more time than classical methods. The slowness of this approach is the consequence of using a general linear programming method, which is not optimized for the kind of instances that we have. It remains, of course, possible to stop the process of optimization before its end, and we can also imagine optimizing the linear programming algorithm for working with the instances of our problem, but these two perspectives have not been yet investigated.

16.6 Experiments

The experiments are based on a phantom acquired by the Center of Nuclear Medicine of Clermont-Ferrand. The projections were acquired by single photon electron computer tomography (SPECT) on a lattice of 64×64 detectors with a step angle of $12°$ along an arc of $180°$ (Fig. 16.4).

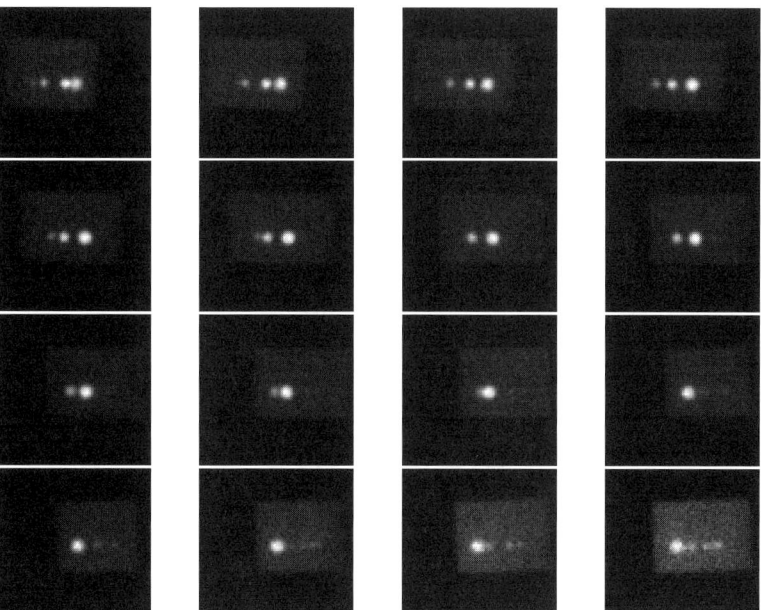

Fig. 16.4. The 16 measurements of the Phantom with a step angle of $12°$. Thus, the first and the last images are projections in opposite directions.

The phantom is composed of a surrounding envelope in plexiglas that does not interfere too much with the measurements. Inside the plexiglas structure, six balls containing radioactive liquids are placed in the same horizontal plane. The balls have varying radii and concentrations. The smallest ball has a size close to the resolution of the measurement device. Since we only use 16 projections instead of the usual 64 projections, it is very improbable that the smallest could be visible in the reconstructions.

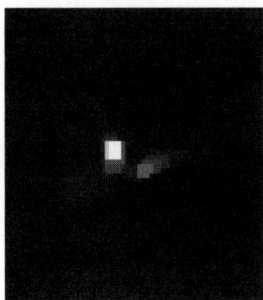

Fig. 16.5. Reconstruction using the $||.||_\infty$ norm.

The first reconstruction was done with the $||.||_\infty$ norm (Fig. 16.5). We have done many tests with varying K to see if a better image could be obtained but without success. We obtain a poor-quality image because of the noise present in the projections. If we suppress completely the entropy by setting $K = 0$, we obtain a worse image with a complete disorder. Due to all these reasons, we decided to focus only on the $||.||_1$ norm with edge entropy and a factor $K = 0.4$. It is clear that in some experiments better images could be obtained based on a careful analysis of the K-value but, for comparison purposes, we chose to impose the value of K such that direct comparisons are possible.

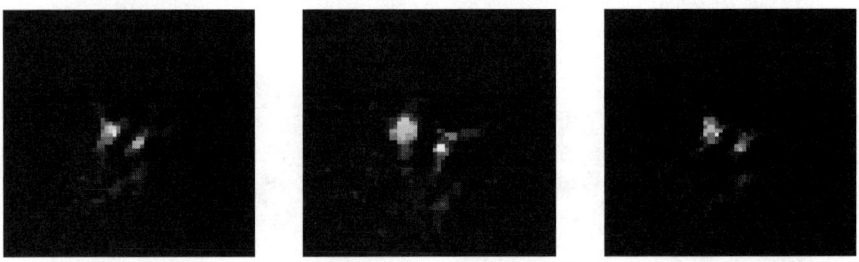

Fig. 16.6. Reconstruction with the naive digital lines model, the standard digital lines model, and the digital lines model ($\delta = \sqrt{a^2 + b^2}$). The third model is the so-called (basic) Dirac model with digital lines.

We tested reconstruction when using the basic Dirac model with digital lines (their thickness $\delta/||(u, v)||$ is equal to the width of the detectors so that the set of digital lines in each direction tiles the lattice), and we tried the two corrections suggested to improve the model by using the naive and the standard digital lines. The corresponding results are given in Fig. 16.6. The basic model provides the best reconstructed image with better localizations of the objects. When using standard lines, the objects are less localized and several artifacts appear in the reconstruction. The result with naive lines is not so bad, but since all directions are not of equal geometric thickness, some directional artifacts appear. It should be noted that the result with naive lines is less spread out than with standard lines. It is a consequence of the smallest geometrical thickness of naive lines.

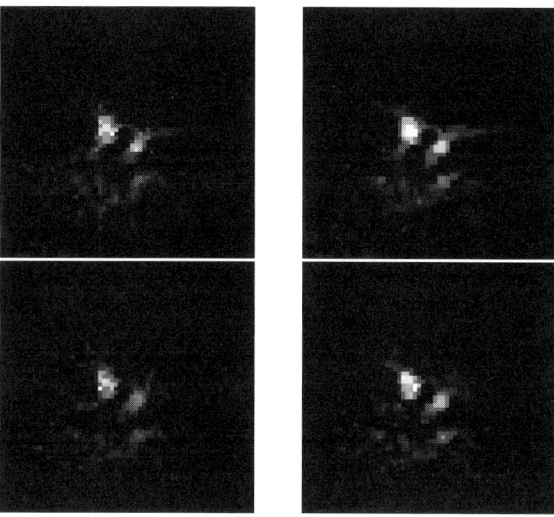

Fig. 16.7. Reconstruction: (top left) original, (top right) with cardinal correction only, (bottom left) with normalization correction only, (bottom right) with both corrections.

Following these reconstructions, we focused on other corrections with the (basic) Dirac model with digital lines. The first correction is a *normalization* that modifies the measurements in order to give them the same mean value in all directions. The second correction is the cardinal correction, introduced for counterbalancing the variations of numbers of pixels in neighboring digital lines. Experiments with or without these two corrections (Fig. 16.7) show that they are both efficacious. The cardinal correction results in images that are less spread out. The normalization correction leads to images with more localized objects. Finally, we applied both corrections so that both effects are cumulated. Contrary to what we thought first, this does not lead to a better image. In fact, this last image does not have a good localization property and has more artifacts. Due to this cumulative effect, we have chosen to use only the normalization correction in next experiments.

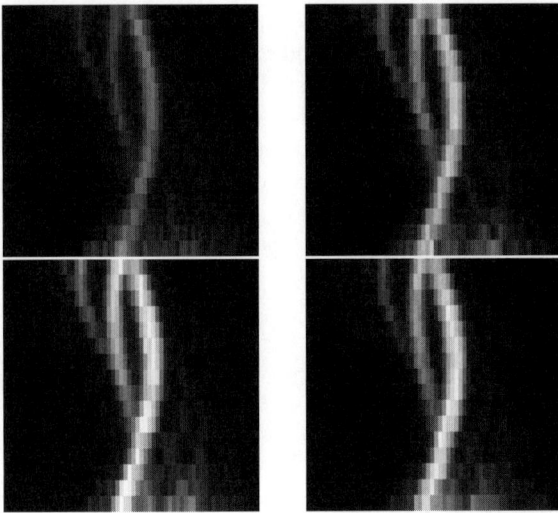

Fig. 16.8. Sinograms for the slices numbered from 31 to 34 with normalization only (order is from top to bottom and left to right).

A careful look at the reconstruction shows that merely three balls are correctly reconstructed. We always used slice 33 in the projections, which corresponds to the plane passing through the center of the balls. To understand the intrinsic complexity of reconstructing more than three balls, we provide the sinograms for the slices 31 to 34 in Fig. 16.8.

Clearly, three balls are visible. One of the other three can be seen in only two projections (see top of Fig. 16.8), and the two smallest ones are not visible at all. This explains why we cannot reconstruct more than three balls. Since all projections have equal importance, the fourth one is not present enough to be reconstructed by our method. It should be noted that this ball could be visible if the contrast in the sinogram was better (a contrast correction could be applied before reconstruction).

As shown in the sinograms above, the location of the plane containing the center of the balls is not clear. Thus, we reconstructed all slices between the levels 31 and 34. The results are presented in Fig. 16.9. Level 32 is the level with the minimum number of artifacts. However, the contrast of the reconstructed balls is less than in level 33. This is why we have chosen to do all our experiments with level 33. Besides this, a careful look at the image of level 32 shows that the shadow of the fourth ball is perhaps present in the reconstruction. The position of the concentration of high values is consistent with the geometry of the phantom and the regular placement of the balls. This is obviously not sufficient for a firm conclusion, but we believe it to be in favor of the quality of discrimination of our reconstruction method.

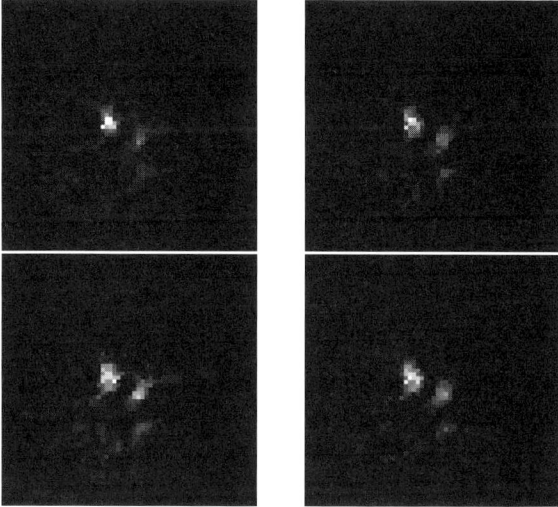

Fig. 16.9. Reconstruction for the slices numbered from 31 to 34 with normalization only (order is from top to bottom and left to right).

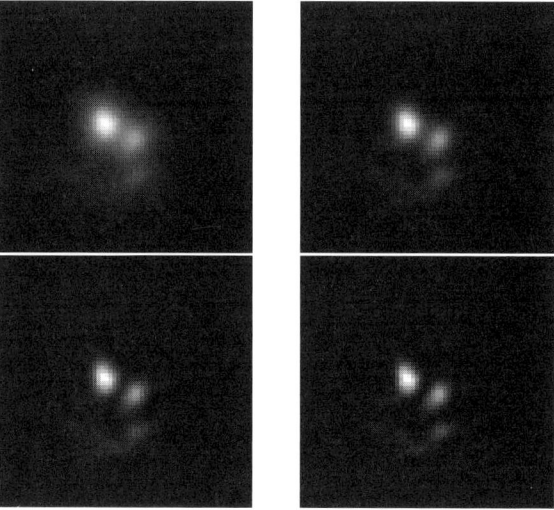

Fig. 16.10. Butterworth post-filtering with varying f in $\{3, 5, 7, 9\}$ and $n = 2$ (order is top to bottom and left to right).

In common clinical use, pre- and postfiltering are used to provide more readable images for the clinicians. One standard filtering is the Butterworth filter, given in the frequency domain by

$$B(w) = \frac{1}{1 + \left(\frac{w}{f}\right)^{2n}} \, , \tag{16.1}$$

where f is the cut-off frequency, which limits the influence of the filter, and n is the order of the filter. We provide two types of experiments by fixing of the parameters f or n and modifying the other one. We first present the impact of the cut-off frequency with a fixed order in Fig. 16.10.

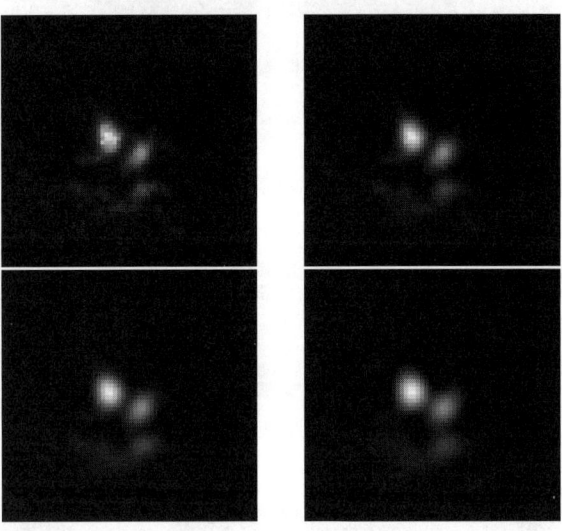

Fig. 16.11. Butterworth postfiltering with varying n in $\{1, 2, 3, 5\}$ and $f = 7$ (order is top to bottom and left to right).

The impact of f is clear. Smaller values lead to fewer frequencies preserved in the frequency domain. Thus, the images tend to be overblurred and details are simply removed. When f is increasing, we tend to the original image. Thus, f must be chosen not too low (to retain details), but not too high (to filter artifacts). The value of f thus depends on the relative frequencies between the details and the artifacts.

In a second sequence of experiments, we fixed $f = 7$ and modified n. Intuitively, n governs the speed of the decay of the influence of the filter. This is confirmed in Fig. 16.11 by the fact that the balls become more blurry with high n, corresponding to the fact that fewer frequencies are kept by the filter.

To investigate the impact of postfiltering, we searched for a compromise between f and n to provide the nice filtered image that is presented in Fig. 16.12.

We now compare our reconstruction with the two standard methods: FBP and OSEM. In Fig. 16.13, we provide the reconstructions made by FBP and OSEM from 16 projections.

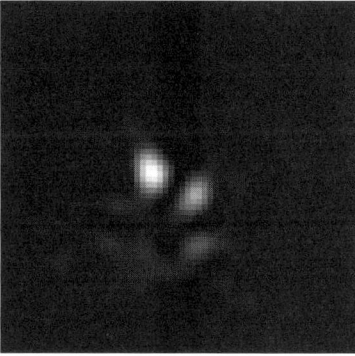

Fig. 16.12. Butterworth filtering with $f = 10$ and $n = 4$.

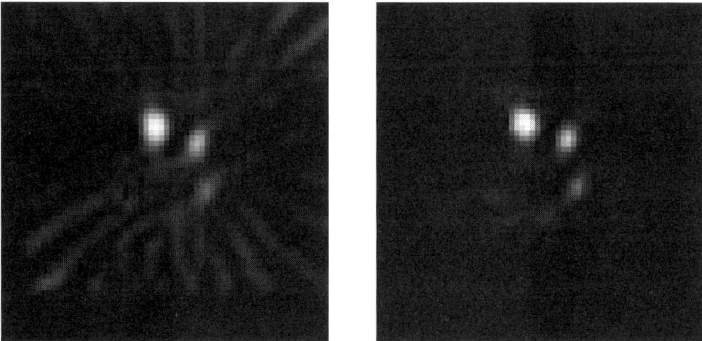

Fig. 16.13. (Left) FBP reconstruction, (right) OSEM reconstruction.

The FBP reconstruction is usually performed with 64 projections. When the number of projections is reduced, the star artifacts become too noticable. Hence the reconstructed image is polluted by this effect and is not suitable for automatic inspection. However, the three main balls are clearly visible on the reconstruction.

The image reconstructed by OSEM is of good overall quality. As we can see, the three main balls are clearly visible and the shadow of the fourth one is present. Moreover, very few artifacts are present in the reconstructed image.

When comparing the OSEM reconstruction with our reconstruction, we can clearly see that the quality of our method is close to the one of OSEM in this experiment. There is still a little bit more artifact in our reconstruction, but the discrimination power toward the different balls is almost similar.

To end this experimental part, we provide in Fig. 16.14 the reconstruction using only eight projections and no postfiltering. Note that this reconstruction was impossible with both the FBP and the OSEM methods, since the software of the machine does not accept less than 16 projections.

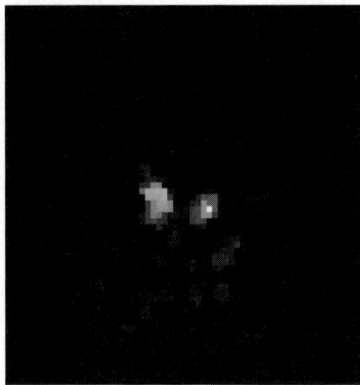

Fig. 16.14. Reconstruction using LP and only 8 projections.

The quality of the reconstruction with only eight projections is not so bad. The three main balls are still clearly visible. Of course, having fewer projections provides more artifacts, but we hope that our approach can be robust toward the number of projections.

16.7 Conclusion

The three features of our method are

(a) a Dirac model with digital lines,
(b) an expression of the likelihood as sum of a smoothness prior and the norm $||Ax - b||_1$ of the error between the simulated measurements Ax and the real measurements b,
(c) and a LP method of optimization.

This approach comes directly from the algebraic model used in classical ART, with the difference that it guarantees the optimality of the likelihood of the result.

A comparison of the experimental results with ART should be the next step of our investigations as well as the comparison with iterative least-squares algorithms. What are the relative benefits of the $||.||_1$ minimization of the error and of the Dirac model with digital lines toward these classical approaches? Is there really a difference and does it justify such an increase in the time of computation?

Whatever the real practical interest of our approach, it is not completely surprising that its principle comes from DT, because the small number of directions used in this framework requires us to make the most of the measurements. It is in such conditions that our method can find its application. If the measurements are very accurate, the use of such an optimal method is not necessary, but it becomes interesting only in the case of noisy projections in only a few directions. Unfortunately, this kind of instance is less uncommon than we could hope, and it clearly appears that if a method admits a decrease in the quality of the measurements without impairing the reconstructed image, it would allow us to improve the productivity of some very expensive equipments.

Acknowledgments

We thank D. de Freitas, F. Cachin, and J. Maublant from the Center of Nuclear Medecine Jean-Perrin of Clermont-Ferrand for their interest in this work, their fruitful discussions, and the images they provided to us.

References

1. Aharoni, R., Herman, G.T., Kuba, A.: Binary vectors partially determined by linear equation systems. *Discr. Math.*, **171**, 1–16 (1997).
2. Censor, Y., Matej, S.: Binary steering of nonbinary iterative algorithms. In: Herman, G.T., Kuba, A. (ed.), *Discrete Tomography, Foundations, Algorithms, and Applications*. Birkhaüser, Boston, MA, pp. 285–296 (1999).
3. Feschet, F., Gerard, Y.: Computerized tomography with digital lines and linear programming. In: Andres, É., Damiand, G., Lienhardt, P. (eds.), *Discrete Geometry in Computed Imagery*, pp. 126–135 (2005).
4. Fishburn, P., Schwander, P., Shepp, L., Vanderbei, R.: The discrete Radon transform and its approximate inversion via linear programming. *Discr. Appl. Math.*, **75**, 39–61 (1997).
5. Gerard, Y., Feschet, F.: Application of a discrete tomography algorithm to computerized tomography. *Electr. Notes Discr. Math.*, **20**, 501–517 (2005).
6. Gordon, R.: A tutorial on ART (algebraic reconstruction techniques). *IEEE Trans. Nucl. Sci.*, **21**, 31–43 (1974).
7. Gordon, R., Bender, R., Herman, G.T.: Algebraic reconstruction techniques (ART) for three-dimensional electron microscopy and X-ray photography. *J. Theor. Biol.*, **29**, 471–481 (1970).
8. Gritzmann, P., de Vries, S., Wiegelmann, M.: Approximating binary images from discrete X-rays. *SIAM J. Optimization*, **11**, 522–546 (2000).
9. Herman, G.T.: *Image Reconstruction from Projections*. Academic Press, New York, NY (1980).
10. Herman, G.T.: Reconstruction of binary patterns from a few projections. In: Gunther, A., Levrat, B., and Lipps, H. (eds.), *International Computing Symposium*, North-Holland, Amsterdam, The Netherlands, pp. 371–378 (1974).
11. Herman, G.T., Lent, A.: Iterative reconstruction algorithms. *Comput. Biol. Med.*, **6**, 273–274 (1976).
12. Herman, G.T., Lent, A.: A computer implementation of a Bayesian analysis of image reconstruction. *Information and Control*, **31**, 364–384 (1976).
13. Herman, G.T., Meyer, L.B.: Algebraic reconstruction techniques can be made computationally efficient. *IEEE Trans. Med. Imag.*, **12**, 600–609 (1993).
14. Kaufman, L.: Maximum likelihood, least squares and penalized least squares for PET. *IEEE Trans. Med. Imag.*, **12**, 200–214 (1993).

15. Kaufman, L., Neumaier, A.: PET regularization by envelope guided conjugate gradients. *IEEE Trans. Med. Imag.*, **15**, 385–389 (1996).
16. Matej, S., Vardi, A., Herman, G.T., Vardi, E: Binary tomography using Gibbs priors. In: Herman, G.T., Kuba, A. (ed.), *Discrete Tomography, Foundations, Algorithms, and Applications*. Birkhäuser, Boston, MA, pp. 191–211 (1999).
17. Radon, J.: Über die Bestimmung von Funktionen durch ihre Integralwerte langs gewisser Mannigfaltigkeiten. *Ber. Verh. Sächs. Akad. Wiss. Leipzig, Math.-Nat. Kl.*, **69**, 262–277 (1917).
18. Reveillès, J.P.: *Géométrie discrète, calcul en nombres entiers et algorithmique*. M.A. thesis, ULP University, Strasbourg, France (1991).
19. Schrijver, A.: *Theory of Linear and Integer Programming*. John Wiley and Sons, New York, NY (1986).
20. Shepp, L.A., Vardi, Y.: Maximum likelihood reconstruction for emission tomography. *IEEE Trans. Med. Imag.*, **1**, 113–122 (1982).
21. Vardi, Y., Zhang, C.H.: Reconstruction of binary images via the EM algorithm. In: Herman, G.T., Kuba, A. (ed.), *Discrete Tomography, Foundations, Algorithms, and Applications*. Birkhäuser, Boston, MA, pp. 297–316 (1999).
22. Weber, S., Schnörr, C., Hornegger, J.: A linear programming relaxation for binary tomography with smoothness priors. *Electr. Notes Discr. Math.*, **12** (2003).
23. Weber, S., Schüle, T, Hornegger, J., Schnörr, C.: Binary tomography by iterating linear programs from noisy projections. In: Klette, R, Zunic, J.D. (eds.), *Combinatorial Image Analysis*, Springer, Berlin, Germany, pp. 38–51 (2004).
24. Wunderling, R., *Paralleler und Objektorientierter Simplex-Algorithmus*, Ph.D. thesis, ZIB TR 96-09, Berlin, Germany (1996).
25. Ye, Y: *Interior Points Algorithms: Theory and Analysis*. John Wiley and Sons, New York, NY (1997).

Index

Applied and Numerical Harmonic Analysis

J.M. Cooper: *Introduction to Partial Differential Equations with MATLAB* (ISBN 0-8176-3967-5)

C.E. D'Attellis and E.M. Fernández-Berdaguer: *Wavelet Theory and Harmonic Analysis in Applied Sciences* (ISBN 0-8176-3953-5)

H.G. Feichtinger and T. Strohmer: *Gabor Analysis and Algorithms* (ISBN 0-8176-3959-4)

T.M. Peters, J.H.T. Bates, G.B. Pike, P. Munger, and J.C. Williams: *The Fourier Transform in Biomedical Engineering* (ISBN 0-8176-3941-1)

A.I. Saichev and W.A. Woyczyński: *Distributions in the Physical and Engineering Sciences* (ISBN 0-8176-3924-1)

R. Tolimieri and M. An: *Time-Frequency Representations* (ISBN 0-8176-3918-7)

G.T. Herman: *Geometry of Digital Spaces* (ISBN 0-8176-3897-0)

A. Procházka, J. Uhlíř, P.J.W. Rayner, and N.G. Kingsbury: *Signal Analysis and Prediction* (ISBN 0-8176-4042-8)

J. Ramanathan: *Methods of Applied Fourier Analysis* (ISBN 0-8176-3963-2)

A. Teolis: *Computational Signal Processing with Wavelets* (ISBN 0-8176-3909-8)

W.O. Bray and Č.V. Stanojević: *Analysis of Divergence* (ISBN 0-8176-4058-4)

G.T Herman and A. Kuba: *Discrete Tomography* (ISBN 0-8176-4101-7)

J.J. Benedetto and P.J.S.G. Ferreira: *Modern Sampling Theory* (ISBN 0-8176-4023-1)

A. Abbate, C.M. DeCusatis, and P.K. Das: *Wavelets and Subbands* (ISBN 0-8176-4136-X)

L. Debnath: *Wavelet Transforms and Time-Frequency Signal Analysis* (ISBN 0-8176-4104-1)

K. Gröchenig: *Foundations of Time-Frequency Analysis* (ISBN 0-8176-4022-3)

D.F. Walnut: *An Introduction to Wavelet Analysis* (ISBN 0-8176-3962-4)

O. Bratteli and P. Jorgensen: *Wavelets through a Looking Glass* (ISBN 0-8176-4280-3)

H.G. Feichtinger and T. Strohmer: *Advances in Gabor Analysis* (ISBN 0-8176-4239-0)

O. Christensen: *An Introduction to Frames and Riesz Bases* (ISBN 0-8176-4295-1)

L. Debnath: *Wavelets and Signal Processing* (ISBN 0-8176-4235-8)

J. Davis: *Methods of Applied Mathematics with a MATLAB Overview* (ISBN 0-8176-4331-1)

G. Bi and Y. Zeng: *Transforms and Fast Algorithms for Signal Analysis and Representations* (ISBN 0-8176-4279-X)

J.J. Benedetto and A. Zayed: *Sampling, Wavelets, and Tomography* (ISBN 0-8176-4304-4)

E. Prestini: *The Evolution of Applied Harmonic Analysis* (ISBN 0-8176-4125-4)

O. Christensen and K.L. Christensen: *Approximation Theory* (ISBN 0-8176-3600-5)

L. Brandolini, L. Colzani, A. Iosevich, and G. Travaglini: *Fourier Analysis and Convexity* (ISBN 0-8176-3263-8)

W. Freeden and V. Michel: *Multiscale Potential Theory* (ISBN 0-8176-4105-X)

O. Calin and D.-C. Chang: *Geometric Mechanics on Riemannian Manifolds* (ISBN 0-8176-4354-0)

J.A. Hogan and J.D. Lakey: *Time-Frequency and Time-Scale Methods* (ISBN 0-8176-4276-5)

C. Heil: *Harmonic Analysis and Applications* (ISBN 0-8176-3778-8)

K. Borre, D.M. Akos, N. Bertelsen, P. Rinder, and S.H. Jensen: *A Software-Defined GPS and Galileo Receiver* (ISBN 0-8176-4390-7)

G.T. Herman and A. Kuba: *Advances in Discrete Tomography and Its Applications* (ISBN 0-8176-3614-5)

Printed in the United States of America